HEALTH
PROMOTION
IN CANADA

HEALTH PROMOTION IN CANADA

New Perspectives on Theory, Practice, Policy, and Research

Fourth Edition

Edited By:
Irving Rootman, Ann Pederson,
Katherine L. Frohlich, and Sophie Dupéré

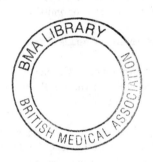

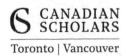

CANADIAN
SCHOLARS

Toronto | Vancouver

Health Promotion in Canada: New Perspectives on Theory, Practice, Policy, and Research, Fourth Edition
Edited by Irving Rootman, Ann Pederson, Katherine L. Frohlich, and Sophie Dupéré

First published in 2017 by
Canadian Scholars
425 Adelaide Street West, Suite 200
Toronto, Ontario
M5V 3C1

www.canadianscholars.ca

Library and Archives Canada Cataloguing in Publication

Health promotion in Canada : new perspectives on theory, practice, policy, and research / edited by: Irving Rootman, Ann Pederson, Katherine L. Frohlich, and Sophie Dupéré. -- Fourth edition.

Subtitle of previous edition: Critical perspectives on practice.
Includes bibliographical references and index.
Issued in print and electronic formats.
ISBN 978-1-77338-006-3 (softcover).--ISBN 978-1-77338-007-0 (PDF).--ISBN 978-1-77338-008-7 (HTML)

1. Health promotion--Canada--Textbooks. 2. Textbooks.
I. Pederson, Ann P., editor II. Rootman, I., editor III. Frohlich, Katherine L., editor IV. Dupéré, Sophie, editor

RA427.8.H43 2017   613.0971   C2017-905706-5
                                            C2017-905707-3

Cover and text design by Elisabeth Springate
Cover image: Photo by Marcus Christensen

Printed and bound in Canada by Webcom

MIX
Paper from
responsible sources
FSC® C004071

Table of Contents

PART III—CRITICAL REFLECTIVE PRACTICE IN HEALTH PROMOTION

Dedication

The editors of this edition would like to honour the past and celebrate the future by dedicating this book to people near and dear to us. Irv would like to dedicate this book to Barb Rootman, his wife and life partner, as well as to the memory of Debra Karby, beloved wife of his son Adam and mother of his grandsons Tobyn and Sacha, who died on November 15, 2012, and to the memory of his colleague and friend Barbara Ronson McNichol who died tragically on March 22, 2017. Ann would like to thank her co-editors for their long-standing friendship and the generosity of spirit that has characterized their partnership. She would like to dedicate this work to her life partner, Barry, and to thank him for his steadfast support and love. Kate would like to dedicate this book to Anita Pratt, past executive director of the Native Women's Shelter of Montréal, from whom she learned many things including First Nations' notions of health, notions that influence her thinking to this day. Sophie would like to thank her co-editors for their constant support and confidence through the ups and downs of her parental leave. She is also grateful to Michel O'Neill who has truly inspired her to become more involved in the health promotion field. He has been a supportive and inspirational mentor and she dedicates the book to him.

Acknowledgements

As was the case for the three previous editions of this book, we relied on the collaboration of a large number of contributors in preparing this edition. Their enthusiasm and willingness to work with our deadlines, as well as the quality of their work, were both exceptional and inspirational. We clearly found the right people to help us with this book. We are grateful and would like to thank them sincerely for their commitment to this project and to health promotion. We are also grateful for the help that we received from Jim Frankish and Natasha Prodan-Bhalla in reviewing specific chapters.

We had the good fortune of working with Natalie Garriga, who managed this project on behalf of Canadian Scholars with professionalism, responsiveness, and flexibility, which we appreciated greatly. We would also like to thank the other staff of Canadian Scholars who worked on this book for their help in facilitating its timely publication.

In addition, we would like to gratefully acknowledge the support that we received from various institutions: British Columbia Centre of Excellence for Women's Health, which supported Ann Pederson's involvement, the Faculté des sciences infirmières de l'Université Laval, which supported the involvement of Sophie Dupéré, and both the École de Santé Publique de l'Université de Montréal and the IUMSP at the Université de Lausanne, where Kate was on sabbatical during the writing of this book.

We would also like to thank the external reviewers that provided us with feedback on the draft manuscript and the reviewers who commented on the third edition; all their suggestions have helped us to reflect more critically upon our work and clearly have improved the quality of the final product.

Preface to the Fourth Edition

This is the fourth edition of *Health Promotion in Canada*. These books were written over a span of more than 20 years, and the contents of each reflect a distinct orientation, indicated by the unique subtitle of each edition, showing how our approach has evolved over time and how we remain committed to looking at health promotion from a variety of perspectives. In this preface, we review the intent of the three previous editions and then describe our vision of this new edition.

In brief, the first edition was framed as a historical and sociological examination of health promotion as a field in Canada. The second built on this theme, but recognized contributions to theory and practice that had emerged within the field since the first edition. The third edition extended the focus on health promotion practice, offering a review of theory, methods, and promising practices in health promotion in Canada. This edition further extends the focus on practice as well as elaborates some new themes such as the role of digital media, collaboration with other sectors, participatory practice, intervention research, and the role of health promotion in relation to the physical environment.

HEALTH PROMOTION IN CANADA: PROVINCIAL, NATIONAL, AND INTERNATIONAL PERSPECTIVES

The first edition, published in 1994 (Pederson, O'Neill, & Rootman, 1994), was mainly a socio-historical analysis of the development of health promotion in Canada over the 20 years following the release of the Lalonde Report (Lalonde, 1974).[1] We looked at health promotion in Canada with a critical eye over those 20 years, particularly the period following the release of the *Ottawa Charter for Health Promotion* in 1986 at the First International Conference on Health Promotion in Ottawa, sponsored by the World Health Organization, the Canadian Public Health Association, and Health and Welfare Canada (WHO, 1986). Contrary to most books in the field at that time, we decided to prepare one that reflected "on" health promotion (Pederson, O'Neill, & Rootman, 1994, p. 1) rather than preparing another manual "in" health promotion that provided suggestions on how to design programs or conduct research in the field. With the help of experienced academics and professionals in Canada and elsewhere, we thus analyzed the development of the field from conceptual, national, provincial, and international perspectives.

Based on the discussions in the book, we concluded, among other things, that there was a consensus about what health promotion was and how to go about implementing it; that Canada was an international leader in the field; and that, while health promotion was beginning to enter the mainstream of health discourse and activity, it remained marginal in health care and was more of a professional movement than a social movement.

HEALTH PROMOTION IN CANADA: CRITICAL PERSPECTIVES

Although the first edition of the book was intended for people working in health promotion or related fields in Canada and other countries, it turned out that the largest group of readers was undergraduate students in health sciences in Canada. As a consequence, the second edition, which included Sophie Dupéré as a fourth editor, was specifically directed at this audience, using a style and format appropriate for undergraduate courses while maintaining an orientation that was also designed to interest other readers in Canada and elsewhere. We maintained the approach of analyzing the health promotion field in Canada by adopting a critical perspective. We tried to identify what was critical in the field at the beginning of the twenty-first century, in the sense of what was important or crucial in Canada and abroad 13 years after the first edition, with the "inclination to criticize" characteristic of "critical social science" (O'Neill, Pederson, Dupéré, & Rootman, 2007, p. 12). In addition, based on feedback about the first edition suggesting that we should be more explicit about how and why reflecting on the field is crucial for practice, we added a new section on practical perspectives that encouraged readers to apply reflexive thinking to their own practice. We also made a deliberate effort to include a team combining newer and more experienced contributors from a variety of backgrounds, including practitioners, policy makers, and academics, because we wanted the book to showcase a new generation of people doing health promotion work. In the final count, the second edition involved a total of 93 authors from 22 countries. In that edition, the authors from other countries, for the most part, contributed information about health promotion in their countries and the extent to which Canada's experience in health promotion affected what was done there.

Thus, the 2007 edition of *Health Promotion in Canada* was an entirely new book relative to the 1994 edition. We also worked on a slightly different version that was published in French at almost the same time (O'Neill, Dupéré, Pederson, & Rootman, 2006). In 2007 we concluded that among other things, health promotion, although resilient, was still marginal in the Canadian health care system and that day-to-day health promotion practice in Canada remained lifestyle-oriented and focused on individuals' behavioural changes. In addition, Canada continued to have a good international reputation and to play an important role internationally in the field.

HEALTH PROMOTION IN CANADA: CRITICAL PERSPECTIVES ON PRACTICE

The third edition, published in 2012, strengthened the emphasis on practice with a focus mainly on the development and status of health promotion in Canada, linking it to health promotion theory, research, evaluation, and ethics. This approach built upon an important development introduced in the second edition, namely the introduction of a discussion of critical reflective practice. Consequently, about half of the chapters in this edition were updated versions of chapters from the second one and the rest were new, covering topics that we felt were central for health promotion practice. This edition, however, maintained a critical interdisciplinary perspective and continued to insert Canadian health promotion within the global context. Its main purpose was to reflect upon health promotion as currently practised in Canada, which at that time was still perceived internationally as a hotbed of innovation and exemplary practices. The third edition provided practitioners with an improved understanding of the forces that shape their practice, as well as concrete examples of what we called "promising practices" (i.e., practices that might or might not have been evaluated enough to reach the status of "best practice," but that are nevertheless illuminating and inspiring).

HEALTH PROMOTION IN CANADA: NEW PERSPECTIVES ON THEORY, PRACTICE, POLICY, AND RESEARCH

In the second edition of *Health Promotion in Canada*, Ilona Kickbusch suggested that health promotion was becoming more like a "rhizome" than a "tree." In the third edition, she defined a rhizome as "a root system that some plants ... use to spread themselves about" (Kickbusch, 2012, p. 309) and presented several international examples of how this metaphor characterized the development of health promotion as a field that "influenced how societies think about health and its determinants, but also its ability to give rise to innovation and its capacity to respond to changes in the context by moving into new conceptual territories" (Kickbusch, 2012, p. 309). We noted the relevance of this metaphor to what had happened in Canada since the second edition in 2007. In the current edition, we also use this metaphor in describing what has happened in health promotion in Canada since 2012 to suggest the acceleration of the "rhizome effect" in Canada as well as elsewhere.

This edition attempts to convey a number of key messages about the current practice of health promotion in Canada. As was the case in the previous editions, it is guided by some values and principles, many of which are embodied in the *Ottawa Charter for Health Promotion* (WHO, 1986). Deciding to explore promising practices across Canada 30 years later is a way to celebrate the accomplishments in the field since the release of the *Ottawa Charter*, which obviously does not preclude looking at it today with a critical eye. Although this edition will appear only in English, in order to show the diversity as well as the similarities of what happens in such a large country, we have again made efforts to include anglophone and francophone authors from different provinces, sometimes working in pairs, as well as newer and more experienced contributors from a variety of backgrounds.

The book has 24 chapters and is divided into three parts, each with a short introduction to establish the context. Part I, "The Context and Foundations of Health Promotion in Canada," is organized into five chapters, of which one is new (Behavioural Theories) and the others are updated versions of chapters in the third edition. Part II, "Health Promotion Practice in Canada," contains eleven chapters, of which eight are new (Gender-Transformative Health Promotion; Promoting Mental Health and Wellbeing; Identifying Appropriate Health Promotion Practices for Immigrants; Healthy Cities and Communities; Promoting Educational Success; Health Promoting Universities; Health Promotion in Clinical Care; and Digital Media and Health Promotion Practice). Part III, "Critical Reflective Practice in Health Promotion," contains eight chapters, seven of which are new (Health in All Policies; Learning from Population Health Intervention Research; Health Promotion Ethics; Participatory Practice; Population Health Promotion in the Anthropocene; Globalization; and Reflections on the Future of Health Promotion in Canada). The book closes with a brief afterword written by Ronald Labonté, who has had a long and distinguished career in health promotion in Canada and globally. All of the other chapters are updated from the third edition.

There are a few things to keep in mind when reading the book. First, the manuscript was sent to the publisher in January 2017; as the field is constantly evolving, some things might have changed by the time the book is released. Second, as noted above, the main audience for this book is students, especially undergraduate students in Canadian health sciences. Each chapter thus includes pedagogical elements such as learning objectives, critical thinking questions, and resources. We are nevertheless convinced that in addition to students, people already working in the field will be interested in reading this book to update themselves on current developments by reflecting critically on their practice and health promotion as a whole.

Finally, as editors we are once more heartened by the continuing support of the numerous colleagues who have written contributions to this edition or previous editions of this book. We see health promotion as a collective enterprise of working together to improve health. That so many people are willing to work with us, some of them for the fourth time, to maintain an active dialogue about health promotion in Canada is evidence that, despite the erosion of official support for health promotion in many jurisdictions, there remains an enthusiastic and thoughtful community of scholars and practitioners engaged in the field. For us, it has also been a pleasure to continue the collaboration we've enjoyed as co-editors, and to have the experience of working with Katherine L. Frohlich. She joined the editorial team as a replacement for Michel O'Neill, who decided to pursue new interests in his retirement, but was nevertheless able to make a contribution to several of the chapters. We hope that the readers of this edition will be inspired by its content and contribute to the continuing development of health promotion thinking and action in Canada and globally.

Irving Rootman, Ann Pederson, Katherine L. Frohlich, and Sophie Dupéré
Vancouver, Québec City, and Montréal, January 2017

NOTE

1.   The Lalonde Report is a key publication in the field of health promotion. Some dates, events, and key documents such as this one will be constantly referred to throughout the book. They are presented in detail in chapter 1.

REFERENCES

Kickbusch, I. (2007). Health promotion: Not a tree but a rhizome. In M. O'Neill, A. Pederson, S. Dupéré, & I. Rootman (Eds.), *Health promotion in Canada: Critical perspectives* (2nd ed.) (pp. 363–366). Toronto: Canadian Scholars' Press.

Kickbusch, I. (2012). Understanding the rhizome effect. In I. Rootman, S. Dupéré, A. Pederson, & M. O'Neill (Eds.), *Health promotion in Canada: Critical perspectives on practice* (3rd ed.) (pp. 308–313). Toronto: Canadian Scholars' Press.

Lalonde, M. (1974). *A new perspective on the health of Canadians.* Ottawa: Health and Welfare Canada.

O'Neill, M., Dupéré, S., Pederson, A., & Rootman, I. (Eds.). (2006). *Promotion de la santé au Canada et au Québec: Perspectives critiques.* Québec: Les Presses de l'Université Laval.

O'Neill, M., Pederson, A., Dupéré, S., & Rootman, I. (Eds.). (2007). *Health promotion in Canada: Critical perspectives* (2nd ed.). Toronto: Canadian Scholars' Press.

Pederson, A., O'Neill, M., & Rootman, I. (Eds.). (1994). *Health promotion in Canada: Provincial, national, and international perspectives* (1st ed.). Toronto: W. B. Saunders Canada.

Rootman, I., Dupéré, S., Pederson, A., & O'Neill, M. (Eds.). (2012). *Health promotion in Canada: Critical perspectives on practice* (3rd ed.). Toronto: Canadian Scholars' Press.

World Health Organization (WHO). (1986). *Ottawa charter for health promotion.* Ottawa: World Health Organization, Health and Welfare Canada, Canadian Public Health Association.

PART I

THE CONTEXT AND FOUNDATIONS OF HEALTH PROMOTION IN CANADA

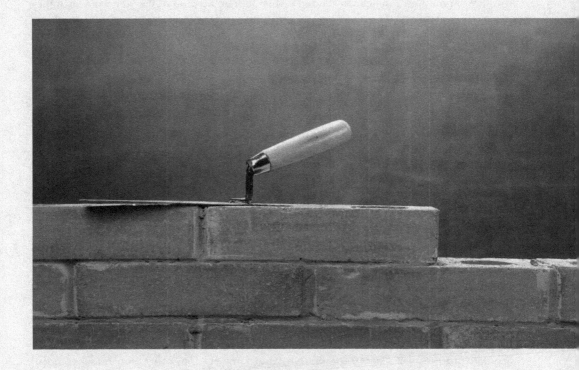

This first part of the book contains five chapters that provide basic building blocks for the reader to reflect critically on health promotion as it is currently practised in Canada, 30 years after the famous *Ottawa Charter for Health Promotion* was released.

Chapter 1 provides *contextual* elements to understanding how the field developed and is positioned in Canada and globally. In this chapter, we build on several chapters of the previous editions and offer a historical analysis of how health promotion has emerged out of the field of health education, both in Canada and internationally. We also look at how it has evolved since the third edition of the book in 2012 and assess whether or not Canada's positive reputation on the global health promotion scene, which has been unquestioned for several decades, is still current.

The other chapters in Part I offer *conceptual* and *theoretical* elements that are important for health promotion practice. Practitioners tend to be action-driven and often are dubious about the usefulness of conceptual and theoretical elements, which some think belong to the academic world and have no practical use. In the introduction to Part I of the second edition, two sentences were used that were true in 2007 and are still true today: "Ce qui se conçoit clairement s'énonce facilement et les mots pour le dire arrivent aisément" ("What is clearly conceived is easily said and words to say it come easily"), by French preacher Jacques-Bénigne Bossuet; and "There is nothing more practical than a good theory," by American social psychologist Kurt Lewin. Indeed, practitioners' capacity to intervene successfully in health promotion is significantly shaped by their understanding of the world in which they operate and of the elements they should work on. For this, concepts and theories are extremely useful tools.

Thus, in chapter 2, Rootman and O'Neill present some of the *central concepts* that frame the field of health promotion: health; health promotion and its distinction from health education; the special place of the social determinants of health within the array of factors that influence health and illness; the notion of empowerment as a key element of interventions; and, finally, the important role played by the notions of health literacy and quality of life as outcomes of health promotion actions. As will be seen, even if there will always be debates, significant consensus exists on all the concepts discussed.

Chapters 3 to 5 address the issue of *theory* in relation to health promotion practice. In chapter 3, Carroll addresses at a more general level the ways in which, in health promotion as a field, theory can be used for the production of scientific knowledge and its use in practice. He focuses particularly on the contribution of social theory. In chapter 4, Gauvin and Bélanger-Gravel provide an overview of behavioural theories commonly used in health promotion and suggest a model that includes structural and environmental factors. In chapter 5, Richard and Gauvin show how ecological models can concretely help to plan interventions, noting some of the issues and dilemmas still challenging this approach.

At the end of this part, the reader should be equipped to better understand what the field of health promotion is, where it comes from, what some of its key conceptual and theoretical elements are, and how theory can be applied to practice.

CHAPTER 1

The Continuing Evolution of Health Promotion in Canada

*Ann Pederson, Irving Rootman, Katherine L. Frohlich,
Sophie Dupéré, and Michel O'Neill*

LEARNING OBJECTIVES

1. Understand how health promotion evolved in Canada
2. Understand the relationship between health promotion and population health
3. Understand the factors that influence the current context for health promotion in Canada

This chapter critically reviews the evolution of health promotion in Canada in the global context. Health promotion formally emerged in the 1980s, evolving from a focus on individually oriented health education practices—providing information on "appropriate" health-related behaviours such as tobacco abstinence, diet, physical activity, and so on—to encompass environmental and policy concerns. Thirty years later, the debate continues on the extent to which health promotion practice has embraced structural and policy concerns and whether it can, positioned as a function of the public health system as it so often is, address the critical health challenges of the twenty-first century, including climate change, migration, inequity, substance use, urbanization, and aging.

In this chapter, we trace the evolution of health promotion in Canada, starting with a discussion of health education and the introduction of the term *health promotion* with the publication of the Lalonde Report in 1974. We outline key activities leading up to the release of the *Ottawa Charter for Health Promotion* and *Achieving Health for All: A Framework for Health Promotion* in 1986. Then we note the emergence of the field of population health and discuss its impact on health promotion as a field, scholarly discipline, and policy direction. We reflect on changes to funding, the structures supporting education and training in health promotion, and the shifting political climate of support for the field. We end with some thoughts on the contemporary context and state of the field, and suggest some of the challenges and opportunities ahead.

Throughout we pay attention to how national and global developments, crises, and opportunities shape the nature of health promotion. In particular, we emphasize that the evolution of health promotion in Canada cannot be understood as simply the product of local and national events and policy decisions but rather it has been—and will continue to be—shaped by global circumstances and developments. To address the health challenges facing us today, health promotion in Canada must embrace responsibility for acting at the local, national, and global levels, for the levers of change operate at all three.

PRIOR TO 1974—THE HEALTH EDUCATION ERA

Badgley (1994) argued that the "dissemination of sanitary information" became a concern for the newly established government of the Dominion of Canada in the 1880s. He suggested that missionary zeal among so-called sanitary reformers rather than scientifically grounded and well-evaluated interventions dominated the field for several decades up to the end of World War II. During this period, a small cadre of public health personnel produced pamphlets, posters, books, and newspaper columns, and later film strips and radio messages, to relay health information.

Similar endeavours were underway in most advanced capitalist countries (see Green &

Box 1.1: Some Key Milestones in the Evolution of Health Promotion in Canada

- **1951**: Founding and 1st World Conference of the International Union for Health Education (IUHE) in Paris
- **1974**: Release of *A New Perspective on the Health of Canadians*, the Lalonde Report
- **1978**: Alma-Ata conference on Primary Health Care, co-organized by the World Health Organization and UNICEF, and release of the *Alma-Ata Declaration*
- **1979**: World Health Assembly of the WHO adopts *Health for All by the Year 2000* resolution
- **1986**: 1st World Health Organization Global Conference on Health Promotion held in Ottawa; release of the *Ottawa Charter for Health Promotion* and *Achieving Health for All* (the Epp Report)
- **2004**: Creation of the Public Health Agency of Canada
- **2007**: 19th World Conference of the IUHPE held in Vancouver
- **2008**: Global economic crisis and release of WHO Commission on Social Determinants of Health report
- **2011**: 25th Anniversary of *Ottawa Charter*
- **2016**: 30th Anniversary of *Ottawa Charter*; 22nd IUHPE conference in Curitiba, Brazil; 6th Global Forum on Health Promotion, Charlottetown, PEI; 9th Global Conference on Health Promotion, Shanghai, China

Kreuter, 1999, for a discussion of developments in the United States) until the late 1940s and early 1950s, when a more systematic and scientific approach to educating the public on health began to emerge. In 1951, two Frenchmen, Léo Parisot and Lucien Viborel, led the creation of the International Union for Health Education (later to become the International Union for Health Promotion and Education or IUHPE) to promote the exchange of experience and information on these new ways of working (Modolo & Mamon, 2001). The IUHPE was to become the most important international non-governmental organization in the field and remains so today.

From the 1950s until the mid-1970s, the focus of health education in the industrialized world was the health professional–patient encounter (understood as the doctor–patient relationship) to ensure that patients understood and used the information provided by health care providers. Then the general, healthy public became the target of health education campaigns, initially to encourage the proper use of the health services—including preventive ones—that governments were establishing post–World War II.

With the epidemiological transition in Western countries, and the advent of lifestyle/ chronic diseases, attention turned towards the behavioural risk factors associated with these new sources of morbidity and mortality (e.g., cardiovascular diseases, cancers, accidents)—smoking, sedentary lifestyles, and unhealthful diets. Thus, health promotion turned its focus to these factors as the prime targets of health education.

The 1950s and 1960s also witnessed the greater involvement of social scientists and communication specialists both in the development of models to try to understand and predict health-related behaviour, and in the design of health education campaigns. This type of psychosocial theorizing continued to develop in the 1970s and 1980s and still is widely used in health education and health promotion (see chapter 4). Such models are premised on the understanding that individuals are rational actors who engage in actions based upon their knowledge of health benefits and risks, and perceive themselves as capable of action to change their personal situation. Context tends to be limited to immediate social relations such as the family or workplace. Based on these models, the focus of health promotion interventions became changing perception of risk or self-efficacy, increasing people's knowledge, and creating reinforcing interpersonal relations to support behaviour change. This approach gradually infiltrated the practice of health educators in Canada (Badgley, 1994) and was reflected in programs, manuals (e.g., Gilbert, 1963, 1967), and training.

These practices were built upon a deeply rooted, virtually unquestioned belief that educating the public was intrinsically good (and sufficient) and the hope that health would improve with the help of science and a more systematic way of conducting health education (Pinder, 1994, p. 95). With the incapacity in the late 1960s and the 1970s of large public health interventions (MRFIT, COMMIT, Pawtucket, Stanford Five City, and others) to change lifestyle behaviours through education at the level that was expected, it became evident that health education was not having the desired effects; individuals—even if better informed—did not necessarily adopt the healthful behaviours expected of them.

Events then took place that produced changes to the way health education was conceived, leading to its transformation into health promotion.

1974–1994: THE EMERGENCE OF HEALTH PROMOTION

The mid-1970s marked the end of 30 years of sustained growth in the Western post-war economies. This period of growth had allowed the welfare state to flourish. Governments were sufficiently wealthy—and the public was sufficiently supportive—to engage in ensuring the welfare of their populations through the provision of health and social services. However, the "oil shocks" of 1973 and 1976 initiated 20 years of economic stagnation and/or minimal growth, thereby depriving governments of tax revenues and forcing them to borrow heavily to maintain public services.

It was in this context that *A New Perspective on the Health of Canadians* was released in 1974 (Lalonde, 1974). The so-called Lalonde Report received immediate worldwide attention because it was the first document by a central government of a major developed country that advocated for investing resources beyond health services to improve the health of the population (Pinder, 1994, p. 96). The core of the report, the "health field concept," identified four sets of factors that contributed to the health of populations: human biology, environment, lifestyle, and health care organization. The report also introduced the term *health promotion* to the world in a manner that drew attention to its importance.

Given the deteriorating macro-economic context, almost every Western industrialized country subsequently produced its own version of the Lalonde Report in the years that followed—all encouraging investment in areas other than health care systems as ways to improve the population's health. Extending this thinking, delegates to the Alma-Ata conference in 1978 suggested a return to "primary health care" (PHC) and to addressing the set of factors described in the Lalonde Report and its counterparts (see UNICEF, 1978).

Box 1.2: Lalonde Calls for Shift to Illness Prevention

Health Minister Marc Lalonde tabled a green paper calling for a dramatic shift in health-policy thinking: an emphasis on prevention of illness to mitigate soaring medical costs. Titled *A New Perspective on the Health of Canadians*, the document influenced policy-making around the world, but was greeted in Ottawa largely with mocking indifference. Tory Heath MacQuarrie dismissed it as "solidly in the motherhood realm," and joked that everyone knows it's better to be slim than fat. The same spring, parliamentary debate was dominated by legislation—also tabled by Lalonde—to ensure the Canadian Football League's monopoly over pro football in Canada. The CFL is alive and kicking, but most of the recommendations in the public health report remain unfulfilled.

Source: Picard, André. (2014). Moment in time: May 1, 1974—Lalonde calls for shift to illness prevention. *The Globe and Mail,* May 1, p. A2..

The conference centrepiece, the *Alma-Ata Declaration*,[1] foreshadowed ideas that were to become foundational to health promotion, such as an emphasis on evidence-based services reflective of national context, multi-sectoral responsibility, and multi-disciplinary care providers. It articulated the importance of basic nutrition, sanitation, and access to potable water as foundations for health and encouraged involving the community in health plan-ning and decision-making. Mindful of these developments, the World Health Assembly approved the *Global Strategy for Health for All by the Year 2000* resolution in 1979, which proposed a set of measures in keeping with the spirit of both the Lalonde Report and the *Alma-Ata Declaration* (WHO, 1981), both incontrovertibly linking health to social and economic development.

The Canadian–European Connection

Lavada Pinder (1994) argued that little happened in Canada following the release of the Lalonde Report until the federal government established a Health Promotion Directorate (thought to be the first national body of its kind in the world) in 1978. The Directorate focused initially on the lifestyle component of the health field concept. Although a more comprehensive strategy directed at both lifestyles and policy measures was developed in 1982, it was never fully funded or implemented (Pinder, 1994).

At about the same time, under the leadership of Ilona Kickbusch, the World Health Organization Regional Office for Europe (WHO/Europe) in Copenhagen articulated a redirection of health education in a small discussion document on health promotion (WHO/Europe, 1984), written in collaboration with international leaders in the field such as David McQueen, Kimmo Leppo, John Catford, Bernard Badura, and Lowell Levin. This paper predated the *Ottawa Charter*, which ultimately formalized the earlier statement.

Collaboration between Canada's Health Promotion Directorate and the WHO/Europe team led to the first International Conference on Health Promotion in 1986, co-sponsored by WHO/Europe, Health and Welfare Canada, and the Canadian Public Health Association. Both the *Ottawa Charter* itself (WHO, 1986) (see figure 1.1) and a Canadian document, *Achieving Health for All* (Epp, 1986) (which came to be known as the Epp Report), were released at the conference. Both documents shared the same definition of health promotion and identified a common set of principles and values, although they differed in other respects. While the *Ottawa Charter* was intended for an international audience, *Achieving Health for All* was intended for a Canadian one.

As a field, the health education community itself had begun to articulate an internal critique at the end of the 1970s (e.g., Brown & Margo, 1978; Freudenberg, 1978; Labonté & Penfold, 1981), conscious that providing health information alone and focusing on individual behaviour could lead to "blaming the victim" (Ryan, 1976). Critics argued that changing the environment should become as great a focus for promoting health as chang-ing individual behaviour, and the aim became to make "the healthiest choice the easiest choice" (Milio, 1986). Critics argued that social, political, economic, cultural, and physical environments needed to support individual changes if people were going to change how they lived, worked, studied, aged, and played.

The Golden Age of Health Promotion?

Within Canada, the *Ottawa Charter* initially had little impact, whereas the Epp Report became an important policy document disseminated and discussed in workshops across Canada organized by Health and Welfare Canada. Additional resources were given to the Health Promotion Directorate, programs and initiatives were started, and a knowledge

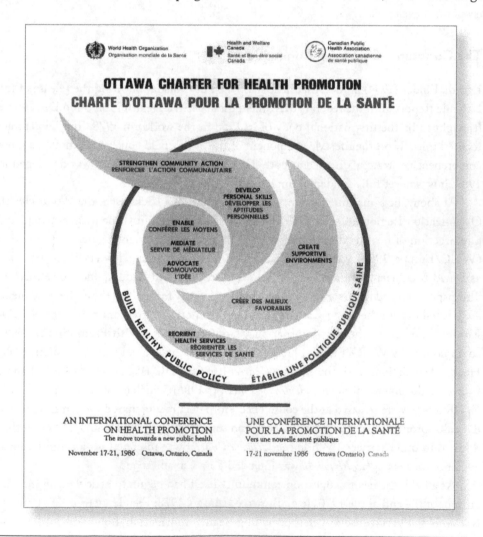

Figure 1.1: The *Ottawa Charter*

Source: WHO. (1986). *Ottawa Charter for Health Promotion* cover. Ottawa: World Health Organization, Health and Welfare Canada, Canadian Public Health Association.

development (KD) strategy was undertaken. The KD strategy involved commissioning literature reviews on the major elements of the Epp framework, developing a national health promotion survey, and supporting national and regional conferences and training events related to health promotion (Rootman & O'Neill, 1994, pp. 139–151). In addition, two important national initiatives were undertaken, the Strengthening Community Health project (Hoffman, 1994) and the Healthy Communities initiative (Manson-Singer, 1994), both of which aimed to stimulate health-enhancing community mobilization processes. A national Health Promotion Contribution Program was established that funded numerous community-based, health-promoting initiatives. The federal government also published a regular report on health promotion activities across the country.

At the provincial level—the level of government with constitutional responsibility for health services in Canada—various initiatives took place that embraced the discourse of health promotion and healthy public policy. These are described in detail in the first edition of *Health Promotion in Canada* (Pederson, O'Neill, & Rootman, 1994, pp. 154–311). In Ontario, for example, an association called Health Promotion Ontario was formed one year after the conference, and health promotion academics and practitioners collaborated with colleagues in Belgium the following year to establish a francophone health promotion network; both of these are still active. It was also during this period that the University of Toronto established a master's program in health promotion that still exists (now known as the MPH in Social and Behavioural Health Sciences).

1994–2007: THE POPULATION HEALTH ERA

Support for health promotion began to weaken—both in Canada and abroad—around 1994 (O'Neill, Pederson, & Rootman, 2000; Pederson, Rootman, & O'Neill, 2005). This shift arose from changes in the global and Canadian economic environment and institutions, as well as the emergence of "population health" as a new perspective on health and health care in Canada.

International Developments

From the mid-1990s on, the shift away from the welfare state that had begun in the late 1980s became clearer. A rhetoric of balanced government budgets, deficit reduction, a diminished role for the state, an increased one for the market, and the necessity of global economic competition in a neo-liberal era dominated political-economic discourse. This shift had numerous consequences. For example, United Nations system organizations (such as the WHO) lost influence while transnational corporations and economic global institutions, such as the World Bank, the International Monetary Fund, and the World Trade Organization, became increasingly powerful (Clift, 2013). This context contributed to the WHO no longer holding its international health promotion conferences on a regular schedule and needing to align the conference with topics that addressed the interests of the host country. Accordingly, the Jakarta (1997), Mexico (2000), and Bangkok (2005) conferences (and their respective policy statements) each reflected this new order of things.[2]

Indeed, some members of the global health promotion community publicly voiced their concern about the WHO's lack of commitment at the Mexico conference (Mittelmark et al., 2001) and about the inclusion of the private sector as a key partner in the *Bangkok Charter* (see the debate in the electronic journal *Reviews of Health Promotion and Education Online* [RHP&EO]).[3] Critics feared that if governments—the main mechanism through which health-enhancing policies were adopted—put health promotion in the hands of private corporations, the common good and the public's health would be at risk.

These global tendencies, in conjunction with the demise of the former communist world (set into motion with the collapse of the Berlin Wall in 1989), had important consequences for the evolution of health promotion. Reflecting on that era, Ron Labonté (2007, p. 93) suggested, for example, that the field needed to align itself with global social movements for health and justice, build empowering partnerships linking poorer nations with wealthier ones, and participate in debates on how globalization affects global health equity. He stressed that health promoters needed to acknowledge and address economic practices that undermine health.

The Rise of Population Health in Canada

In 1994, a book edited by Canadian and American health economists entitled *Why Are Some People Healthy and Others Not?* (Evans, Barer, & Marmor, 1994) was published. This book, and an earlier paper (Evans & Stoddard, 1990), helped to position the concept of "population health" on the health policy agenda, first in Canada and then elsewhere. Through the influence of these publications and skilled presentations to federal/provincial/territorial meetings in Canada, the federal government abandoned its leadership in health promotion. The F/P/T Advisory Committee on Population Health was established in 1992 and the Health Promotion Directorate was replaced by a Population Health Directorate in 1995. The federal Cabinet formally adopted the population health approach to guide health policy in 1997.

According to John Frank (1995), the population health approach focused on the social determinants of population differences rather than individual differences in disease. Accordingly, population health approaches advocate policy interventions, ignoring many aspects of health promotion practice—such as community development and mutual aid.

Yet health promotion did not disappear in Canada. Health Canada made a serious effort to integrate population health and health promotion thinking into a common framework (Hamilton & Bhatti, 1996; see figure 1.2), though some argued the two frameworks were incommensurable (Labonté, 1995). The federal department maintained and produced programs built on the foundation established throughout the first two decades of health promotion. Health promotion concepts and approaches were also integrated into federal, provincial, and territorial strategies, and at least two provinces established ministries or departments of health promotion.

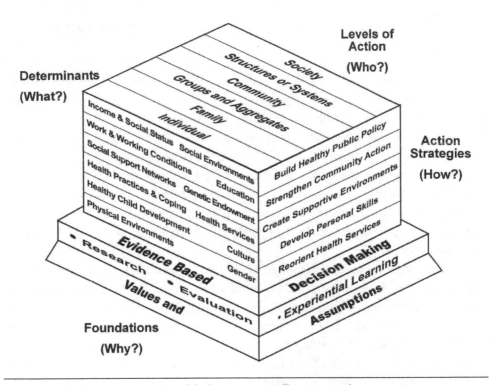

Figure 1.2: Population Health Promotion Framework

Source: Adapted from Hamilton, N. & Bhatti, T. (1996). *Population health promotion: An integrated model of population health and health promotion.* Ottawa: Public Health Agency of Canada.

In addition, Health Canada provided funding for a network of university-based research centres, the Canadian Consortium for Health Promotion Research, to facilitate shared projects and to organize the 19th world conference of the IUHPE in Vancouver in 2007. The Consortium members were very successful in obtaining funding for health promotion research projects from the Canadian Institutes of Health Research (CIHR) (established in 2001) and other research-funding programs and agencies. Indeed, by 2007, leadership of the field had shifted from the government to the academic sector. In fact, there were reasons for optimism about the future of health promotion at the time, particularly given the visibility and opportunities afforded by hosting the IUHPE global conference in Vancouver that year. However, shortly after the 2007 conference, the Canadian Consortium for Health Promotion Research was dissolved, leaving the field without the leadership that it had provided for the previous decade. Over the past decade, several of the university-based centres have closed, leading to a reduction in some forms of research as well as in the number of pan-Canadian research collaborations (Rootman, Jackson, & Hills, 2007). Nevertheless, the academy remains important to health promotion, providing a space for students and researchers to reinvent health promotion for a new era, and fostering a new generation of policy makers, researchers, and practitioners.

2007–2017: HEALTH PROMOTION IN AN ERA OF COMPLEXITY

Internationally, the collapse of the sub-prime mortgage market in the United States led to a global economic crisis in 2008 and forced virtually all countries to radically re-evaluate their commitments to social programs and activities, such as health promotion (CPH, 2008). This was notably visible in the Euro monetary zone, where countries like Greece had to be repeatedly saved from bankruptcy from 2010 on, and where severe public spending cuts have continued, leading to general strikes, massive unemployment, and significant social unrest. In addition, in Europe, there were changes to public funding for the health system in many countries, as well as cuts in prevention and health promotion.[4] Not surprisingly, some research suggests that population health suffered following the global crisis (e.g., Thomson et al., 2014), although the full scale of the impact may not be apparent for years.[5]

In the midst of the global recession, the WHO released the Commission on Social Determinants of Health report (CSDH, 2008), which had taken three years to complete and involved commissioners from both developing and developed countries, including Canada. The Commission relied on support from country partners including the Public Health Agency of Canada as well as from global knowledge networks, two of which were located in Canada (Early Childhood Development and Globalization). Titled *Closing the Gap in a Generation: Health Equity through Action on the Social Determinants of Health*, the report called on countries to address inequities associated with the social determinants of health by various means, including health promotion. Upon its release, Ilona Kickbusch argued that the report was "steeped in health promotion thinking, highlighted by the focus on 'daily living conditions' and reinforced by the statement that health depends on the 'conditions in which people are born, grow, live, work and age'" (Kickbusch, 2012, p. 308).

Further support for health promotion was evident at the IUHPE conference in Geneva in 2010, when then–Director General of the WHO, Dr. Margaret Chan, described herself as a strong ally of the field and renewed the commitment of her organization to health promotion. Furthermore, the Canadian delegation was the second-largest contingent of participants—suggesting the strength, depth, and capacity for health promotion in Canada.

In the past decade, health promotion and population health advocates alike have stressed the need for action to reduce health inequities. There have also been several high-profile reports produced in Canada that were influenced by health promotion practitioners and researchers and reflect health promotion thinking, including one by a subcommittee of the Canadian Senate (Keon, 2009) and another by the Health Council of Canada (HCC, 2010). Both reports reaffirmed the value of working at the level of the political economy and stressed the need for intersectoral action to promote the health of Canadians. However, a key part of the argument was that "unless governments change their approach to addressing the needs of poorer and socially disadvantaged Canadians, we are destined to continue paying handsomely for the consequent demands on our health care system" (Poland, 2012, p. 301). The argument was that health disparities were not only unfair, they were one of the major cost drivers of health care. Consistent with the arguments put forward two decades earlier, the report concluded that health is not only the responsibility of the health ministry, but must involve action across government and investment in the material factors that affect the health of Canadians (Poland, 2012, p. 301).

There have also been encouraging signs in relation to research, education, and training. For example, the five graduate programs in health promotion (at Dalhousie University, University of Montréal, Université Laval, University of Toronto, and University of Alberta) continue to provide training for practitioners and researchers (Potvin, Gauvin, Frohlich, & Richard, 2012). In addition, across the country, students in the more than 40 public health master's programs have access to health promotion training.

The 25th anniversary of the *Ottawa Charter* in 2011 spawned much reflection and discussion about the impact of the Charter and Canada's legacy in the field. At the annual Canadian Public Health Association (CPHA) conference, Trevor Hancock challenged those attending to "Catch the Health Promotion torch" (Hancock, 2011). A series of meetings followed at subsequent CPHA conferences, culminating in June 2016 with a session titled "Catching the Health Promotion Torch." Aimed at the next generations of practitioners and researchers, the session helped strengthen relationships between the practitioner and researcher communities in Canada by encouraging them to work together to support the development of a new pan-Canadian organization called Health Promotion Canada.[6]

As part of the celebration of the 30th anniversary of the *Ottawa Charter*, leaders in the field hosted the 6th Global Forum on Health Promotion in Charlottetown, Prince Edward Island, in October 2016. Traditionally held in Geneva and sponsored by the Alliance for Health Promotion (www.alliance4healthpromotion.org), the Global Forum was a gathering of civil society and non-governmental organizations. Close to 300 people attended, from 25 countries. A *PEI Declaration on Health Promotion* was generated and shared with the organizers of the WHO's 9th Global Conference held in Shanghai in November. The latter conference produced its own declaration on health promotion, known now as the *Shanghai Declaration*.

In spite of these positive developments, we need to recognize that health promotion and public health in general remain under siege in Canada. To quote an editorial in the *Canadian Journal of Public Health*, "Over the past few months, we have seen numerous attacks that directly target the ability of Canadian public health to fulfill its mandate, namely to prevent illness and to monitor, protect and promote the health of Canadians" (Potvin, 2014, p. 401). According to Potvin, these attacks come from a "growing number and variety of organizations" and were "widely echoed in the press" (Potvin, 2014, p. 401). For example, in an article in *The Globe and Mail*, one of Canada's two national newspapers, an author stated that "It is not the job of public health to have an opinion on taxes, economic policy, free-trade or corporate control. Neither should it be their business to interfere in the freely made choices of adults" (Taylor, 2014)—a view contrary to the very essence of health promotion. These attacks contribute to a climate that permits governments to reduce funding to public health initiatives and to reduce the power of trained public health leaders and practitioners.

CONCLUSION

Health promotion is not dead in Canada, though its infrastructure has fluctuated considerably over the past 40 years. Government and academic departments seldom use the term any longer, although courses are still offered in it, and a new association of practitioners is emerging. There is also a generational shift underway in the field. As more and more of the researchers, advocates, and leaders of the 1980s and 1990s retire, we see increasing numbers of younger leaders taking over the provincial public health associations, sitting on the board of directors of CPHA and the North American Regional Committee of the IUHPE, developing the Health Promotion Canada association and other non-governmental organizations (e.g., Bridge for Health), and engaging in health promotion research, policy-making, and practice.

Opportunities continue for "health promoters" to emerge in other sectors—indeed they must. Fields such as engineering, environmental science, education, economics, political science, and social work have much to offer with respect to addressing the social, political, and economic barriers to health and health equity in Canada. Moreover, the future of health promotion in Canada is tied, as it has always been, to challenges within Canada as well as to the global context. Social movements such as Black Lives Matter, fourth-wave feminism, LGBTQI rights, and Indigenous health will be critical to ensuring that Canada contributes to the commitment of the global Sustainable Development Goals and ensuring that "no one is left behind."

How do we account for the resilience of health promotion in Canada? We would suggest that its values base remains meaningful to discussions of globalization, migration, minority rights, and the unfairness of health inequities; that its evidence base supports action on environmental degradation, climate change, and social cohesion; and that its advocates—those who align themselves with its progressive agenda—continue to act through fluid, evolving networks of individuals and organizations, both in and beyond the state.

CRITICAL THINKING QUESTIONS

1. Can the *Ottawa Charter for Health Promotion* be considered a Canadian document? Why or why not?
2. Why did the Lalonde Report receive so much international attention?
3. Do you think 2007 was the beginning of a new era in Canadian health promotion? Why or why not?
4. Do you think that Canada is an international leader in health promotion? Why or why not?

RESOURCES

Further Readings

Critical Public Health. (2008). *Critical public health*. Special issue on *Health Promotion, 18*(4), 431–540.

In this special issue, the situation of health promotion is addressed with a critical eye at the global level, as well as in several countries (Canada, Australia, England) or continents (Africa).

Pederson, A., & Rootman, I. (2017). From health care to the promotion of health: Establishing the conditions for healthy communities in Canada. In E. de Leeuw & J. Simos (Eds.), *Healthy cities: The theory, policy, and practice of value-based urban planning* (pp. 43–61). London: Springer.

This chapter identifies and examines the conditions that led to the development of the healthy communities movement in Canada.

Relevant Websites

International Union for Health Promotion and Education (IUHPE)

www.iuhpe.org/index.php/en/

The International Union for Health Promotion and Education is the only global professional organization entirely devoted to advancing public health through health promotion and health education. This site is an important source for news and events in health promotion in three languages (English, Spanish, French). IUHPE has seven regional offices around the globe including a North American Regional Office (NARO) that includes Canada, the United States, and the Caribbean.

Reviews of Health Promotion and Education Online

www.iuhpe.org/rhpeo/

The website of IUHPE'S electronic journal, the *Reviews of Health Promotion and Education Online* (RHPEO).

World Health Organization

www.who.int/healthpromotion/en/

WHO's website on global health promotion conferences, including charters, declarations, etc., as well as the complete text of the *Alma-Ata Declaration on Primary Health Care* and the report of the Commission on the Social Determinants of Health (2009).

NOTES

1. See www.who.int/publications/almaata_declaration_en.pdf
2. See www.who.int/healthpromotion/conferences/en/
3. See www.iuhpe.org/rhpeo/reviews/2007/index.htm
4. For example, government spending on prevention and public health services was cut by about 13 percent even though this sector was already underfinanced in Greece between 2009 and 2012 (the latest year for which data are currently available). See www.euro.who.int/__data/assets/pdf_file/0007/266380/The-impact-of-the-financial-crisis-on-the-health-system-and-health-in-Greece.pdf
5. For more information, see: www.euro.who.int/__data/assets/pdf_file/0008/257579/Economic-crisis-health-systems-Europe-impact-implications-policy.pdf; www.thelancet.com/journals/lancet/article/PIIS0140-6736(09)61124-7/abstract; www.thelancet.com/journals/lancet/article/PIIS0140-6736(13)60102-6/abstract; www.thelancet.com/journals/lancet/article/PIIS0140-6736(11)61079-9/fulltext?rss%3Dyes
6. See www.healthpromotioncanada.ca

REFERENCES

Badgley, R. (1994). Health promotion and social change in the health of Canadians. In A. Pederson, M. O'Neill, & I. Rootman (Eds.), *Health promotion in Canada* (pp. 20–39). Toronto: W. B. Saunders.

Brown, R. E., & Margo, G.E. (1978). Health education: Can the reformers be reformed? *International Journal of Health Services, 8*(1), 3–26.

Clift, C. (2013). *The role of the World Health Organization in the international system.* London, Chatham House: Centre on Global Health Security Working Group Papers.

Commission on Social Determinants of Health (CSDH). (2008). *Closing the gap in a generation: Health equity through action on the social determinants of health.* Geneva: World Health Organization.

Critical Public Health (CPH). (2008). *Critical public health.* Special issue on *Health Promotion, 18*(4), 431–540.

Dupéré, S., Ridde, V., Carroll, S., O'Neill, M., Rootman, I., & Pederson, A. (2007). Conclusion: The rhizome and the tree. In M. O'Neill, A. Pederson, S. Dupéré, & I. Rootman (Eds.), *Health promotion in Canada* (2nd ed.) (pp. 371–389). Toronto: Canadian Scholars' Press.

Epp, J. (1986). *Achieving health for all: A framework for health promotion.* Ottawa: Health and Welfare Canada.

Evans, R. G., Barer, M. L., & Marmor, T. R. (1994). *Why are some people healthy and others not? The determinants of health of populations (social institutions and social change).* New York: Aldine de Guyter.

Evans, R. G., & Stoddard, G. L. (1990). Producing health, consuming health care. *Social Science and Medicine, 31*(12), 1347–1363.

Frank, J. W. (1995). Why 'population health'? *Canadian Journal of Public Health, 86*, 162–164.

Freudenberg, N. (1978). Shaping the future of health education: From behaviour change to social change. *Health Education Monographs, 6*(4), 372–377.

Gilbert, J. (1963). *L'éducation sanitaire*. Montréal: Presses de l'Université de Montréal.

Gilbert, J. (1967). The grandeur and decadence of health education. *Canadian Journal of Public Health, 58*, 355–358.

Green, L. W., & Kreuter, M. (1999). *Health promotion planning: An educational and ecological approach* (3rd ed.). Mountain View: Mayfield.

Hamilton, N., & Bhatti, T. (1996). *Population health promotion: An integrated model of health and health promotion*. Ottawa: Health Promotion Development Division, Health Canada.

Hancock, T. (2011). The Ottawa Charter at 25. *The Canadian Journal of Public Health, 102*(6), 404–406.

Health Council of Canada (HCC). (2010). *Stepping it up: Moving the focus from health care in Canada to a healthier Canada*. Toronto: Health Council of Canada.

Hoffman, K. (1994). The strengthening community health program: Lessons for community development. In A. Pederson, M. O'Neill, & I. Rootman (Eds.), *Health promotion in Canada* (pp. 123–139). Toronto: W. B. Saunders.

Keon, W. (2009). *A healthy productive Canada; A determinant of health approach*. Ottawa: Senate Sub-committee on Population Health.

Kickbusch, I. (2012). Understanding the rhizome effect: Health promotion in the twenty-first century. In I. Rootman, S. Dupéré, A. Pederson, & M. O'Neill (Eds.), *Health promotion in Canada: Critical perspectives* (2nd ed.) (pp. 308–313). Toronto: Canadian Scholars' Press.

Labonté, R. (1995). Population health and health promotion: What do they have to say to each other? *Canadian Journal of Public Health, 86*, 165–168.

Labonté, R. (2007). Promoting health in a globalizing world: The biggest challenge of all? In M. O'Neill, A. Pederson, S. Dupéré, & I. Rootman (Eds.), *Health promotion in Canada* (2nd ed.) (pp. 207–222). Toronto: Canadian Scholars' Press.

Labonté, R., & Penfold, S. (1981). Canadian perspectives in health promotion: A critique. *Health Education, 19*(3–4), 4–10.

Lalonde, M. (1974). *A new perspective on the health of Canadians*. Ottawa: Government of Canada.

Manson-Singer, S. (1994). The Canadian healthy communities project: Creating a social movement. In A. Pederson, M. O'Neill, & I. Rootman (Eds.), *Health promotion in Canada* (pp. 107–122). Toronto: W. B. Saunders.

Milio, N. (1986). *Promoting health through public policy* (2nd ed.). Ottawa: Canadian Public Health Association.

Mittelmark, M. B., Akerman, M., Gillis, D., Kosa, K., O'Neill, M., Piette, D., … Wise, M. (2001). Mexico conference on health promotion: Open letter to WHO director general, Dr. Gro Harlem Brundtland. *Health Promotion International, 16*(1), 3–4.

Modolo, M. A., & Mamon, J. (2001). *A long way to health promotion through IUHPE conferences (1951–2001)*. Perugia: University of Perugia, Inter-university Experimental Center for Health Education.

O'Neill, M., Pederson, A., & Rootman, I. (2000). Health promotion in Canada: Declining or transforming? *Health Promotion International, 15*(2), 135–141.

O'Neill, M., Pederson, A., Rootman, I., & Dupéré, S. (Eds.). (2007). *Health promotion in Canada: Critical perspectives.* Toronto: Canadian Scholars' Press.

Pederson, A., O'Neill, M., & Rootman, I. (Eds.) (1994). *Health promotion in Canada: Provincial, national and international perspectives.* Toronto: W. B. Saunders Canada.

Pederson, A., Rootman, I., & O'Neill, M. (2005). Health promotion in Canada: Back to the past or towards a promising future? In A. Scriven & S. Garman (Eds.), *Promoting health: Global perspectives* (pp. 255–265). London: Palgrave Macmillan.

Pinder, L. (1994). The federal role in health promotion: Art of the possible. In A. Pederson, M. O'Neill, & I. Rootman (Eds.), *Health promotion in Canada* (pp. 92–105). Toronto: W. B. Saunders.

Pinder, L. (2007). The federal role in health promotion: Under the radar. In M. O'Neill, A. Pederson, S. Dupéré, & I. Rootman (Eds.), *Health promotion in Canada* (2nd ed.) (pp. 92–106). Toronto: Canadian Scholars' Press.

Poland, B. (2012). A healthier Canada is not just the responsibility of health ministries. In I. Rootman, S. Dupéré, A. Pederson, & M. O'Neill (Eds.), *Health Promotion in Canada* (3rd ed.). Toronto: Canadian Scholars' Press.

Potvin, L. (2014). Editorial: Canadian health promotion under siege. *Canadian Journal of Public Health, 105*(6), e401–403.

Potvin, L., Gauvin, L., Frohlich, K. L., & Richard, L. (2012). Health promotion at the University of Montreal: The legacy of an option in a graduate training program. In I. Rootman, S. Dupéré, A. Pederson, & M. O'Neill (Eds.), *Health Promotion in Canada* (3rd ed.). Toronto: Canadian Scholars' Press.

Rootman, I., Jackson, S., & Hills, M. (2007). Developing knowledge for health promotion. In M. O'Neill, A. Pederson, S. Dupéré, & I. Rootman (Eds.), *Health promotion in Canada* (2nd ed.) (pp. 123–138). Toronto: Canadian Scholars' Press.

Rootman, I., & O'Neill, M. (1994). Developing knowledge for health promotion. In A. Pederson, M. O'Neill, & I. Rootman (Eds.), *Health promotion in Canada: Provincial, national, and international perspectives* (pp. 139–153). Toronto: W. B. Saunders.

Ryan, W. (1976). *Blaming the victim* (rev. ed.). New York: Vintage Books Edition.

Taylor, P. S. (2014, November 17). Public health officials should focus on disease, not politics. *The Globe and Mail.* Retrieved from www.theglobeandmail.com/opinion/public-health-officers-should-focus-on-disease-not-politics/article21610596/

Thomson, S., Figueras, J., Evetovits, T., Jowett, M., Mladovsky, P., Maresso, A., … Kluge, H. (2014). *Economic crisis, health systems and health in Europe: impact and implications for policy.* Copenhagen: European Office of the World Health Organization.

UNICEF. (1978). *The declaration of Alma-Ata.* International Conference on Primary Health Care. Alma-Ata: United Nations Children's Fund and World Health Organization.

World Health Organization (WHO). (1981). *November 19, 1981 64th plenary meeting, Resolution 36/43.* Retrieved from www.un-documents.net/a36r43.htm

World Health Organization (WHO). (1986). *Ottawa charter for health promotion*. Ottawa: World Health Organization, Health and Welfare Canada, Canadian Public Health Association.

WHO/Europe. (1984). *Health promotion: A discussion document on the concept and principles. ICP/HSR 602 (m01)*. Unpublished manuscript, Copenhagen. Retrieved from heapro.oxfordjournals.org/content/1/1/73.citation

CHAPTER 2

Key Concepts in Health Promotion

Irving Rootman and Michel O'Neill

LEARNING OBJECTIVES

1. Understand key concepts in health promotion
2. Understand the role of concepts in health promotion
3. Understand variations in definitions of concepts
4. Understand conceptual issues in health promotion

INTRODUCTION

A concept is "an abstract idea."[1] Concepts are critical for both research and practice, help to define what a field is about, stimulate theory-building, and are the primary elements of the theories that are then built. In addition, they reflect the values that guide a field. All of this is certainly true for health promotion. Thus, this chapter discusses some of the key concepts that help to define the field and its practice, given, as the old saying from social psychologist Kurt Lewin goes, "there is nothing more practical as a good theory" (Lewin, 1952, p. 169). In particular, it covers the following: health, health promotion, determinants of health, empowerment, health literacy, and quality of life. In doing so, it draws on some chapters from the previous three editions of *Health Promotion in Canada* and adds new material from other sources. It reflects the evolution in thinking about health promotion over the years and the dynamic nature of this field of study and practice.

THE CONCEPT OF HEALTH

Health is a fundamental concept for many fields, including medicine, nursing, public health, and health promotion. There are many competing concepts of health (Rootman & Raeburn, 1994; Raeburn & Rootman, 2007). Examples of different views of health

Box 2.1: Some Definitions of Health

WHO definition: "Health is a state of complete physical, mental and social well-being and not merely the absence of disease and infirmity" (WHO, 1946, p. 1).

Medical definition: "The normal physical state, i.e., the state of being whole and free from physical and mental disease or pain, so that the parts of the body carry on their proper function" (Critchley, 1978, p. 784).

Combined medical and non-medical definition: "[H]ealth is much more than the measurement of death, disease and disability, it also encompasses mental and social well-being, quality of life, life satisfaction and happiness" (Hancock, Labonté, & Edwards, 1999, p. S21).

Academic definition: Health "involves the interplay of biological, psychological and social aspects of the person's life" (Sarafino, 1990, p. 16).

Bangkok Charter definition: [Health promotion] "offers a positive and inclusive concept of health as a determinant of the quality of life and encompassing mental and spiritual well-being" (WHO, 2005, p. 1).

Holistic definition: "[A]n on-going sense of finely tuned wellness, which involves not only excellent care of the physical body but also care of ourselves in such a way that we nurture our capacity to be mentally alert and creative as well as emotionally stable and satisfied ..." (quoted in Alster, 1989, p. 78).

Ottawa Charter definition: "[A] resource for everyday life, not the objective of living. Health is a positive concept emphasizing social and personal resources, as well as physical capacities" (WHO, 1986, p. 1).

Public conceptions: 1. Not being ill; 2. Fitness; 3. Sense of wellbeing; 4. Ability to carry out tasks; 5. Resource for living; 6. Asset to be managed (summarized in Segall & Fries, 2011, p. 238–240).

Sociological conception: "Today, health is increasingly seen as a resource that is shaped not only by lifestyle activities but also by structural factors ... health as a resource for living consists of a combination of physical fitness, a sense of psychological healthiness or wellbeing, and a social capacity to perform well expected roles, and all three are necessary for the pursuit of health and wellness" (Segall & Fries, 2011, p. 240).

from different perspectives are shown in box 2.1. Probably the most influential in general, as well as for health promotion, has been the definition of health in the World Health Organization's *Constitution* as "a state of complete physical, mental and social wellbeing and not merely the absence of disease and infirmity" (WHO, 1946). However, some critics have questioned the use of the term *state* rather than *process*, and others have argued that it puts no boundaries on what is encompassed and therefore no limits on expenditures to deal with it (Rootman & Raeburn, 1994). Nevertheless, it strongly influenced the definition of health included in the *Ottawa Charter for Health Promotion* (WHO, 1986), which in turn has had and continues to have significant influence on health promotion practice in Canada and throughout the world.

As mentioned in chapter 1, another internationally influential concept of health for health promotion was developed in Canada: "the health field concept" (Lalonde, 1974). It suggested that health was determined by more than just health services. As noted, it listed four broad contributory categories of factors or "elements," later to be called determinants, making up the "health field": human biology, environment, lifestyle, and health care organization.

For health promoters, it was the introduction of lifestyle and environment into the health discourse that was memorable, especially the notion of "lifestyle," a concept that dominated Canadian and international health promotion thinking and action for at least a decade after the Lalonde Report, and still lingers on. However, as also mentioned in chapter 1, during the 1980s there was a move away from individualistic behavioural views of health promotion to more social and policy views. In Canada, the mid-1980s were important for the influential introduction of concepts like the "Mandala of Health" (Hancock & Perkins, 1985). In 1986, the *Ottawa Charter for Health Promotion* proposed to view health as a "resource for living" and did put an emphasis on a broad social determinants model of health (WHO, 1986). This model was echoed in the Canadian government document *Achieving Health for All: A Framework for Health Promotion*, released at the same conference as the *Ottawa Charter* (Epp, 1986), albeit with a more personal tone (using concepts like "self-help" and "mutual aid") and a strong emphasis on equity. In 1989, Raeburn and Rootman combined the health concepts of the Lalonde health field and the *Ottawa Charter* (Raeburn & Rootman, 1989), and in 1993, Labonté (1993) took up the issue of subjective and objective views of health.

Specifically, as shown in figure 2.1, Labonté suggested that health is not on a continuum, but rather a domain that overlaps with two other domains—illness and disease. According to him, the circle of health/wellness represents persons who would say that they are healthy. Those falling into area A would have a commitment to important values, sense of control over their life, and ability to see change as a challenge; they would not be experiencing illness or have a medically diagnosed condition. On the other hand, the illness circle represents feeling ill or "out-of-sorts," the white area being illness that cannot be explained by conventional medicine. The "disease" circle represents diagnosed or diagnosable pathologies, the white area covering undiagnosed disease such as high blood

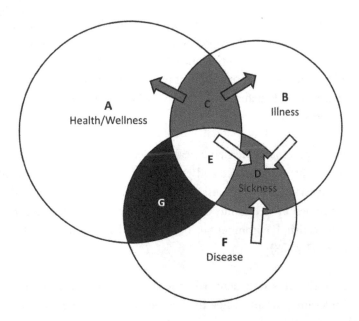

Figure 2.1: Relationships between Health, Illness, and Disease

Source: Labonté, R. (1993). *Community health and empowerment.* Toronto: Centre for Health Promotion.

pressure. The shaded area D represents a situation in which people are diagnosed as having disease and actually feel sick. E is where people feel sick as a result of having been given the diagnosis and the shaded area G refers to people diagnosed with diseases but who consider themselves to be healthy. Finally, shaded area C is the grey zone of feeling "so-so" where it doesn't take much to be tipped into feeling well or unwell.

Even if there are many ways of looking at health, the common conceptual feature to them all is that it relates to a broad domain of life that can be differentiated from other broad domains, such as economics, politics, justice, and education. The distinctive feature of this domain is that it relates to the integration of the human organism's condition, wellbeing, and functioning. Thus, it was suggested in 1994 (in the first edition of *Health Promotion in Canada*) that the following statement describes a concept of health that could be of use to Canadian health promoters:

> Health as perceived in a Canadian health promotion context has to do with the bodily, mental and social quality of life of people as determined in particular by psychological, societal, cultural and policy dimensions. Health is seen by Canadian health promoters as being enhanced by a sensible lifestyle and the equitable use of public and private resources to permit people to use their initiative individually and collectively to maintain and improve their own well being, however they may define it. (Rootman & Raeburn, 1994, p. 69)

Thirteen years later (in the second edition of *Health Promotion in Canada*), the same authors took a further look at the concept and at the dilemmas that it generated. They concluded that a new concept was necessary for the twenty-first century, to reinvigorate health promotion and make it more relevant to the present and the future. The following was suggested as a possible definition, underpinning and giving direction to health promotion practitioners:

> In the health promotion domain, health is equivalent to healthiness and is related to concepts of resilience and capacity. It refers primarily to mental and physical dimensions of healthiness, has strong experiential and social aspects, and is determined by many internal and external factors, including those of a personal, collective, environmental, political, and global nature. (Raeburn & Rootman, 2007, p. 28)

It was hoped that this statement would lead to the articulation of a strong, positive, exciting, and relevant concept of health that would take the field of health promotion forward at that point in time.

A step leading in this direction was a paper published about the same time in *Health Promotion International* (Eriksson & Lindström, 2008), which argued that Antonovsky's salutogenic theory of health should become a key one for the field. The authors suggested that the focus on factors supporting wellbeing, in contrast to ones that cause disease, could make an important contribution to health promotion theory and practice. The high profile that salutogenesis (see box 2.2) received at the 20th Global Conference on Health Promotion, held in Geneva in 2010,[2] indicated that the idea of emphasizing salutogenesis was encouraged by the international health promotion community. However, a search of Google Scholar found that the number of mentions of the concept of salutogenesis from 2005 to 2010 as compared to 2011 to 2016 declined from 71 to 22, perhaps

Box 2.2: Salutogenesis

The term *salutogenesis* was put forward by Aaron Antonovsky in the early 1980s to describe an approach to human health emphasizing the factors supporting health and wellbeing, rather than those that cause disease. He developed this concept from his research on how people survive, adapt, and overcome even the most difficult life-stress experiences, such as living in a concentration camp. He hypothesized that a stress factor will be either pathogenic, neutral, or salutary, depending on what he called *generalized resistance resources* (GRRs). According to him, these GRRs help people make sense of and manage events. He postulated that a person's sense of coherence determines whether stress will harm them.

Source: Lindström, B., & Eriksson, M. (2010). *The hitchhiker's guide to salutogenesis: Salutogenic pathways to health promotion.* Helsinki: Folkhälsan Research Centre.

suggesting that scholars were, if anything, less interested in studying the concept rather than more interested. Nevertheless, a recent publication in the journal *Health Promotion International* continued to argue that salutogenesis "provides a theoretical frame in which suffering is presented as a potential positive source of learning" (Oliveira, 2014, p. 222). Moreover, a handbook on salutogenesis edited by leaders in health promotion, and to be released as this book goes to press, may renew interest in the concept in Canada and around the world (Mittelmark et al., 2017).

On the other hand, as suggested above, there has been increasing interest in the concept of "wellbeing" in health promotion as well as in the concept of "wellness." According to Segall and Fries (2011, p. 65), the latter is "much broader than health and actually subsumes good health."

In summary, although there is yet no unanimously accepted definition of health, and perhaps will never be one, it appears as if Canadian scholars and practitioners in health promotion recognize that health has physical, mental, and social components; is related to "wellbeing"; and can been seen as a *resource for life* (Segall & Fries, 2011, pp. 238–240; Raeburn & Rootman, 2007, p. 28).

THE CONCEPT OF HEALTH PROMOTION

As is the case for "health," there are also many different concepts of "health promotion" and, not surprisingly, much confusion among them (O'Neill & Stirling, 2007). In order to sort this out, it is important to distinguish between two ways in which the words *health promotion* are used: (1) as a *discourse* on the place of health in societies, and (2) as a *specialized field of intervention* within the broader field of public health. Thus, it has been suggested that the expression *the promotion of health* be used for the discourse that can be undertaken by anybody and that the expression *health promotion* be restricted to the specialized field of practice (O'Neill & Stirling, 2007).

This distinction is well illustrated by contrasting two of the best-known definitions of the field. The first is from the *Ottawa Charter for Health Promotion*: "The process of enabling people to increase control over, and improve, their health" (WHO, 1986, p. 1), whereas the other is by Green and Kreuter, whose PRECEDE-PROCEED model dominated the field for decades: "any planned combination of educational, political, regulatory and organizational supports for actions and conditions of living conducive to the health of individuals, groups or communities" (2005, p. 462).

The Promotion of Health

The *Ottawa Charter* definition, as well as most governmental health policy documents in Canada or around the world since the mid-1970s, are typical of the reflections on what health is or should be; on the place health should have in societies; and on who should undertake health-promoting, health-restoring, or health-maintaining endeavours—hence

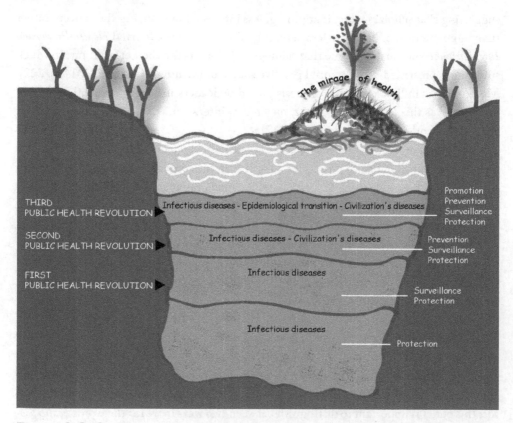

Figure 2.2: Sedimentation Approach to Public Health throughout Human History

Source: Adapted from Potvin, L. (2005). Présentation dans le séminaire doctoral SAC-66008, Université Laval, October 17, 2005; and Breslow, L. (1999). From disease prevention to health promotion. *JAMA, 281*(11), 1030–1033.

the idea of naming this a discourse on *the promotion of health*, which is nothing but the old public health discourse that has been around for centuries (Fassin, 2000). This reflects upon what health is in societies or populations; what produces or hinders it; and what can be done to improve it, reduce the risk of losing it, or restore it when compromised. It is in this perspective that health promotion (as symbolized by the *Ottawa Charter*) was identified as the "third public health revolution" of humankind (Breslow, 1999) after the first, which tackled infectious diseases, and the second, which addressed chronic illnesses. The health promotion era, according to Breslow, embarks on the journey toward health rather than engaging in a battle against diverse types of diseases. This shift in thinking is illustrated in figure 2.2, where we can see that with the evolution of humankind, of the epidemiological patterns of disease, and of the technological means available, the various functions of public health have successively developed in a series of layers like sediments. Each successive layer builds on top of, rather than displacing, the former one, which still needs support from the previous ones to continue to function properly.

The discourse on the promotion of health in *modern* societies, which is symbolized by the *Ottawa Charter*, has been referred to as the "new" (Ashton & Seymour, 1988; Martin & McQueen, 1989) or the "ecological" public health (Chu & Simpson, 1994; Kickbusch, 1989) in order to differentiate it from the more classical discourse of "hygiene" or "old" public health. We thus argue that population health, as it emerged in Canada in 1994 and as discussed in chapter 1, was but a variation of this new public health discourse on *the promotion of health* and that "in general, the proponents of population health can be seen as allies [of health promotion] in the move towards the new public health, particularly since overall, neither framework has significantly challenged the dominance of biomedicine in the health field" (O'Neill, Pederson, & Rootman, 2000, p. 141).

Health Promotion

Conversely, Green and Kreuter's definition is more in line with the idea that *health promotion* is a specialized sub-area, or essential function, of the public health sector of health systems. According to the Pan-American Health Organization, health promotion aims at "the promotion of changes in lifestyle and environmental conditions to facilitate the development of a culture of health" (2002, p. 67). We thus argue that what really defines health promotion is its focus on the *planned change* of lifestyles and life conditions having an impact on health, using a variety of specific strategies including health education, social marketing, and mass communication on the individual side, as well as political action, community organization, and organizational development on the collective side.

Given this view, the planned-change skills and other specific competencies of properly trained health promoters can be used at whatever stage in the natural history of any illness or health problem (thus in primary or secondary prevention, in acute care, in rehabilitation, or in tertiary prevention) and at any level, from the individual to the societal, including the family and the community. Moreover, even if the value base (empowerment and participation of populations, social justice, etc.) of the *Ottawa Charter* can be used to work with these *health promotion* skills, they can also be used by other groups, working with other value bases. Finally, in order to be as effective as possible, planned-change *health promotion* interventions must apply strategies that are knowledge-based or evidence-based when that type of information is available. The relationship between *the promotion of health* and *health promotion* is illustrated in figure 2.3.

We thus propose that the words *new public health* or *ecological public health* should be used when we talk about the discourse on the promotion of health, and the expression *health promotion* reserved to designate the specific planned-change skills needed to achieve the results desired by the "new public health" discourse.

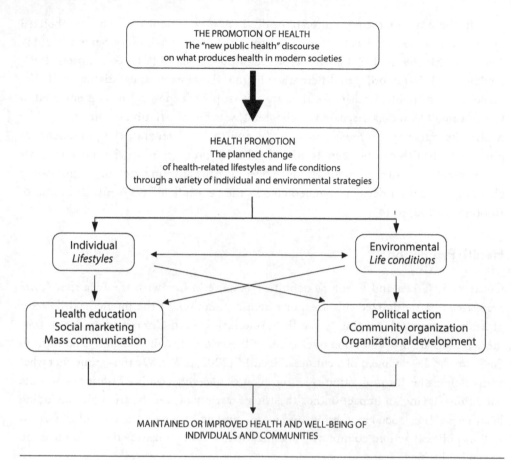

Figure 2.3: The Promotion of Health versus Health Promotion

Source: Adapted and modified from O'Neill, M., & Stirling, A. (2007). The promotion of health or health promotion? In M. O'Neill, S. Dupéré, A. Pederson, & I. Rootman (Eds.), *Health promotion in Canada: Critical perspectives* (p. 42). Toronto: Canadian Scholars' Press.

Health Promotion versus Health Education

Furthermore, in trying to clarify the boundaries of health promotion as a field, it is helpful to compare it with another closely related field, namely, health education (O'Neill & Stirling, 2007). As noted in chapter 1, health promotion emerged as an evolution of health education, which had formalized itself at the beginning of the 1950s and worked from then on to influence individual health-related behaviours. However, during the 1970s, many health educators realized that trying to influence individual behaviours without altering the environments in which they occurred produced limited results. In the mid-1980s, the field as a whole thus re-labelled itself "health promotion" to signify that from then on, just working to change individual lifestyles was no longer a viable option. A much broader way of looking at things, soon to be called "ecological" (see chapter 5 of this book), was suggested to be required to understand and influence health-related behaviours.

For many, the transition from traditional individualistic health education towards a more ecologically oriented health promotion, requiring practitioners to intervene at a variety of levels, was difficult (Green & Raeburn, 1988). For instance, it was only in 1993, several years after the adoption of the *Ottawa Charter*, that the main professional and scientific global organization in the field, the International Union for Health Education (IUHE), decided to follow the trend and rename itself the International Union for Health Promotion and Education (IUHPE), keeping the two expressions within its new title.

In several countries such as the US and France, the words health education had more currency than health promotion, the former being sometimes used to designate the old version of individualistic health education, and sometimes used to designate the new enlarged field called "health promotion" elsewhere. According to Nutbeam: "Health education comprises consciously constructed opportunities for learning involving some form of communication designed to improve health literacy, including improving knowledge, and developing life skills which are conducive to individual and community health" (Nutbeam, 1998, p. 354).

Box 2.3 was co-authored for the second edition of this book by Keith Tones and Jackie Green, the former editors of one of the most important journals in the field, *Health Education Research*. It shows that the debate was then far from over. Nevertheless, most people working in health promotion currently take the view that health education is one strategy within the larger field of health promotion (see figure 2.2).

Box 2.3: Health Education: Resurrection and Reinvention

By K. Tones and J. Green

The following simple equation encapsulates a "revitalized" definition of health education: *Health promotion = Health education × healthy public policy.*

An essential weakness of pre-Ottawa health education was its apparent lack of awareness of the importance of the social and environmental determinants of disease in its blinkered emphasis on the individual. However, health promotion's justifiable attempts to remedy this myopic view have tended to ignore the importance of education in overcoming political barriers in pursuit of *Healthy Public Policy*. Education without policy is emasculating; on the other hand, policy without education is virtually unattainable. Technically, Health Education involves a planned attempt to provide the conditions necessary for efficient learning, including those learning outcomes centrally involved in empowering communities. Accordingly, we assert the importance of providing community members, through health education, with specific skills (e.g., assertiveness), recognize that it is highly desirable for them to enlist the support of coalitions, and, finally, believe in media advocacy in order to generate indignation and community action.

OTHER KEY CONCEPTS IN HEALTH PROMOTION

There are a number of other key concepts in health promotion and a discussion of some is presented below. The specific concepts presented are determinants of health, empowerment, health literacy, and quality of life. They were selected because they are considered by many to be core to the practice of health promotion and are frequently used by people working in the field.

Determinants of Health

Although the term *determinants of health* is now widely used in population health and in health promotion, it is seldom, or never, defined. However, according to the *Oxford English Dictionary*, a determinant is "a factor that decisively affects the nature or outcome of something." As noted above, the *Health Field Concept* identified four elements or "factors" that contribute to health: human biology; environment; lifestyle; and health care organization.

Subsequently, as a result of the work of the Population Health Group at the Canadian Institute for Advanced Research, in 1994 the federal and provincial minsters of health in Canada endorsed a list of "Determinants of Health" that included the four elements of the *Health Field Concept* as well as some others. Specifically, the so-called determinants were income and social status; social support networks; education; employment and working conditions; physical environments; biology and genetic endowment; personal health practices and coping skills; healthy child development; and health services (FPT ACPH, 1994). Subsequently, Health Canada added gender and culture to the list.

Since then, among the various sets of determinants that have an impact on health, the "social" ones have gained significant currency in health promotion, partly as a result of work done in Canada. The history of the importance of social determinants has been traced to the political economist Friedrich Engels (see chapter 3) and to the physician and politician Rudolf Virchow in the nineteenth century (Raphael, 2016), both of whom drew attention to the links between social conditions and health. Other contributions have been made over the years by British politicians and researchers, as well as Canadian politicians (Lalonde, 1974; Epp, 1986) and public health officials (Canadian Public Health Association, 2000, 2001).

The term *social determinants of health* made its debut in a book by British researchers (Blane, Brunner, & Wilkinson, 1996) that expanded on the environmental determinants of health in the health field concept of the Lalonde Report; the authors considered that the environment was not just physical, but social as well. As noted above, work was also done by the Canadian Institute for Advanced Research (Evans, Barer, & Marmor, 1994) and Health Canada (1998) to outline various determinants of health, many of which are social in nature. A pivotal national conference in 2002 on the social determinants of health identified 12 key social determinants (see box 2.4) and led to the definition of social determinants of health as "the economic and social conditions that shape the health of individuals, communities, and jurisdictions as a whole" (Raphael, 2009, p. 2).

Attention has been drawn internationally to the social determinants of health by the World Health Organization's Commission on Social Determinants of Health (CSDH, 2008). Although it does not provide a simple declarative definition of social determinants of health in its report, a WHO backgrounder on the work of the commission defines it as "the circumstances in which people are born, grow up, live, work and age, and the systems put in place to deal with illness" (WHO, 2010, p. 2).

In addition to the focus on the social determinants, in Canada and elsewhere the interest of people working in health promotion has also been drawn to implications of the physical environment for health promotion. For example, in the third edition of *Health Promotion in Canada*, Trevor Hancock discussed the issue of "sustainable development," particularly in relation to the physical environment (e.g., global climate and atmospheric changes, depletion of renewable and non-renewable resources, and exotoxicity), as one that people working in health promotion should be more concerned about (Hancock, 2012, pp. 128–130). He expands on the challenge of addressing the physical-environment determinants of health in chapter 22 of this edition.

Thus, the concept of "determinants of health" has evolved; it is still very much alive in health promotion work in Canada and internationally and is discussed in a number of places in this book, especially in chapters 5, 8, 18, 19, 22, and 23. In addition, the concept of "inequities" is an important concept linked to the determinants of health and is thoroughly discussed in chapter 8.

Box 2.4: The Social Determinants of Health Framework

The following 12 social determinants of health were identified by the organizers of the York University conference on the social determinants of health (Raphael, 2009):

- Aboriginal status
- Early life
- Education
- Employment and working conditions
- Food security
- Gender
- Health care services
- Housing
- Income and its distribution
- Social exclusion
- Social safety net
- Unemployment and employment security

The following four other social determinants have been added since then by Raphael and colleagues: disability; geography; immigrant status; and race (Raphael, 2016, p. 11).

Empowerment

Empowerment is another key concept and value for health promotion. In fact, it has been suggested that "the primary criterion for determining whether or not a particular initiative should be considered to be health promoting, ought to be the extent to which it involves the process of enabling, or empowering individuals or communities" (Rootman, Goodstadt, Potvin, & Springett, 2001, p. 14). Similarly, the authors of this statement suggested that "health promotion is fundamentally about ensuring that the individuals and communities are able to assume the power to which they are entitled" (pp. 13–14). Although some people working in the field do not routinely apply the criterion of empowerment to their work, perhaps because they often have constraints that limit their capacity to act in empowering ways, it is widely acknowledged by many, if not most, as a cardinal principle and value of health promotion. This is, in part, because of its relevance as a mechanism for reducing inequities in health, which is a fundamental goal of health promotion.

The concept of empowerment was developed in the field of community psychology in the 1980s, where it was defined by Rappaport as "a mechanism by which people, organizations and communities gain mastery over their lives" (1987, p. 122). It was also picked up in the field of nursing with a similar definition (Gibson, 1991). Rissel (1994) added to the concept in health promotion by distinguishing between psychological and community empowerment. He defined the former as "a feeling of greater control over their own lives which individuals experience following active membership in groups or organizations, and may occur without participation in collective political action" (Rissel, 1994, p. 41). He suggested that "community empowerment" "includes a raised level of psychological empowerment among its members, a political action component in which members have actively

Box 2.5: A Pioneer in Empowerment

Paulo Freire was a twentieth-century pioneer in empowerment even though he probably never used the term in his lifetime. Although he grew up in poverty himself in Brazil, he managed to empower himself though education and never forgot his humble beginnings when he became Director of Education and Culture of one of the Brazilian states. Working primarily among poor people, he adopted a form of "liberation theology" that ultimately formed the basis for what is now called "critical pedagogy." In his most influential book, *Pedagogy of the Oppressed*, he stated: "No pedagogy which is truly liberating can remain distant from the oppressed by treating them as unfortunates and by presenting for their emulation models from among the oppressors. The oppressed must be their own example in the struggle for their redemption" (Freire, 1970, p. 54). This statement still stands as an inspirational definition of the essence of empowerment and has had an important impact on the way in which empowerment is viewed in health promotion today (see chapter 21).

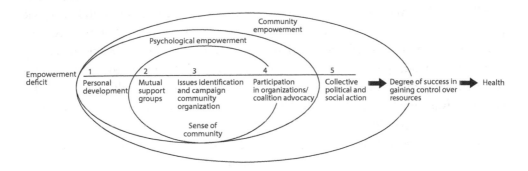

Figure 2.4: Model of the Critical Components of Community
Empowerment and the Process by Which It May Be Achieved

Source: Rissel, C. (1994). Empowerment: The holy grail of health promotion. *Health Promotion International, 9*(1), 43.

participated, and the achievement of some redistribution of resources or decision-making favourable to the group or community in question" (Rissel, 1994, p. 41). He further added to the understanding of the concept by putting forward a conceptual framework (figure 2.4) outlining a process through which psychological and community empowerment can lead to health, both at the individual and community levels.

Subsequently, empowerment has been defined as a "social action process for people to gain mastery over their lives in the context of changing their social and political environment to improve equity and quality of life" (Wallerstein, Minkler, Cater-Edwards, Avila, & Sanchez, 2015, p. 285). As did Rappaport, the authors of this definition added "organizational empowerment," located between "individual" and "community empowerment," as another level to consider (Wallerstein et al., 2015, p. 285).

Health Literacy

Health literacy is increasingly becoming a core concept in health promotion (Rootman, Frankish, & Kaszap, 2007). Although it first appeared in the health education literature in 1974 (Simonds, 1974), it wasn't picked up by health promotion until the late 1990s in a paper by Kickbusch (1997), as well as in a glossary of health promotion terms by Nutbeam (1998) and in a paper in which he argued (Nutbeam, 2000) that health literacy is a key outcome of health education activity for which people in health promotion and health education should be held accountable.

The concept of health literacy made its appearance in Canada in 2000 at the first Canadian Conference on Literacy and Health. It has become a focus of increased research and practice since the second Canadian conference in 2004 and the report of the Canadian

Expert Panel on Health Literacy (Rootman & Gordon-El-Bihbety, 2008). Although there is still some controversy over the definition of health literacy, elements of the following one put forward by the British Columbia Health Literacy Research team in 2006 are becoming more widely used in this country, and in others: "The degree to which people are able to access, understand, appraise and communicate information to engage with the demands of different health contexts in order to promote and maintain good health across the life-course" (Kwan, Frankish, & Rootman, 2006). In particular, most recent definitions include the elements of accessing, understanding, appraising, and communicating information although many also include the element of "using" it. In addition, they usually refer to the idea that health literacy is "contextual" and varies over the "life-course."

Chapter 5 in the second edition of *Health Promotion in Canada* discussed the development of health literacy work in Canada and issues it raised in relation to health promotion (Rootman, Frankish, & Kaszap, 2007, pp. 61–74). In addition, a section of a chapter on issues as a point of intervention in health promotion in the third edition also discussed health literacy (Gillis & Kaszap, 2012, pp. 125–127). Since the current edition does not have a specific chapter or section about it, we will briefly comment here on the evolution of the concept since the publication of the last edition of this book.

Over the past five years, some progress has been made on the development of a suitable definition of health literacy that addresses some of the limitations of previous ones. This progress is captured in a discussion paper recently published by the US National Academy of Medicine (Pleasant et al., 2016). Entitled "Considerations for a New Definition of Health Literacy," it suggests four necessary components for such a definition: (1) include system demands and complexities as well as individual skills and abilities; (2) include measurable components, processes, and outcomes; (3) recognize potential for an analysis of change; and (4) demonstrate linkage between informed decisions and action. The authors concede that there is still much to be done to reach a practical consensus on a definition that includes the above components, but think that it is achievable.

In the meantime, Canadian researchers and practitioners have been contributing to the development of the field of health literacy in areas like health promotion, health care, education, and many other fields. For example, a Canadian think tank sponsored by the Public Health Agency of Canada produced a discussion paper that stressed the need for an intersectoral approach (Mitic & Rootman, 2012). Such an approach has been taken up in British Columbia through the establishment of a network of networks, organizations, and individuals involved in health literacy work. In addition, the Province of Ontario has also recently developed a health literacy strategy that involves many sectors. Finally, three books on health literacy edited by Canadians have been published in the last five years (Begoray, Gillis, & Rowlands, 2012; Hoffman-Goetz, Donelle, & Ahmed, 2014; Begoray & Banister, 2015). Thus, the concept continues to develop and guide practice in health promotion and other fields in Canada and elsewhere. Most recently, health literacy featured prominently in declarations from the 2016 Global Forum on Health Promotion in PEI[3] and the 9th WHO Global Conference on Health Promotion in Shanghai.[4]

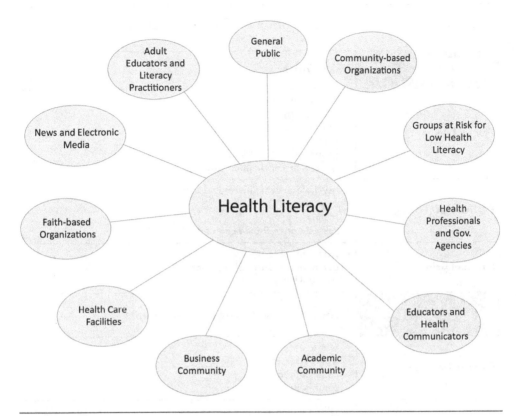

Figure 2.5: Major Stakeholders Involved in Health Literacy

Source: Mitic, W., & Rootman, I. (2012). *An intersectoral approach for improving the health literacy of Canadians: Discussion paper.* Victoria, BC: Public Health Association of British Columbia.

Quality of Life

Another key concept that was mentioned in the *Ottawa Charter* and is used in health promotion research and practice is "quality of life," which is often seen as the ultimate outcome of health promotion work. Although again, there are many definitions of quality of life, the one developed by the University of Toronto's Centre for Health Promotion research unit on this topic is: "The degree to which a person enjoys the important possibilities of his or her life."[5] This vision of quality of life is represented in nine life sectors grouped into Being, Belonging, and Becoming, as shown in table 2.1.

In this model, "Being" consists of physical, psychological, and spiritual components; "Belonging" of physical, social, and community ones; and "Becoming" of practical, leisure, and growth elements.

The concept of quality of life fits well in health promotion because it is both positive and inclusive (Raeburn & Rootman, 2007). Possibly for these reasons, it was included explicitly in the *Bangkok Charter for Health Promotion* (WHO, 2005).

Table 2.1: Centre for Health Promotion Quality of Life Model

Being	Who One Is
Physical Being	• physical health • personal hygiene • nutrition • exercise • grooming and clothing • general physical appearance
Psychological Being	• psychological health and adjustment • cognitions • feelings • self-esteem, self-concept, and self-control
Spiritual Being	• personal values • personal standards of conduct • spiritual beliefs
Belonging	**Connections with One's Environments**
Physical Belonging	• home • workplace/school • neighbourhood • community
Social Belonging	• intimate others • family • friends • co-workers • neighbourhood and community
Community Belonging	• adequate income • health and social services • employment • educational programs • recreational programs • community events and activities
Becoming	**Achieving Personal Goals, Hopes, and Aspirations**
Practical Becoming	• domestic activities • paid work • school or volunteer activities • meeting health or social needs
Leisure Becoming	• activities that promote relaxation and stress reduction
Growth Becoming	• activities that promote the maintenance or improvement of knowledge and skills • adapting to change

Source: Quality of Life Research Unit. (n.d.). *Quality of life model.* University of Toronto website. Retrieved from http://sites.utoronto.ca/qol/qol_model.htm

CONCLUSION

This chapter has discussed a number of key concepts in health promotion. Others could have been included, such as "life-course," which has long been a concept in the field of gerontology and is increasingly being used in health promotion research and practice. For example, Segall and Fries, in their book on health and wellness, draw on a life-course perspective that they define as "an approach that investigates how social factors (such as class, gender and ethnicity) operate at different stages of the life cycle and contribute to the creation of health disparities" (Segall & Fries, 2011, p. 369). That is, they link it with the concept of "determinants of health" and other related concepts such as "inequities in health" and "intersectional theory," which are discussed in other chapters of this book (see chapters 7 and 8). Dupéré, O'Neill, and De Koninck's (2012) work on the poor and underserved men in the Montréal area is another example of the fruitful use of the life-course perspective in health promotion.

Additional concepts will be introduced in other chapters, especially in those about theories relevant to health promotion such as the three chapters that follow. However, we believe that this chapter has presented a sufficient number of key ones to provide the reader with a good sense of what the central concepts and conceptual issues of the field are.

CRITICAL THINKING QUESTIONS

1. What concept of health do you prefer? Why do you think it is an appropriate concept for health promotion?
2. If you had to explain what "health promotion" is to the following people, what would you say to: your mother; your uncle Jack, a plumber, at a family gathering; a graduate student in physics; or Ms. Jones, a client at the neighbourhood community centre?
3. Explain the difference between the promotion of health and health promotion. Do you believe it is a useful distinction or not? Why?
4. What is the relationship between health education and health promotion? Do you think they should be separate fields or integrated into one?
5. Which of the other concepts discussed in this chapter do you think are most important in health promotion? Why?

RESOURCES

Further Readings

Antonovsky, A. (1979). *Health stress and coping.* San Francisco: Jossey Bass; and Antonovsky, A. (1987). *Unravelling the concept of health.* San Francisco: Jossey Bass.
These two books raise the question of what creates "health" rather than "disease." Antonovsky suggests and discusses the term *salutogenesis* to encourage more thinking and

research about the determinants of health rather than of disease. Lindström and Eriksson (2010) have published a book on the concept and Lindström has also established a research centre in Finland built around salutogenic research.

Contandriopoulos, A. P. (2005). A "topography" of the concept of health. In R. Lyons (Ed.), *Social sciences and humanities health research* (pp. 13–15). Ottawa: Canadian Institute of Health Research.
This is an interesting article about the concept of health that considers contributions from the social sciences and humanities to thinking about the concept. Also in the same volume is a one-page article (p. 120) by Contandriopoulos and other Canadian colleagues on a proposed project to integrate approaches and perspectives about the concept of health from the social and life sciences.

Hoffman-Goetz, L., Donelle, L., & Ahmed, R. (2014). *Health Literacy in Canada.* Toronto: Canadian Scholars' Press.
This book, mainly intended for students but of interest to researchers and practitioners as well, presents a comprehensive overview of health literacy from a Canadian perspective, but also contains examples from other countries. It discusses topics relevant to health promotion such as determinants of health, social justice, and health equity as they relate to health literacy.

Mittelmark, M., Sagy, S., Eriksson, M., Bauer, G. F., Pelikan, J. M., Lindstrom, B. & Espnes, G. A. (Eds.). (2017). *The handbook of salutogenesis.* Switzerland: Springer Nature, Springer International Publishing.
This recent book shows the breadth and strengths of the concept of salutogenesis in relation to health promotion, health care, and wellness. Background and historical chapters trace the development of the concept and flesh out its components, most notably generalized resistance resources and the sense of coherence, that differentiate it from pathogenesis. It also describes a range of real-world applications.

Raphael, D. (Ed.). (2010). *Health promotion and quality of life in Canada.* Toronto: Canadian Scholars' Press.
This book contains a series of papers produced by the University of Toronto Centre for Health Promotion's Quality of Life Unit, as well as other papers written for the volume. It explores the integral link between quality of life and public policy choices.

Raphael, D. (Ed.). (2016). *Social determinants of health: Canadian perspectives* (3rd ed.). Toronto: Canadian Scholars' Press.
This latest edition discusses key issues related to the social determinants of health in Canada and elsewhere, income security, employment, education (including literacy and health literacy), food, shelter, social exclusion, and public policy.

Ronson McNichol, B., & Rootman, I. (2016). Chapter 12: Literacy and health literacy: New understandings about their impact on health. In D. Raphael (Ed.), *Social Determinants of Health* (3rd ed.) (pp. 261–290). Toronto: Canadian Scholars' Press.
This chapter is an updated version of the chapters in the first and second editions of *Social Determinants of Health* and adds new material on literacy and health literacy in the context of Indigenous cultures drawing on Barbara Ronson McNichol's work on Indigenous Health as well as her experience in living in an Indigenous community for the last few years of her life.

Segall, A., & Fries, C. (2017). *Pursuing health and wellness: Healthy societies, healthy people* (2nd ed.). Toronto: Oxford University Press.
This book explores the structural and behavioural factors that affect health and wellbeing over the life-course using a sociological approach. It uses strong theoretical frameworks such as "intersectional" theory as well as current and historical examples.

Relevant Websites

Quality of Life Research Unit

sites.utoronto.ca/qol/qol_model.htm
The Quality of Life Research Unit at the University of Toronto is currently located in the Department of Occupational Science and Occupational Therapy. Since its establishment in 1991, it has done research and developed tools and initiatives in relation to various topics having to do with quality of life in relation to different population groups including children, adolescents, families, people with developmental disabilities, communities, people with disabilities, and seniors.

Relevant Listservs

Click4HP

www.lsoft.com/scripts/wl.exe?SL1=CLICK4HP&H=YORKU.CA
Click4HP is a listserv that was established by the Ontario Health Promotion Clearinghouse in 1996 and is operated by York University. It has an archive of discussions that have taken place since it was established on a wide range of health promotion topics, including the concept of health.

SDOH

listserv.yorku.ca/archives/sdoh.html
SDOH is a listserv that discusses issues related to the social determinants of health. Located at York University and moderated by Professor Dennis Raphael, SDOH is very active and committed to action related to the social determinants of health. Archives go back to January 2004.

CHLPEN

www.symplur.com/healthcare-hashtags/chlpen/

CHLPEN (Canadian Health Literacy and Patient Education Network) is a listserv that discusses issues related to health literacy, especially issues associated with patient education.

NOTES

1. Retrieved from oxforddictionaries.com/definition/concept
2. Retrieved on November 23, 2016, from www.iuhpe.org/index.php/en/
3. Retrieved on November 23, 2016, from globalforumpei-forummondialipe.com/en2016/pei-declaration/
4. Retrieved on November 23, 2016, from www.who.int/healthpromotion/conferences/9gchp/shanghai-declaration/en/
5. Retrieved on November 24, 2016, from sites.utoronto.ca/qol/qol_model.htm

---

REFERENCES

Alster, K. B. (1989). *The holistic health movement.* Tuscaloosa: University of Alabama Press.

Ashton, J., & Seymour, H. (1988). *The new public health.* Philadelphia: Open University Press.

Begoray, D., & Banister, E. (2015). *Adolescent health literacy,* New York: Nova Science Publishers.

Begoray, D., Gillis, D., & Rowlands, G. (Eds.). (2012). *Health literacy in context: International perspectives.* New York: Nova Science Publishers.

Blane, D., Brunner, E., & Wilkinson, R. (Eds.). (1996). *Health and social organization.* London: Routledge.

Breslow, L. (1999). From disease prevention to health promotion. *JAMA, 281*(11), 1030–1033.

Canadian Public Health Association (CPHA). (2000). *Reducing poverty and its negative effects on health: Resolution passed at the 2000 CPHA Annual Meeting.* Retrieved from www.cpha.ca/uploads/resolutions/2000_e.pdf

Canadian Public Health Association (CPHA). (2001). *CPHA policy statements.* Retrieved from www.cpha.ca/uploads/policy/conditions_e.pdf

Chu, C., & Simpson, R. (1994). *Ecological public health: From vision to practice.* Toronto: Centre for Health Promotion, University of Toronto.

Commission on Social Determinants of Health (CSDH). (2008). *Closing the gap in a generation: Health equity through action on the social determinants of health.* Geneva: World Health Organization.

Critchley, M. (Ed.). (1978). *Butterworth's medical dictionary.* London: Butterworth's.

Dupéré, S., O'Neill, M., & De Koninck, M. (2012). Why poor men in Montreal do not use health and social services in times of crisis. *Journal of the Poor and the Underserved, 23*(2), 781–796.

Epp, J. (1986). *Achieving health for all: A framework for health promotion.* Ottawa: Health and Welfare Canada.

Eriksson, M., & Lindström, B. (2008). A salutogenic interpretation of the Ottawa Charter. *Health Promotion International, 23*(2), 190–199.

Evans, R. G., Barer, M. L., & Marmor, T. R. (1994). *Why are some people healthy and others not? The determinants of health of populations.* New York: Aldine de Guyter.

Fassin, D. (2000). Comment faire de la santé publique avec des mots. Une rhétorique à l'œuvre. *Ruptures, revue transdisciplinaire en santé, 7*(1), 58–78.

Federal, Provincial and Territorial Advisory Committee on Population Health (FPT ACPH). (1994). *Strategies for population health.* Ottawa: Health Canada.

Freire, P. (1970). *Pedagogy of the oppressed.* New York: Continuum.

Gibson, C. H. (1991). A concept analysis of empowerment. *Journal of Advanced Nursing, 16,* 354–361.

Gillis, D., & Kaszap, M. (2012). Health literacy. In I. Rootman, S. Dupéré, A. Pederson, & M. O'Neill (Eds.), *Health Promotion in Canada: Critical perspectives on practice* (3rd ed.) (pp. 125–127). Toronto: Canadian Scholars' Press.

Green, L. W., & Kreuter, M. W. (2005). *Health program planning: An educational and ecological approach* (4th ed.). Boston & Toronto: McGraw-Hill Higher Education.

Green, L. W., & Raeburn, J. M. (1988). Health promotion: What is it? What will it become? *Health Promotion, 3*(2), 151–159.

Hancock, T. (2012). (Un)sustainable development. In I. Rootman, S. Dupéré, A. Pederson, & M. O'Neill (Eds.), *Health promotion in Canada: Critical perspectives on practice* (pp. 127–130). Toronto: Canadian Scholars' Press.

Hancock, T., Labonté, R., & Edwards, R. (1999). Indicators that count! Measuring population health at the community level. *Canadian Journal of Public Health, 90,* S22–26.

Hancock, T., & Perkins, F. (1985). The mandala of health: A conceptual model and teaching tool. *Health Education, 24*(1), 8–10.

Health Canada. (1998). *Taking action on population health: A position paper for health promotion and programs branch staff.* Ottawa: Health Canada.

Hoffman-Goetz, L., Donelle, L., & Ahmed, R. (2014). *Health literacy in Canada: A primer for students.* Toronto: Canadian Scholars' Press.

Kickbusch, I. (1989). *Good planets are hard to find.* Copenhagen: FADL Publishers.

Kickbusch, I. (1997). Think health: What makes the difference? *Health Promotion International, 12,* 265–272.

Kwan, B., Frankish, J., & Rootman, I. (2006). *The development and evaluation of measures of health literacy in different populations.* Vancouver: Institute of Health Promotion Research.

Labonté, R. (1993). *Community health and empowerment.* Toronto: Centre for Health Promotion.

Lalonde, M. (1974). *A new perspective on the health of Canadians.* Ottawa: Government of Canada.

Lewin, K. (1952). *Field theory in social science: Selected theoretical papers by Kurt Lewin.* London: Tavistock.

Lindström, B., & Eriksson, M. (2010). *The hitchhiker's guide to salutogenesis: Salutogenic pathways to health promotion.* Helsinki: Folkhälsan Research Centre.

Martin, C. J., & McQueen, D. V. (Eds.). (1989). *Readings for a new public health.* Edinburgh: Edinburgh University Press.

Mitic, W., & Rootman, I. (2012). *An intersectoral approach for improving the health literacy of Canadians: Discussion paper.* Victoria, BC: Public Health Association of British Columbia.

Mittelmark, M., Sagy, S., Eriksson, M., Bauer, G. F., Pelikan, J. M., Lindstrom, B. & Espnes, G. A. (Eds.). (2017). *The handbook of salutogenesis.* Switzerland: Springer Nature, Springer International Publishing.

Nutbeam, D. (1998). Health promotion glossary. *Health Promotion International, 13,* 349–364.

Nutbeam, D. (2000). Health literacy as a public health goal: A challenge for contemporary health education and communication strategies into the 21st century. *Health Promotion International, 15,* 259–267.

Oliveira, C. C. (2014). Suffering and salutogenesis. *Health Promotion International, 30*(2), 222–227.

O'Neill, M., Pederson, A., & Rootman, I. (2000). Health promotion in Canada: Declining or transforming? *Health Promotion International, 15*(2), 135–141.

O'Neill, M., & Stirling, A. (2007). The promotion of health or health promotion? In M. O'Neill, S. Dupéré, A. Pederson, & I. Rootman (Eds.), *Health promotion in Canada: Critical perspectives* (pp. 32–45). Toronto: Canadian Scholars' Press.

Pan-American Health Organization (PAHO). (2002). *Public health in the Americas.* Technical publication no. 589. Washington: Pan-American Health Organization.

Pleasant, A., Rudd, R., O'Leary, C., Pasche-Orlow, M. K., Allen, M. P., Alvarado-Little, W., … Rosen, S. (2016). Consideration for a new definition of health literacy. Washington: National Academy of Medicine.

Quality of Life Research Unit. (2016). *Concepts.* Retrieved from sites.utoronto.ca/qol/

Raeburn, J., & Rootman, I. (1989). Towards an expanded health field concept: Conceptual and research issues in a new era of health promotion. *Health Promotion International, 3*(4), 383–392.

Raeburn, J., & Rootman, I. (2007). A new appraisal of the concept of health. In M. O'Neill, S. Dupéré, A. Pederson, & I. Rootman (Eds.), *Health promotion in Canada: Critical perspectives* (pp. 1–16). Toronto: Canadian Scholars' Press.

Raphael, D. (Ed.). (2009). *Social determinants of health* (2nd ed.). Toronto: Canadian Scholars' Press.

Raphael, D. (2016). *Social determinants of health: Canadian perspectives* (3rd ed.). Toronto: Canadian Scholars' Press.

Rappaport, J. (1987). Terms of empowerment/exemplars of prevention: Toward a theory for community psychology. *American Journal of Community Psychology, 15*(2), 121–148.

Rissel, C. (1994). Empowerment: The holy grail of health promotion. *Health Promotion International, 9*(1), 39–47.

Rootman, I., Frankish, J., & Kaszap, M. (2007). Health literacy: A new frontier. In M. O'Neill, S. Dupéré, A. Pederson, & I. Rootman (Eds.), *Health promotion in Canada: Critical perspectives on practice* (pp. 61–74). Toronto: Canadian Scholars' Press.

Rootman, I., Goodstadt, M., Potvin, L., & Springett, J. (2001). A framework for health promotion evaluation. In I. Rootman et al. (Eds.), *Evaluation in health promotion: Principles and perspectives* (pp. 7–38). Copenhagen: European Regional Office of the World Health Organization.

Rootman, I., & Gordon-El-Bihbety, D. (2008). *A vision for a health literate Canada: Report of the expert panel on health literacy.* Ottawa: Canadian Public Health Association.

Rootman, I., & Raeburn, J. (1994). The concept of health. In A. Pederson, M. O'Neill, & I. Rootman (Eds.), *Health promotion in Canada: Provincial, national, and international perspectives* (pp. 139–152). Toronto: W. B. Saunders Canada.

Sarafino, E. P. (1990). *Health psychology: Biopsychosocial interactions*. New York: John Wiley & Sons.

Segall, A., & Fries, C. J. (2011). *Pursuing health and wellness*. Toronto: Oxford University Press.

Simonds, S. K. (1974). Health education and social policy. *Health Education Monographs, 2*(Suppl. 1), 1–10.

Wallerstein, N., Minkler, M., Cater-Edwards, L., Avila, M., & Sanchez, V. (2015). Improving health through community engagement, community organization, and community building. In Glanz, K., Rimer, B. K., & Viswanath, K. (Eds.), *Health behaviour: Theory, research and practice* (pp. 277–300). San Francisco: Jossey-Bass,

World Health Organization (WHO). (1946). *Constitution*. Geneva: World Health Organization.

World Health Organization (WHO). (1986). *Ottawa charter for health promotion*. Ottawa: Canadian Public Health Association.

World Health Organization (WHO). (2005). *Bangkok charter for health promotion*. Geneva: World Health Organization. Retrieved from www.who.int/healthpromotion/conferences/6gchp/bangkok_charter/en/index.html

World Health Organization (WHO). (2010). *Backgrounder 3: Key concepts*. Retrieved from www.who.int/social_determinants/final_report/key_concepts_en.pdf

CHAPTER 3

Social Theory and Health Promotion

Simon Carroll

LEARNING OBJECTIVES

1. Understand the role of social theory in health promotion
2. Understand how health promotion is a critical social theory perspective on public health
3. Understand how the central themes in social theory are foundationally related to the central themes in health promotion

INTRODUCTION

Embarking on a chapter with such an ambitious title is perilous. To pretend to adequately cover the breadth of developments in the field of health promotion relevant to "social theory" and vice versa, even over the past ten years, would be to overreach. Nevertheless, ironically, to get to the bottom of what needs to be considered, we have to start on a tangent that has even more risk at its heart.

I start with the end, by prefacing the chapter with what I take to be its central conclusion: What marks health promotion as an ambiguous, contradictory, and at times even nebulous field of thought and practice is its problematic relationship with its own theoretical basis. Health promotion has and uses many "theories," yet it is nearly silent, though less so recently (McQueen & Kickbusch, 2007) on just what should constitute its own theoretical basis. As we shall see, this is partly due to a conception of "theory" handed down from a narrowly positivistic empiricism that sees "theories" exclusively as analytical devices constructed to help *explain* specific empirical phenomena. There is nothing inherently wrong with this narrowly empiricist interpretation of "theory," and certainly health promotion, in practice, has need of understanding and using all sorts of specific empirical theories (e.g., epidemiological theories about the causes of disease in populations; psychological theories of behaviour change; theories of community coalition-building). Indeed, other publications have taken this approach to theory very seriously (DiClemente, Crosby, & Kegler, 2002). However, we must begin with a deeper issue: What is theory and how should health promotion relate to it?

A corollary to the conclusion prefaced above is that health promotion is—unlike medicine, disease prevention, or even population health (see Hancock, 1994, chapter 2 for conceptual distinctions)—almost exclusively about *social action* broadly interpreted. Of course, all the other activities are or involve *social* activities; however, for health promotion, it is not just the application of its knowledge that involves understanding the social world, it is the theoretical core of its knowledge that is *essentially social in nature*. The argument here is that health promotion is about social change, and that even when it is concerned with individuals, it is about individuals as social beings. Health is produced socially; individual health behaviours can only be understood, never mind changed, within a social context (Kickbusch, 1989). In this guise, this chapter takes a position close to the perspective on theory offered by McQueen and Kickbusch in their book, *Health & Modernity: The Role of Theory in Health Promotion* (McQueen & Kickbusch, 2007).

The implication of this perspective for health promotion is that we have to think very differently about "theory" than is typical within the received tradition of empirical science. In fact, the type of theorization necessary for health promotion is more akin to the traditions of philosophical and social theory than to theory as it is often interpreted within the sciences. Such a departure from the orthodox scientific[1] understanding of "theory" is difficult to manage, particularly for a field so institutionally dominated by its relations with the biomedical sciences and epidemiology, and even the positivistic orthodoxy of certain psychological and sociological approaches to social science.[2] Yet, if we cannot move from this narrow interpretation of theory, then the hopes of understanding what health promotion is really about—and, even more so, what it *should* be about—will be unrealized.

Before delving more deeply into the vexing problem of how theory relates to health promotion, something should be said about how "methodology" fits into this picture. There is an unfortunate tendency to think of "methods" and "theories" as separate entities that operate independently in the grand enterprise of science. Nothing could be further from the truth. All scientific methods are built on theoretical presuppositions. We can use thermometers to "read" temperature only because we assent to a series of theoretical suppositions concerning the material arrangements used to construct the thermometer, among many other considerations. Similarly, we use instruments such as a social survey based on a series of theoretical assumptions about people's responses to questions, how language works, their intentions and behaviours, along with broader conceptions of "society, the individual and the relationship between them" (Ackroyd & Hughes, 1992, p. 8). In fact, the important distinction (though often conflated) between *methodology* and *methods* is built upon this insight. A *methodology* is the logical or "theoretical" justification for the use of a specific method or methods to answer particular types of research questions. Thus, when we talk about different ways to theorize about health promotion, we are at the same time talking about what kind of methodological implications these different theoretical

Box 3.1: Key Philosophical Terms: Ontology

Ontology is the study of "being," "existence," or "reality." In other words, it is the study of that which "is." However, ontology is the abstract conceptualization of being, meaning that it is not concerned with the facts pertaining to a particular thing, but rather to the nature of existence itself. That is, it wants to know what kind of things exist in general, and whether there are certain fundamental beings. It is interested in questions such as: What things are essential and what things are merely accidental or contingent? What does it mean for something to have an *identity*, and when does a thing cease to be, as opposed to merely changing? It also asks other general questions, such as: Is reality eternal or is it in constant flux? Is reality stratified into different levels and, if so, what are they? To understand why these very abstract questions can be important, even in such concrete subject areas as health promotion, we have to be aware that how we think the world is structured has a profound influence on how we think about the world and how we act in it. For example, if you see the essence of the social world as fundamentally unchanging and eternal (e.g., "The poor will always be with us," "People are basically greedy"), you approach social problems and whether and how to solve them in a very different way than someone who sees even basic aspects of social life as open to change.

Box 3.2: Key Philosophical Terms: Epistemology

Epistemology is the study of the nature of "knowledge," including how we attain it and the extent of its scope and limitations. Epistemology addresses three fundamental questions: What is knowledge? How is knowledge acquired? How do we know what we know? The first question is concerned mainly with defining knowledge and establishing criteria for whether a person can be said to have knowledge of something. The second question concerns where knowledge comes from and how it is attained, with the main traditional dividing line being between those who accept that knowledge can come from *a priori* reasoning or "intuition," and those who believe that the only reliable knowledge has to come from experience. Many further divisions have developed over time in philosophy concerning this question, but it is important to know that the vast majority of what we call "empirical science" is based on the assumption that we can gain knowledge only through experiencing the world, particularly by way of perceiving "sense impressions." The final question addresses the problem of skepticism, or how any of our claims to knowledge can be warranted. For the purpose here, it is important to understand that epistemology is influenced by our ontological assumptions and vice versa. If you do not believe in the existence of an ontological level of reality where ideas have an independent existence (as Plato did), then it is very hard to admit that one can derive knowledge from ideas alone; conversely, if the only way to access knowledge is through sense impressions, then any talk of different levels of reality makes no sense, as the only level we can rationally access is the world of empirical experience. Furthermore, as shown in box 3.3, how we understand both ontology and epistemology has much to do with the type of *methodology* we might use to discover new knowledge.

Box 3.3: Key Philosophical Terms: Methodology

Methodology is the logic or reasoned justification for following certain principles or rules of inquiry and for the use of particular methods for collecting and analyzing data. Methodology is not simply a description of the various *methods* available to the inquirer; rather, it is the philosophically coherent combination of theory and method that is required to answer a particular sort of researchable question. To understand how methodology is connected to ontology and epistemology, imagine one starts with a particular research question. First, one has to know what we are assuming about the nature of the phenomenon under inquiry: What type of thing(s) is it? Second, we have to know how we might come to know about this phenomenon: What is the source of knowledge we will need to access in order to better understand it? Finally, given our answers to these questions, we can construct a rationale for using specific procedures for attaining this knowledge that are consistent with our ontological and epistemological assumptions. Is this how every inquiry is actually constructed? Rarely. However, without this type of reflection, we often proceed with methodological strategies that incorporate these ontological and epistemological assumptions without us consciously acknowledging them.

---

conceptions have for the field. This chapter will directly address certain methodological issues that have recently captured the imagination of health promoters. Nevertheless, the reader should keep in mind that there is a constant dialectic between theoretical and methodological concerns, and that in many ways, the real distinction is within a broader understanding of "theory" that considers both *ontological* and *epistemological* questions, with both these concepts being more directly connected to issues of methodology. In other words, "theory" in health promotion is about what health promotion's object or field (ontological) is, and how we know about it (epistemological), and thus what the rationale or (methodological) justification is for using a particular set of methods for acquiring this knowledge. Having now introduced two quintessentially philosophical terms (ontology and epistemology), we can move to what theory is about from a philosophical perspective.

PHILOSOPHY AND SOCIAL THEORY

"Theory" is a loaded term in philosophy. In fact, it represents the key distinguishing feature of the being, knowledge, and activity of the philosopher. It constitutes the ground upon which philosophers, since Plato and Aristotle, have defined the essence of what it is to be a philosopher or "lover of wisdom"; it is what distinguishes philosophical knowledge from other forms of knowledge; and it is what marks the difference between philosophical activity and practical or, as Aristotle put it, "utilitarian" activity. It is "loaded" because, as Plato and Aristotle knew very well, the possibility of an activity with no immediate practical utility, that could be carried out only by people with the leisure and thus support provided by the rest of society, was in desperate need of justification. So, what was this justification? Well, it wasn't just that theoretical or "contemplative" activity was worthwhile; it was that it was superior to all other forms of activity! Thus, from its very beginnings, "theory" was an essentially hubristic and condescending occupation (as Socrates found to his cost). Nevertheless, what has been handed down from the Greeks is the notion that theory is about understanding the first principles or "causes" of phenomena. It was about discovering "why" things worked the way they did, as opposed to just that they worked. Yet, it also set up a lasting, and in many ways damaging, hierarchical contrast between superior "theory" on the one hand, and inferior "practice" on the other. It is no coincidence that these great philosophers had political theories that favoured the aristocracy, given their penchant for denigrating practical work as a lower form of existence (Meiksins Wood, 2008). It is a good warning to health promoters enamoured (as I am) with "theory," particularly in a field dominated by practitioners (and ones who have often been historically subordinated to a distinctly aristocratic medical caste), to be mindful and reflectively critical of theory's pretensions.

Nevertheless, what lessons can health promotion derive from the philosophical tradition, the originators of the "theoretical attitude"? First, we have to briefly consider the development of the conception of "theory," and reason itself, within the philosophical tradition; then we can trace how social theory is really a further development of, and originated from, philosophical reflection, and in particular, out of the tradition of "critical reason" as it was fully formed in the Enlightenment and post-Enlightenment. This genealogy is important because another basic argument made in this chapter is that health promotion is constituted as a *social critique* of public health. That is, health promotion's basic orientation is as an emancipatory project in the tradition of critical social theory. This is not an original insight, as some health promotion researchers have long argued something analogous (Eakin, Robertson, Poland, Coburn, & Edwards, 1996). However, too often what gets articulated as "concepts and principles" of health promotion, such as those found in the *Ottawa Charter for Health Promotion* (WHO, 1986), are not understood as foundational *theoretical* positions; this is problematic as these positions make very specific philosophical assumptions linked to important traditions in post-Enlightenment thought.

It should be made clear that what is argued here is *not* that all people identifying themselves as health promoters would recognize the peculiar genealogy of thought I am about to reconstruct as *the* theoretical basis for health promotion. Rather, what is argued is that if one follows through on certain foundational premises of health promotion, as set out in the *Ottawa Charter* (a declared bias to begin with, but one that I think is both compatible with this book and with Canadian health promotion generally), one is led, logically, to a very particular tradition of thought. If health promotion is essentially tied to the tradition of thought we call "critical social theory," what does that mean? The tradition of critical reason, since Kant, is the story of a constantly evolving, dialectical movement of reason, aimed at a critique of existing society, with the goal of the emancipation of human beings from a variety of arbitrary and (collectively) self-imposed restrictions on their ability and capacity to flourish and express themselves equitably, freely, and authentically. How and why is health promotion a part of this, admittedly grandiose, project?

First, it takes some historical perspective to understand how deeply embedded health promotion is in modernity. Following many others, health promotion can best be seen as a kind of "third revolution" of public health (Breslow, 1999; Potvin & McQueen, 2007). Key to understanding this revolution is to follow the shift within public health from a focus on individual behaviour change to a focus on the social context of health and on the levers of societal change that are necessary if one wants to transform the lives of populations for the better. Now, there is little doubt that public health, particularly as a societal movement, but also as a field of knowledge, is deeply embedded in the whole historical development of modern society. In fact, many of the most prominent theorizations of modernity give a pride of place to public health in the narrative of how a self-consciousness of the possibility of societal "improvement" came into being (Porter, 2000). For thinkers like Foucault, the appearance of "society" as an object of reflection is itself coincident with the development of the concepts of "population," "statistics," "political arithmetic," and many others that inaugurate reflections on how to manage the state, as not simply bounded territories with certain resources, but as containing populations with specific, measurable characteristics, such as wealth and health (Foucault, 1980, 2000, 2008). John Graunt's famous "Bills of Mortality," epidemiological science's prototype, is at once a precursor to public health and a peculiar mode of societal self-consciousness, premised on the notion that societies were objects that could be strengthened and improved with the use of reason. At the core of public health's story is an almost perfect embodiment of the dilemmas and contradictions at the heart of the development of modern societies; public health is a grand tradition that is driven by the great Enlightenment themes of improvement, progress, freedom, and reason, while at the same time being caught up with all the less positive modern tropes,[3] such as bureaucratization, rationalization, domination, and a hubristic scientism. The modern health promotion movement arrives with a series of other "second wave" critical social movements, such as environmentalism, feminism, and the peace movement, as part of a general trend of "postmodern" critique that puts advanced, industrial societies under intense scrutiny and, in many cases, finds the modern experiment wanting (cf. Labonté, 1994). Although health promotion itself is probably less a social movement and more a kind of para-bureaucratic tendency (Stevenson & Burke, 1991), it shares with the zeitgeist a deep suspicion of the social engineering approach to an increasingly administered society, and a strong attachment to participatory democratic principles. Yet despite its attachment to these more postmodern themes, health promotion is still tied to some fundamental commitments that one can identify only with the values of the Enlightenment and modernity. It is how it negotiates the ambiguous legacy of modernity that frames health promotion from a social-theoretical perspective.

To more carefully consider how this tradition of critical thought unfolds in relation to our contemporary situation, we need to move more directly to an analysis of some of the guiding thematic disputes within the realm of critical social theory understood broadly.[4] Some of these guiding themes, it will be seen, constitute central problems for health promotion theory and the appropriate methodological strategies that are necessary to meet these challenges.

SOCIAL THEORY AND HEALTH PROMOTION

In this section, I begin to address some of the central animating themes in social theory and demonstrate how they are connected to core dilemmas for health promotion research and practice. The three key themes that I explore are (1) class and status; (2) the dialectic of rationalization; and (3) the duality of structure and agency. These themes all have strong relevance to health promotion and the point is not to resolve these debates or contradictory perspectives for health promotion, but to explore their dialectical development in order to give the reader a deeper sense of the types of theoretical tensions that drive social theory, and thus the types of theoretical questions that should drive, at least an important part of, future debates within the field of health promotion.

Class and Status

Ironically, although contemporary health promotion is awash with references to the link between social inequality and inequitable health outcomes, there is little, if any, direct confrontation with one of the central questions of social theory: What are the main causal mechanisms underlying social inequality? Within the sociological tradition in particular, this constitutes the main differences between followers of Marx and followers of Weber, along with further substantial disputes within these two social theoretical traditions. Why is this important to health promotion? Well, if health promotion aims to change society in order to reduce social inequity and thereby health inequity (surely one of its main goals and, arguably, increasingly the central goal), it requires a clear-headed approach to understanding what causes these inequities in the first place, in order to be effective at changing them for the better. This inquiry is a different one from social epidemiological disputes concerning which types of social variables (e.g., income, education, SES, Gini coefficients [measure of inequalities], etc.) have the most impact on health, although these empirical findings are complementary and informative. Rather, what is at stake is to understand the underlying, dynamic mechanisms that create and reproduce relatively stable group differences in income, wealth, housing, education, health, and many other characteristics.

For Marx, it was clear that the basic driving force of social inequalities was the division of societies into antagonistic "classes," defined by their relationship to the means of the material reproduction of those societies (Marx, 1976, 1981). In Western societies in particular, stages of social development were divided into different sets of class relations of production, from classical ancient societies based on the relationship between slave owners and slaves, to feudal societies based on the relationship between landlords and serfs, to modern capitalist societies based on the relationship between the bourgeois owners of capital and the free wage labourers forced to sell their labour for subsistence. Marxist theory has developed in many forms since Marx, and there have been many different approaches to interpreting his concept of class (Olin Wright, 2009), yet key to understanding this perspective is to avoid identifying classes primarily using different brackets of income or different occupational strata. For Marxists, it is the *dynamic* of class struggle in capitalist societies over the division of surplus value between capital and labour that is the most powerful force underlying the generation of social inequalities more broadly. What does this mean? When we look only at different snapshots of income differentials or other social inequalities, we may miss some underlying trends and tendencies that form the main tectonic shifts in social relations and cause ripple effects throughout the social structure. A prime example is how over the past 40 years there has been a steady yet massive shift of wealth and power to the capitalist class, and at the same time a receding set of public institutions and resources (often collectively referred to as the "welfare state") that acted as a bulwark against rampant inequality in the previous post-World War II era. The Marxist explanation for this inexorable trend is based on two mutually reinforcing tendencies: one, the objective pressures on capital accumulation and the rate of profit, causing a need for the system to undergo several crises of "creative destruction" in order to restore profitability; second, a subjective defeat of working-class institutions, particularly labour unions, that had acted as resources to defend working-class gains and a share in the expansion of social productivity.[5] In other words, the capitalist class has been relatively successful in passing on the costs of various economic crises to the workers and to come out the other end of these crises in a strengthened position for renewed profitability. One need not look far from current news headlines to find ample evidence that substantiates some of these insights.

To summarize, Marxists see class, and a particular version of that concept, as the key driving force behind the generation of social inequality. There are certain features of this perspective that are important to keep in mind in relation to health promotion. First, taking a Marxist or Marx-inspired perspective on social inequality means taking a medium- to long-term view because it focuses on what are seen as the fundamental underlying economic forces that affect all other levels of society. How deterministic a view this is depends on how you conceptualize and theorize the relationship between these basic economic drivers and other levels and spheres of the social world. However, for health promoters, the message is that having a real impact on social inequality may require some basic shifts in the relationships between owners of capital and those employed by them. This does not mean that nothing positive can be done short of social revolution, but it does mean having a more sanguine view of the possibilities of social change within a system that so powerfully drives those very inequalities we aim to ameliorate.

While the Weberian approach to class and status differs substantially from the Marxist approach (though not as much as many think: Sayer, 1991), both share a common characteristic that is missing from the more familiar social epidemiological conception of class and status as the hierarchical stratification of social *attributes* and *conditions* (Olin Wright, 2009). Both Marx's and Weber's conceptions of class and Weber's concept of status are deeply connected to *relations of power*. For Marx, the power relations are domination and exploitation, whereas for Weber they are relations of exclusion and distinction. This is a key theoretical point as this *relational* aspect of class and status underlies both the inherent antagonism and the dynamism of class and status-divided societies. Marxist analysis demonstrates the antagonism between the overall distribution of economic surplus between profits and wages, and the relations of domination within the workplace between employers and employees; Weberian analysis points to the forms of closure and exclusion that privileged classes impose on subordinate classes in the marketplace, along with the forms of authority established through social distinction between different status groups in the population. Both approaches tell us about fundamental social forces that drive change and conserve power in modern society, as well as expose deep rifts and contradictions at the heart of those societies. While for Marx the fundamental axis of power was the ownership and control of the means of production, for Weber it was control of property and marketable assets or services.

In order to understand how these classic sources of social theory are still relevant to contemporary health promotion, we can look briefly at health promotion researchers' attempt to apply the work of more recent social theorists working from within the broad tradition of class and status analytical frameworks. One of the more interesting problems that health promotion has confronted in trying to think through the *social* aspect of its revolution in public health is how to deal with so-called lifestyles. It is indisputable that there is a direct causal relationship between certain individual health-related behaviours (e.g., poor diet, lack of exercise, smoking) and negative health outcomes. However, health promotion, since the *Ottawa Charter*, has recognized that there is a connection between these behaviours and social stratification; in other words, there is consistent evidence that negative health-related behaviours are associated disproportionately with lower socioeconomic strata. This has led to two reciprocal conclusions: (1) that more has to be done to understand the *social* causation of these "risk factors"; and, conversely, more has to be done to understand how to effectively intervene to change those behaviours.[6] Many health promoters have become disenchanted with the traditional, individual-psychological focus of many behaviour change strategies, along with the tendency for these approaches to implicitly endorse a narrative of victim-blaming. An alternative approach is to reconsider the notion of "lifestyles" from a sociological or social theory perspective (Kickbusch, 1989; Frohlich, Corin, & Potvin, 2001; Abel, 2007). Kickbusch's article was prescient, but mainly outlined a framework to start thinking in different terms about how so-called lifestyles had to be conceptualized as socially produced, and therefore understanding what those social mechanisms were was part of health promotion's agenda. Over the past 10 years, Frohlich, Abel, and other colleagues have separately and together started to flesh out in more specific theoretical terms just what approaches to social theory might be most helpful in understanding what they have come to call "collective lifestyles." This approach is more concretely addressed in the Frohlich et al. chapter in this volume; however, here we will examine more closely the theoretical arguments behind this move and place them in the historical context of social theory that has been discussed above.

These health promotion researchers used Pierre Bourdieu, a key thinker and famous sociologist, to develop the notion of collective lifestyles. While Bourdieu created his own original theoretical perspective, there is no doubt that he was deeply indebted to both Marx and Weber, and perhaps more to the latter. Bourdieu's conception of how classes reproduced themselves in society was a deeply relational one. For Bourdieu, as for Weber, the social field(s), a system of social positions, was a site of constant power struggles over what Bourdieu called economic, social, cultural, and symbolic capital. Like Weber, he was critical of the Marxist tendency to focus solely on the economic sphere of class struggle and subordinate all other levels of society to this struggle. Bourdieu was primarily occupied with a particular question: Why was it that subordinate classes and status groups in society tended to be resigned to their fate in the social hierarchy? Using his concepts of *habitus*, *field*, and *capital*, Bourdieu offered an explanatory framework that allowed us to conceptualize how individuals internalize social structure through the interaction between the fields of action they operate in, the various forms of capital, and their "habitus," which was the set of mainly unreflective dispositions forming both the medium and outcome of their practical activities. For example, Bourdieu demonstrated that musical tastes, diet, sport preference and many other social variables were clearly aligned as inherited dispositions according to what part of the class structure an individual came from, rather than as the result of conscious individual choices.

Abel argues that in terms of thinking about "collective lifestyles," a key concept is that of cultural capital (Abel, 2007). For Bourdieu, cultural capital consisted of educational attainment, clothing, food habits, musical taste, exercise habits, and even bodily comportment. Instead of conceiving all these as a set of individual choices made consciously, Bourdieu understood them as primarily dispositions or habits that one was automatically socialized into as part of being in a particular social strata, group, or class fraction. Crucially, and following Weber and Marx, these forms of capital are the object of relational power struggles, such that their "value" is relative to the scarcity that can be maintained by excluding access through forms of social closure to subordinate social strata. One critical conclusion Bourdieu came to was that subordinate groups or classes suffer from "symbolic violence," where some cultural tastes and habits come to be "valued" as better than others, and also happen to be the tastes and habits of the group that is superior in wealth and status. Oppressed groups accept this valuation and thus legitimize their subordinate status as part of the "natural order" of things. Thus they "refuse what they are denied." The implications this has for generating change in the social habits of disadvantaged and so-called at-risk populations from a health perspective are very far-reaching. As can be seen in a recent study by Frohlich and colleagues, these different attitudes can have drastically divergent implications for policies such as anti-tobacco legislation (Frohlich, Poland, Mykhalovskiy, Alexander, & Maule, 2010).

There are two significant concerns with the theoretical framework of Bourdieu, despite its potentially fruitful line of inquiry for health promotion. First, Bourdieu's theoretical framework tends towards a deeply pessimistic scenario when it comes to emancipatory change due to his social epistemology. According to Bourdieu, we are highly constrained by the fact that much of social inequality is deeply ingrained and internalized through unreflective habit, making it extraordinarily difficult to overcome, as we reproduce these inequalities as a matter of course, even if we consciously intend to reduce them. On the other hand, people would say that Bourdieu offers us a salutary realism that asks us to work that much harder to be reflexive practitioners in developing social change and, furthermore, even if his concept of habitus tends towards the more deterministic end of the structure/agency spectrum we discuss below, we need something like his concept of habitus as a mediating concept between praxis and social structure (Sayer, 2005; Mouzelis, 2007). A more serious critique is that developed by Andrew Sayer (2009), who argues that Bourdieu over-sociologizes human interaction to the extent where a positive empirical focus leaves no room for normative or evaluative questions as all interaction is reduced to strategic manoeuvres to accumulate capital, including the move of moral reasoning itself. One can see how this can become problematic in terms of distinguishing between "symbolic violence" and legitimate moral reasoning. For example, Frohlich et al. (2010) point to serious differences in how anti-smoking legislation in relation to public space affects different social groups, and there is no doubt that a certain amount of symbolic violence is inflicted upon subordinate and marginalized groups. However, does this mean that being identified with this symbolic violence automatically taints all the evaluative reasoning behind the implementation of smoking bans? Don't we methodologically deny subordinate classes a certain universal capacity for moral reflection if we paint them as inevitably incapable of doing anything but taking up their habitual disposition of self-identifying as smokers? In their study, Frohlich et al. have examples that seem to find that middle-class smokers invite the imposition of smoking bans, and this is interpreted as being consistent with their ambiguous relationship to other aspects of their cultural capital that tells them that smoking is incompatible with their lifestyles. However, we don't want to conflate this explanation with situations where the distinction is between a self-interested particularism that is concerned only with "my smoking habit," and an other-oriented moral argument that says that my smoking habit shouldn't harm others who choose not to take that risk with their health, and we certainly don't want to identify one or the other stance exclusively with a particular social class. Health promoters, when citing theorists such as Bourdieu or Anthony Giddens, should be aware and explicit about the context of these theorists' work as part of a long-term continuity of sociological reflection on class. Without this awareness, the inherently political implications of their work, as well as an understanding of the underlying social causes of inequality, will be lost.

The Dialectic of Rationalization

The second major theme of the social theory of modernity is the dialectic of rationalization. Since Immanuel Kant's three *Critiques* (of pure reason; of practical reason; and of judgment), within Western philosophy there has been a tradition of critiquing the limits and boundaries of reason. One constant theme has been the potential or actual contradictions between an instrumental, means-ends calculating reason, a practical-moral reasoning based on a substantive values-based orientation to action, and a rationality of aesthetic judgment based on distinctions of taste. Different thinkers have developed this theme in a variety of ways. Followers of Kant have tended to think of modernity as having become differentiated into different "value-spheres," with each type of reason legislating over its own appropriate societal jurisdiction (with pure theoretical reason governing the sciences and other purely cognitive interests, practical reason governing politics and the law, and aesthetic reason governing the arts and other areas of cultural production). Others have been concerned about the domination of one type of reason over the others, with either more or less pessimistic extrapolations of where modern societies' developmental trajectory is heading (Marcuse, 1991; Horkheimer & Adorno, 2002). Martin Heidegger (1993) and his followers developed the ultimate extreme of the pessimistic approach, where a totalizing domination of instrumental reason is traced back as a fundamental original sin of Western philosophy starting with Plato and ending with the critique of Western reason *in toto* as "logocentrism" by Derrida (1976). Foucault developed his own critique of Western reason in a series of penetrating analyses of different modern institutions, such as the hospital, the prison, and the therapeutic relationship dominated by psychoanalysis, but also more generally he analyzed the relationship between power, knowledge, and what he came to term a "biopolitics of health" (2008). An attempt to develop a more balanced approach to the legacy of the Enlightenment and modernity through a positive reconstruction of the history or modern reason has been the life work of Habermas (1984, 1987, 1998), who also happens to be the philosopher who most closely engaged with the sociological tradition and who most explicitly linked the tradition of critical theory to that discipline. How we understand our relationship with the history of Western rationality can have a deep influence on how we do health promotion. Particularly in relation to instrumental reason, our relative optimism or pessimism about its potential for resolving societal problems will lead us in very specific directions in terms of the types of programs we develop or the types of processes we use in doing our work.

In social theory more directly, many writers have taken up Max Weber's original analysis of what he called contradictions between formal reason (*Zweckrationalitat*) and substantive reason (*Wertrationalitat*). Weber outlined how all the major modern institutions—including capitalism, rational-legal authority, legal systems, bureaucracy, science, and technology—embodied a contradiction between a formal, instrumental reason aimed at intervening in society to make it more efficient and effective through a generic cost-benefit, calculative rationality, and a substantive reason that judges outcomes based on concrete and particular values (Weber, 1978, 2002). Weber argued that there is a constant dialectic of *rationalization* in modern society that makes formal reason's interventions the basis of ambiguous substantive consequences, some of which are judged as negative, which then calls for further instrumental interventions. A typical example relevant to health promotion and public health is the problem of redressing the results of social inequalities by intervening with a variety of programs of social support, only to have the negative unintended consequence of creating dependency and disempowering local communities.

This dilemma is one that is indirectly addressed in Raeburn and Rootman's book *People-Centred Health Promotion* (1998), in which the authors make clear the potential ambiguities of shifting from a focus on individual-level, over-psychologizing interventions to macro-level, over-socializing interventions and end up squeezing people living in communities out of the equation. The question here goes to the core of the stated health promotion values of *participation* and *empowerment*. It is also a key distinguishing feature of health promotion from a much more state-centred, utilitarian tradition in public health (Hills & Carroll, 2009). Two negative consequences of traditional public health approaches to health promotion issues can be seen in both the bureaucratic formal rationality of state-run programs that take little account of local context and often undermine community empowerment and participation, and in the excesses of scientism that appear in the formal rationality of evaluation techniques emerging from the academy. Despite the stated intentions of redressing inequities in many of these programs, often unintended consequences are generated that substantively undermine core values, such as empowerment and participation, never mind those programs that also undermine the value of equity itself. For example, parenting programs that focus on redressing "poor parenting skills" without acknowledging the broader social issues that these parents may be dealing with can both undermine the parents' self-confidence and self-esteem and ignore their potential input and knowledge, thereby doing damage to the value of participation and empowerment; conversely, parents with fewer social barriers who take better advantage of the program's narrow focus on knowledge and skills can have disproportionately positive gains, thereby undermining the value of equity (with the people the most in need receiving the least benefits). As we will pick up in the final section, the Weberian theme of rationalization is also intimately tied to how we consider the dualism of structure and agency for, as Habermas has warned, there is a danger in not recognizing the autonomy of the communicative lifeworld and subsuming it entirely under the rubric of a systems rationality.

Agency and Structure: Dualism or Duality?

The whole history of social theory has been taken up with a cleavage around the issue of what the nature of sociality and social action is: What is its ontology? In other words, what kind of thing is society? What is it made up of? Does it have special "social" substances, or is it just the collective properties of individual people? Philosophically, this is intertwined with several older debates, such as free will (or "voluntarism") vs. determinism, individualistic vs. holistic explanation, and the micro- vs. macro-level opposition and/or linkage. While both Marx and Durkheim tended to defend a structural or functionalist holism, Weber and other more phenomenologically inspired thinkers tended to look at social order as constituted by social interaction, with the "unit act," as Talcott Parsons was to put it, as the foundational concept. Thus, most of social theory's history has been built on a major internal dualism between those who looked to social structure as the primary lever of explanatory value, and those who focused almost entirely on the interaction setting as the locus for the production of social order. Much ink has been spilt on this dualism, with a fair amount of commentary consisting of straw-man caricatures of the opposing position. Structuralists and functionalists are accused of entirely wiping the individual human agent off the face of the social theory map, while interactionists are accused of a myopic, blinkered attitude to structures and in particular of ignoring the powerful constraints they impose on human action. Rather than focus any further on the merits of each polarized position, we can look at a more recent example of an approach that has tried to convert this dualism into a more balanced "duality of structure and agency," as Giddens (1984) has coined the phrase. We will then end by briefly considering how "complexity theory" can add to this debate.

Before moving on to consider Giddens's attempted resolution, we should note why this particular theme is so crucial for health promotion. In order to avoid falling into the trap Raeburn and Rootman warned against in their previously cited text, we have to negotiate carefully how we reconcile the need to integrate insights concerning structural constraints on human agency and choices with the imperative not to treat social actors as "cultural dupes," thereby undermining their autonomy and dignity, and thus destroying the potential for participation and empowerment, which health promoters rightly emphasize. The twin dangers are, on the one hand, acceding to a victim-blaming voluntarism that tragically overemphasizes people's ability to make simple choices concerning their own health-related lifestyles and, on the other, so powerfully developing a narrative of structural constraint that the possibility of change and resistance recedes into some never feasible, impractical utopian future. It also matters a lot how this "dualism" is conceptualized because depending on what pole of the dualism gets emphasized, strategic priorities for intervention and engagement become initiated. For example, if the argument falls on the side of the importance of structure and macro-level institutional phenomena, then a focus will tend to offer prescriptions that advocate for large-scale public policy changes at the expense of more micro-level community engagement; conversely, if the argument focuses on the importance of agency and local action, then we tend to focus on individual behaviour change and community development at the expense of taking into account the need for broader supportive environments and macro-level healthy public policy. In other words, the structure/agency dualism is closely tied in health promotion to whether or not an integrated approach to the *Ottawa Charter* strategies will be implemented: If the dualism holds, then battles over which strategies are more important takes place; if we can truly transcend the dualism and think of it as a duality, then it is much easier to conceptualize the integrated, multi-level, multi-strategy approach that has been consistently advocated for over the past decade or more.

Anthony Giddens's approach to resolving this constitutive dualism is perhaps the best-known contemporary effort to do so, and his theory of "structuration" is still a popular source for those who do not want to choose sides in the old polarizing debates. Giddens's efforts developed out of a long-term concern he had about the cleavages in social theory between those who emphasized an objectivist, often functionalist reading of social structure as the basic causal force in social life, and those who held that social action was really about subjective meaning and understanding. The so-called theory of structuration is not really a substantial social theory at all, but is rather an "ontological framework for the study of human social activities" (Giddens, 1991). It is essentially a conceptual recategorization of classical social thought in an attempt to reconcile the above-mentioned dualism. It is important to grasp this lesson, as health promoters, locked as they are into a deeply applied field of research, may be too quick to jump from the rarified theoretical atmosphere of structuration theory into a definite empirical application of Giddens's conceptual framework. The issue is that Giddens's "theory" works much better as a sort of sensitizing conceptual device that allows us to avoid certain ontological assumptions about how sociality works than as some concrete methodological guide to carrying out health promotion research or, for that matter, any specific social research endeavour at all!

The key conceptual manoeuvre that Giddens employs in his attempt to transcend the dualism of structure and agency is in his use of *time* and *space* as categories that relativize social agency and social structure. For Giddens, the relative durability of social systems and social institutions has to do with systematic patterns of social activity (thus agency) as they are distributed across time and space; hence, social structure is both the medium and outcome of social activity. In acting as a medium, structure is both constraining and enabling in relation to social action. He argues that the process of modernization has built increasingly distanciated societies, where the effects of social action and institutions are spread across larger expanses of time and space, reducing the relative import of face-to-face interactions in the structuring of societies. Conversely, new mediums of communication have also enormously increased the amount of social interaction that is possible across great distances by compressing the amount of time it takes to engage in those interactions. A second innovation of structuration theory was to incorporate the concepts of *power* and *domination* into his theoretical framework. In Giddens's terms, modern societies have both increased the level and effectivity of administrative "power" in terms of its ability to transform and act, along with an increase in the potential for relations of domination, particularly through the use of knowledge.

While Giddens's work is still seen as a substantial contribution, many theorists have suggested that he has failed to fully transcend the dualism of structure and agency at the conceptual level (Mouzelis, 1995; Jessop, 2001), while from the very beginning, empirical researchers have felt there is little positive methodological guidance in structuration theory in how to conduct better research (Storper, 1985). This is not to discourage the use of

Giddens's work; however, health promoters should recognize that within the field of sociology itself, and for social theorists themselves, there is just as little consensus on how to move forward in conceptualizing the ontological and epistemological aspects of the social world as there was when Giddens published his theory. In particular, theorists concerned with producing adequate accounts of social structure are not convinced that Giddens's use of language as the exemplary social institution as the basis for conceptualizing structure was helpful. Nor are theorists of social action satisfied with his account of agency. Following Mouzelis's (1995) critique of Giddens, arguably health promoters should retain the tension in social theory represented by the dualism of structure and agency or, in older terms, between social interaction and social institutions. Many key questions that health promotion must address require *both* an analysis of key patterns of social interaction (such as with "collective lifestyles"), as well as systemic analyses of social institutions, including how governmental institutions, markets, and networks function to coordinate social action on broader scales. The duality of structure is a key insight shared by many contemporary thinkers, but this insight alone will not by itself produce substantive knowledge of important health promotion issues.

One other emerging theoretical approach to resolving the dualism between structure and agency is *complexity theory* (see chapter 6). Originating from work in a variety of fields (general systems theory, cybernetics, chaos theory, non-linear dynamics, information theory), scientists began, in the late 1980s, to coalesce around a series of general propositions concerning how complex systems worked (Waldrop, 1992). While it is impossible here to explicate the full range of theoretical and methodological implications of complexity theory, it is important to grasp the potential insight it can bring to the structure/agency problem. The core dilemma for the social theorist is to offer a persuasive explanation for how it is that relatively enduring social institutions and structural characteristics arise out of the complex interactions of individual human agents (the so-called micro-macro linkage). While almost everyone will accede to the proposition that there is no ontological gap between social institutions and social action (in other words, social activity produces social structure), a key dispute is around whether or not social institutions are *nothing but* the aggregate results of individual human agency. Or, more strongly, can social structure be *reduced* to the properties of individual agents? This is a profound epistemological question. How do we know about social structure? Can we predict what it will look like by examining only the interaction of individuals? Methodological individualists in the social sciences tell us that if you accede to the ontological proposition mentioned above, then there can be nothing left over or extra after you take account of all the individual activities. Yet, methodological holists point out that there clearly are properties that certain social structures or institutions have that an individual human agent does not. Thus far, the methodological individualist has been left with a reductionism that seemed satisfactory in terms of its parsimony, yet wanting in terms of its ability to explain the full development of complex social institutions or systems; conversely, the holist could wax lyrically about the irreducible complexity of social systems, yet be open to legitimate criticism concerning the nebulous extra quality that pertained to social orders that one could not find in the individuals who made it up.

Complexity theory offers a way out of this dilemma or paradox. Through the concept of "emergence" (Sawyer, 2005), it offers a rigorously systematic way of demonstrating how individual components of a system interact to create enduring orders, including social institutions, norms, and role structures, except these orders are created through iterations of interaction that cannot be *reduced* to the original properties of the system in its initial state (including all its individual components). This resolution does not undermine the basic ontological argument of the methodological individualists that social orders are produced by social interaction; rather, it shifts the emphasis to the epistemological failure of the methodological individualist's reductionist program. It argues first that genuinely novel properties are indeed generated by the interaction of individual agents, none of whom have these properties, in part or in whole, prior to the set of relevant interactions. Second, it argues that because this is the case, it has a radical methodological implication: that the static, linear, predictive models that social science has relied so heavily on have to be superseded by new models that *simulate* social systems by allowing artificial, computer-based interactions to take place over time, with changing parameters that attempt to realistically reflect variable social environments.

Interestingly, this new theoretical manoeuvre tends to sidestep the traditional debate over the ontology of the social, turning the question of the "micro-macro linkage" and the agency/structure debate into an epistemological and methodological question to be resolved through experiment with these new forms of modelling. Thus, the question of whether complexity theory solves the grand theoretical dilemmas of social science is turned into the question of whether the findings it produces have some practical relevance to better understanding how the social world works. For that answer we have to wait.

CONCLUSION

To summarize, health promotion must engage much more deeply with social theory in the coming decade as it attempts to turn its original youthful intuitions into a mature and substantial field of inquiry. I have argued here that much of this theoretical reflection will not necessarily translate into immediate empirical results. In fact, the approach to social theory advocated is one that critically embraces its legacy in the philosophical tradition, a tradition that understands the series of conceptual debates outlined above as constitutive oppositions in a dialectical progression that works by deepening our understanding of the social world through rigorous reflection rather than by way of a narrative of positive transcendence of the debates themselves. Thus, instead of seeing social theory as a *cul-de-sac* of endless, stagnant disputation, it is to be seen as a rich resource of conceptual innovation, opening up new vistas of inquiry and reinvigorating old questions and offering novel answers.

Another conclusion is that as health promotion begins to more seriously take up the question of social theory, it needs to connect to its fundamental core as a mode of societal critique, concerned with applying reflexive reason to basic questions of power, equity, values, resources, capabilities, and general human flourishing. In doing so, it can avoid falling into the trap of using social theory in a purely instrumental fashion as just one other argumentative resource in what are largely academic exercises. As health promotion becomes more comfortable using social theory, it will find that it can substantially enhance its intellectual resources for engaging in broader societal debates beyond the narrow health sector, a perspective that will become increasingly necessary if health promoters are to match their research and advocacy to their rhetoric, particularly in relation to social inequality and health inequity.

CRITICAL THINKING QUESTIONS

1. How should we think about the concept of "theory" in relation to health promotion?
2. How do you think class and status affect health inequities and the efforts to reduce or eliminate them?
3. What are the real dangers of "rationalization" for health promotion interventions?
4. Should health promotion be a critical social theory? Why or why not?
5. What are the implications of social theory for the concepts of "empowerment" and "participation"?

RESOURCES

Further Readings

Berman, M. (1988). *All that is solid melts into air: The experience of modernity*. New York: Penguin.
One of the truly great and accessible discussions of the process of modernity and how it has affected social change for over 200 years, this is a key text for understanding the cultural dilemmas at the heart of modern capitalist societies. For health promotion, it offers an example of how to think about the ironic and contradictory aspects of modern social life without falling into despair.

Harvey, D. (2002). Agency and community: A critical realist paradigm. *Journal for the Theory of Social Behaviour, 32*(2), 164–194.
This is a key theoretical article, from a critical realist perspective, that addresses the problem of structure vs. agency. Harvey is one of the most important social theorists of the past 40 years.

Nettleton, S. (2006). *The sociology of health and illness*. Cambridge: Polity Press.
This book is a summary and synthesis of sociological approaches to health and illness. Much
of the book is relevant to health promotion, particularly chapter 9, in which Nettleton directly addresses contemporary sociological critiques of health promotion.

Raeburn, J., & Rootman, I. (1998). *People-centred health promotion*. New York: John Wiley
    & Sons.
As indicated by its title, this book emphasizes the importance of "people" in health promotion. It focuses particularly on the "community" as the key locus for health promotion and
suggests methods to "empower" people where they live. The book also emphasizes the role
of "culture" and "spirituality" in health promotion, but also uses case studies to show how to
translate idealism about health promotion into health-enhancing action. It presents a vision
for a society based on health promotion values.

Thorogood, N. (2002). What is the relevance of sociology for health promotion? In R.
    Bunton & G. Scambler (Eds.), *Health promotion: Disciplines, diversity, and develop-
    ments* (pp. 53–75). London: Routledge.
This is a dedicated chapter on health promotion and sociology in an important collection.
Some key theoretical issues are covered, including social stratification, health promotion
values and ideology, and lay perspectives on health.

Relevant Websites

Health Sociology Review
hsr.e-contentmanagement.com/
    An international scholarly peer-reviewed journal, *Health Sociology Review* explores
the contribution of sociology and sociological research methods to understanding health
and illness; to health policy, promotion, and practice; and to equity, social justice, social
policy, and social work.

International Journal of Health Services
http://journals.sagepub.com/home/joh
    The journal contains articles on health and social policy, political economy and so-
ciology, history and philosophy, and ethics and law in the areas of health and health care.
It provides analysis of developments in the health and social sectors of every area of the
world, including relevant scholarly articles, position papers, and stimulating debates about
the most controversial issues of the day. It is of interest to health professionals and social
scientists interested in the many different facets of health, disease, and health care.

Social Theory & Health
www.palgrave-journals.com/sth/index.html

The theorization of health issues is crucial both for understanding and as a guide for action. By providing a forum for academics and practitioners to engage with the theoretical development of the health debate, *Social Theory & Health* aims to develop the theoretical underpinnings of health research and service delivery. The journal is of interest to scholars of health-related sociology, nursing, health and clinical psychologists, health and public policy analysts, and theorists in related disciplines.

Sociology of Health and Illness
www.onlinelibrary.wiley.com/journal/10.1111/(ISSN)1467-9566
Sociology of Health and Illness is an international journal that publishes sociological articles on all aspects of health, illness, medicine, and health care. This journal is particularly open to theoretical approaches to health and supports diverse methodological perspectives.

NOTES

1.   Though this use of "science" is typically a peculiarity of the English-speaking world, as in German, for example, the word for science, *Wissenschaft*, tends to mean any systematic scholarly inquiry.

2.   In fact, when it comes to empirical research, much of social science is inherently skeptical of the type of theorizing discussed in this chapter, and still trundles along happily, churning out the type of "abstracted empiricism" that Wright Mills (1959) warned of so many years ago.

3.   They are "tropes" in the sense that they have become metaphors for modern society as a whole: as in "the bureaucratic society," "the rationalist society," etc.

4.   In this argument, I do not equate the generic term *critical social theory* with the narrower identification of the former with the specific set of ideas that developed out of the Frankfurt School of critical theory (Jay, 1973; Benhabib, 1986; Bernstein, 1995; Rush, 2004), although the latter is certainly one of the more productive and important traditions to consider.

5.   Interestingly, the fact that these trends have not been universal in either direction or strength adds to the evidence of their effect on social inequality. It is now clear that countries and societies that retained strong working-class institutions and a relatively generous welfare system have endured fewer increases in social inequality than we have seen in societies more heavily influenced by neo-liberalism and attacks on labour and the welfare state (Esping-Anderson, 1990; Pinch, 1997; Pierson, 1999; Goodin, Heady, Muffels, & Dirven, 2000; Jenson & Sineau, 2003).

6.   See Frohlich et al. in this volume for a detailed account of this rationale.

REFERENCES

Abel, T. (2007). Cultural capital in health promotion. In D. McQueen & I. Kickbusch (Eds.), *Health & modernity: The role of theory in health promotion* (pp. 43–73). New York: Springer.

Ackroyd, S., & Hughes, J. (1992). *Data collection in context*. Longman: London.

Benhabib, S. (1986). *Critique, norm, and utopia: A study of the foundations of critical theory.* New York: Columbia University Press.

Bernstein, R. (1995). *Habermas & modernity.* Cambridge: MIT Press.

Breslow, L. (1999). From disease prevention to health promotion. *Journal of the American Medical Association, 281*(11), 1030–1033.

Derrida, J. (1976). *Of grammatology.* G. Spivak (Trans.). Baltimore: Johns Hopkins University Press.

DiClemente, R., Crosby, R., & Kegler, M. (2002). *Emerging theories in health promotion practice and research.* San Francisco: John Wiley & Sons.

Eakin, J., Robertson, A., Poland, B., Coburn, D., & Edwards, R. (1996). Towards a critical social science perspective on health promotion research. *Health Promotion International, 11*(2), 157–165.

Esping-Anderson, G. (1990). *The three worlds of welfare capitalism.* Princeton: Princeton University Press.

Foucault, M. (1980). *Power/knowledge: Selected interviews & other writings.* C. Gordon (Ed.). New York: Pantheon Books.

Foucault, M. (2000). *Aesthetics: Essential works of Foucault 1954–1984*, vol. 2. J. Faubion (Ed.). Penguin Books: London.

Foucault, M. (2008). *The birth of biopolitics: Lectures at the College de France, 1978–1979.* New York: Palgrave MacMillan.

Frohlich, K., Corin, E., & Potvin, L. (2001). A theoretical proposal for the relationship between context and disease. *Sociology of Health & Illness, 23*, 776–797.

Frohlich, K., Poland, B., Mykhalovskiy, E., Alexander, S., & Maule, C. (2010). Tobacco control and the inequitable socio-economic distribution of smoking: Smokers' discourses and implications for tobacco control. *Critical Public Health, 20*(1), 35–46.

Giddens, A. (1984). *The constitution of society: Outline of the theory of structuration.* Cambridge: Polity Press.

Giddens, A. (1991). Structuration theory: Past, present, and future. In C. Bryant & D. Jary (Eds.), *Giddens's theory of structuration: A critical appreciation* (pp. 201–221). London: Routledge.

Goodin, R., Heady, B., Muffels, R., & Dirven, H. (2000). The real worlds of welfare capitalism. In C. Pierson & F. Castles (Eds.), *The welfare state reader, Part II: Debates and issues* (pp. 171–188). Oxford: Blackwell Publishers.

Habermas, J. (1984). *The theory of communicative action*, vol. 1: *Reason and the rationalization of society.* T. McCarthy (Trans.). Boston: Beacon Press.

Habermas, J. (1987). *The philosophical discourse of modernity: Twelve lectures.* Cambridge: MIT Press.

Habermas, J. (1998). *Between facts and norms.* W. Rehg (Trans.). Cambridge: MIT Press.

Hancock, T. (1994). Health promotion in Canada: Did we win the battle but lose the war? In A. Pederson, M. O'Neill, & I. Rootman (Eds.), *Health promotion in Canada: Provincial, national & international perspectives* (pp. 350–373). Toronto: W. B. Saunders.

Heidegger, M. (1993). *Basic writings: From being and time (1927) to the task of thinking (1964).* D. Farrell Krell (Trans.). San Francisco: HarperCollins Publishers.

Hills, M., & Carroll, S. (2009). Health promotion, health education and the public's health. In R.

Detels, M. A. Lansang, & M. Gulliford (Eds.), *Oxford textbook of public health* (5th ed.) (pp. 752–766). Oxford: Oxford University Press.

Horkheimer, M., & Adorno, T. (2002). *Dialectic of enlightenment*. Palo Alto: Stanford University Press.

Jay, M. (1973). *The dialectical imagination: A history of the Frankfurt School and the Institute of Social Research, 1923–1950*. Berkeley: University of California Press.

Jenson, J., & Sineau, M. (2003). *Who cares? Women's work, child care, and welfare state redesign*. Toronto: University of Toronto Press.

Jessop, R. (2001). Institutional re(turns) and the strategic-relational approach. *Environment and Planning A, 33*, 1213–1235.

Kickbusch, I. (1989). Approaches to an ecological base to public health. *Health Promotion International, 4*, 265–268.

Labonté, R. (1994). Death of program, birth of metaphor: The development of health promotion in Canada. In A. Pederson, M. O'Neill, & I. Rootman (Eds.), *Health promotion in Canada: Provincial, national & international perspectives* (pp. 72–90). Toronto: W. B. Saunders.

Marcuse, H. (1991). *One-dimensional man*. London: Routledge.

Marx, K. (1976). *Capital*, vol. 1. London: Penguin Classics.

Marx, K. (1981). *Capital*, vol. 3. London: Penguin Classics.

McQueen, D., & Kickbusch, I. (2007). *Health & modernity: The role of theory in health promotion*. New York: Springer.

Meiksins Wood, E. (2008). *Citizens to lords: A social history of Western political thought from antiquity to the Middle Ages*. London: Verso.

Mouzelis, N. (1995). *Sociological theory: What went wrong?* London: Routledge.

Mouzelis, N. (2007). Social causation: Between social constructionism and critical realism. Available at mouzelis.gr/wp/wp-content/uploads/2010/05/Mouzelis_Social_Causation.pdf

Olin Wright, E. (Ed.). (2005). *Approaches to class analysis*. Cambridge: Cambridge University Press.

Olin Wright, E. (2009). Class patternings. *New Left Review, 60*, 101–116.

Pierson, C. (1999). The welfare state: From Beveridge to Borrie. In H. Fawcett & R. Lowe (Eds.), *Welfare policy in Britain: The road from 1945* (pp. 208–224). London: MacMillan Publishers Ltd.

Pinch, S. (1997). *Worlds of welfare: Understanding the changing geographies of social welfare provision*. London: Routledge.

Porter, R. (2000). *The Enlightenment*. New York: Palgrave.

Potvin, L., & McQueen, D. (2007). Modernity, public health, and health promotion: A reflexive discourse. In D. McQueen & I. Kickbusch (Eds.), *Health & modernity: The role of theory in health promotion* (pp. 12–20). Springer: New York.

Raeburn, J., & Rootman, I. (1998). *People-centred health promotion*. New York: John Wiley & Sons.

Rush, F. (Ed.). (2004). *The Cambridge companion to critical theory*. Cambridge: Cambridge University Press.

Sawyer, R. (2005). *Social emergence: Societies as complex systems*. Cambridge: Cambridge University Press.

Sayer, A. (2005). *The moral significance of class.* Cambridge: Cambridge University Press.

Sayer, A. (2009). Chapter 3: "Bourdieu, ethics, and practice," published by the Department of Sociology, Lancaster University, Lancaster, UK. Retrieved from www.lancs.ac.uk/fass/sociology/papers/sayer_chapter3_bourdieu_ethics_&_practice.pdf

Sayer, D. (1991). *Capitalism and modernity: An excursus on Marx and Weber.* London: Routledge.

Stevenson, H., & Burke, M. (1991). Bureaucratic logic in new social movement clothing. *Health Promotion International, 6,* 281–289.

Storper, M. (1985). The spatial and temporal constitution of social action: A critical reading of Giddens. *Environment and Planning D: Society and Space, 3*(4), 407–424.

Waldrop, M. (1992). *Complexity: The emerging science at the edge of chaos.* New York: Touchstone.

Weber, M. (1978). *Economy and society: An outline of interpretive sociology.* Berkeley: University of California Press.

Weber, M. (2002). *The Protestant ethic and the spirit of capitalism: And other writings.* P. Baehr & G. Wells (Trans.). New York: Penguin Books.

World Health Organization (WHO). (1986). *Ottawa Charter for Health Promotion.* Ottawa: World Health Organization, Health and Welfare Canada, Canadian Public Health Association.

Wright Mills, C. (1959). *The sociological imagination.* New York: Oxford University Press.

CHAPTER 4

Behavioural Theories and Building Health Promotion Interventions: Persistent Challenges and Emerging Perspectives

Lise Gauvin and Ariane Bélanger-Gravel

LEARNING OBJECTIVES

1. Explain why the aim of changing health-related behaviours should be an integral part of health promotion
2. Explain why changing health-related behaviours represents such a unique challenge in health promotion
3. Describe the main components of the most frequently used theoretical models of behaviour change in health promotion
4. Outline the behaviour change wheel and its added value to developing effective health promotion interventions

INTRODUCTION

A substantial body of scientific evidence shows that individual behaviours including but not limited to healthy eating; physical activity; avoidance of smoking; avoidance of alcohol and substance use and abuse; adherence to medications; and use of protective equipment and devices such as bicycle helmets, seat belts, and condoms are associated with favourable health outcomes. Consequently, the goal of fostering either the adoption of health-related behaviours or the avoidance of behaviours leading to deleterious outcomes is often the target of health promotion. In fact, several calls to action have been issued to promote behaviour change at the individual level to improve population health (Michie, 2008; Spring et al., 2013). Interestingly, researchers had already begun to heed this call by developing theories and using these theories to build health promotion interventions (Glanz & Bishop, 2010). Intervention developers can now count on a substantial body of empirical research and several theories to design effective health promotion programs or policies that can result in favourable changes in health-related behaviours.

Towards this end, one important contribution comes from Michie, West, Campbell, Brown, and Gainforth (2014) who reviewed and compared 83 theories emerging from the fields of psychology, anthropology, economics, and sociology. Some of these theories have been and still are being used to build health promotion interventions—and for good reason. Although a debate is still ongoing regarding the link between theory use and effectiveness of interventions (Prestwich et al., 2014), Webb, Joseph, Yardley, and Michie (2010) observed in a review of Internet-based interventions that greater use of theory was linked to better success of interventions in the context of promoting physical activity.

Yet, as mentioned by Kelly and Barker (2016), changing health-related behaviours is notoriously difficult at least in part because behaviour change is often thought to be nothing more than "common sense" or, as defined by the Merriam-Webster dictionary, "sound and prudent judgment based on a simple perception of the situation or facts." Kelly and Barker go on to list five common errors that appear to be widespread among policy makers, practitioners, and the public, notably that changing behaviour is simply about (1) getting the message across because once people know "what to do" they will change their behaviour; (2) delivering knowledge and information about the consequences of health-related behaviours because this is what really drives behaviour change; (3) believing that people act rationally and will simply adopt a rational solution to change their behaviours; (4) believing that people act irrationally and thus that changing behaviour is a hopeless endeavour; and (5) believing that it is possible to predict and control behaviour accurately and thus that a single solution will work for all individuals and populations. Of course, none of these adages constitutes a scientific basis for action in health promotion.

To complicate things just a little further, although there is consensus about how different behaviours are associated with health outcomes, the role of behavioural theories in health promotion has been the object of criticism and debate. As eloquently stated in a recent editorial (Van Den Broucke, 2014, p. 597), "health promotion has always had a somewhat ambivalent relationship with behaviour and behaviour change" because promoting behaviour change without accounting for or acting on the social, cultural, and political factors that influence both behaviours and health leads to ineffective interventions and blaming people for not successfully adopting healthful behaviours. Others (see chapter 8 and Katikireddi, Higgins, Smith, & Williams, 2013) have also argued that behaviour change interventions may disenfranchise segments of the population and hence lead to increased social inequalities in health.

Despite the wealth of theory and evidence about behaviour change, the existing zeitgeist about how to achieve behaviour change and the difficult tasks of accounting for contextual influences and overcoming social inequalities render the development of health promotion interventions uniquely challenging. Therefore, we pursue two goals in this chapter. First, we describe the theories used most often in the field of health promotion to understand and promote behaviour change. In doing so, we briefly discuss some of the significant issues associated with the use of these theoretical models to build health promotion interventions. Second, we outline a new, more encompassing model called the "behaviour change wheel," which is an intervention development framework created with the aim of translating the accumulated scientific knowledge on behaviour change into practice (Michie, van Stralen, & West, 2011). We illustrate the added value of this model by outlining how it might be used to support the design of theory-informed interventions aimed at promoting health-related behaviours and point to useful resources for developing behaviour change interventions.

A FEW BUILDING BLOCKS

Over the past four or five decades, numerous behavioural theories have been developed, empirically tested, and refined to predict the adoption and maintenance of health-related behaviours and orient the development of health promotion interventions. The most frequently used theories in health promotion are the health belief model, the reasoned action approach (including the theories of reasoned action and planned behaviour), the transtheoretical model, and social cognitive theory. As described below, these theories were developed by researchers interested in identifying the intrapersonal factors that allowed people to direct and change their own behaviour.

The Health Belief Model

The health belief model was among the first models introduced in the field of health promotion and was aimed at promoting health-related behaviours from a more theoretical stance. This model was initially developed in the 1950s by the United States Public Health Service to promote preventive screening behaviours (e.g., X-rays to detect tuberculosis) and was formally described in the scientific literature by Rosenstock (1966, 1974) in the 1960s and 1970s. The theory is known as an expectancy-value theory because behaviour is thought to be self-managed through people's understanding of what they will accrue from the behaviour (expectancy) and how much they value this outcome (value). The health belief model suggests that individuals hold different sets of beliefs about a disease or health threats (e.g., tuberculosis) and that these beliefs are likely to influence the uptake of preventive actions (e.g., tuberculosis screening through X-rays). The model outlines perceived severity, perceived susceptibility, perceived benefits, and perceived barriers as some of the main psychological variables involved in predicting behaviour.

Perceived severity is defined as the extent to which an individual believes that a disease will have significant negative consequences (e.g., severe illness, death, economic difficulties, family issues, depression, etc.). Perceived susceptibility is conceived as the extent to which an individual perceives him/herself as being at high risk of developing the disease. Perceived benefits refer to the positive outcomes of taking action and perceived barriers are those obstacles or hurdles that must be overcome to take action. Perceived severity and susceptibility must be prominent in an individual's mind to lead to uptake of a preventive action, while outcomes must be perceived as positive and highly valued and barriers as minimal. The model was updated following its initial description (Rosenstock, Strecher, & Becker, 1988) and notably, the concept of self-efficacy (i.e., one's perceptions of his/her capacities to perform the behaviour, see below for a definition of this concept) was included as an additional factor predicting the uptake of preventive actions. The influence of social, cultural, and environmental cues to action such as mass communication campaigns, social norms, significant others' behaviours or illness, and physician advice were identified as instrumental signals from the person's environment to prompt the adoption of health-related behaviours.

From a more practical standpoint, a practitioner interested in developing a health promotion intervention based on the health belief model would develop activities to ensure that individuals achieve the following: accurately perceiving the severity of the disease or health threat (e.g., "Smoking will lead to the development of a lung cancer that is killing a lot of people"), believing that they can personally be affected by the disease ("It could happen to me because I have been a heavy smoker for 25 years"), believing that the suggested preventive action will be useful ("My counsellor told me that it is never too late to stop and that I can significantly reduce my risk of developing lung cancer even if I have been smoker for many years"), and perceiving that she/he can overcome the barriers required to take this action ("I have tried so many times to stop smoking and have never succeeded, but now I believe that my counsellor and I will succeed because I have all the tools that I need"). One important challenge for intervention developers using this model is that in the absence of all four components, the intervention is not likely to lead to effective behaviour change. Although this model has been helpful in understanding the uptake of preventive actions that occur infrequently (e.g., X-rays for detection, breast cancer screening), it remains unclear whether or not this model is broad enough to fully explain behaviours that occur more frequently (e.g., decisions about food intake) and that unfold in contexts that vary. Also, in a recent review (Jones, Smith, & Llewellyn, 2014), only perceived benefits and barriers consistently predicted preventive behaviours, leaving the role of perceived severity and susceptibility in predicting behaviour uncertain.

The Reasoned Action Approach

The reasoned action approach (Fishbein & Ajzen, 2010) emerged from two theories: the theory of reasoned action (Fishbein & Ajzen, 1975) and the theory of planned behaviour (Ajzen, 1991). These theories are predictive models, as the aim is to explain the adoption and/or the maintenance of behaviours, and are also considered to be expectancy-value theories. The theory of reasoned action was developed in the 1970s and stemmed from the basic idea that behaviours are predominantly driven by people's intentions (i.e., the strength of a person's mental plan for action). In turn, intentions (also called motivation) were thought to be influenced by individuals' attitudes and subjective norms. Attitude refers to the positive or negative value a person ascribes to a given behaviour (i.e., "I like doing this" or "I dislike doing this"). Subjective norms refer to people's perception of the extent to which peers, friends, loved ones, and others approve or disapprove of the behaviour. More favourable attitudes and subjective norms were thought to lead to stronger intentions and then behaviour. To account for the presence of external or internal obstacles that might hamper the adoption or maintenance of behaviours, the notion of perceived behavioural control (or the extent to which people believe they can control situations in which the behaviour is likely to be performed) was integrated and the theory of reasoned action evolved into what is known as the theory of planned behaviour.

In a more recent iteration of this theory—the reasoned action approach—the initial constructs were redefined, and more detailed descriptions of beliefs were integrated into the model. For example, the notion of attitude was stratified into two sub-dimensions in recognition of the distinct instrumental (cognitive) and experiential (affective) features of attitude. Similarly, the idea of subjective norm was further described to account for the perception of support from significant others (called the injunctive aspect of norm) and the perception of how prevalent a given behaviour is in one's immediate social environment (called descriptive norm). Finally, the construct of perceived behavioural control was defined to include two distinct aspects, namely capacity (equivalent to self-efficacy) and autonomy (as initially defined as perception of control over one's situation).

According to the reasoned action approach, attitude (both instrumental and experiential aspects), injunctive norms, and capacity are underpinned by a set of beliefs, that is, any thoughts, perceptions, and evaluations that individuals hold towards a given behaviour. For instance, a man might enjoy the adoption of an active lifestyle (i.e., the experiential aspect of attitude towards the behaviour of active lifestyle) because exercising represents a healthy way of controlling his weight (the instrumental aspect of attitude). Furthermore, beliefs are thought to be formed through direct experience (e.g., believing that exercise will lead to significant weight loss because that occurred in a previous life experience). However, depending on how people perceive and integrate experiences, beliefs may be factually incorrect (e.g., thinking that physical activity can lead to spot reductions in fat). From an intervention standpoint, this implies a prerequisite understanding of beliefs held by a person when attempting to support a behaviour change process. Normative beliefs represent the appraisal of individuals with regard to the approval of specific groups of persons (e.g., a man is adopting an active lifestyle because his wife approves of this behaviour or an older man is not adopting a healthy diet because his wife doesn't want to change her cooking habits). Finally, beliefs about one's capacity to control the situation represent how an individual views his/her capacity to overcome barriers.

From an intervention perspective, although the reasoned action approach and its predecessors are among the most powerful theories allowing for predicting the adoption and maintenance of behaviour, one systematic review (Hardeman et al., 2002) showed that few interventions based on these theories led to significant changes in behaviour. Hence, one of the most important criticisms of these theories is the fact that even though they provide useful guidance for identifying intervention targets (e.g., predictors of intention and behaviour, salient beliefs), the reasoned action approach does not provide clear guidance on *how* to act on these intervention targets. To overcome this limitation, some authors have suggested the integration of the reasoned action approach with other theoretical models to design more effective interventions (Fishbein & Cappella, 2006; Fishbein & Yzer, 2003).

The Transtheoretical Model

The transtheoretical model was first developed in the context of smoking cessation (Prochaska & DiClemente, 1983). This model is generally viewed as a behaviour change theory because specific intervention strategies are included in the model. The basic assumption of this model is that behaviour change represents a long-term and non-linear process. Individuals can be categorized as being in one of five stages of change according to their level of readiness regarding the adoption and maintenance of a given health-related behaviour. These stages are pre-contemplation, contemplation, preparation, action, and maintenance. Individuals in pre-contemplation do not intend to change and any intervention aimed at promoting a given behaviour (e.g., smoking cessation) among individuals in this stage are likely to fail if not carefully tailored to this stage. Individuals in contemplation intend to change, but not in the near future (i.e., within the next six months), while those in preparation stage intend to take actions within the next month. Finally, individuals in the action (having adopted the behaviour for less than six months) and maintenance (having adopted the behaviour for more than six months) stages are trying/performing the behaviour and require substantial support to continue through the achievement of a final stage named termination. To design health promotion interventions, the transtheoretical model suggests tailoring processes of change according to individuals' current stages of change. For instance, informational or educational strategies (e.g., information about the negative consequences of being sedentary or the benefits of being physically active) should be used when individuals are in pre-contemplation to favour the development of motivation toward the adoption of a new behaviour. Once individuals have developed motivation for change and initiated action (action/maintenance stages), self-regulation processes of change (e.g., reinforcement [identify rewards for achieving behaviour goals] and stimulus control [changing cues in the environment]) should be used to favour maintenance (see Prochaska, DiClemente, & Norcross, 1992). Finally, individuals will progress toward stages of change when the pros of adopting the targeted behaviour increase and the cons decrease (i.e., the decisional balance), alongside increases in self-efficacy.

The transtheoretical model is intuitively appealing for designing theory-informed health promotion interventions and several reviews show that application of the transtheoretical model to a variety of health-related behaviours leads to adoption and maintenance of physical activity, smoking cessation, and mammography, to name a few (Marshall & Biddle, 2001; Spencer, Pagell, & Adams, 2005; Spencer, Pagell, Hallion, & Adams, 2002).

However, the basic assumptions of the model have also been criticized. According to Bandura (1998) and West (2005), there are significant weaknesses in this theory that limit the capacity of the transtheoretical model to inform the development of interventions.

One criticism is the arbitrary definition of stages (e.g., the timeline used to categorize individuals into stages is difficult to ascertain) and the absence of qualitative characteristics to define stages per se is viewed as problematic because tailoring an intervention based on these stages may lead to misclassification of individuals into stages and consequent inadequate application of change strategies. Another criticism of the model is the necessary progression through the stages of change, thus discarding the possibility that, for instance, a smoker stops smoking abruptly (i.e., "going cold turkey"). Although authors of the transtheoretical model stipulate that individuals can relapse into previous stages at any time because behaviour change is not a linear process, individuals must progress through all subsequent stages before attaining termination. Despite these critiques, the transtheoretical model, which is still widely used by practitioners, provides a useful intervention framework when the health promotion context requires face-to-face programs tailored to individual needs.

Social Cognitive Theory

The social cognitive theory developed by Albert Bandura is arguably one of the most dominant and useful theories for understanding behaviour change processes and informing the design of health promotion interventions (Bandura, 1986). Accordingly, many behavioural theories that did not include the concept of self-efficacy (one of the core constructs of this theory) were revised in favour of its inclusion. Social cognitive theory is thought of as a behaviour change theory. This theory (as its earlier version, called self-efficacy theory, see Bandura, 1977) revolves around the concept of self-efficacy. According to Bandura, an individual's perception regarding her/his own capacity to undertake specific actions (i.e., self-efficacy or personal mastery) is the cornerstone of any change in human behaviour. In keeping with this basic idea, a recent meta-analysis of interventions has shown that changes in self-efficacy led to the most important behaviour change (Sheeran et al., 2016). Practically speaking, if smokers or heavy drinkers, for example, are not convinced that they have the capacity to overcome cravings, they will not be motivated or will not attempt to stop smoking or drinking. From an intervention perspective, this highlights the inescapable need to ascertain the individuals' level of self-efficacy, to acknowledge barriers hampering self-efficacy, and to implement intervention components to allow individuals to overcome these barriers (finding solutions or problem solving) and strengthen self-efficacy. According to the theory, the most important sources for fostering self-efficacy are the successful performance of behaviours (directly through personal experiences and indirectly through observing similar others being successful, known as vicarious experience) and the development of favourable perceptions of the outcomes of these behaviours (i.e., expectations regarding the outcomes of behaviour). Throughout the years, Bandura further refined social cognitive theory by introducing the notion of goals, perceived environment, and what is known as triadic influence (i.e., behaviour is jointly determined by behavioural, personal, and environmental factors).

According to social cognitive theory, interventions should include a number of components aimed at, mostly, increasing self-efficacy (through mastery experiences, vicarious experiences, social persuasion, the control of somatic and emotional states, and management of environmental contingencies). For instance, a health care practitioner who aims to promote exercising among post-infarct patients might first verbally encourage his/her patients by telling them that they are still able to exercise and that it is never too late to start (i.e., social persuasion). Second, they might support patients by setting progressive (and attainable) goals to ensure that patients will experience a challenge while ensuring a success (mastery experiences). According to Bandura, sense of mastery depends extensively on past successes and, inversely, failure will hamper future attempts to change. Third, the practitioner may think of a way to expose the patients to others with similar health conditions who are successfully performing the target behaviour (i.e., vicarious experience; for example, planning a few group sessions of exercise in a cardiac rehabilitation setting). Finally, the health care practitioner may wish to investigate how the patients are feeling or in which mood they are during or after exercising to investigate anxiety or negative moods, among others, that patients might misleadingly interpret as personal failure to cope with the disease and/or the exercise program. Other techniques associated with the social cognitive theory might also include the provision of information regarding the health problem and/or the health benefits of the health-related behaviours (outcomes expectancies) as well as self-monitoring, feedback on performance, and problem solving (finding ways to overcome barriers).

TOWARDS AN INTEGRATIVE FRAMEWORK: THE COM-B SYSTEM AND THE BEHAVIOUR CHANGE WHEEL

Given the significant number of constructs and possible overlap in concepts across theories (e.g., attitude from the reasoned action approach, outcome expectancies from the social cognitive theory, perceived benefits from the health belief model), selected researchers attending a scientific meeting held in the 1990s suggested the need to integrate accumulated scientific knowledge about theories into one overarching framework accounting for the most important determinants of behaviour adoption and/or maintenance (Fishbein et al., 2001). More recently, and at least partly in response to this previous consensus, Michie et al. (2011) proposed the COM-B system. According to this system, behavioural adoption/maintenance can be viewed as the result of interactions between perceived capabilities, motivation, perceived opportunities, and behaviours (see figure 4.1). Perceived capabilities are akin to social cognitive theory's self-efficacy construct; that is—similarly to reasoned action approach and social cognitive theory—motivation and behaviours are thought to be influenced by the extent to which individuals perceive themselves as being capable of adopting any given behaviour. According to Michie and West (2013), capabilities can be either in the physical realm (e.g., physical strength, absence of physical limitations or handicaps) or the psychological

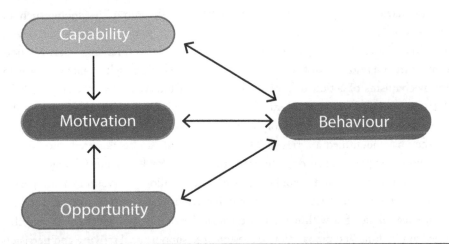

Figure 4.1: The COM-B System: A Framework for Understanding
Behaviour

Source: Michie, S., van Stralen, M. M., & West, R. (2011). The behaviour change wheel: A new method for characterising and designing behaviour change interventions. *Implementation Science*, 6, 42, figure 1. doi:10.1186/1748-5908-6-42

realm (e.g., knowledge, cognitive skills, self-confidence). Opportunity refers to the social
(e.g., culture, norms, media environment) and physical (e.g., infrastructures, resources in
communities, health services accessibility) environment, thus integrating the notion of
triadic influence from social cognitive theory as well as emerging ecological perspectives
(see chapter 5). Motivation, in the COM-B system, involves two processes: a reflexive or
thought-out process (involving mostly cognitive processes as conceived in previously described behavioural theories) and an automatic process that accounts for impulsive and/
or emotional motivational drives (i.e., habits, urges) to adopt or avoid a given behaviour.
This latter type of motivation is often neglected in behavioural theories.

Based on PRIME theory of motivation (West, 2006), human motivation is viewed
as a chaotic, complex, and changing system. From this perspective, the most proximal
influence on behavioural responses (i.e., health-related behaviours) is thought to include
automatic processes that involve competing or countering impulses (e.g., addictive urges), competing wants (e.g., self-presentation), and needs (e.g., satiety) as well as habits.
Consequently, the more distal influences on behavioural responses are governed by reflexive processes involving beliefs, attitudes, self-efficacy, and planned behaviour. Hence,
from an intervention perspective, the development of a positive attitude or a greater sense
of self-efficacy (mostly associated with reflexive processes) will require substantial strength
to overcome competing impulses or needs (e.g., urges to smoke during a tobacco cessation
process) through, among others, the development of a greater self-regulation capacity (e.g.,
abilities to manage cravings to attain the goal of smoking cessation).

In parallel to the work around synthesizing theories and developing the COM-B system, Abraham and Michie (2008) developed a taxonomy to inform and harmonize the

use of behaviour change techniques in interventions. The aim of developing such a taxonomy was to "break down" interventions into their smallest components (i.e., the specific behaviour change techniques) to allow researchers and practitioners to clearly understand what an intervention consists of. Another aim of developing such a taxonomy was to identify mechanisms of action to explain the effects of interventions on changing behaviour. With the support and involvement of an international advisory board, Michie et al. (2013) embarked upon the task of inventorying and classifying behaviour change techniques. Thus far, they have identified a series of 93 techniques that can be clustered into 16 categories according to expert evaluations. Recently, the Centre for Behaviour Change developed an online training system and a mobile app (see below) to allow intervention developers to learn the techniques and understand their role in behaviour change interventions. The behaviour change techniques fall within the broad categories of being either motivation enhancing, aimed at planning and preparation, or designed to support goal striving and persistence.

Furthermore, in addition to the COM-B system and the behaviour change techniques, an intervention design framework was subsequently developed to support practitioners in the development of theory-driven interventions: the "behaviour change wheel" (Michie, Atkins, & West, 2014; Michie et al., 2011, see figure 4.2). This framework is eliciting extensive excitement (see Spence & Dinh, 2015, and Foley & Fairmichael, 2015, for major policy briefs that recommend its use) because, as described below, it overcomes many of the limitations of existing theories and allows for behaviour change interventions to be cast within the broader perspective of population health.

The behaviour change wheel emerged from an integration of the numerous theories of behaviour change and intervention development frameworks proposed across a variety of disciplines. Michie and colleagues (2011, 2014) introduced this framework to support the design of interventions specifically aimed at promoting the adoption and/or maintenance of health-related behaviours. That is, the behaviour change wheel is a comprehensive guide that integrates constructs from 19 intervention development frameworks or models and that was developed through an extensive review of the literature and consultations with an international team of experts. Two important features of the preliminary work consisted of defining intervention functions and identifying policy options for implementation. According to the approach, intervention functions represent the aim of the activities that can be implemented to change behaviours. These are education, persuasion, incentivization, coercion, training, restriction, environmental restructuring, modelling, and enablement. Policy options represent the means by which an intervention function can be operationalized. These include developing communication/implementing social marketing strategies, developing guidelines, implementing fiscal measures, applying new or different regulations, developing or modifying legislation, conducting environmental/social planning, and creating or modifying service provision.

To design health promotion interventions using the behaviour change wheel, three broad steps are proposed: (1) a sound and detailed understanding of the behaviour that is the object of the intervention, including an outline of the contexts in which the behaviour

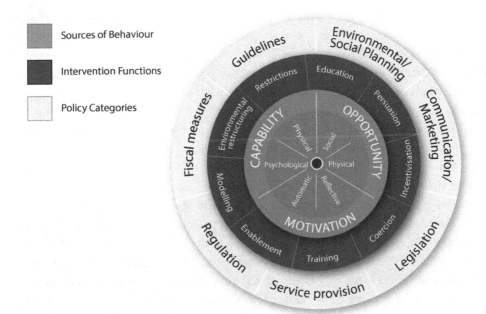

Figure 4.2: Behaviour Change Wheel

Source: Michie, S., van Stralen, M. M., & West, R. (2011). The behaviour change wheel: A new method for characterising and designing behaviour change interventions. *Implementation Science*, 6, 42, figure 2. doi:10.1186/1748-5908-6-42

will unfold and some of the barriers involved. This step involves identifying which specific aspects of the COM-B model should be targeted to change the behaviour (i.e., capacity, motivation, or environment); (2) the identification of optimal intervention aims through a matching between components of the COM-B model identified and the intervention functions that can allow for change in these components; and (3) the identification of the specific implementation options that can be enacted in the context wherein the health promotion intervention will unfold. For example, in an effort to improve quality of life among patients with type 2 diabetes, a health care practitioner might first identify a specific behavioural target (e.g., medication adherence, healthy diet, physical activity, foot care) that has a good potential to improve quality of life and then examine major sources of influence on the behaviour from the individual (e.g., perceived capacities, barriers, motivation) and the contextual constraints (environmental opportunities or limitations). Once the major influences on behaviour change are identified in step 1, the practitioner might identify one or more intervention functions that would allow for action on the behaviour and its determinants. For example, if, during the first step, the practitioner observed that patients with type 2 diabetes lack knowledge regarding the need to carefully monitor their feet and toes (the identified behavioural target), he/she might choose to educate (intervention function: education) patients about this problem and its causes as well as ensure that patients have the appropriate skills to perform the behaviour accurately (intervention function: training).

At this step, the intervention developer might do as suggested in the behaviour change wheel and identify specific behaviour change techniques to unequivocally operationalize intervention functions. Finally, the practitioner might identify the service provision policy option and attempt to develop and deliver a manualized intervention within a health care system. From this example, the reader should realize that applying the behaviour change wheel requires appropriate training and experience as well as an interdisciplinary team that can ensure the feasibility of its application (see end of chapter for appropriate resources and references). A manual outlining how to develop behaviour change interventions according to the behaviour change wheel was recently published (Michie & West, 2016) and an Internet site also supports intervention development.

Although the behaviour change wheel is a recent development, the scientific literature includes evidence suggesting that this new approach is likely to be very useful. For example, a quick search of the scientific literature or the online grey literature shows that numerous interventions are currently applying the behaviour change wheel to develop interventions aimed at a variety of health-related behaviours. Furthermore, a recent review of digital apps aimed at changing physical activity showed that only a few of the 93 behaviour change techniques were integrated into the apps (Conroy, Yang, & Maher, 2014), highlighting the need to strengthen and improve behaviour change interventions. A similar content analysis of digital behaviour change interventions aimed at medication adherence showed that interventions studied did not systematically include appropriate behaviour change techniques (Morrissey, Corbett, Walsh, & Molloy, 2015).

CONCLUSION

There is no doubt that changing health-related behaviours should be an integral part of health promotion interventions. However, ensuring that health promotion interventions are evidence-informed poses unique challenges because of the omnipresence of common-sense views of behaviour change and of the diversity and complexity of theories, models, and scientific literature relevant to behaviour change. The challenge of identifying how to apply behavioural theories in specific contexts has been remarkably elusive.

Fortunately, there have been very significant strides achieved in integrating models and in developing intervention frameworks that account for how intrapersonal and environmental/social factors may interact in promoting individual and population patterns of behaviour. To achieve the promise of these scientific advancements, beginner and seasoned intervention developers may wish to reinvest in acquiring and practising a new set of competencies aimed at conceptualizing, building, implementing, and evaluating behaviour change interventions based on the most recent scientific evidence. An equally important task will consist of performing evaluations of interventions developed through these new models and broadly sharing under which conditions and in which populations they achieve greater and lesser outcomes. In this way, Canadians across the country may reap the benefits of health promotion efforts.

CRITICAL THINKING QUESTIONS

1. What are some specific examples of the five common errors about behaviour change that you have encountered in your professional experience?
2. What are some of the key targets for health promotion interventions that can be derived from behavioural theories?
3. How much time and resources must be invested into developing a theory-informed intervention?
4. What are the benefits of using theory and research to build health promotion interventions aimed at changing health-related behaviours?

RESOURCES

Further Readings

Glanz, K. M. (n.d.). Social and behavioral theories. *e-Source Book*. Bethesda, MD: Office of Behavioral and Social Sciences Research.
www.esourceresearch.org/portals/0/uploads/documents/public/glanz_fullchapter.pdf
This link provides access to a chapter wherein different theories of behaviour change are described and illustrated in a very succinct manner.

Glanz, K. M., Rimer, B. K., & Viswanath, K. (Eds.). (2015). *Health behavior and health education: Theory, research and practice* (5th ed.). San Francisco, CA: Jossey-Bass.
This book, now in its fifth edition, presents a detailed overview of theories and approaches for changing health behaviours. The reader can access further information regarding the theories described in this chapter but also examples of their potential application in health promotion.

Michie, S., Atkins, L., & West, R. (2014). *The behaviour change wheel: A guide to designing interventions*. London, England: Silverback Publishing.
www.behaviourchangewheel.com/
This website provides online access to a book and other online training resources to master the behaviour change wheel.

Michie, S., West, R., Campbell, R., Brown, J., & Gainforth, H. (2015). *ABC of behaviour change theories: An essential resource for researchers, policy makers and practitioners*. London, England: Silverback Publishing.
www.behaviourchangetheories.com/online-book#11
This website provides online access to a book describing and comparing 83 theories of behaviour change.

Nutbeam, D., Wise, M., & Harris, E. (2010). *Theory in a nutshell: A practical guide to health promotion theories.* Sydney: McGraw-Hill.

This book, now in its third edition, allows the reader to appreciate the role of theory for developing health promotion interventions. Different types of theories aimed at different phenomena relevant to health promotion are outlined and illustrated.

Relevant Websites

Behaviour Change Technique Taxonomy

www.bct-taxonomy.com/

This website provides information about the newly developed behaviour change taxonomy. There is also a link to an app (both Android and Apple) that outlines, describes, and illustrates each of the 93 behaviour change techniques.

Davidson Films

www.davidsonfilms.com/products/bandura-s-social-cognitive-theory-an-introduction with-albert-bandura-ph-d

This link provides access to a brief video clip of Albert Bandura discussing his work on social cognitive theory. There is also access to a longer film (for purchase) with the famous author, in which he provides further details and insights.

Pro-Change

www.prochange.com/

This website describes a set of services provided by a company founded by the developers of the transtheoretical model of behaviour change. The website provides numerous graphs and examples of interventions.

University College London Centre for Behaviour Change

www.ucl.ac.uk/behaviour-change

This website showcases the newly founded UCL Centre for Behaviour Change. The centre provides numerous training resources to learn about behaviour change, hosts a variety of seminars and meetings, and links to different resources relevant to behaviour change.

REFERENCES

Abraham, C., & Michie, S. (2008). A taxonomy of behavior change techniques used in interventions. *Health Psychology, 273,* 379–387.

Ajzen, I. (1991). The theory of planned behavior. *Organizational Behavior and Human Decision Processes, 502,* 179–211.

Bandura, A. (1977). *Social learning theory* (1st ed.). Englewood Cliffs, NJ: Prentice-Hall.

Bandura, A. (1986). *Social foundations of thought and action: A social cognitive theory.* Englewood Cliffs, NJ: Prentice-Hall.

Bandura, A. (1998). Health promotion from the perspective of social cognitive theory. *Psychology & Health, 134*, 623–649.

Conroy, D. E., Yang, C.-H., & Maher, J. P. (2014). Behavior change techniques in top-ranked mobile apps for physical activity. *American Journal of Preventive Medicine, 46*(6), 649–652.

Fishbein, M., & Ajzen, I. (1975). *Belief, attitude, intention and behavior: An introduction to theory of research.* Reading, MA & Don Mills, ON: Addison-Wesley.

Fishbein, M., & Ajzen, I. (2010). *Predicting and changing behavior: The reasoned action approach.* New York: Taylor and Francis Group.

Fishbein, M., & Cappella, J. N. (2006). The role of theory in developing effective health communications. *Journal of Communication, 56*, S1–S17.

Fishbein, M., Triandis, H. C., Kanfer, F., Becker, D. M., Middlestadt, S., & Eichler, A. (2001). Factors influencing behaviour and behaviour change. In A. Baum, T. Revenson, & J. Singer (Eds.), *Handbook of health psychology* (pp. 3–17). Mahwah, NJ: Lawrence Erlbaum Associates.

Fishbein, M., & Yzer, M. C. (2003). Using theory to design effective health behavior interventions. *Communication Theory, 132*, 164–183.

Foley, T., & Fairmichael, F. (2015). *The potential of learning healthcare systems.* Report to the Health Foundation, UK: The Learning Healthcare Project.

Glanz, K., & Bishop, D. B. (2010). The role of behavioral science theory in development and implementation of public health interventions. *Annual Review of Public Health, 31*, 399–418.

Hardeman, W., Johnston, M., Johnston, D. W., Bonetti, D., Wareham, N. J., & Kinmonth, A. (2002). Application of the theory of planned behaviour in behaviour change interventions: A systematic review. *Psychology & Health, 172*, 123–158.

Jones, C. J., Smith, H., & Llewellyn, C. (2014). Evaluating the effectiveness of health belief model interventions in improving adherence: A systematic review. *Health Psychology Review, 83*, 253–269.

Katikireddi, S. V., Higgins, M., Smith, K.E., & Williams, G. (2013). Health inequalities: The need to move beyond bad behaviours. *Journal of Epidemiology & Community Health, 67*(9), 715–716.

Kelly, M. P., & Barker, M. (2016). Why is changing health-related behaviour so difficult? *Public Health, 136*, 109–116.

Marshall, S. J., & Biddle, S. J. (2001). The transtheoretical model of behavior change: A meta-analysis of applications to physical activity and exercise. *Annals of Behavioral Medicine, 234*, 229–246.

Michie, S. (2008). Designing and implementing behaviour change interventions to improve population health. *Journal of Health Services Research & Policy, 13 Suppl*, 364–369.

Michie, S., Atkins, L., & West, R. (2014). *The behaviour change wheel: A guide to designing interventions.* London, England: Silverback Publishing.

Michie, S., Richardson, M., Johnston, M., Abraham, C., Francis, J., Hardeman, W., … Wood, C. E. (2013). The behavior change technique taxonomy (v1) of 93 hierarchically clustered techniques: building an international consensus for the reporting of behavior change interventions. *Annals of Behavioral Medicine, 461*, 81–95.

Michie, S., van Stralen, M. M., & West, R. (2011). The behaviour change wheel: A new method for characterising and designing behaviour change interventions. *Implementation Science, 6*, 42.

Michie, S., & West, R. (2013). Behaviour change theory and evidence: A presentation to Government. *Health Psychology Review, 71*, 1–22.

Michie, S., & West, R. (2016). *A guide to development and evaluation of digital behaviour change interventions in healthcare*. London, England: Silverback Publishing.

Michie, S., West, R., Campbell, R., Brown, J., & Gainforth, H. (2014). *ABC of behaviour change theories: An essential resource for researchers, policy makers and practitioners*. London, England: Silverback Publishing.

Morrissey, E. C., Corbett, T. K., Walsh, J. C., & Molloy, G. J. (2015). Behavior change techniques in apps for medication adherence: A content analysis. *American Journal of Preventive Medicine, 50*(5), e143–e146.

Prestwich, A., Sniehotta, F. F., Whittington, C., Dombrowski, S. U., Rogers, L., & Michie, S. (2014). Does theory influence the effectiveness of health behavior interventions? Meta-analysis. *Health Psychology, 335*, 465–474.

Prochaska, J. O., & DiClemente, C. C. (1983). Stages and processes of self-change of smoking: Toward an integrative model of change. *Journal of Consulting and Clinical Psychology, 513*, 390–395.

Prochaska, J. O., DiClemente, C. C., & Norcross, J. C. (1992). In search of how people change: Applications to addictive behaviours. *American Psychologist, 47*, 1102.

Rosenstock, I. M. (1966). Why people use health services. *Milbank Memorial Fund Quarterly, 44*(3), 94–127.

Rosenstock, I. M. (1974). Historical origins of the health belief model. *Health Education Monographs, 2*(4), 328–335.

Rosenstock, I. M., Strecher, V. J., & Becker, M. H. (1988). Social learning theory and the health belief model. *Health Education Quarterly, 152*, 175–183.

Sheeran, P., Maki, A., Montanaro, E., Avishai-Yitshak, A., Bryan, A., Klein, W. M., … Rothman, A. J. (2016). The impact of changing attitudes, norms, and self-efficacy on health-related intentions and behavior: A meta-analysis. *Health Psychology, 35*(11), 1178–1188.

Spence, J. C., & Dinh, T. (2015, May). *Moving ahead: Taking steps to reduce physical inactivity and sedentary behaviour*. Ottawa, ON: The Conference Board of Canada.

Spencer, L., Pagell, F., & Adams, T. (2005). Applying the transtheoretical model to cancer screening behavior. *American Journal of Health Behavior, 291*, 36–56.

Spencer, L., Pagell, F., Hallion, M. E., & Adams, T. B. (2002). Applying the transtheoretical model to tobacco cessation and prevention: A review of literature. *American Journal of Health Promotion, 171*, 7–71.

Spring, B., Ockene, J. K., Gidding, S. S., Mozaffarian, D., Moore, S., Rosal, M. C., … Lloyd-Jones, D. (2013). Better population health through behavior change in adults: A call to action. *Circulation, 12819*, 2169–2176.

Van Den Broucke, S. (2014). Needs, norms and nudges: The place of behaviour change in health promotion. *Health Promotion International, 29*(4), 597–599.

Webb, T. L., Joseph, J., Yardley, L., & Michie, S. (2010). Using the Internet to promote health behavior change: A systematic review and meta-analysis of the impact of theoretical basis, use of behavior change techniques, and mode of delivery on efficacy. *Journal of Medical Internet Research, 121*, e4.

West, R. (2005). Time for a change: Putting the transtheoretical (stages of change) model to rest. *Addiction, 1008*, 1036–1039.

West, R. (2006). *Theory of addiction*. Oxford: Blackwell.

CHAPTER 5

Building and Implementing Ecological Health Promotion Interventions

Lucie Richard and Lise Gauvin

LEARNING OBJECTIVES

1. Understand the ecological approach and its origins
2. Describe examples of health promotion ecological initiatives
3. Identify challenges to the design, implementation, and evaluation of health promotion ecological initiatives

INTRODUCTION

This chapter provides examples of innovative, contemporary health promotion programs that effectively translate social ecological conceptions into tangible health promotion interventions. The ecological approach continues to generate much enthusiasm among theorists, planners, and practitioners in health promotion and public health. As an innovation, this approach offered a vision and models congruent with the new public health and thus an increased potential of translating interventions into gains in terms of population health. However, despite this ongoing high level of interest, proponents continue to lament its poor level of integration into programming efforts. In most fields of professional practice, there is often a lag between the emergence of an innovation and its integration into professional actions. This may be the case in health promotion, where professionals have not been in a position to fully adopt and implement ecological health promotion practices. In an effort to contribute to the integration of the ecological approach into practice, the aim of this chapter is to describe programs deemed as exemplary in their degree of integration of the ecological approach. Accordingly, after having briefly described the ecological approach and the historical context of its emergence in public health, we illustrate some applications by describing three highly ecological health promotion initiatives from Canada and how they have evolved since their initial launch. Finally, we identify some emerging challenges to the design, implementation, and evaluation of such innovative initiatives.

THE ECOLOGICAL APPROACH

Derived from ecology, a subfield of biology, the ecological approach offers a research and action framework that emphasizes the complex interactions between people, groups, and their environments. Contrary to traditional ecology, which highlighted the physical features of environment, the ecological approach used in health promotion is more social-ecological in nature and focuses more centrally on the social, organizational, and cultural components of the environment, although in this book in chapter 22, Trevor Hancock notes its importance in relation to the physical and built environment. Within such a vision, planners and practitioners are urged to design interventions and programs that will integrate people-focused efforts to modify health behaviours with interventions that will enhance the numerous dimensions of the environment: physical, social, and cultural. Such complex intervention packages are touted as having the potential for greater success than traditional individual-focused health education interventions (Richard, Gauvin, & Raine, 2011; Sallis & Owen, 2015; Trickett & Beehler, 2015).

The Rise of the Ecological Perspective

Ecological thinking has a long history in disciplines such as biology and psychology. An emphasis on socio-environmental determinants of health was also at the root of public health at the turn of the nineteenth century. However, the ecological discourse re-emerged only recently in public health with the World Health Organization Regional Office for Europe (WHO, 1984) presenting its new conceptualization of health issues as recently as the mid-1980s. This conceptualization reiterated the importance of environmental determinants of health and ecological approaches in promoting population health. Besides the WHO, several Canadian organizations played a leadership role in the emergence of the ecological approach and of the health promotion discourse (Epp, 1986; Kickbusch, 2003; WHO, Health and Welfare Canada, & Canadian Public Health Association, 1986).

Oddly enough, because of its emphasis on complexity and wide-scale system influences, the ecological approach has often been seen as intimidating and difficult to operationalize (Green, Richard, & Potvin, 1996). One way to address this problem has been to stratify the environment as, for example, psychologists have done: Bronfenbrenner (1979) stratified the environment into micro-, meso-, exo-, and macrosystems, whereas Moos (1979) proposed a four-stratum classification revolving around physical settings, organizational factors, human aggregate factors, and social climate. Similar efforts have been undertaken in health promotion (see McLeroy, Bibeau, Steckler, & Glanz, 1988; Simons-Morton, Simons-Morton, Parcel, & Bunker, 1988; Stokols, 1992).

More contemporary ecological models in health promotion depart from earlier contributions in that they integrate new analytic dimensions or provide increased emphasis on conceptualizations emanating from other disciplines. For example, Stokols, Grzywacz, McMahan, and Phillips (2003) supplemented Stokols's earlier notion of a health-supportive environment by emphasizing the concept of community capacity for health improvement. Similarly, Best et al. (2003) proposed an overarching framework integrating not only a community-partnering axis but also a temporal dimension highlighting the centrality of life-course processes. Other theoretical approaches draw upon concepts from the field of behaviour analysis (Hovell, Wahlgren, & Adams, 2009) or sociology and anthropology (Burke, Joseph, Pasick, & Barker, 2009) in order to shed light on processes through which environmental influences result in behaviour adoption and maintenance. Besides these theoretical contributions, application of the ecological approach for intervention planning was undertaken by Stokols (1996), Green and Kreuter (2005), and Bartholomew Eldredge, Markham, Ruiter, Fernandez, Kok, and Parcel (2015). The availability of these theoretical and planning models has paved the way for applications of the approach to a wide variety of health and disease problems (see Richard et al., 2011).

Despite these efforts, the materialization of an ecological approach in health promotion is still often perceived as "a work in progress" (Trickett & Beehler, 2015, p. 1232). Yet, the health promotion literature, reports from the field, and testimonials of dozens of planners and practitioners indicate that descriptions of innovative programs aimed at a variety of health determinants are available as exemplars. In order to promote greater integration of the ecological approach into professional practices, we describe selected examples of successful Canadian applications of the ecological approach in health promotion programs and outline how they evolved following their initial launch. The selection was strategic, covering a variety of target populations, intervention areas, and geographical regions. We now turn to a description of these three evolving success stories.

THREE EXAMPLES OF PROGRAMS

Promoting Healthy Living and Health-Supportive Environments: Inception of a "Possibility Framework" through the PATH Project

Promoting Action toward Health (PATH) was a five-year, federally funded health promotion research project. It was implemented in a relatively disadvantaged area of a medium-sized city in western Canada. It involved a partnership between a community centre, a regional health authority, and a university. PATH was initially aimed at preventing type 2 diabetes among middle-aged adults (35–64 years) of the target area. However, in acknowledging that many medical and non-medical causes of diabetes (e.g., obesity, poverty) are also at the root of several other chronic diseases, the need to include other age groups and to adopt a population health approach were recognized (Chappell, Funk, Carson, MacKenzie, & Stanwick, 2006). It was also evident at the start of the project that involvement of the broader community would be desirable for the project to facilitate community development and health goals (Carson, Chappell, & Knight, 2007). Gradually, a stronger emphasis on reducing social inequalities in health became apparent:

> PATH's goal is to support healthy living through addressing social determinants; that is, the focus is on barriers and obstacles, and making the healthy choices the easy choices. Recognizing the difficulties if not impossibility of changing root socioeconomic conditions in a time-limited research project, PATH seeks to promote healthy living and health supportive environments via initiatives at multiple levels that identify and respond to resident concerns. (Chappell et al., 2006, p. 4)

In line with the ecological approach that the promoters explicitly adopted as a theoretical underpinning (Chappell et al., 2006), a central criterion guiding the choice of initiatives for the project was the capacity to address one or more determinants of health and to effect change at multiple levels. To help ensure this multi-level focus, a planning tool allowing for the charting of project activities by level of change was used. Labelled the "Possibility Framework" (see table 5.1), this tool "lists specific initiatives in the project by their current level of focus, and includes 'possible' examples of initiatives and activities at other levels of intervention" (Chappell et al., 2006, p. 11). Obviously, the list of initiatives shown in table 5.1 is not exhaustive (non-listed initiatives such as health fairs, community gardens, and history and heritage activities are also mentioned by Chappell et al.), but the information illustrates the strong ecological breadth of the PATH project.

As seen in table 5.1, initiatives implemented had potential for reaching the target population in a variety of settings—at an arts centre or community kitchens, for example. PATH also included a variety of intervention targets and strategies. At the organizational level, interorganizational networks and linkages were established "to enhance collaboration among organizations and across sectors" (Chappell et al., 2006, p. 355). For instance, community kitchens that were developed in partnership with a local community centre also involved professionals from the health authority to provide education to participants. Such a networking of two organizations not only facilitated the implementation of the community kitchens, but it also contributed to creating community capacity in that this new partnership bore the potential of developing additional community and advocacy initiatives. Other PATH strategies were aimed at developing and reinforcing personal competencies. For example, among its objectives, the community arts centre explicitly aimed to enhance personal competencies, including participants' self-esteem, creative development, artistic skills, and knowledge.

A final strength of the PATH project pertains to the strong emphasis directed toward community participation (Carson et al., 2007; Chappell et al., 2006). For example, consistent with a community activation strategy, community residents and local organizations were involved in planning, design, and management of activities. Accordingly, it

Table 5.1: Multi-level "Possibility Framework" for Initiatives

	Individual Level	Group Level	Organizational Level	Community Level	Macro/Policy Level
Community kitchens	Kitchen participants learn low-cost, healthy food-preparation skills	Friendships and social activities are promoted among those in support groups	Health authority becomes involved in providing training and education for kitchen participants	Kitchen group promotes sense of community via holding cooking events, publishing recipes	Potential for food-costing training, which can influence policy development around food issues
Facilitating interorganizational networks and linkages	Enhanced individual willingness to work with individuals from other organizations with different perspectives	New relationships and trust formed among those facing similar challenges in their work roles	Enhanced organizational capacity to work with one another for mutual benefit	Community capacity is enhanced through increased organizational networking	Possibility of coordinated, more powerful, co-operative interorganizational efforts to change policy affecting local residents
Community arts centre	Arts centre participants gain increased self-esteem, creative development, artistic skills, and knowledge	Promoting group bookings and events, encouraging social support and sharing of artistic ideas and experiences	School capacity for delivering art programs is enhanced	A sense of community is promoted through community art shows, outreach programs, and neighbourhood beautification through art	School board policies may become more flexible to alternate space uses and partnering with community groups for mutual benefit
Participation in city's greenways initiative	Participants in related mapping events gain renewed appreciation of local green spaces	Formation of new groups in the area to protect local spaces; meeting people with similar interests	Capacity of existing organizations may be strengthened, i.e., with increased resources and information	Improved neighbourhoods through creation of green spaces enhance community life	Local groups gain increased public support and effectiveness regarding local land-use policies

Source: Adapted from Chappell, N., Funk, L., Carson, A., MacKenzie, P., & Stanwick, R. (2006). Multilevel community health promotion: How can we make it work? *Community Development Journal*, 41(3): 352–366. doi:10.1093/cdj/bsi061

was believed that initiatives ought to come from residents rather than professionals and researchers. For this reason, the project started at the individual level; "this strategy [...] helped avoid a potential paralysis of action due to multiple simultaneous commitments" (Chappell et al., 2006, p. 4). As discussed below, there is often a tension between the comprehensive focus of an ecological approach and the ideal of participation inherent in health promotion (Chappell et al., 2006; Stokols, 1996). The PATH project is a good demonstration of how such a large-scale approach can thrive with an agenda involving community participation and capacity-building.

The PATH project is now concluded. Several of the initiatives such as the community gardens, community kitchens, and a community newsletter begun within the project are still ongoing today, as they were taken over by members of the community (Chappell, personal communication, September 5, 2016). An interesting avenue for research would be to investigate the ecological dimensions of such initiatives as well as the conditions and dynamics that facilitated their maintenance after research funding ended.

Getting Kids on the Move and Eating Well: Impact of the Annapolis Valley Health Promoting School Project and Implementation of the Alberta Project Promoting active Living and healthy Eating in Schools

Another interesting example of the application of the ecological approach is found in the Annapolis Valley Health Promoting School Project (AVHPSP, 2010) which is an application of comprehensive school health (Deschênes, Martin, & Hill, 2003; Veugelers & Schwartz, 2010). It is one of the few initiatives that have been evaluated in terms of behaviour and health outcomes (Veugelers & Fitzgerald, 2005). More importantly, it served as the inspiration for another large-scale, successful project called the Alberta Project Promoting active Living and healthy Eating in Schools (APPLE Schools). Both projects appear on the Public Health Agency of Canada's Best Practices Portal (cbpp-pcpe. phac-aspc.gc.ca/).

Similar to the PATH project, the AVHPSP revolved around the theme of making the healthy choice the easy choice, but focused more specifically on promoting healthy eating and daily physical activity to fight overweight and obesity among elementary school children in Nova Scotia. Program promoters believed that "multiple strategies occurring simultaneously to promote healthy eating and physical activity enhances the acceptance and ability to deliver the programmes at the school, school board, and community level. These strategies include policy, education, awareness, leadership development, programme development, programme implementation, and advocacy (AVHPSP, 2010). Activities were organized in six sets: (1) mobilizing people around the idea of changing environments and policies to effect change by identifying a program champion, creating links with the community, and developing leadership among school staff; (2) conducting school surveys and sharing school-specific information with schools; (3) developing a business plan for healthy food and physical activity in each participating school; (4) implementing a healthy eating strategy including changes to food offerings and in presentation of new types of food; (5) implementing physical activity on a daily basis through non-competitive running, playground games, "kids teaching kids" coaching clinics, equipment loans, etc.; and (6) creating links between schools and the community by building partnerships with local stakeholders. An effectiveness evaluation of the AVHPSP showed that children attending intervention schools had significantly lower rates of obesity and overweight, had healthier diets, and reported more physical activities (Veugelers & Fitzgerald, 2005).

The APPLE schools initiative was inspired by the AVHPSP (www.appleschools. ca/). However, in addition to creating healthy environments, each of the APPLE schools included a full-time school health facilitator whose main role was to adapt the intervention to the unique features of the context of each school. Towards this end, facilitators created liaisons with school and community partners, promoted ongoing training of school personnel, and engaged in curriculum and policy development within schools. A two-year follow-up of APPLE schools showed that children ate more fruits and vegetables, cumulated fewer calories, were more physically active, and were less likely to be obese in comparison to children at other Alberta schools (Fung et al., 2012). In addition to these compelling findings, the team of researchers also explored how the program served to decrease social inequalities in physical activity, what could be done to train school facilitators, the role of the principal in supporting intervention success, and the determinants of sustainability.

The AVHPSP and APPLE schools are examples where successful integration of ecological principles led to measurable changes in indicators of population health. In addition to demonstrating effectiveness, it is noteworthy to mention that the projects have been maintained and blended in with other federal (i.e., AVHPSP into Canada Get Active) and provincial (i.e., Strive for 5 in Nova Scotia, Comprehensive School Health in Alberta) initiatives aimed at improving eating and activity practices among children and youth.

The Fight against Tobacco: Shaping the Web of Determinants in Montréal

An earlier edition of this chapter presented, as an example of ecological programming, the anti-smoking program of one of Québec's regional public health departments (Richard & Gauvin, 2012), which was based on Québec's first major action plan in this sector, which was launched in 1994 (MSSS, 1994). Analysis of the overall program showed it included several previously existing intervention approaches deployed in a variety of settings—a characteristic illustration of the ecological approach.

Much has transpired since these initial efforts. Several provincial action plans have been enacted, and the Tobacco Act was adopted in 1998 (reinforced in 2010 and 2015). This law provided Québec with strong leverage in matters related to tobacco control, protection of non-smokers, and the creation of an anti-smoking standard. The law and its accompanying action plans provide for a broad cross-section of actions to guide prevention, protection, and smoking-cessation activities at the regional and local levels. Globally, such benchmarks have been very influential in orienting the development of truly ecological programs and initiatives across all Québec regions. We outline here the example of Montréal's 2012 anti-smoking plan, entitled Montréal sans tabac (Smoke-free Montreal) (www.group eentreprisesensante.com/wp-content/uploads/2016/04/plan-tabac-mtl-2012-15.pdf).

The plan targets seven objectives, which include lowering smoking prevalence in different population subgroups (i.e., children, adolescents, adults, pregnant women), reducing children's and adolescents' exposure to second-hand smoke, and improving rates of smoking cessation among smokers. Underlying the actions proposed in the plan is a concern about reducing smoking-related social inequalities in health. The plan's actions are structured around six areas of intervention. Three of these are cross-cutting:

- Mobilization and consultation of key actors in the health and social services, education, and early childhood networks. This component also involves supporting the planning and implementation of activities in local organizations (health and social services centres, community organizations).
- Knowledge acquisition and dissemination. This involves observation, research and evaluation, monitoring, knowledge updating, and supporting the use of evidence by various actors involved in planning and implementing activities.
- Influencing public policies. Activities in this area are aimed at influencing decision-making on policies at various levels: policy emergence, formulation, and implementation at all levels (federal, provincial, regional, local).

Three other areas relate to specific anti-smoking interventions:

- Preventing smoking among adolescents. Interventions proposed here are geared toward complementing and supporting fiscal, legislative, and media strategies implemented province-wide. They involve reaching out to young people in their own settings: family, school, and social milieux. They include a variety of strategies: raising awareness and mobilizing partners in the education and health sectors; supporting adolescents' social action and involvement in projects in their environments (e.g., "la Gang Allumée"); and fostering other activities to encourage the creation of smoke-free school environments. The latter involves not only schools, but also other locations in the community (e.g., points of sale, leisure services).
- Protection against environmental tobacco smoke (ETS) or second-hand smoke. Here the focus is on guarding against ETS in private settings. Actions include raising awareness among workers at the local level (education, health, and childcare services) and supporting measures developed at the provincial level (e.g., Smoke-Free Family campaign).
- Smoking-cessation interventions. The plan incorporates a variety of strategies and settings to develop and strengthen actions including short-term counselling

in clinical settings (training professionals, setting up communities of practice, etc.), increasing access to smoking-cessation services and tools (Quit Smoking Centres, telephone lines, access to medications, etc.), and promoting smoking cessation through campaigns targeting both the general population and specific groups (e.g., workers). The plan includes a section devoted specifically to smoking cessation among adolescents.

The *Montréal sans tabac* plan is an excellent example of an ecological intervention (Richard, Potvin, Kishchuk, Prlic, & Green, 1996). First, it integrates environmental and individual targets across a variety of settings. Second, these targets translate into a diversity of strategies, some of which are aimed directly towards the target population itself and others at the environment. It is noteworthy to mention that smoking was among the first contemporary public health issues to be redefined from a broader social perspective that extended well beyond personal behaviour, thus calling for a comprehensive ecological response from the public health community (Brownson, Eriksen, Davis, & Warner, 1997). The anti-smoking plan described above is a good example of such a response.

WHERE TO FROM HERE?

We view the ecological approach as a contemporary and practicable framework within which to orient health promotion interventions. However, we also note several challenges that threaten the reach it might have for future practice and research.

The first challenge is conceptual and pertains to the role of community participation in the development and implementation of programs. Although we highlighted the fact that ecological health promotion programming is founded on a broad conception of health determinants, we also note that less emphasis has been devoted to the role of community participation even though it is seen as pivotal in health promotion and population health (Butterfoss & Kegler, 2009; Rootman, Goodstadt, Potvin, & Springett, 2001) and even more so in recent years (George, Mehra, Scott, & Sriram, 2015). A first explanation pertains to the inherent challenge of conciliating objectives related to multi-level community outcomes and maximizing community participation, often fuelled by more proximal preoccupations. For example, Chappell et al. (2006) suggest that "residents may be seen to want their kitchens to remain at the individual and group level of intervention, whereas PATH may seek expansion to more macro levels. This demonstrates potential conflicting priorities for PATH facilitators between being responsive to community desires on the one hand while on the other hand seeking changes at broader levels" (p. 13). Another explanation relates to ecological models, which have traditionally emphasized the notions of environmental determinants and their interaction with behaviour and health at the expense of other key dimensions of the ecological approach. In a recent analysis of contributions emanating from community psychologists (e.g., Kelly, 2006; Trickett, 2009), Richard et al. (2011) pointed out that central to the ecological approach are features pertaining to the building of community capacity and resources. Although these concepts have always ranked highly among core orientations and central concepts of health promotion, particularly in planning models (Bartholomew Eldredge et al., 2015; Green & Kreuter, 2005), they still remain to be fully integrated in ecological models, as they are disseminated in public health in general and health promotion in particular. In their review of contemporary ecological models in health promotion, Richard et al. (2011) indeed noted that among such models, a limited number have included a dimension related to community capacity or participation, with models recently proposed by Stokols et al. (2003) and Best et al. (2003) being two exceptions. There is still a need to further develop a community capacity dimension, thus rendering work conducted on the ecological approach more integrated with the health promotion vision.

A second challenge pertains to the apparent unwillingness of practitioners to advocate for legislative and policy changes, partly because they find themselves in the awkward position of trying to influence the very people who employ them. Similarly, they are in the difficult position of interfering with the daily business of very powerful corporations (e.g., the tobacco or fast-food industries). As a result, existing health promotion programs understandably display timid efforts towards influencing the political sphere.

Nevertheless, as described above, actions at the political level have been successfully undertaken. Public policy advocacy is one of the six intervention areas of the Montréal anti-tobacco action plan, with public health professionals being involved at different steps of the development and implementation of legislative changes. Indeed, a study of the process having led to the adoption of the tobacco law showed that one way of facilitating political action involved the public health sector supporting coalitions and other collaborative networks that then acted as leaders in political action and advocacy (Breton, Richard, Gagnon, Jacques, & Bergeron, 2008). Similarly, in the "Possibility Framework" of the PATH project, activities were aimed at cooperative interorganizational efforts to change policy affecting local residents.

Finally, although not directly related to the AVHPSP, there have been recent efforts aimed at the development of practical tools that might facilitate advocacy and political action on physical activity. For example, the Toronto Charter for Physical Activity (Bull et al., 2010) outlines four actions based on nine guiding principles to promote health-enhancing physical activity at the population level. Significant results in health promotion programming are likely to be achieved only if practitioners, in addition to working at the individual level, are able to influence political targets (Breton, Richard, Gagnon, Jacques, & Bergeron, 2013) and scale-up intervention efforts (Milat, Bauman, & Redman, 2015).

A third challenge pertains to the evaluation of the complex and multi-level health promotion programs that integrate the ecological approach. First, there is a need for appropriate designs and methods to deal with the complexity of multi-target, multi-settings interventions (Trickett & Beehler, 2015). With regards to the evaluation of efficacy and effectiveness, we note that AVHPSP promoters deployed unusual efforts to produce evidence of the impact of the program in preventing obesity and in changing eating and activity patterns (Fung et al., 2012; Veugelers & Fitzgerald, 2005). As noted by several authors, though, randomized clinical trials, which still represent the gold standard for evidence, are difficult to apply in evaluating complex community programs (Craig et al., 2008; Moore et al., 2015; Victora, Habicht, & Bryce, 2004) and numerous interesting alternatives exist: clustered randomized trials, quasi-experimentation, and case studies (see also Shadish & Cook, 2009). Yet, efficacy/effectiveness is not the only focus of evaluation, as health promotion efforts must also address reach, adoption, implementation, and maintenance (e.g., Glasgow, Klesges, Dzewaltowski, Bull, & Estabrooks, 2004). Given continued efforts in promoting knowledge transfer and exchange, as well as evidence-based practice, and the fact that practitioners are getting more involved in stimulating community participation and political action, we anticipate that conducting evaluations will become increasingly complex.

A final challenge pertains to resources. Implementing large-scale programs and multi-pronged interventions requires a high level of material, financial, and time resources. Studies have indeed confirmed that the presence of plentiful resources was a critical factor in helping regional public health organizations to successfully implement ecological health promotion programs (Richard et al., 2008). It is crucial that health promotion planners and practitioners access the resources required to achieve their ambitions.

CONCLUSION

As shown above, integrating ecological principles in practice is possible. We anticipate that further advances will occur at an accelerated pace if researchers and practitioners devote continued efforts to comprehensive evaluation of ecological programs and to knowledge transfer and exchange activities. Research on the identification of factors associated with greater levels of integration of the ecological approach in real-world programming is also a promising avenue for future efforts.

CRITICAL THINKING QUESTIONS

1. How can the ideal of increased community participation in the health promotion process be reconciled with ecological intervention in health promotion?
2. How can public health interventionists further integrate advocacy and legislative action into their repertoire of action?
3. What are the most appropriate research designs for evaluating health promotion interventions that are ecological?
4. Why is the ecological approach often qualified as intimidating and difficult to operationalize? What would facilitate its integration into programs?
5. What are other examples of programs and interventions that have successfully integrated the ecological approach?

RESOURCES

Further Readings

Bauman, A. (2005). The physical environment and physical activity: Moving from ecological associations to intervention evidence. *Journal of Epidemiology and Community Health, 59*, 535–536.
This editorial provides a provocative view on how evidence can be translated into interventions.

Kelly, J. G. (2006). *Becoming ecological: An expedition into community psychology*. New York: Oxford University Press.
A collection of landmark papers by J. G. Kelly, a founder of community psychology. Kelly formulated the "ecological metaphor," which transposes principles from biological ecology to the investigation of relationships between individuals and their environment. The ecological perspective in community psychology has inspired research and action in many disciplines.

McLaren, L., & Hawe, P. (2005). Ecological perspectives in health research. *Journal of Epidemiology and Community Health, 59*, 6–14.
A glossary of terms pertaining to an ecological approach in health research.

Richard, L., Cargo, M., & Lévesque, L. (2015). *An ecological analysis procedure to assess health promotion programs: An instruction manual*. E-Valorix: evalorix.com/wp-content/uploads/2015/11/481-Ecological_Approach_Codebook.pdf.
A methodological guide that outlines a model of the ecological approach. It also presents a grid and coding instructions for assessing the ecological dimension of programs.

Smedley, B. D., & Syme, S. L. (Eds.). (2000). *Promoting health: Intervention strategies from social and behavioral research*. Washington: National Academy Press.
A landmark report from the Institute of Medicine Committee on Capitalizing on Social Science and Behavioral Research to Improve the Public's Health, which emphasizes the role of social and behavioural factors in influencing health and disease throughout the lifespan. Many chapters are devoted to public health interventions.

Relevant Websites

Health Nexus
en.healthnexus.ca
Health Nexus (formerly Ontario Prevention Clearinghouse) offers consultations, referrals, opportunities for networking, educational events like workshops and conferences, and resources (both electronic and print) on health promotion priorities.

Health Promotion Clearinghouse (Nova Scotia)

www.hpclearinghouse.ca

An online resource to find out more about what's happening in health promotion in Nova Scotia.

Institut national de santé publique du Québec

www.inspq.qc.ca/english

The mandate of the institute is to support the minister and regional agencies in fulfilling their public health mission. The institute's mission includes development, updating, dissemination, and implementation of knowledge. The website provides information and resources related to a variety of health issues and interventions.

Public Health Agency of Canada

www.phac-aspc.gc.ca

With the mandate of promoting and protecting the health of Canadians, the agency is involved in various activities such as program delivery, research and knowledge development, and public and professional education. Its website includes information and resources related to key health issues and interventions in Canada.

RE-AIM

www.re-aim.org

RE-AIM provides a framework to systematically evaluate health behaviour interventions. RE-AIM stands for Reach, Efficacy/Effectiveness, Adoption, Implementation, and Maintenance. The website provides links to several resources useful for researchers and interventionists.

REFERENCES

AVHPSP. (2010). *Annapolis Valley health promoting school project: Making the healthy choice the easy choice*. See: www.avdha.nshealth.ca/sites/default/files/avh_promoting_school_project_1.pdf

Bartholomew Eldredge, K. L., Markham, C. M., Ruiter, R. A. C., Fernandez, M. E., Kok, G., & Parcel, G. S. (2015). *Planning health promotion programs: An intervention mapping approach* (4th ed.). San Francisco: Jossey-Bass.

Best, A., Stokols, D., Green, L. W., Leischow, S., Holmes, B., & Buchholz, K. (2003). An integrative framework for community partnering to translate theory into effective health promotion strategy. *American Journal of Health Promotion, 18*, 168–176.

Breton, E., Richard, L., Gagnon, F., Jacques, M., & Bergeron, P. (2008). Health promotion research and practice require sound policy analysis models: The case of Quebec's Tobacco Act. *Social Science and Medicine, 67*, 1679–1689.

Breton, E., Richard, L, Gagnon, F., Jacques, M., & Bergeron, P. (2013). Coalition advocacy action and research for policy development. In C. Clavier & E. De Leeuw (Eds.), *Health Promotion and the Policy Process* (pp. 43-62). Oxford, UK: Oxford University Press.

Bronfenbrenner, U. (1979). *The ecology of human development: Experiments by nature and design.* Cambridge: Harvard University Press.

Brownson, R. C., Eriksen, M. P., Davis, R. M., & Warner, K. A. (1997). Environmental tobacco smoke: Health effects and policies to reduce exposure. *Annual Review of Public Health, 18,* 163–185.

Bull, F. C., Gauvin, L., Bauman, A., Shilton, T., Kohl, H. W., & Salmon, A. (2010). The Toronto Charter for Physical Activity: A global call for action. *Journal of Physical Activity and Health, 7,* 421–422.

Burke, N. J., Joseph, G., Pasick, R. J., & Barker, J. C. (2009). Theorizing social context: Rethinking behavioral theory. *Health Education and Behavior, 36,* 55S–70S.

Butterfoss, F. D., & Kegler, M. C. (2009). The community coalition action theory. In R. J. DiClemente, R. A. Crosby, & M. C. Kegler (Eds.), *Emerging theories in health promotion practice and research* (pp. 237–276). San Francisco: Jossey-Bass.

Carson, A., Chappell, N. L., & Knight, C. J. (2007). Promoting health and innovative health promotion practice through a community arts centre. *Health Promotion Practice, 8*(4), 366–374.

Chappell, N., Funk, L., Carson, A., MacKenzie, P., & Stanwick, R. (2006). Multilevel community health promotion: How can we make it work? *Community Development Journal, 41*(3), 352–366.

Craig, P., Dieppe, P., Macintyre, S., Michie, S., Nazareth, I., & Petticrew, M. (2008). Developing and evaluating complex interventions: The new Medical Research Council guidance. *BMJ, 29*(337), a1655.

Deschêsnes, M., Martin, C., & Hill, A. J. (2003). Comprehensive approaches to school health promotion: How to achieve broader implementation? *Health Promotion International, 18,* 387–396.

Epp, J. (1986). *Achieving health for all: A framework for health promotion.* Ottawa: Health and Welfare Canada.

Fung, C., Kuhle, S., Lu, C., Purcell, M., Schwartz, M., Storey, K., & Veugelers, P. J. (2012). From "best practice" to "next practice": The effectiveness of school-based health promotion in improving healthy eating and physical activity and preventing childhood obesity. *International Journal of Behavioral Nutrition and Physical Activity, 9,* 27.

George, A. S., Mehra, V., Scott, K., & Sriram, V. (2015). Community participation in health systems research: A systematic review assessing the state of research, the nature of interventions involved and the features of engagement with communities. *PLoS ONE, 10*(10), e0141091.

Glasgow, R. E., Klesges, L. M., Dzewaltowski, D. A., Bull, S. S., & Estabrooks, P. (2004). The future of health behavior change research: What is needed to improve translation of research into health promotion practice? *Annals of Behavioral Medicine, 27,* 3–12.

Green, L. W., & Kreuter, M. W. (2005). *Health program planning: An educational and ecological approach.* New York: McGraw-Hill.

Green, L. W., Richard, L., & Potvin, L. (1996). Ecological foundation of health promotion. *American Journal of Health Promotion, 10*(4), 270–281.

Hovell, M., Wahlgren, D., & Adams, M. (2009). The logical and empirical basis for the behavioral ecological model. In R. J. DiClemente, R. A. Crosby, & M. C. Kegler (Eds.), *Emerging theories in health promotion practice and research* (pp. 415–449). San Francisco: Jossey-Bass.

Kelly, J. G. (2006). *Becoming ecological: An expedition into community psychology*. New York: Oxford University Press.

Kickbusch, I. (2003). The contribution of the World Health Organization to a new public health and health promotion. *American Journal of Public Health, 93*(3), 383–387.

McLeroy, K. R., Bibeau, D., Steckler, A., & Glanz, K. (1988). An ecological perspective on health promotion programs. *Health Education Quarterly, 15*(4), 351–377.

Milat, J., Bauman, A., & Redman, S. (2015). Narrative review of models and success factors for scaling up public health interventions. *Implementation Science, 10*, 113.

Ministère de la santé et des services sociaux (MSSS). (1994). *Plan d'action de lutte au tabagisme* [Anti-tobacco action plan]. Québec: Gouvernement du Québec.

Moore, G. F., Audrey, S., Barker, M., Bond, L., Bonell, C., Hardeman, W., ... Baird, J. (2015). Process evaluation of complex interventions: Medical Research Council guidance. *British Medical Journal, 350*, h1258.

Moos, R. H. (1979). Social-ecological perspectives on health. In G. Stone, F. Cohen, & N. Alder (Eds.), *Health psychology—a handbook: Theories, applications, and challenges of a psychological approach to the health care system* (pp. 523–547). San Francisco: Jossey-Bass.

Richard, L., & Gauvin, L. (2012). Building and implementing ecological health promotion interventions. In I. Rootman, A. Pederson, S. Dupéré, & M. O'Neill (Eds.), *Health promotion in Canada: Critical perspectives on practice* (pp. 67–80). Toronto: Canadian Scholars' Press.

Richard, L., Gauvin, L., Gosselin, C., Ducharme, F., Sapinski, J. P., & Trudel, M. (2008). Integrating the ecological approach in health promotion for older adults: A survey of programmes aimed at elder abuse prevention, falls prevention, and appropriate medication use. *International Journal of Public Health, 53*, 46–56.

Richard, L., Gauvin, L., & Raine, K. (2011). Ecological models revisited: Their uses and evolution in health promotion over two decades. *Annual Review of Public Health, 32*, 307–326.

Richard, L., Potvin, L., Kishchuk, N., Prlic, H., & Green, L. W. (1996). Assessment of the integration of the ecological approach in health promotion programs. *American Journal of Health Promotion, 10*(4), 318–328.

Rootman, I., Goodstadt, M., Potvin, L., & Springett, J. (2001). A framework for health promotion evaluation. In I. Rootman, M. Goodstadt, B. Hyndman, D. V. McQueen, L. Potvin, J. Springett, & E. Ziglio (Eds.), *Evaluation in health promotion: Principles and perspectives* (pp. 7–38). Copenhagen: World Health Organization.

Sallis, J. F., & Owen, N. (2015). Ecological models of health behaviors. In K. Glanz, B. K. Rimer, & K. Viswanath (Eds.), *Health behavior and health education: Theory, research, and practice* (5th ed.) (pp. 43–64). San Francisco: Jossey-Bass.

Shadish, W. R., & Cook, T. D. (2009). The renaissance of field experimentation in evaluating interventions. *Annual Review of Psychology, 60*, 607–629.

Simons-Morton, D.-G., Simons-Morton, B. G., Parcel, G. S., & Bunker, J. F. (1988). Influencing personal and environmental conditions for community health: A multilevel intervention model. *Family and Community Health, 11*(2), 25–35.

Stokols, D. (1992). Establishing and maintaining healthy environments: Toward a social ecology of health promotion. *American Psychologist, 47*(1), 6–22.

Stokols, D. (1996). Translating social ecological theory into guidelines for community health promotion. *American Journal of Health Promotion, 10*, 282–298.

Stokols, D., Grzywacz, J. G., McMahan, S., & Phillips, K. (2003). Increasing the health promotive capacity of human environments. *American Journal of Health Promotion, 18*(1), 4–13.

Trickett, E. J. (2009). Community psychology: Individuals and interventions in community context. *Annual Review of Psychology, 60*, 395–419.

Trickett, E. J., & Beehler, S. (2015). The ecology of multilevel interventions to reduce social inequalities in health. *American Behavioral Scientist, 57*(8), 1227–1248.

Veugelers, P. J., & Fitzgerald, A. L. (2005). Effectiveness of school programs in preventing childhood obesity: A multilevel comparison. *American Journal of Public Health, 95*(3), 432–435.

Veugelers, P. J., & Schwartz, M. E. (2010). Comprehensive school health in Canada. *Canadian Journal of Public Health 2010, 101*(Suppl. 2), S5–S8.

Victora, C. G., Habicht, J. P., & Bryce, J. (2004). Evidence-based public health: Moving beyond randomized trials. *American Journal of Public Health, 94*, 400–405.

World Health Organization (WHO). (1984). *Health promotion: A discussion document on the concept and principles*. Copenhagen: World Health Organization, Regional Office for Europe.

World Health Organization (WHO), Health and Welfare Canada, & Canadian Public Health Association. (1986). Ottawa Charter for Health Promotion. *Canadian Journal of Public Health, 77*, 425–430.

PART II

HEALTH PROMOTION PRACTICE IN CANADA

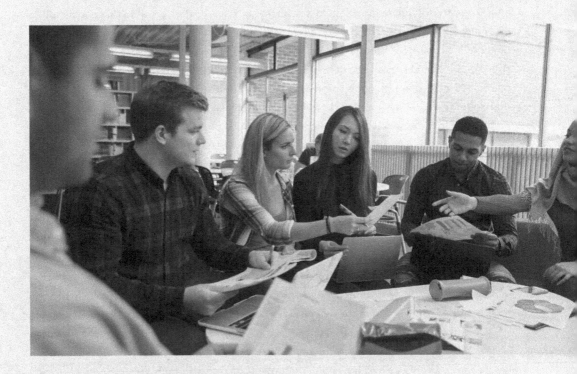

This part of the book considers the "practice" of health promotion in Canada. As indicated in Part I, health promotion has been an evolving field in Canada and globally. And as will be suggested in other chapters in this book, particularly those in Part III, it is likely to continue to evolve in terms of practice. This part covers the current state of health promotion practice in Canada and provides examples of practices that are supported by substantial research and experience as well as what can be called "promising practices" that are supported by less research and experience but that, nevertheless, appear to be worth trying and studying in other circumstances.

As was the case in the last edition of this book, we have organized this part based on a chapter written by Frohlich, Poland, and Shareck that suggested there were three classical entry points used to develop interventions in health promotion, namely *issues*, *populations*, and *settings*—which proved to be a reasonable and successful way of presenting the material on practice. Among other things, we discovered that the three entry points were interrelated in that successful interventions "encompass all three aspects in its design and implementation to some degree" (Pederson, 2012, p. 151). We also learned that through focusing on the entry points, it was possible to identify "promising practices" in health promotion. In addition, we discovered that using these entry points, it was possible to apply certain theories to provide an "organized framework useable in a variety of health promoters' real-life work situations" (O'Neill, 2012, p. 185). Chapter 6 is an updated and expanded version of the chapter in the last edition by Frohlich, Poland, and Shareck. It has been expanded mainly by emphasizing the importance of theory for practice. For example, it starts by taking the position that "social context matters." It then moves on to a definition of *social context* drawing on critical realism and complexity science. The chapter describes the three classical points of entry for intervention, outlines how each has grappled with the notion of the social context, and discusses their strengths and weaknesses. As was the case in the third edition, it concludes with a suggestion of a fourth entry point for health promotion research and practice, namely *collective lifestyles*, and presents a current example of how the collective lifestyles framework was used as an entry point to explore the social context of physical activity.

The next three chapters focus on specific *issues* relevant to health promotion as entry points to interventions. Chapter 7, written for this edition of the book by Pederson, focuses on the important issue of *violence against women* (VAW). The first section of the chapter defines VAW and applies a gender lens to the issue using the concept and theory of *intersectionality*. The chapter then moves on to present statistics on VAW in Canada, followed by a discussion of who is vulnerable (this includes men in certain social categories as well as disabled persons) and the known health effects of VAW. The next section explains the causes of VAW using an ecological framework and suggests that gender inequality and discrimination are key determinants. The rest of the chapter discusses how health promotion and public health in general have begun to, and can continue to, effectively address the issue of violence against women.

Chapter 8 by Raphael is an updated version of his chapter in the third edition focused on the issue of *inequities*. After defining the issue, he presents seven ways to address inequities, followed by three ways that health promoters can do so, namely through education and knowledge transmission; professional association and agency network action; and political engagement. In concluding, he suggests that the best way for health promoters and their agencies to reduce health inequities is to inform citizens about the political and economic forces that shape the health of society.

Chapter 9, a new chapter by Ardiles, considers the issue of *mental health* from the perspective of *mental health promotion*. She starts by reviewing the development of mental health promotion as an area of focus in Canada and proceeds to identify barriers and facilitators to integrating mental health into health promotion and vice versa. She suggests that one of the key barriers is "lack of a common agenda" between these two fields. She then presents three relatively successful Canadian initiatives that demonstrate that integrating mental health into health promotion research, policy, and practice and vice versa is possible and that policy support and engagement are key enablers to make this work effective and impactful.

The next two chapters focus on two *populations* of concern in health promotion, mainly because they are subject to serious social inequities. The first is the Indigenous community discussed in chapter 10 by Loppie, who drafted a similar chapter in the third edition of this book with Reading. As was the case with the previous chapter, after providing a background regarding Indigenous populations and concepts, this one outlines an Indigenous peoples' approach to health promotion to complement the Western approach that dominates in Canada. Loppie then illustrates an Indigenous approach in action through four promising initiatives grounded in the distinct cultural concepts, contexts, and approaches of their respective communities. These are KSDPP, a diabetes prevention program in Kahnawake (also considered in the third edition); a garden project in the Coast Salish community in BC (new); a day camp program for children and youth in Nunavut (new); and an intensive parenting program in Victoria (new). Among other things, she concludes that "success of these programs can be attributed, at least in part, to the appreciation and application of Indigenous concepts, contexts, and processes."

The second "population-based" chapter (chapter 11) focuses on immigrants. Authored by Khan and Kobayashi, this new chapter attempts to answer the following questions: What are the determinants of immigrant health? What are the barriers to the uptake of health promotion practices among immigrants? and How can we optimize the uptake of health promotion practices among immigrants? The authors use a social determinants of health approach to respond to these questions. In relation to the first question, among other things, they suggest that the status of "foreign-born" and markers of identity may preclude immigrants from accessing and effectively using health promotion resources and may intersect to produce conditions of "multiple jeopardy." With regard to the barriers to uptake, they suggest that the following factors are key: migration; socio-economic status; language proficiency; visible minority status; gender; cultural perceptions around health and disease prevention; and age. As for optimizing uptake of health promotion practices, they present two case studies, namely the South Asian Exercise Trial and Mental Health Promotion within Immigrant Communities— both of which suggest promising practices. They conclude with the suggestion that policy makers at multiple levels need to develop health promotion strategies targeted and tailored to meet the unique needs of an increasingly diverse immigrant population, and they make suggestions for specific interventions.

Part II continues with five new chapters focusing on various *settings* for health promotion. The first of these is chapter 12 on healthy cities and communities, authored by Hancock, one of the originators of the "healthy city" concept. He sets the stage by noting that currently, more than half of the world's population lives in urban areas and the concentration is likely to grow significantly in the future. Thus, in his view, "health promotion is now largely an urban-based and urban-focused concern." Given this, he suggests that an attempt to create healthier cities and communities is extremely important for health promotion. He then reviews the development of the Healthy Cities and Communities movement. In the rest of the chapter, he stresses the need to find common ground and shared purpose between health promotion and municipalities and stresses the need for improving urban governance to improve health, suggesting that "participatory democracy" would be helpful. In concluding he suggests that "together, we can and must create a vision of a more just, sustainable, and healthy future and then co-create the cities, towns, and villages that are compatible with that vision."

Chapter 13, authored by McCall and Laitsch, reviews the development of school health initiatives in Canada and internationally and suggests that the "absence of a consistent, comprehensive, and systems-based understanding and concomitant planned approach ... is the greatest challenge for school health promotion in Canada and most other parts of the world." The authors acknowledge Canada's international leadership in school health and cite two recent Canadian initiatives to develop a "systems-based" approach focused on disadvantaged and Indigenous communities as well as the development of Canadian and international approaches to monitoring systems. However, the authors conclude that despite the progress, "our work in school-based and school-linked health promotion and social development is still occurring in silos separated by topic expertise, structures, and boundaries" and they express the hope that the next generation of leaders in school health will accept the challenge to "not only make the paradigm shift to systems-based approaches, but to implement and maintain that shift in policy and practice."

Chapter 14, authored by Ardiles and several colleagues from Simon Fraser University and the University of British Columbia, focuses on the university setting. The authors start by noting that Canada has been a major contributor to developing the concept of a "Healthy University" through releasing two charters for a healthy university, the first at a conference in Edmonton in 2005, and the second ten years later at a conference in Kelowna (called the *Okanagan Charter*). In addition, they provide several examples of healthy university initiatives in Canada that use a *whole-systems approach* and discuss the enablers and barriers that facilitate or impede the implementation of such an approach, as well as the importance of measurement and monitoring. They conclude by challenging Canadian higher education institutions to focus on building an evidence base for healthy university initiatives and on key principles of implementation as well as "development of students and other campus members with the capacity to act as change agents for health promotion action beyond campuses."

Chapter 15, by Bertoni and Dubé, considers the clinical care setting for health promotion. In contrast to other discussions of health promotion in the clinical care setting, the authors stress the importance of taking the determinants of health into account in clinical practice and suggest some means of doing so at the level of the *patient*, the *practice*, and the *community*. They also discuss health literacy in the context of clinical practice and suggest several strategies that health care practitioners can use to address health literacy issues among patients. In addition, they consider the implications of family theory and family-centred care in relation to addressing determinants of health in clinical practice, and discuss the role of nurses and nurse practitioners as well as advanced nursing practice. The chapter concludes with a discussion of trends and issues in translating health promotion into clinical practice and strategies for the future.

Chapter 16, by Struik, Haines-Saah, and Bottorff, considers digital media and the Internet, which are increasingly being used as a setting for health promotion. The authors note that although digital media has become ubiquitous in health promotion over the past few years and is promising, it has created unique challenges for the field and has some limitations. The chapter discusses both the positive and negative attributes of digital media in relation to health promotion using examples drawn from the authors' own research and elsewhere. One of the main conclusions is that although digital media provide health promotion with new technologies to engage "hard to reach" populations, digital health promotion strategies have mainly focused on the behavioural change of individuals and may be drawing attention away from strategies such as strengthening communities and focusing upstream on the social determinants of health and health inequities.

At the end of this second part of the book, the reader should have a good idea of how the practice of health promotion is currently organized in Canada, as well as of the positive but also problematic sides of such a situation. The numerous "promising practices" described should also have provided inspiring ideas and examples to develop or modify future health promotion interventions.

REFERENCES

O'Neill, M. (2012). Introduction: Part III. In I. Rootman, S. Dupéré, A. Pederson, & M. O'Neill (Eds.), *Health promotion in Canada: Critical perspectives on practice* (3rd ed.) (pp. 193–195). Toronto: Canadian Scholars' Press.

Pederson, A. (2012). Conclusions from chapter: Bringing people back in. In I. Rootman, S. Dupéré, A. Pederson, & M. O'Neill (Eds.), *Health promotion in Canada: Critical perspectives on practice* (3rd ed.) (pp. 149–151). Toronto: Canadian Scholars' Press.

CHAPTER 6

Contrasting Entry Points for Intervention in Health Promotion Practice: Situating and Working with Context

Katherine L. Frohlich, Blake Poland, and Martine Shareck

LEARNING OBJECTIVES

1. Articulate the difference between interventions intended to change risk factors, improve the status of population groups, and change settings
2. Understand some social theory explanations for group-level health-related social practices (behaviours)
3. Understand health behaviour as more than an individual, rational choice

INTRODUCTION

Historically there have been three main entry points for intervention in health promotion practice: (1) issues/risk factors; (2) population groups (at-risk groups); and (3) settings. Entry points matter because they influence how a "problem" is framed and thus what is done about it (intervention). Each approach reflects different assumptions about what shapes health, what is most important, and what can most feasibly be changed. Concomitantly, each has singled out different aspects of analysis and intervention. In all three approaches the social context has some relevance and importance to what they do, albeit in different ways.

We take the position that social context matters. Context, we argue, is not just background "noise" to be factored out (statistically or otherwise) in the search for generalizable, best practice, or one-size-fits-all interventions. As health promotion seeks to create and sustain change through increasingly complex interventions characterized by intersectoral collaboration, cross-jurisdictional scope, multi-level and multi-component programming (seeking individual, familial, social network, organizational, community-based, and policy-level change), the importance of context is heightened. Furthermore, interest in the development of a robust evidence base for health promotion intervention under circumstances of complexity and multi-site variability impels us to take fuller account of the determinative role of context for intervention impact, scalability, and cross-jurisdictional relevance.

While context is frequently invoked in public health intervention research, it remains ill-defined and under-theorized. Lip service is paid to the widely recognized need to take social, political, economic, and other aspects of context into account, but few authors go beyond a listing of "factors" to unpack which aspects of context matter most, how, and why. Following Poland, Frohlich, and Cargo (2008), for reasons that will become clear later in this chapter, drawing on critical realism and complexity science, we define social context as follows:

> The local mix of conditions and events (social agents, objects and interactions) which characterise open systems ... whose unique confluence in time and space selectively activates (triggers, blocks or modifies) causal powers (mechanisms) in a chain of reactions that may result in very different outcomes depending on the dynamic interplay of conditions and mechanisms over time and space. (Poland et al., 2008)

To situate our discussion, we begin this chapter with a brief description of each entry point for intervention and outline how each has grappled with the notion of the social context, discussing its strengths and weaknesses. We conclude with a suggestion of a fourth potential entry point for health promotion research and practice: collective lifestyles.

ISSUES, POPULATION GROUPS, AND SETTINGS AS POINTS OF HEALTH PROMOTION INTERVENTION

Issues/Risk Factors

The *Ottawa Charter for Health Promotion* (WHO, 1986) set the stage for health promotion practice as we understand it today. The scope of the *Ottawa Charter* was broad, covering five large areas of action and multiple conditions and resources for health. Progressives within the movement lauded the expanded focus and attention to prerequisites to health, foundational social determinants, and community involvement. Nevertheless, for reasons (of perceived feasibility, political expediency, vested interests, etc.) that remain poorly articulated, the emerging personal wellness industry, large bureaucracies oriented to health education, and (in the main) the North American public were not so easily dissuaded from a deep cultural and institutional commitment to individualism. As a result, "developing personal skills" was one of the areas identified in the *Charter* that continued to receive the lion's share of funding, research, and public attention in the decades that followed its release. Within the *Charter*, developing personal skills was described as being possible through "providing information, education for health, and enhancing life skills. By so doing, it increases the options available to people to exercise more control over their own health and their environments, and to make choices conducive to health" (WHO, 1986, p. 3).

Prior to the *Ottawa Charter*, and definitively since then, health promotion practice has been dedicated to developing these personal skills in three major ways: (1) by focusing on a reduction in the prevalence and incidence of those *diseases* seen to be burdening the population the most (cardiovascular disease, cancer, diabetes, and HIV/AIDS); (2) by focusing on the reduction of *risk factors*, especially health behaviours linked to prevalent health problems facing the population (such as smoking, poor eating habits, lack of exercise, lack of condom use); and (3) by reducing *risk conditions* such as homelessness, which is neither a disease nor a health behaviour. Even so, the overwhelming focus since the *Ottawa Charter* has continued to be on the reduction of health lifestyle habits such as smoking, poor diet, lack of exercise, and risky sexual behaviour, through information and education programs and more recently through health literacy (Rootman & Gordon-El-Bihbety, 2008; see chapter 2), albeit with an expanded focus on increasing the options available to people to exercise more control over their own health and their environments in order to reduce disease prevalence, incidence, and risk conditions.

The focus on risk factors in health promotion interventions has a protracted history stemming from health promotion's historical roots in epidemiology and health education, as well as the influence of the Lalonde Report (Lalonde, 1974). It is well known that what we measure (and how) at the problem identification and needs assessment stage has a profound impact on subsequent phases of program development, implementation, and evaluation. Tannahill (1992) describes the fundamental role that epidemiology plays for health promotion in identifying and prioritizing prevalent health problems and their causes. First, and most obviously, programs and interventions are oriented to address the problems highlighted in epidemiological studies. So, for instance, the focus on cardiovascular disease, cancer, diabetes, or HIV/AIDS, driven by epidemiological studies, has created great impetus for health promotion programs to address these issues. Second, epidemiologists derive categories of risk factors associated with these health problems, which, if prevented, are presumed to reduce illness and death (Frohlich & Potvin, 1999). These risk factors are then often directly translated into health promotion programs. Because many of these risk factors (high blood pressure, overweight, and risky sexual behaviour) are seen to be modifiable through behaviour change (e.g., diet, exercise, condom use), the focus of health promotion has often been more on the proximal (those factors most directly related to the health outcome in question), and supposedly most modifiable, individual-level risk factors.

Lalonde's contribution to the framing of health promotion interventions is also significant (Lalonde, 1974). Lalonde's report recommended that public health interventions focus attention on the segment of the population with the highest level of risk exposure as indicated by health risk behaviours (e.g., smoking, alcohol consumption) or biological markers (e.g., body mass index, blood pressure). In this way, interventions became focused on what were termed populations "at risk" or groups showing elevated risk for some disease.

As a result of both epidemiology's and Lalonde's focus on individual-level risk factor reduction, health promotion drew on individual-level theories to guide the creation of its intervention programs. These understandings come largely from models of social psychology such as the health belief model (Becker, 1974), Bandura's social cognitive theory (Bandura, 1986), and Ajzen and Fishbein's theory of reasoned action (1980). All focused attention on the major biomedical and behavioural risk factors for developing the major health problems of concern at the time. Underlying these models is the assumption that population prevalence of adverse risk conditions is modifiable by providing education and behaviour-change tools to individuals to help them achieve lifestyle changes (Barnett, Anderson, Blosnich, Halverson, & Novak, 2005) (see chapter 4).

With regard to an issue-based approach, one of the most substantiated critiques of the "developing personal skills" approach to health promotion practice has been that individually based models of behaviour change have often yielded disappointing results. For example, in the Multiple Risk Factor Intervention Trial (MRFIT), 6,000 men, who were all in the highest 10 to 15 percent risk group in the United States due to their high rates of cigarette smoking, hypertension, and hyper-cholesterol levels, were enrolled in a six-year intervention program. The intervention was state-of-the-art: well-funded, well-staffed, and used the best behaviour-change techniques available. Even so, the results were disappointing: 62 percent of the men were still smoking after the six-year period, 50 percent still had hypertension, and few men had changed their dietary patterns (Multiple Risk Factor Intervention Trial Research Group, 1981, 1982).[1]

Among the many reflections on the MRFIT experience, one has been that the gains are short-lived because new smokers are continually being recruited into lifelong addiction by a combination of tobacco industry tactics, media, and structural conditions of poverty and hardship. The underlying problem with the high-risk behaviour modification approach, if one is truly interested in sustained population change, is that it does not address what has been termed the "fundamental causes" (Link & Phelan, 1995). The concept of fundamental causes posits that one has to understand the factors, as well as the mechanisms, that put people at risk in the first place—that is, the social context—and not focus on risk factors alone.

Population Groups

A second major entry point of intervention in health promotion, focusing on population groups, has largely sought to target particular groups thought to share certain key characteristics. These characteristics are frequently thought to predispose certain groups to be at greater risk for "sub-optimal" health outcomes. The main advantage of this approach is that it provides an opportunity to see how behaviours cluster within populations. This approach also fits structurally with how many organizations (governmental and non-governmental) and funding bodies are organized, with separate structures for organizations working with the elderly, children, women, and so on.

An important critique of interventions concerned with specific populations is that they focus on the higher exposure of these populations to a specific risk factor or disease outcome, thus dealing only with one risk factor or disease at a time. For instance, with children it may be cognitive development, or in the current context, issues of obesity. For the elderly, organizations may be concerned with fall prevention and long-term care. But some groups at higher risk of some diseases are typically at higher risk of others also. At issue are not just the specific risk factor exposures for a single disease, but the patterning of exposure across many factors that predispose some groups to be routinely more vulnerable or disadvantaged than others. In other words, the question to be asked is, Why are these groups more at risk for a wide range of risk factors and diseases than others?

To address this, it has been suggested that interventions be developed using the heuristic of "vulnerable" populations (Frohlich & Potvin, 2008). "Vulnerable" populations differ from specific population groups in that, due to their position in the social strata, they are commonly exposed to contextual conditions that distinguish them from the rest of the population. As such, what defines vulnerable populations are shared social characteristics generated by non-random distributions of material and social conditions. These characteristics have their roots in power relations structured in society to create cleavages along race, class, and gendered lines (Grabb, 2002) as key enduring features of the social context (Poland et al., 2006, 2008). This involves the structured relationships between what Saul Alinsky (1971) would call the "haves" and the "have-nots" and involves the power that operates through control over material, ideological, and human resources (Grabb, 2002). In this sense, the label of *vulnerable* could be seen to be blaming the victim (vulnerability is understood as a property of those so labelled), whereas the term *marginalized* or *disadvantaged* more clearly names the issue of marginalization (shifts the implied blame to those responsible for marginalization).

A particularly poignant example of a vulnerable or marginalized population in the current Canadian context is the example of Indiginous peoples (Adelson, 2005; Frohlich, Ross, & Richmond, 2006). Indiginous people are diverse in language and culture, but they all share a common experience of colonization and all that this has entailed (forced resettlement, residential schools, removal of ancestral lands, violations of treaty rights, rights to minimum services defined according to governmental arbitration of who qualifies as status or non-status Indians, and so forth). Indiginous leaders have long fought against the dominant Western cultural paradigm's tendency to blame the victim (labelling Indigenous peoples as lazy, stupid, backwards, or uneducated) and have advocated instead for an understanding that places current community health problems in their proper historical context (as impacts of colonization, institutional racism, etc.). The resultant cultural upheaval, family and community breakdown, sedentarization, disrupted connection to the land, etc., has had severe consequences in terms of community and individual mental, social, spiritual, and physical health. As a result, the vast majority of Indiginous communities find themselves at a much higher risk, and with much higher prevalence, of many of the most important markers of morbidity and mortality, such as addictions, suicide, diabetes, HIV/AIDS, cancer, cardiovascular disease, and the list goes on.

Settings

Settings where people live, work, play, and otherwise spend time are a third entry point for intervention in health promotion practice (Poland, Green, & Rootman, 2000). Settings can be defined as the physical place and social space in which people engage in daily activities, and where personal, organizational, and environmental factors interact to affect health and wellbeing (Nutbeam, 1998; Rice & Hancock, 2016). Common examples of settings include schools, workplaces, hospitals, sports clubs, and prisons; geographical areas such as neighbourhoods and cities; as well as more loosely bounded communities. In practice, two different conceptualizations of settings, and of what related interventions might look like, have emerged.

The first one views settings as physically bounded entities with a clear organizational structure, within which "captive" populations, the targets for health promotion intervention, can be found. This conceptualization of settings has largely been associated with individually focused health promotion activities such as mass media campaigns, health education, and personal skills development aimed at directly changing people's behaviours (Richard, Potvin, Kishchuk, Prilic, & Green, 1996; Whitelaw et al., 2001; Dooris, 2004). Examples include stress reduction interventions in the workplace or nutritional education programs in schools to promote healthy eating among pupils.

This approach has administrative appeal since it allows one to reach conveniently captive audiences for intervention (Whitelaw et al., 2001) and also benefits from more straightforward negotiation for entry through organizational leaders, compared to the messier dynamics of outreach in community settings. Important limitations of interventions based on this conceptualization, however, reside in their generally targeting individual health issues (such as stress or healthy eating) in one setting (such as the workplace or school) at a time, and in promoting individual behaviour change without attending to the healthfulness of the setting itself (Poland et al., 2000). This can lead to blaming the victim or to interventions that potentially aggravate health inequalities if they fail to reach the worst off (Frohlich, Poland, Mykhalovskiy, Alexander, & Maule, 2010). It is widely acknowledged that behaviour change needs to be supported by environmental conditions that favour its emergence and maintenance. If a setting's structures are not modified to accommodate change, it may be difficult for individuals to sustain behaviour change once they are outside the targeted setting (Dooris, 2004).

The second conceptualization of settings attempts to address the above limitations by harnessing the social context defined through both a setting's structure and the individuals found within it (Poland et al., 2008). This conceptualization is based on an ecological model of health that assumes that differences in health are influenced by interactions between personal, interpersonal, organizational, community, and policy factors that unfold over the life-course of individuals, families, and communities (McLeroy, Bibeau, Steckler, & Glanz, 1988; Stokols, 1996; Smedley & Syme, 2000; see also chapters 13–15). It also involves a systems perspective whereby settings comprise individuals and structures that constantly interact with one another, creating a whole that is more complex than the sum of its parts (Dooris, 2006; Dooris et al., 2007). Finally, it puts forth a whole-system development and change approach that entails focusing on changing the setting's organization and structure rather than only aiming to change the individuals found within it (St. Leger, 1997; Dooris, 2006, 2009). An example of an intervention to promote healthy eating rooted in this conceptualization of settings would involve nutritional education and cooking classes in schools, workplaces, and communities combined with policies to improve access to affordable healthy foods in these same settings. Health-promoting schools initiatives increasingly adopt this broader perspective (www.who.int/school_youth_health/gshi/hps/en/).

A major advantage of this perspective on settings is that interventions focus not so much on individuals changing their behaviour but on changing the settings themselves to be more health-enhancing. In addition, by altering the social and structural conditions that shape individual health behaviours, such interventions assist in reducing the risk for those currently at risk, as well as for those still to come (Smedley & Syme, 2000). They also show great potential in addressing social inequalities in health if they focus on the social determinants of health, address the needs of marginalized groups, effect change in a setting's structure, and involve key stakeholders (Shareck, Frohlich, & Poland, 2013). However, action on settings, even action that seeks to make settings themselves more health-enhancing, is rarely informed by a deeper social analysis of the intersectionality of race/class/gender/ableism, by the myriad ways in which inequity is sustained and repro-duced in and through interpersonal and institutional practices, or by extra-local policy and practice (see chapter 8).

Complexity theory and critical realism are two established theoretical approaches that offer particularly useful insights into these issues. Complexity theory provides us with change theories that go beyond those of planned and structured change by considering complex systems' emerging properties (Norman, 2009; Holman, 2010). For instance, it could help us understand how neighbourhood physical decay might lead to social dis-organization, which could then trigger behavioural pathologies such as crime, thereby engendering a vicious cycle of more decay and disorganization (Gatrell, 2005).

In turn, critical realism moves attention to the lived experiences of people within the social context (Dooris et al., 2007) and encourages us to uncover *how* interventions work and through what *mechanisms*, rather than solely focusing on whether or not interventions have an *effect* (Porter, 1993; Poland et al., 2008; Kontos & Poland, 2009). The potential that these theories offer to a settings approach to health promotion is discussed in Dooris et al. (2007), Poland et al. (2008), and Shareck et al. (2013), but we invite you to see also Holman (2010) for an excellent understanding of engaging emergence. Several methodological approaches are also particularly helpful in grasping the social context of settings-related interventions. These include community-based participatory intervention and research (see chapter 17), arts-enabled approaches, joined-up approaches, and whole-of-government or health in all policies (Shareck et al., 2013; chapter 16).

Despite these helpful tools, we acknowledge that this more complex conceptualization of settings and related interventions remains challenging to translate into practice and may not always have the expected results. For example, two years after the New Deal for Communities program was implemented in socio-economically disadvantaged areas in the United Kingdom, the more-educated residents had benefited more from training opportunities and smoking cessation programs than the less-educated ones, and educational differences in income and smoking had widened (Stafford, Nazroo, Popay, & Whitehead, 2008). Poland, Krupa, and McCall (2009) offer a more detailed rubric of guiding analytic questions for operationalizing a more holistic settings approach to inform program design, implementation, and evaluation.

Shortcomings: A Summary

All three main entry points for health promotion intervention have, in various ways, fallen short in taking into account the social context. We suggest that to improve the situation we need to know more specifically how social inequities in health are (re)produced, and thus, what it is about the social environment that contributes to ill health; not only *which* factors are important, but *how* and *why* they are important. We are fully cognizant, however, that even in the face of the growing recognition of the importance of addressing inequities in health, it is enormously difficult to change institutional practices and that most public health practitioners' room to innovate is significantly limited by questions of funding, politics, and human resources. Despite institutional limitations, we make the plea for a greater understanding of how individuals, their behaviours, and their social circumstances interact to bring about the health problems faced by Canadian society today. We maintain that this knowledge can help us intervene more appropriately.

WHAT CAN BE DONE DIFFERENTLY?

The Structure/Agency Debate

Studies of the social context of health behaviours and outcomes bring us inevitably to a critical discussion as old as Western philosophy—that of individual free will versus structural determinism, or what is today referred to as the structure/agency debate (see chapter 3). Proponents of structural explanations emphasize the power of structural conditions in shaping individual behaviour (Cockerham, 2005). So, for instance, if one were to take a structural position to understanding tobacco consumption, one might be particularly concerned with the role of social class (which is one manifestation of the social structure) in shaping smoking. Advocates of agency, on the other hand, accentuate the capacity of individual actors to choose and influence their behaviour regardless of structural influences. This structure/agency dichotomy was also defined in terms of "life chances" and "life choices" by Max Weber (1922), who was the first theorist to discuss the term *lifestyle* (see chapter 3). Weber viewed life chances as the opportunities that people encounter due to their social situation (their position within the social structure). Choices, on the other hand, are the decisions people make. So, whereas health-related choices are (more or less) voluntary, life chances either enable or constrain choices, as choices and chances interact to shape behavioural outcomes. What Weber highlighted, then, is that both chances and choices are socially determined, and thus choices cannot simply be individually controlled. In so doing, Weber also underscored the collective nature of behaviours by associating lifestyles with status groups, and not solely with individuals; that is, choices are shaped by one's position within the social field. What Weber witnessed was that people from different social classes tended to have certain behaviours and practices in common.

French sociologist Pierre Bourdieu, 60 years later, went further, arguing that "choices" are an expression of a habitus that itself is a dynamic, evolving inculcation of structuring structures (or "chances," to use Weber's term) (Bourdieu, 1980, 1992). The habitus, according to Bourdieu, is produced by the objective conditions of existence combined with positions in the social structure, and it generates practices and tastes that together result in a lifestyle. While there is an element of choice with regard to one's lifestyle, people are predisposed by their habitus toward a certain choice of lifestyle. Bourdieu therefore viewed it as being entirely misleading to separate, analytically, "choices" and "chances" (see chapter 3).

One especially promising approach to understanding the social nature of routinized behaviours as well as learning and socio-technical transitions is *practice theory*. Informed by the work of Giddens (1984), Bourdieu (1990), Foucault (1970), Latour (1991), Taylor (2004), and Schatzki (1996, 2002; Schatzki, Knorr Cetina, & Von Savigny, 2001), and more recently Harrison (2009) and Shove (Shove, Pantzar, & Watson, 2012; Shove & Walker, 2010), practice theory (less a unified theory than an approach associated with the "practice turn" in social and cultural theory; Reckwitz, 2002; Schatzki et al., 2001) conceives of practices as "assemblages of images (meanings, symbols), skills (forms of competence, procedures) and stuff (materials, technology) that are dynamically integrated into daily life by skilled practitioners through regular and repeated performance" (Hargreaves, 2011, p. 83; Schatzki et al., 2001) under relations of power characterized by "strong inequalities in the availability of requisite elements, or in the capacity to promote, mobilize and configure" (Shove & Walker, 2010, p. 474).

Collective Lifestyles as a Useful Heuristic Device to Address Social Context Issues in Health Promotion

Considerations of the role of lifestyle are far from new in health promotion practice. Green and Kreuter (1999), for instance, paid particular attention to the important role that lifestyle played in permitting health promotion to move away from its earlier emphasis on health behaviour alone. While these authors were mindful of the collective aspect to lifestyles, they tended to consider them more in terms of practice and behavioural patterns, rather than situating these practices within the broader social structure as Weber and Bourdieu do.

We maintain that a theoretically informed approach to understanding "collective life-styles" (Frohlich, Corin, & Potvin, 2002), building on the ideas of Weber and Bourdieu, has the potential to offer more to health promotion practice than simply existing as a synonym for patterns of individual risk behaviours and packages of variables. Instead it takes into account both behaviours and social circumstances (Abel, Cockerham, & Niemann, 2000). Collective lifestyles comprise interacting patterns of health-related behaviours, orientations, and resources adopted by groups of people in response to their social, cultural, and economic environment (Abel et al., 2000, p. 63). Viewed in this way, collective lifestyles are akin to the social environmental approach in that they take into consideration the social, cultural, and economic environments in which people live, get sick, and die. There are a number of important differences, however, between these two approaches that make the collective life-styles option particularly attractive to health promoters hungry for change.

First, the collective lifestyles framework develops further the issue of choices and chances by situating them in current sociological theory. Within this framework, there-fore, we speak of *social* practices (Bourdieu, 1980, 1992; Giddens, 1984) (or behaviours) and *social* structure (or social conditions). Social practices are routinized and socialized behaviours common to groups. Social structure is defined as the way in which society is organized, involving norms, resources, policy, and institutional practices. Similarly to choices, social practices are understood as emerging from the structure, and thus the relationship between structure and practices is always explicit and recursive. In this way, an individual behaviour, or social practice, is never divorced from its position within the social structure. Further, this relationship is not unidirectional; the structure is seen to shape people's social practices, but in turn, people's social practices impact structure by either reproducing or transforming it.

Second, social practices are not considered purely in terms of health behaviours. An empirical example of the usefulness of considering social practices beyond health behaviours themselves comes from Hargreaves et al. (2010), who employed the collec-tive lifestyles framework to help understand the social and cultural contexts of change in tobacco consumption following the implementation of smoke-free legislation in England between 2007 and 2008. Conducting a qualitative longitudinal study using systematic observations in six localities across the North and South of England, pre- and post-legislation, these researchers concluded that there were inequitable struc-tural opportunities to "comply" with the new legislation across localities. Also, in spite of the apparent impact of structural influences on smoking, people who smoke rarely attributed the changes they made to their smoking to the legislation. Instead, participants cited their own capacity as agents of change or the dual effects of struc-ture and agency. As such, the key contextual mediators and moderators of outcomes were the local structural opportunities and individual agency. While the structural opportunities for change were the same across England, due to the new legislation being population-based, people's abilities to actually conform with the legislation were shaped by the social and cultural contexts in which they lived, with some areas being less tolerant of smoking, and others being smoking-friendly. By examining smoking rates alone, pre- and post-legislation, one would be unable to understand why the rates differ so widely across localities.

A third feature of a collective lifestyles framework, therefore, is a focus on the constraints on, and opportunities for, individual agency and what implications they have for true empowerment. People's position within the social structure clearly shapes their agency. Approaches that focus on changing health behaviours give attention to agency, but what is often missing is a well-developed analysis of the structural constraints to individual agency (McLaren, McIntyre, & Kirkpatrick, 2010), that is, a direct link established between structure and agency. While the *Ottawa Charter* initially suggested focusing on increasing the options available to people to exercise more control over their health, in practice this has been addressed mostly through environmental change, that is, changing the conditions rather than focusing on how these changes might increase individual control. The collective lifestyles framework suggests that agency needs to be understood in relation to the social context of the health problem of concern.

Ivory et al. (2015) recently used the collective lifestyles framework to explore the social context of physical activity in Auckland, New Zealand, revealing the essential role that agency plays in shaping people's abilities to be physically active. The framework was used to understand how residents in Auckland talked about and made sense of physical activity with regard to place. While they found that not all residential settings provided equal opportunities to undertake physically and socially active lifestyles at the most proximal level, many residents were able to actively construct what they considered their neighbourhood by engaging in physical activity in many non-local places. They conclude that despite the inequitable environments that people found themselves in with regard to ability to be physically active, many residents, despite coming from more socially deprived areas, revealed agency in how they managed the limitations within their immediate residential setting in order to seek out opportunities to be active elsewhere.

Fourth, an implicit but underdeveloped aspect to the collective lifestyles framework is the issue of power. Power relations are central to shaping the uneven social distribution of health behaviours and disease outcomes among groups and ultimately in creating and sustaining the social structure. A focus on power relations draws attention to the ways in which the social patterning of health behaviours and disease outcomes mirrors the patterning of other processes of marginalization and disadvantage through both the social structure and social practices. A focus on power further invites us to consider our role, within health promotion practice, as actors within systems of power and relative privilege or marginality. We are, of course, active participants in the social context of health promotion as we influence, through our research and interventions, the way disease, health, and behaviours are understood (Frohlich, Mykhalovskiy, Poland, Haines-Saah, & Johnson, 2012). Reflections and action on such issues are vital for a true focus on social context to be realized (Frohlich et al., 2010).

An important aspect of a collective lifestyles framework for understanding the social context is therefore reflexivity with respect to the social location of health promotion as a field (see also chapter 18). By reflexivity, we mean the maintenance of a self-critical attitude and a questioning of the taken-for-granted assumptions regarding the political nature of our work and its intended and unintended effects, as well as the social distribution of these effects (Caplan, 1993; Poland et al., 2006). More concretely this could include (1) attention to the tacit knowledge and perspectives that practitioners bring to their work; (2) an openness to being transformed by the experience of engaging with individuals who may question the practice of health promotion; (3) a questioning of "received knowledge" (what we hold to be self-evident and true); (4) a curiosity about and openness towards other perspectives and ways of seeing; and (5) an awareness of power relations and one's own social location and positionality (how we fit into class and gender relations and how this affects the work we do individually and as a group performing health promotion) (Poland et al., 2006; Bisset, Tremblay, Wright, Poland, & Frohlich, 2016).

CONCLUSION

Health promotion has come a long way since the *Ottawa Charter* in its position on where the entry points of intervention in health promotion practice could and should be. We have learned much in health promotion practice and research by focusing on issues, specific population groups, and settings. As we have seen, however, each falls short in addressing the full complexity and social embeddedness of health determinants and the recursive relationship of structure and agency. We offer an approach to addressing social context as a potential fourth point of intervention using the collective lifestyles framework, as well as issues relating to power and reflexivity. In so doing, we address a number of the critiques discussed throughout this chapter using the application of the framework to urban health inequities.

The consideration of collective lifestyles, as opposed to behaviours alone, has three important implications for health promotion and the study of urban area effects. First, it suggests that when studying area effects on behaviour we must move beyond an individually based high-risk behaviour focus to one that considers both the structural barriers and opportunities in areas and how these conditions structure, and are structured by, behaviours. Second, it suggests that these barriers and opportunities may affect groups differentially based on their position within the social structure; it is a socially shaped group phenomenon. These group effects are often termed ecological, in reference to group-level exposures. In better understanding these ecological effects we might be better able to intervene on a population level, rather than on one individual at a time. Lastly, a focus on collective lifestyles introduces a social justice agenda; if these barriers and opportunities for healthy behaviour are inequitably distributed throughout areas, and we view the social structure to be mutable, health promotion should be addressing this issue as one of injustice.

CRITICAL THINKING QUESTIONS

1. What are the advantages and disadvantages to the points of intervention discussed in this chapter?
2. Are there other ways in which we could intervene in health promotion that would better take into account the social context?
3. Do current interventions in health promotion stand to be improved and, if yes, why?
4. Is there a danger of increasing inequalities in health by intervening through health promotion? If yes, how so? What can be done to prevent this?
5. What theories can we draw on to help improve our interventions in health promotion? Which theories do you like best? Why?

RESOURCES

Further Readings

Dooris, M. (2013). Expert voices for change: Bridging the silos—Towards healthy and sustainable settings for the 21st century. *Health & Place, 20*, 39–50.
This paper reports on a qualitative study undertaken through in-depth interviews with key individuals widely acknowledged to have been the architects and pilots of the settings movement. Exploring the development of the settings approach, policy and practice integration, and connectedness "outwards," "upwards," and "beyond health," it concludes that the settings approach has much to offer—but will only realize its potential impact on the wellbeing of people, places, and the planet if it builds bridges between silos and reconfigures itself for the globalized twenty-first century.

Frohlich, K. L., Corin, E., & Potvin, L. (2002). A theoretical proposal for the relationship between context and disease. *Sociology of Health and Illness, 23*, 776–797.
This article develops the notion of collective lifestyles drawing on the work of Pierre Bourdieu, Anthony Giddens, and Amartya Sen.

Global Health Promotion, supplement issue on Approaches to Health-Promoting Settings around the World: ped.sagepub.com/content/23/1_suppl.toc.
The 11 papers included in this supplement issue of *Global Health Promotion* provide rich insights into how health-promoting settings have been envisioned, created, and sustained, both in Taiwan and around the world.

Poland, B., Frohlich, K. L., Haines, R. J., Mykhalovskiy, E., Rock, M., & Sparks, R. (2006). The social context of smoking: The next frontier in tobacco control? *Tobacco Control, 15*, 59–63.
This article moves beyond the discussion developed in this chapter to include the exploration

of social context through the sociology of the body as it relates to smoking, collective patterns of consumption, the construction and maintenance of social identity, the ways in which desire and pleasure are implicated in these latter two dimensions in particular, and smoking as a social activity rooted in place.

Poland, B., Krupa, E., & McCall, D. (2009). Settings for health promotion: An analytic framework to guide intervention design and implementation. *Health Promotion Practice*, *10*(4), 505–516.

This paper, selected as "best of the year" by the Society for Public Health Education (SOPHE) in the US, provides a detailed framework for guiding the design, implementation, and evaluation of settings-based health promotion interventions.

Scriven, A., & Hodgins, M. (Eds.). (2012). *Health promotion settings: Principles and practice.* London: Sage.

This book outlines the history, content, and utility of the settings approach in health promotion interventions.

Shareck, M., Frohlich, K., & Poland, B. (2013). Reducing social inequities in health through settings-related interventions: A conceptual framework. *Global Health Promotion*, *20*(2), 39–52.

This paper reports findings from a scoping review of the literature on theoretical bases and practical applications of the settings approach focused on addressing social inequalities in health.

Williams, G. (2003). The determinants of health: Structure, context, and agency. *Sociology of Health and Illness, 25*, 131–154.

Williams reviews the ways in which the concept of social structure has been deployed within medical sociology, paying particular attention to its role in the debate over health inequalities and the role of the social context in shaping these inequalities.

Relevant Websites

A Critique of the Settings Approach, hosted by University of New South Wales School of Public Health

www.ldb.org/setting.htm

Health promotion recognizes the idea that people live in social, cultural, political, economic, and environmental contexts. This acknowledgement may have been new for public health, although sociologists and social psychologists have been aware of the embeddedness of behaviour into larger contexts for a longer period of time. However, the acknowledgement by public health practitioners that health is developed in the context of everyday life, which itself is structured by its related social system, has not led to a fundamental reconsideration of the social science basis of public health concepts and its incorporation into planning and activity.

World Health Organization—Settings Approach
www.who.int/healthy_settings/en/

This multi-lingual site describes the history of the WHO Healthy Settings approach. Specifically, Healthy Settings emphasizes practical networks and projects to create healthy environments such as healthy schools, health-promoting hospitals, healthy workplaces, and healthy cities. Healthy Settings builds on the premise that there is a health development potential in practically every organization and/or community.

NOTE

1. Although a 38 percent quit rate would be phenomenal if generalized to the entire population, focused "best practice" intervention trials are typically so resource-intensive that the costs of doing so would be prohibitive (and would compete politically with other determinants of health, programs, and service priorities).

REFERENCES

Abel, T., Cockerham, W. C., & Niemann, S. (2000). A critical approach to lifestyle and health. In J. Watson & S. Platt (Eds.), *Researching health promotion* (pp. 54–77). London: Routledge.

Adelson, N. (2005). The embodiment of inequity: Health disparities in Aboriginal Canada. *Canadian Journal of Public Health, 96*, S45–S61.

Ajzen, I., & Fishbein, M. (1980). *Understanding attitudes and predicting social behaviour.* Englewood Cliffs: Prentice-Hall.

Alinsky, S. D. (1971). *Rules for radicals: A realistic primer for realistic radicals.* New York: Random House.

Bandura, A. (1986). *Social foundations of thought and action: A social cognitive theory.* Englewood Cliffs: Prentice-Hall.

Barnett, E., Anderson, T., Blosnich, J., Halverson, J., & Novak, J. (2005). Promoting cardiovascular health: From environmental goals to social environmental change. *American Journal of Preventive Medicine, 29*, 107–112.

Becker, M. H. (1974). The health belief model and personal health behaviour. *Health Education Monographs, 2*, 324–508.

Bisset, S., Tremblay, M-C., Wright, M., Poland, B., & Frohlich, K. L. (2016). Can reflexivity be learned? An experience with tobacco control practitioners in Canada. *Health Promotion International.* doi: 10.1093/heapro/dav080

Bourdieu, P. (1980). *Le sens pratique.* Paris: Les Éditions de Minuit.

Bourdieu, P. (1990). *The logic of practice.* Stanford, CA: Stanford University Press.

Bourdieu, P. (1992). *Réponses: Pour une anthropologie réflexive.* Paris: Éditions du Seuil.

Caplan, R. (1993). The importance of social theory for health promotion: From description to re-flexivity. *Health Promotion International, 8*, 147–157.

Cockerham, W. (2005). Health lifestyle theory and the convergence of agency and structure. *Journal of Health and Social Behavior, 46*, 51–67.

Dooris, M. (2004). Joining up settings for health: A valuable investment for strategic partnerships? *Critical Public Health, 14*(1), 49–61.

Dooris, M. (2006). Health promoting settings: Future directions. *Promotion and Education, 23*(2), 1–4.

Dooris, M. (2009). Holistic and sustainable health improvement: The contribution of the settings-based approach to health promotion. *Perspectives in Public Health, 129*(1), 29–36.

Dooris, M., Poland, B., Kolbe, L., de Leeuw, E., McCall, D., & Wharf-Higgins, J. (2007). Healthy settings: Building evidence for the effectiveness of whole systems health promotion—challenges and future directions. In D. V. McQueen & C. M. Jones (Eds.), *Global perspectives on health promotion effectiveness* (pp. 327–352). New York: Springer.

Foucault, M. (1970). *The order of things: An archaeology of the human sciences.* New York: Vintage Books (Random House).

Frohlich, K. L., Corin, E., & Potvin, L. (2002). A theoretical proposal for the relationship between context and disease. *Sociology of Health and Illness, 23*, 776–797.

Frohlich, K. L., Mykhalovskiy, E., Poland, B., Haines-Saah, R., & Johnson, J. (2012). "Creating" the socially marginalized smoker: The role of tobacco control. *Sociology of Health and Illness, 34*(7), 978–993.

Frohlich, K. L., Poland, B., Mykhalovskiy, E., Alexander, S., & Maule, C. (2010). Tobacco control and the inequitable socio-economic distribution of smoking: Smokers' discourse and implications for tobacco control. *Critical Public Health, 20*, 35–46.

Frohlich, K. L., & Potvin, L. (1999). Health promotion through the lens of population health: Toward a salutogenic setting. *Critical Public Health, 9*(3), 211–222.

Frohlich, K. L., & Potvin, L. (2008). The inequality paradox: The population approach and vulnerable populations. *American Journal of Public Health, 98*, 216–221.

Frohlich, K. L., Ross, N., & Richmond, C. (2006). Health disparities in Canada today: Evidence and pathways. *Health Policy, 79*, 132–143.

Gatrell, A. C. (2005). Complexity theory and geographies of health: A critical assessment. *Social Science and Medicine, 60*, 2661–2671.

Giddens, A. (1984). *The constitution of society.* Cambridge: Polity Press.

Grabb, E. G. (2002). *Theories of social inequality: Classical and contemporary perspectives* (4th ed.). Toronto: Harcourt Brace.

Green, L. W., & Kreuter, M. W. (1999). *Health promotion planning: An educational and ecological approach* (3rd ed.). Mountain View: Mayfield Publishing Company.

Hargreaves, K., Amos, A., Highet, G., Martin, C., Platt, S., Ritchie, D., & White, M. (2010). The social context of change in tobacco consumption following the introduction of "smokefree" England legislation: A qualitative, longitudinal study. *Social Science and Medicine, 71*, 459–466.

Hargreaves, T. (2011). Practice-ing behaviour change: Applying social practice theory to pro-environmental behaviour change. *Journal of Consumer Culture, 11*(1), 79–99.

Harrison, P. (2009). In the absence of practice. *Environment & Planning D: Society & Space, 27*(6), 987–1009.

Holman, P. (2010). *Engaging emergence: Turning upheaval into opportunity.* San Francisco: Berret-Koehler.

Ivory, V. C., Russell, M., Witten, K., Hooper, C. M., Pearce, J., & Blakely, T. (2015). What shape is your neighbourhood? Investigating the micro geographies of physical activity. *Social Science & Medicine, 133*, 313–321.

Kontos, P. C., & Poland, B. D. (2009). Mapping new theoretical and methodological terrain for knowledge translation: Contributions from critical realism and the arts. *Implementation Science, 4*(1), 1–10.

Lalonde, M. (1974). *A new perspective on the health of Canadians.* Ottawa: Government of Canada. Retrieved from www.phac-aspc.gc.ca/ph-sp/pdf/perspect-eng.pdf

Latour, B. (1991). *Nous n'avons jamais été modernes. Essai d'anthropologie symétrique.* Paris: La Découverte.

Link, B. G., & Phelan, J. (1995). Social conditions as fundamental causes of disease. *Journal of Health and Social Behavior,* Extra Issue, 80–94.

McLaren, L., McIntyre, L., & Kirkpatrick, S. (2010). Rose's population strategy of prevention need not increase social inequalities in health. *International Journal of Epidemiology, 39*(2), 372–377.

McLeroy, K. R., Bibeau, D., Steckler, A., & Glanz, K. (1988). An ecological perspective on health promotion programs. *Health Education Quarterly, 15*, 351–377.

Multiple Risk Factor Intervention Trial Research Group. (1981). Multiple risk factor intervention trial. *Preventive Medicine, 10*, 387–553.

Multiple Risk Factor Intervention Trial Research Group. (1982). Multiple risk factor intervention trial: Risk factor changes and mortality results. *Journal of the American Medical Association, 24*, 1465–1476.

Norman, C. D. (2009). Health promotion as a systems science and practice. *Journal of Evaluation in Clinical Practice, 15*(5), 868–872.

Nutbeam, D. (1998). Health promotion glossary. *Health Promotion International, 13*(4), 349–364.

Poland, B., Frohlich, K. L., & Cargo, M. (2008). Context as a fundamental dimension of health promotion program evaluation. In L. Potvin & D. V. McQueen (Eds.), *Health promotion evaluation practices in the Americas values and research* (pp. 299–317). New York: Springer.

Poland, B., Frohlich, K. L., Haines, R. J., Mykhalovskiy, E., Rock, M., & Sparks, R. (2006). The social context of smoking: The next frontier in tobacco control? *Tobacco Control, 15*(1), 59–63.

Poland, B. D., Green, L. W., & Rootman, I. (Eds.). (2000). *Settings for health promotion: Linking theory and practice.* Thousand Oaks: Sage Publications.

Poland, B., Krupa, E., & McCall, D. (2009). Settings for health promotion: An analytic framework to guide intervention design and implementation. *Health Promotion Practice, 10*(4), 505–516.

Porter, S. (1993). Critical realist ethnography: The case of racism and professionalism in a medical setting. *Sociology, 27*(4), 591–665.

Reckwitz, A. (2002). Toward a theory of social practices: A development in culturalist thinking. *European Journal of Social Theory, 5*(2), 243–263.

Rice, M., & Hancock, T. (2016). Equity, sustainability and governance in urban settings. *Global Health Promotion, 23*, 94–97.

Richard, L., Potvin, L., Kishchuk, N., Prilic, H., & Green, L. W. (1996). Assessment of the integration of the ecological approach in health promotion programs. *American Journal of Health Promotion, 10*(4), 318–328.

Rootman, I., & Gordon-El-Bihbety, D. (2008). A vision for a health literate Canada: Report of the Expert Panel on Health Literacy. Ottawa: CPHA. www.cpha.ca/uploads/portals/h-l/report_e.pdf

Schatzki, T. (1996). *Social practices: A Wittgensteinian approach to human activity and the social.* Cambridge: Cambridge University Press.

Schatzki, T. R. (2002). *The site of the social: A philosophical account of the constitution of social life and change.* University Park: Pennsylvania State University Press.

Schatzki, T. R., Knorr Cetina, K., & Von Savigny, E. (Eds.). (2001). *The practice turn in contemporary theory.* London & New York: Routledge.

Shareck, M., Frohlich, K. L., & Poland, B. (2013). Reducing social inequities in health through settings related interventions—A conceptual framework. *Global Health Promotion, 20*(2), 39–52.

Shove, E., Pantzar, M., & Watson, M. (2012). *The dynamics of social practice: Everyday life and how it changes.* London: Sage.

Shove, E., & Walker, G. (2010). Governing transitions in the sustainability of everyday life. *Research Policy, 39*(4), 471–476.

Smedley, B. D., & Syme, S. L. (Eds.). (2000). *Promoting health: Intervention strategies from social and behavioral research.* Washington: National Academy Press.

Stafford, M., Nazroo, J., Popay, J. M., & Whitehead, M. (2008). Tackling inequalities in health: Evaluating the New Deal for Communities initiative. *Journal of Epidemiology and Community Health, 62*, 298–304.

St. Leger, L. (1997). Health promoting settings: From Ottawa to Jakarta. *Health Promotion International, 12*(3), 99–101.

Stokols, D. (1996). Translating social ecological theory into guidelines for community health promotion. *American Journal of Health Promotion, 10*, 282–298.

Tannahill, A. (1992). Epidemiology and health promotion: A common understanding. In R. Bunton & G. Macdonald (Eds.), *Health promotion: Disciplines and diversity* (pp. 42–65). London: Routledge.

Taylor, C. (2004). *Modern social imaginaries.* Durham, NC: Duke University Press.

Weber, M. (1922). *Wirschaft und Gesellschaft (Economy and society).* Tübingen: Mohr Siebeck.

Whitelaw, S., Baxendale, A., Bryce, C., Machardy, L., Young, I., & Witney, E. (2001). 'Settings' based health promotion: A review. *Health Promotion International, 16*(4), 339–353.

World Health Organization (WHO). (1986). *Ottawa Charter for Health Promotion.* Ottawa: Canadian Public Health Association.

CHAPTER 7

Gender-Transformative Health Promotion as an Approach to Addressing Violence against Women

Ann Pederson

LEARNING OBJECTIVES

1. Understand the concepts of sex and gender
2. Explain in what ways violence against women is a gendered issue
3. Identify potential opportunities for health promotion action on violence against women

Let us commit as a country to stopping violence against women and girls. Each of us can do something. Together we will make a real difference.

—The Right Honourable Justin Trudeau, Prime Minister of Canada[1]

INTRODUCTION

Since 1989, Canada has recognized December 6th as the National Day of Remembrance and Action on Violence against Women. The day honours the lives of 14 young women who were murdered while attending l'École Polytechnique de Montréal in what has been described as "an act of gender-based violence that shocked the nation."[2] The young women who died are understood to have been killed because they were women. Events such as this provide a chilling annual reminder of the persistence of violence against women (VAW) in Canada (and around the globe) and invite those working in health promotion to reflect upon VAW as a health issue and what can be done to reduce and prevent it.

Over the past 35 years, the women's movement in Canada (and elsewhere) has transformed the discourse of VAW as a personal problem into an issue of human rights and social justice (Abraham & Tastsoglou, 2016). Through research, education, and activism, women's organizations created shelters, challenged legislation and the lack of evidence on VAW, and educated one another, the justice system, and the state about the nature of VAW. In time, institutionalized structures were established within the state apparatus to formalize and support government, state systems, and civil society action to address VAW. Yet VAW persists.

As part of the social system that conveys and reproduces social norms, whether in research, policy, or care (Sen & Ostlin, 2010), the health sector needs to strengthen the health system response to identifying VAW, supporting women with experiences of violence, and raising overall awareness of violence as a health issue (García-Moreno et al., 2015; Provincial Health Officer, 2011; UN Women, 2015; Wilkinson, 2013). Though findings are just emerging and more research is needed, there is some evidence that interventions that address the root causes of violence against women, including gender norms that support, perpetuate, and normalize some forms of violence, including sexual assault and relationship violence, can contribute to preventing and reducing it. Such gender-transformative interventions (Dworkin, Treves-Kagan, & Lippman, 2013; Pederson, Greaves, & Poole, 2014) address the underlying and structural causes of violence against women, particularly biased and harmful norms that limit and disempower women and girls while fostering stifling notions of masculinity (Dworkin, Kambou, Sutherland, Moalla, & Kapoor, 2009).

Violence is the leading cause of death and disability among women at all ages and it has multiple health and social consequences (Fulu, Kerr-Wilson, & Lang, 2014), many of which are not quantifiable (Morrow & Varcoe, 2000). In 2016, the Chief Public Health Officer (CPHO) of Canada's annual report focused on family violence, cementing the significance of violence as a public health problem in Canada. The CPHO noted that family violence affects health

> beyond just immediate physical injury, and increases the risk for a number of conditions, including depression, anxiety, post-traumatic stress disorder, as well as high blood pressure, cancer and heart disease. Despite the work of many researchers, health care professionals, organizations and communities, we still do not have a good understanding of why family violence happens, nor do we know how best to intervene. (Public Health Agency of Canada, 2016)

Building on the 2016 CPHO report, this chapter discusses violence against women, with a particular focus on intimate partner violence and sexual assault, as a health issue in Canada and how gender-transformative health promotion—health promotion interventions that address both gender equity and health—may offer some promising directions for prevention.

BACKGROUND

Defining Violence against Women

As a UN organization, the World Health Organization (WHO) uses the definition of violence against women embraced by the UN General Assembly in 1993 as "any act of gender-based violence that results in, or is likely to result in, physical, sexual or mental harm or suffering to women, including threats of such acts, coercion or arbitrary deprivation of liberty, whether occurring in public or private life."[3] And while violence against women exists on a "continuum from name-calling to homicide"[4] (see box 7.1), worldwide there is a distinct pattern of violence against women. Unlike violence against men, violence against women (and girls) is more likely than not to involve an assailant or perpetrator who is known to or is an acquaintance of the survivor (though of course men and individuals across the gender spectrum are also subject to intimate partner violence). That is, VAW commonly involves intimate partner or family violence and/or non-partner sexual violence by a person known to the woman.

The nature of VAW changes with time and social conditions. For example, new crimes such as cyber-violence, which has had tragic consequences in Canada,[5] have yet to be incorporated adequately into monitoring systems (Sinha, 2013) and data gaps persist for activities such as trafficking and female genital mutilation in many jurisdictions. Moreover, in Canada, both official (police) and self-reported (population-based survey) rates of offences such as intimate partner violence are assumed to be underestimates, given the stigma

Box 7.1: What Constitutes Violence against Women?

Violence against women manifests in various forms, including

- Intimate partner violence
- Non-partner sexual assault
- Dating violence
- Economically coerced sex
- Forced pregnancy and/or abortion
- Sex-selective abortion
- Trafficking
- So-called honour crimes
- Sexual harassment and exploitation
- Intimidation
- Stalking
- Witchcraft/sorcery-related violence
- Gender-related killings/female infanticide/femicide
- Female genital mutilation
- Child, early, and forced marriage
- Forced and child prostitution and pornography
- Dowry-related violence
- Online/cyberbullying

Source: Adapted from UN Women (2015); World Health Organization (1997, 2013).

and risks associated with disclosure (Sinha, 2013; Wathen & MacMillan, 2014). Thus it is fair to say that what is officially known about VAW is likely the proverbial tip of the iceberg. However, generating a picture of violence against women is critical to understanding its nature, distribution, trends over time, and whether any populations of women and girls are particularly vulnerable.

Benoit, Shumka, Phillips, Kennedy, & Belle-Isle (2015) argue that determining the scope of sexual violence against women—which is a broader lens than what is used in this chapter—is difficult because there are numerous terms used to discuss the issues, ranging from *domestic violence/abuse* (which prioritizes the setting) to *family violence* (a gender-neutral term) to *intimate partner violence/abuse* (which prioritizes the relationship) to *dating violence* (which suggests it involves younger people). What they contend, however, is that a consistent thread through all of these terms is the "implicit recognition that violence is gendered" (p. 4). However, "what is not always clear is whether or not the violence being referred to is sexual" (p. 4). This discussion reminds us that in order to compare data sources, terminology needs to be clear and consistent, which is part of the challenge when analysts look at estimates of VAW in Canada.

A Gender Lens on VAW

What does it mean to say that there is an implicit understanding that violence is "gendered"? It means, in part, that with respect to some forms of violence there are distinct patterns such that women are more likely to be victimized and men are more likely to victimize (Benoit et al., 2015). In this way, gender is a fundamental determinant of health—or, as in this case, determinant of a risk to health (Benoit & Nuernberger, 2007; Doyal, 2001). Whereas *sex* refers to one's biology (anatomy and physiology) and is typically labelled according the external genitalia one has at birth (i.e., penis, vulva), *gender* refers to socially constructed roles and norms typically ascribed to people based on the two, binary sex categories of male and female. Sex can be found on a continuum and includes individuals who are intersexed. Gender too has typically been ascribed on the basis of the two sex categories although it is increasingly understood to exist on a very wide continuum of diverse gender expressions (Johnson, Greaves, & Repta, 2009). Gender, however, is not limited to individual experiences and expressions of identity. Johnson, Greaves, & Repta (2009, para. 10), for example, distinguish between "gender identity at the individual level, gender relations at the interpersonal or group level, and institutional gender at the macro level," all of which have implications for patterns of gender-based violence.

Taking this discussion a step further, it is important to recognize that not only are there differences between women and men in patterns of violence, there are also differences among women such that not all women are equally likely to be victimized. The concept of intersectionality helps to explain such differences between women by highlighting the interactions of a woman's identity with other aspects of her social location such as age, disability, income, education, ethnicity/race, sexual orientation, employment status, residence, immigration status, and so on (Hankivsky et al., 2010; Mullings & Schulz, 2006; Reid, Pederson, & Dupéré, 2012). Intersectional theory contends that "different dimensions of social life cannot be separated into discrete or pure strands" (Brah & Phoenix, 2004, p. 76). Social categories of difference, such as those arising from income, race, education, and age, are complex, fluid, and flexible, yet may intersect to reduce or increase the likelihood of victimization, as might be the case for newcomer women who are undocumented and therefore dependent on family and a partner for security, shelter, and income (Guruge & Khanlou, 2004) or, for example, for Indigenous women who work in the sex industry (Benoit et al., 2015).

For the purposes of health promotion research, policy, and practice, intersectionality is an analytic tool and framework that is useful at both the micro and macro levels. At a micro level it aims to understand the effects of structural inequities on individual lives; it focuses on the interaction between social categories and (multiple) sources of power and privilege—arising from gender, race, and class, for example. At a macro level it seeks to understand how multiple power systems (i.e., institutions) are implicated in the production, organization, and maintenance of inequities (Hankivsky et al., 2010; Mullings & Schulz, 2006; Reid, Pederson, & Dupéré, 2012). In the case of the health sector, an intersectional analysis asks about how the systems within health care structure, limit, erase, or highlight certain health issues and particular types or groups of patients rather than others. With respect to VAW, we can ask how the health sector constructs some women as more likely to be victimized than others, silences patients from disclosing particular experiences of violence, and/or creates conditions that reproduce structural and interpersonal violence.

GRIM STATISTICS

Violence against women is difficult to measure, as much goes unreported (Provincial Health Officer, 2011), yet grasping the nature and scale of VAW is an essential part of any policy and action agenda.

Prevalence Estimates

In 2013, the WHO, London School of Hygiene and Tropical Medicine, and South African Medical Research Council released "the first global systematic review and synthesis of the body of scientific data on the prevalence of two forms of violence against women— violence by an intimate partner (intimate partner violence) and sexual violence by someone other than a partner (non-partner sexual violence)" (WHO, 2013, p. 2). The findings are disturbing; worldwide, it is estimated that 35 percent of women have experienced some form of physical and/or sexual violence from either an intimate partner or non-partner. The most common form of VAW is intimate partner violence (IPV).

Estimating the prevalence of violence against women in Canada is challenging. Analysts note that there is likely tremendous underreporting due to the reluctance of women to disclose their experience, whether to police, health workers, or surveyors (Sinha, 2013) (though the WHO suggests that health care workers are the most likely to receive reports of disclosure). Estimates based on police-reported administrative surveys, captured in the Uniform Crime Reporting Survey and Homicide Survey, reflect only those events that come to the attention of the justice system, while population-based surveys, such as the General Social Survey (GSS), attempt to capture self-reported victimization rates (Sinha, 2013; Statistics Canada, 2016).

Both police reports and survey data suggest that women and men tended to be victims of similar offences, including common assault, uttering threats, serious assault, sexual assault, and criminal harassment, but women were more likely than men to be victims of a sexual offence, and offences against women were more likely to be committed by intimate partners, including spouses and dating partners (Sinha, 2013). Indeed, intimate partners represented "45% of all those accused of victimizing women, followed by acquaintances or friends (27%), strangers (16%) and non-spousal family members (12%)" (Sinha, 2013, p. 14). In contrast, the perpetrators of violent crimes against men were least likely to be intimate partners (only 12%). This distinct pattern means that the men closest to a woman pose the greatest threat to her safety and wellbeing.

Self-reported spousal violence has declined since 2004 (Statistics Canada, 2016) but remains a significant problem. Risk of violence escalates following the breakup of relationships; both women and men report being victimized more than six months after a separation, with women were more likely than men to report serious forms of spousal violence such as sexual assault or being threatened with a gun or knife (Statistics Canada, 2016).

Others can also be affected by spousal violence in which women are the victims. Some 11 percent of female spousal victims reported in the 2009 GSS that they were pregnant and a similar number reported that the perpetrator had physically or sexually abused another family member (Sinha, 2013). In addition to direct harm, children can also witness violence against women; nearly 60 percent of female spousal victims with children reported that the children had witnessed violence against them, compared to 43 percent of male spousal victims (Sinha, 2013).

Women are vastly more likely than men to be sexually assaulted. According to police-reported data, 92 percent of sexual assault survivors aged 15 and older in 2009 were women. While police data estimate there were 15,500 victims of sexual assault in 2009, this compared to self-reported survey data from the 2009 GSS, in which women reported 472,000 sexual assaults, a rate of 34 sexual assault incidents per 1,000 women (this contrasts with a rate of approximately 15 sexual assaults reported per 1,000 men) (Sinha, 2013). The extent of underreporting of sexual assault to police challenges our understanding of the extent of this problem and has implications for service providers in multiple sectors, including health.

Who Is Vulnerable?

While VAW occurs throughout the life-course, women aged 18 to 44, the prime reproductive years, are particularly vulnerable (UN Women, 2015). And while violence is a problem for women in all social classes, certain groups of women are especially vulnerable, including women with a disability; women from minority ethnic or Indigenous communities; refugees and asylum seekers; lesbian, bisexual, transgender, or intersex individuals (who are particularly at risk of non-partner sexual assault); low-income women; women living with HIV infection; and those living in rural and remote communities (WHO, 2013). Data from the GSS suggest that individuals who self-identify as Aboriginal were two times as likely as non-Aboriginal people to report having experienced spousal violence in the previous five years (Statistics Canada, 2016). Current research also suggests that there is a strong link between childhood experiences of maltreatment and subsequent spousal victimization later in life—a reminder of the importance of supports for families and parenting and for interventions that support young children (MacMillan, 2010; Statistics Canada, 2016) and for attention to the intergenerational effects of colonization, discrimination, and residential schooling (Bombay, Matheson, & Anisman, 2014). The 2014 GSS also documented "that individuals who described themselves as gay, lesbian, or bisexual were twice as likely as heterosexuals to report having been the victim of spousal violence during the previous 5 years" (Statistics Canada, 2016, p. 14)—especially lesbian or bisexual women.

Benoit et al. (2015) note that there is "sparse literature addressing elevated sexual violence among women with disabilities" though there is some Canadian evidence that people with activity limitations are victims of both sexual and physical assault about twice as often as those without such limitations (Perreault, 2009). Those with severe disabilities, living in institutions, and those with mental disorders seem to be at more risk. DisAbled Women's Network of Canada (DAWN Canada) suggests that although 20 percent of women in Canada live with a disability, in one study, 40 percent of respondents reported having experienced some form of violence in their lifetime. Notably, researchers seldom assess intimate partner violence among women with disabilities so it often is not detected or recorded. Finally, disabled women also experience barriers to reporting victimization that women without disabilities do not necessarily experience.[6] Other women who are more likely to experience sexual violence, including sexual assault, include women working in the sex industry, particularly outdoor sex workers (Benoit et al., 2015).

VAW Is a Health Promotion Issue

Globally, research has documented that VAW can have serious and lasting health impacts (WHO, 2013). It is the leading cause of death and disability among women worldwide (Fulu et al., 2014). IPV may result in death; data suggest that in 2012 almost half of female murder victims were killed by family members or intimate partners (United Nations Office on Drugs and Crime, 2014). For those who are not murdered, the effects of violence and abuse include alcohol and substance use disorders and anxiety or depression (WHO, 2013). Reproductive impacts include low birth-weight babies, pre-term birth, and higher rates of induced abortion (WHO, 2013).

As mentioned, Canada's Chief Public Health Officer has identified family violence as a public health issue, noting that the health impacts of family violence "extend far beyond physical injuries and include poor mental health, psychological and emotional distress, suicide, and increased risk of chronic diseases and conditions such as cancer, heart disease and diabetes." Also, taking a public health view of IPV, the PreVAiL Network reports that it has direct physical, mental, and emotional harms but also leads to health risk behaviours such as alcohol and drug abuse, smoking, unsafe sexual practices, and physical inactivity—many of the areas of core public health concern (Wathen & MacMillan, 2014).

Some of the physical consequences of IPV exposure include chronic pain; disability; fibromyalgia; gastrointestinal disorders; irritable bowel syndrome (IBS); sleep disorders; generally low health-related quality of life; and possibly cardiac problems (Wathen, 2013). IPV is also associated with reproductive issues (e.g., pelvic inflammatory disease [PID]; pregnancy complications; miscarriage; sexual dysfunction) and psychological, social, behavioural, and emotional difficulties including depression; anxiety; substance use disorders; sleep disorders; suicidal behaviour; self-harm; and post-traumatic stress disorder (PTSD) (Wathen, 2013). Sexual assault tends to produce fewer physical injuries but also has gynecological and reproductive impacts such as bleeding, fibroids, pain, and sexually transmitted diseases, including HIV. The mental health impacts are similar to IPV and include depression, anxiety, and PTSD—the latter being particularly strongly associated with sexual assault (Wathen, 2013). In short, the impact of VAW can be diverse, dramatic, and chronic—damaging lives for a lifetime.

EXPLAINING VIOLENCE AGAINST WOMEN

Ecological models suggest that there is no single factor that causes violence, no "single pathway to perpetration" (Fulu et al., 2014, p. 4), however, it is generally agreed that the root causes of VAW are gender inequality and discrimination and recognized that these are shaped by social norms, practices, and structures that act and interact at the individual, relationship/family, community/organizational, and societal levels (UN Women, 2015). Economic, political, and social factors, including legislation, policy, and legal frameworks, can contribute to a context of respect for gender equality, while historical factors such as environmental disaster, conflict, colonization, and economic restructuring can foster gender inequalities and increase vulnerability risk (UN Women, 2015). In sum, VAW emerges through the interaction of multiple factors, from genetic endowment to developmental experience to household structures and dynamics to relationship interactions, all within a context of forces that "shape prevailing norms, access to resources, and the relative standing of men versus women" (Fulu et al., 2014, p. 4).

ADDRESSING VIOLENCE AGAINST WOMEN

UN Women (2015, p. 4) suggests that

> To prevent violence before it happens or reoccurs means that our work has to demonstrate and teach what inequality is, and how its continued existence is preventing progress. We know that community mobilization, group interventions for both women and men, educational programmes and empowerment of women are some of the interventions that have impact.

These actions recognize that VAW is "rooted in gender inequality, discrimination and harmful cultural and social norms" (UN Women, 2015, p. 8). Accordingly, interventions to prevent, reduce, or address the impact of violence against women need to acknowledge and address these root causes. This entails addressing the social, political, and economic structures that influence violence, as well as social norms and practices that condone or ignore it, such as through interventions that raise awareness of violence and try to change social norms with regard to its acceptability, through interventions to enhance the social and economic empowerment of women, and through prevention interventions that engage men and boys in addition to girls and women in school-based, peer, or relationship interventions (Fulu et al., 2014). There is also evidence to suggest that interventions to promote healthy early childhood development and reduce substance use and depression are part of the spectrum of actions to reduce and prevent VAW (Fulu et al., 2014).

A Gender-Transformative Health Promotion Approach

Framing VAW through the lens of public health makes the call for prevention appear clear, visible, and feasible—though evidence is desperately needed for each stage of the continuum; for the various levels of the ecological model of violence against women; and to address the features, mandates, and responsibilities of the different sectors involved (e.g., justice, policing, education, health, social services, post-secondary education) (Wathen & MacMillan, 2014). A prevention lens also identifies opportunities for intervention. Alberta's *Family Violence Hurts Everyone* document (Government of Alberta, 2013) identifies six levels on the spectrum of prevention of family violence that range from action with individuals to policy change—classic health promotion interventions.

1. Strengthening individual knowledge and skills
2. Promoting community education
3. Educating service providers and practitioners
4. Fostering coalitions and networks
5. Changing organizational practices
6. Influencing policy and legislation

These different levels of prevention align with the key strategies of the *Ottawa Charter for Health Promotion* (WHO, 1986).

Introducing Gender-Responsiveness

While these approaches reflect traditional health promotion approaches, recent evidence suggests that the most effective interventions to prevent VAW are ones that seek to transform root causes such as fostering gender equity, for example, by challenging assumptions about caregiving and economic contributions to the household, and which focus not only on attitudinal but behavioural change (UN Women, 2015). Gender-transformative interventions have their origins in the fight against HIV (Gupta, 2000) and the concept has been adopted by the WHO (2009) and USAIDS (Boender et al., 2004). More recently, Canadians have examined how health promotion could be more gender-responsive (Fang, Gerbrandt, Liwander, & Pederson, 2014; Greaves, Pederson, & Poole, 2014; Pederson et al., 2014) and evidence has been accumulating on the effectiveness of gender-responsive approaches in adolescent health (WHO, 2011a, 2011b) and physical activity in men (Bottorff et al., 2015).

Gender-transformative interventions specifically seek to shift gender norms and relations to enhance gender equity. They can be envisioned as one end of a continuum of action on gender and health (see figure 7.1). Moving from gender-unequal approaches through those that are gender-sensitive to those that are gender-transformative moves the intervention from exploitation to accommodation to transformation. Gender-sensitive approaches, such as some of the physical activity interventions that accommodate and work with men's interest in professional sports as a way to support their engagement in physical activity, are showing success in influencing health practices and outcomes

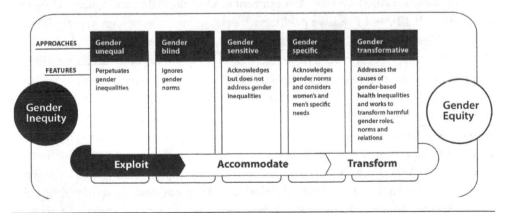

Figure 7.1: A Continuum of Approaches to Action on Gender and Health

Source: Greaves, L., Pederson, A., & Poole, N. (Eds.). (2014). *Making it better: Gender-transformative health promotion* (pp. 22). Toronto: Canadian Scholars' Press/Women's Press.

(Bottorff et al., 2015; Hunt, McCann, Gray, Mutrie, & Wyke, 2013). In contrast, gender-transformative approaches challenge the very social norms that underpin sports as principally an activity for men or question the portrayal of women and girls in health education on substance use during pregnancy (Poole, Bopp, & Greaves, 2014).

In the context of reducing or preventing violence against women, there are some encouraging findings regarding approaches and interventions that address men's and boys' discriminatory attitudes towards women and girls, and support both genders to engage in healthy relationships, manage alcohol abuse, and balance domestic responsibilities.

Select Examples of Gender-Transformative Health Promotion and Addressing Violence against Women in Canada

Policy Supports

Canada is a signatory to the Convention on the Elimination of All Forms of Violence Against Women (CEDAW) a key document that recognizes violence against women as a human rights violation (Abraham & Tastsoglou, 2016), which sends an important signal to other countries as well as to anti-violence advocates within Canada. In addition, the federal government has made numerous policy commitments to address VAW including a recent strategy on gender-based violence (Status of Women Canada, 2017) and funding for the Family Violence Initiative, which brings together over a dozen departments and agencies to prevent and respond to family violence; the Public Health Agency of Canada coordinates this initiative.

All provinces and territories have made commitments to address violence against women including Alberta (Government of Alberta, 2013), British Columbia (Government of British Columbia, 2015), Ontario (Government of Ontario, 2015), and Québec (Province of Québec, 2012), and five have published specific plans of action on sexual violence: Ontario, New Brunswick, Nova Scotia, Manitoba, and Québec (Benoit et al., 2015). In Atlantic Canada, cyberbullying has received significant attention; Nova Scotia was the first province in the country to establish a special cyberbullying investigative unit. In addition, the Atlantic Ministers Responsible for the Status of Women launched the cybersafegirl.ca website in the fall of 2012, a joint initiative to support girls and young women. The three territorial governments fund victim services and cyber-exploitation awareness for children (Yukon) as aspects of their actions on violence but do not currently have comprehensive action plans.[7] A thorough analysis is needed to shed light on the extent to which these various policies are explicit about the gendered nature of some of these forms of violence. Are young women, for example, more at risk for cyberbullying than young men, particularly as a result of sexual exploitation? Thus while the gendered nature of violence may not be sufficiently visible, policy statements such as these create the context for health promotion practitioners and researchers to engage in efforts to address VAW and, ideally, to explore interventions to prevent it.

National Inquiry into Missing and Murdered Indigenous Women and Girls

A particularly important initiative currently underway, which will undoubtedly set direction for important restorative and preventive initiatives, is the two-year National Inquiry into Missing and Murdered Indigenous Women and Girls, established in 2016[8] in response to national alarm over the 1,181 "missing and murdered" women and girls identified in a police report in 2014 (Royal Canadian Mounted Police, 2014) and by numerous Canadian and international Indigenous and women's advocacy groups (e.g., Committee on the Elimination of Discrimination against Women, 2015; Native Women's Association of Canada, 2010). The disproportionate vulnerability of Indigenous women and girls to violence calls for thoughtful discussion, analysis, and engagement with issues such as poverty, homelessness, racism, sexism, education, and limited economic opportunities, and the legacies of colonization, residential schools, and systemic racism (Daoud, Smylie, Urquia, Allan, & O'Campo, 2013; Pearce et al., 2015).

Health promoters can contribute to addressing the conditions that foster violence against Indigenous women and girls as well as join in efforts to prevent these conditions from continuing. As individuals, we need to educate and inform ourselves on the history of colonization and its repercussions in Indigenous communities. This could mean participating in Indigenous Cultural Safety training for those working in the health sector (see www.sanyas.ca) or reading about reconciliation to explore one's own understanding of the issues (see Metcalfe-Chenai, 2016). It may mean confronting one's own understandings and feelings about being Indigenous or a settler in this country. It can involve becoming an ally to Indigenous communities through education and support for action[9] and taking training on Indigenous health. Organizationally, it may mean conducting analyses to ensure that data on Indigenous people are represented in general public data and reporting; ensuring that Indigenous workers are hired and supported to flourish; and working together to ensure that health promotion practices are not further colonizing or discriminating. Finally, it may mean tailoring interventions to be acceptable, appropriate, and accessible to Indigenous people, in partnership with those who can guide us on how to do so.

Improving the Health Sector Response

Recent reviews (Ellsberg et al., 2015; García-Moreno et al., 2015) suggest that low- and middle-income countries have paid greater attention to preventing VAW, often through actions to prevent HIV infection, whereas high-income countries have focused on clinical and community responses to VAW. There are actions underway in Canada to improve the health care response to VAW such as the PreVAiL team on the Violence, Evidence, Guidance and Action (VEGA) project (www.projectvega.ca). The aim of this work is to provide curricula for different provider groups in various settings, based on the principles of trauma- and violence-informed care, cultural safety and competence, and sex- and gender-based analysis principles. Another concrete example is the development of online education regarding gender-based violence to be made available to those working in the health sector across British Columbia, an estimated 170,000 workers. The challenge remains, however, to move the health sector from responding to violence to contributing to its prevention. This means, for example, bridging the divide between seeing violence as "intentional" or "unintentional" and shifting our thinking toward seeing it as preventable; this would mean including action on violence in social marketing campaigns such as those run in British Columbia and Alberta.[10]

Meeting the Sustainable Development Goals

It has been suggested that the 17 Sustainable Development Goals (SDGs) offer an important new opportunity for both Canada's domestic and international agendas to incorporate actions to improve human health, wellbeing, and quality of life through integrating economic, social, and environmental policies.[11] Goal 5 of the SDGs is "achieve gender equality and empower all women and girls."[12] This goal identifies VAW as a violation of girls' and women's human rights that "hinders development," linking the issue of addressing VAW to other pressing economic, social, and environmental priorities.

For example, research into natural disasters—which are understood to be more common and severe as a result of climate change—has illustrated that there are important sex/gender considerations to be managed in disaster preparation and relief efforts in Canada (Enarson, 2008). "Gender influences who is vulnerable to which impacts of a natural disaster."[13] Disasters strain social networks, introduce uncertainty, and increase demands on services. There was just such a concern following the wildfire that forced the evacuation of Fort McMurray, Alberta, in the spring of 2016. In Fort McMurray, clients of the city's only emergency shelter had to be relocated along with the rest of the community; the clients lost access to dedicated domestic violence support immediately and observers worried about what the crisis would do to displaced survivors.[14] Reports of gender-based violence after Hurricane Katrina rose significantly, from an estimated 4.6 per 100,000 people per day before the hurricane to 16.3 per 100,000 people per day a year after the disaster (Hunt et al., 2013). Following a systematic review of the literature, Rezaeian (2013) confirmed that, though the evidence is still limited, higher rates of rape and sexual abuse against girls and women have been documented following natural disasters such as hurricanes, tsunami, floods, and earthquakes. Among the strategies for mitigating this risk, he suggests active efforts to quickly reunite children who are separated from their official guardians; creating safe, secure places for women and girls who are on their own; providing proper health services that include reproductive care; and offering counselling and legal support for survivors. Others suggest ensuring that women are involved as leaders in disaster responses (Ha-Redeye, 2009) and ensuring that greater recognition is given to the needs of diverse gender minorities who, by virtue of their marginalization in society, have their specific vulnerabilities in the context of disaster (Gaillard et al., 2016). These and other gender-sensitive responses would go a long way to reducing the risks of violence and its many consequences. And while clearly Goal 5 also involves activities such as addressing the gender wage gap, differences in access to education for various gender groups, and participation in leadership/governance roles, addressing violence against women is inextricably linked to the SDGs in complex ways and could bring new actors into sustainable development activities.

Programming with Men and Boys

Globally, evidence is accumulating regarding the value of working with men and boys to prevent and reduce violence against women and girls:

> interventions have been motivated by a desire to address the role of men in violence perpetration, and recognition that masculinity and gender-related social norms are implicated in violence. Although not all men are violent, all men and boys have a positive part to play to help stop violence against women. (Jewkes, Rachel, Michael, & James, 2015, p. 1580)

While in high-income countries many interventions over the past 20 years addressed only women or consisted of establishing key sectoral responses to violence such as emergency health services, shelters, and housing (Ellsberg et al., 2015), work with men and boys emerged from interventions to reduce HIV infection, often in low- and middle-income countries.

Today in Canada, there are many initiatives that involve men and boys as change agents to reduce violence against women and girls. In BC, for example, the Ending Violence Association of BC (EVA BC) established the Be More than a Bystander campaign in 2011 in partnership with the BC Lions football club, with support from Status of Women Canada, the BC Ministry of Children and Family Development, and Encana Corporation. Campaigns such as this one aim to raise awareness of violence against women and encourage men to be allies in preventing violence. This particular initiative includes having members of the football team deliver training to coaches of boys' football teams about VAW and how to speak about VAW and respectful relationships.[15] Evaluation of this initiative suggests it has reached vast numbers of individuals including coaches, players, students, and fans, and has successfully increased understanding of VAW (Deyer, 2014). Other initiatives to raise awareness include It Starts with You, It Stays with Him, an initiative of the White Ribbon Canada group (see www.whiteribbon.ca), which works to challenge "harmful ideas of manhood that lead to violence against women"; and the Moose Hide Campaign (moosehidecompaign.ca), a grassroots movement of Aboriginal and non-Aboriginal men who are standing up and speaking out against violence towards Aboriginal women and children. A very recent initiative of the First Nations Health Authority in BC is the Commitment Stick Initiative, which involves the use of Commitment Sticks as individual expressions of a commitment to live violence-free and to actively stop violence against Indigenous girls and women (see www.fnha.ca/wellness/commitment-stick).

Home Visiting Programs

There is emerging evidence of the value of in-home visiting by health care professionals as a means of identifying and reducing VAW. For example, British Columbia and Ontario have both implemented versions of the Nurse-Family Partnership (NFP), which was not originally designed to address intimate partner violence (IPV) but was later modified to include content on identifying and responding to IPV (Jack et al., 2012). The NFP is a home-visiting program in which public health nurses establish therapeutic relationships with first-time young mothers to help foster parenting skills and improve both the mother's and child's health and wellbeing. The findings from a pilot study by Jack et al. (2012) suggest that, among other things, the relationship between the nurse and mother make disclosure of IPV safer. The findings of the BC version of the program (the British Columbia Healthy Connections program) are just emerging but look promising (Jack et al., 2015).

Supporting Healthy Relationships

Supporting young people to learn about healthy relationships is another strategy that is being employed to help reduce violence in relationships. This is one dimension of the Be More than a Bystander program described above, which targeted men and boys, but it can be a focus of other types of interventions as well. For example, there are programs specific to Indigenous girls, such as the Ask Auntie project piloted in BC (see www.indigenousyouthwellness.ca/ask-auntie), that ground the discussion of healthy relationships in culture and traditional practices, and emphasize that healthy relationships are not limited to "dating" relationships. A national organization devoted to supporting girls, the Girls Action Foundation (www.girlsactionfoundation.ca), has conducted extensive programming with girls across the country and produced supports to help prevent violence, such as an infographic.[16] Girls-only programming may be a critical aspect of violence prevention as it offers girls and young women a safe physical and social space to learn, connect with others, explore their identity, and meet older girls and women.

CONCLUSION

This chapter has introduced VAW as a health promotion issue and argued that health promotion has the potential to contribute to reducing and preventing it. None of the initiatives described in this chapter are sufficient in themselves to stop VAW in Canada, but might they, in combination, create the tipping point (Gladwell, 2000)? What combination of policies, education, training, and structures will create the conditions for change that is so needed? What supports for healthy relationships, community wellness, and self-care can health promoters develop, assess, and share? How can we shift from gender-blind programming to gender-transformative?

The prime minister of Canada[17] recently stated that "Violence against women is not a women's issue. Men must boldly challenge the attitudes and behaviours that allow this violence to exist, and that allow disrespect for and abuse of women to become commonplace."

Will statements like this mobilize the health promotion community to also step up and engage on this issue, applying its ethics, methods, and resourcefulness to improving gender equity while addressing the health effects of violence against women? May it be so.

CRITICAL THINKING QUESTIONS

1. How can health promotion contribute to preventing violence against women?
2. What do you think are the barriers to violence prevention?
3. What does gender-transformative health promotion mean?

RESOURCES

Further Readings

Greaves, L., Pederson, A., & Poole, N. (2014). *Making it better: Gender transformative health promotion*. Toronto: Women's Press.
This book offers a substantial introduction to the theory and practice of gender-transformative health promotion, with particular attention to case studies and topics relevant to Canada.
    Available from Canadian Scholars/Women's Press at womenspress.canadianscholars.ca/books/making-it-better.

UN Women. (2015). *A framework to underpin action to prevent violence against women*. New York: Author.
    www.unwomen.org/en/digital-library/publications/2015/11/prevention-framework
This framework outlines an ecological approach to preventing violence against women and links action on VAW to the 2020 Agenda for Sustainable Development. The publication is available in English, French, and Spanish.

Relevant Websites

Gender Equity through Health Promotion
promotinghealthinwomen.ca/
    This website was developed to share practical tools, offer online training, and provide information on gender-transformative health promotion.

Preventing Violence Across the Lifespan Research Network, PreVAiL
prevailresearch.ca/
    PreVAiL is an international research collaboration of over 60 researchers and partners from Canada, the US, the UK, Asia, Europe, and Australia, funded by the Canadian Institutes of Health Research's Institute for Gender and Health (2009–2017). This website contains useful resources and research briefs.

Stop Family Violence, Public Health Agency of Canada
www.phac-aspc.gc.ca/sfv-avf/index-eng.php

This website is a useful entry point to the PHAC's activities to address family violence, including violence against women.

Infographics

Violence against Women: The Health Sector Responds
www.who.int/violence_injury_prevention/publications/pvl_infographic.pdf

Violence against Women: Global Picture Health Response
www.who.int/reproductivehealth/publications/violence/VAW_infographic.pdf

Girls Action on Violence Prevention
girlsactionfoundation.ca/en/infographics/girls-action-on-violence-preventions

NOTES

1. www.swc-cfc.gc.ca/commemoration/vaw-vff/index-en.html
2. www.swc-cfc.gc.ca/commemoration/vaw-vff/remembrance-commemoration-en.html
3. www.un.org/documents/ga/res/48/a48r104.htm
4. The exact origin of this phrase is difficult to determine but it was used in Sinha (2013) and in a recent LNG Canada Export Terminal Environmental Assessment Certificate Application (see a100.gov.bc.ca/appsdata/epic/documents/p398/d38157/1415047927217_KGyFJXmP1x2sG8wCmyvdfS27j60hvHtwhPJZxGRMqpgdrdszwXMw!-1038573416!141504683147.pdf). A significantly earlier use of the same words can be found in Boyle's (1992) paper entitled "School's a rough place: Youth gangs, drug users, and family life in Los Angeles," available at files.eric.ed.gov/fulltext/ED360435.pdf
5. This is a reference to the case of Amanda Todd, a 15-year-old girl who committed suicide following cyberbullying and sexual exploitation. See www.theglobeandmail.com/news/national/multiple-vigils-celebrate-bc-teen-amanda-todd-condemn-bullying/article4625976/
6. DisAbled Women's Network of Canada. Factsheet: Women with Disabilities and Violence. www.dawncanada.net/main/wp-content/uploads/2014/03/English-Violence-January-2014.pdf
7. Policy Centre for Victim Services. www.justice.gc.ca/eng/rp-pr/cj-jp/victim/news-bulit/iss13-bul13.html
8. Government of Canada webpage on the National Inquiry into Missing and Murdered Indigenous Women and Girls. www.aadnc-aandc.gc.ca/eng/1448633299414/1448633350146
9. See Indigenous Issues 101 at apihtawikosisan.com/aboriginal-issue-primers/
10. See *The British Columbia Casebook for Injury Prevention* at www.injuryresearch.bc.ca/wp-content/uploads/2015/08/BCIRPU-Casebook-2015.pdf and www.preventable.ca

11. This is a blog entry by Livia Bizikova and Darren Swanson on the International Institute for Sustainable Development website dated April 20, 2016. See www.iisd.org/blog/towards-strategy-implementing-2030-agenda-sustainable-development-canada

12. See sustainabledevelopment.un.org/sdg5

13. This a blog entry by Barbara Clabots, on *The Seattle Globalist*, posted May 11, 2016. See www.seattleglobalist.com/2016/05/11/climate-change-violence-against-women-connection/51105

14. See www.cbc.ca/news/canada/edmonton/domestic-abuse-concerns-in-aftermath-of-fort-mcmurray-fire-1.3629228

15. endingviolence.org/prevention-programs/be-more-than-a-bystander/

16. Girls Action on Violence Prevention infographic. girlsactionfoundation.ca/en/infographics/girls-action-on-violence-preventions

17. Statement by the Prime Minister of Canada on the International Day for the Elimination of Violence Against Women. pm.gc.ca/eng/news/2016/11/25/statement-prime-minister-canada-international-day-elimination-violence-against-women

REFERENCES

Abraham, M., & Tastsoglou, E. (2016). Addressing domestic violence in Canada and the United States: The uneasy co-habitation of women and the state. *Current Sociology, 64*(4), 568–585. doi: 10.1177/0011392116639221

Benoit, C., & Nuernberger, K. (2007). *Health determinants and women's health.* Paper presented at the Women's Health Research Network Workshop, Victoria, BC.

Benoit, C., Shumka, L., Phillips, R., Kennedy, M. C., & Belle-Isle, L. (2015). *Issue brief: Sexual violence against women in Canada.* Ottawa: Federal-Provincial-Territorial Senior Officials for the Status of Women.

Boender, C., Santana, D., Santillan, D., Hardee, K., Greene, M. E., & Shuler, S. (2004). *The "so what?" report. A look at whether integrating a gender focus into programs makes a difference in outcomes.* Washington, DC: Interagency Gender Working Group & USAIDS.

Bombay, A., Matheson, K., & Anisman, H. (2014). The intergenerational effects of Indian Residential Schools: Implications for the concept of historical trauma. *Transcultural Psychiatry, 51*(3), 320–338. doi: 10.1177/1363461513503380

Bottorff, J. L., Seaton, C. L., Johnson, S. T., Caperchione, C. M., Oliffe, J. L., More, K., … Tillotson, S. M. (2015). An updated review of interventions that include promotion of physical activity for adult men. *Sports Medicine (Auckland, N.z.), 45*(6), 775–800. doi: 10.1007/s40279-014-0286-3

Brah, A., & Phoenix, A. (2004). Ain't I a woman? Revisiting intersectionality. *Journal of International Women's Studies, 5*(3), 75.

Committee on the Elimination of Discrimination against Women. (2015). *Report of the inquiry concerning Canada of the Committee of the Elimination of Discrimination against Women under article 8 of the Optional Protocol to the Convention on the Elimination of All Forms of Discrimination against Women.* New York: Author.

Daoud, N., Smylie, J., Urquia, M., Allan, B., & O'Campo, P. (2013). The contribution of socio-economic position to the excesses of violence and intimate partner violence among Aboriginal versus non-Aboriginal Women in Canada. *Can J Public Health, 104*(4), e278–e283.

Deyer, C. (2014). *Be More than a Bystander Program evaluation report: No ordinary win!* Vancouver, BC: Ending Violence Association of BC.

Doyal, L. (2001). Sex, gender, and health: The need for a new approach. *BMJ: British Medical Journal (09598138), 323*(7320), 1061–1063.

Dworkin, S. L., Kambou, S. D., Sutherland, C., Moalla, K., & Kapoor, A. (2009). Gendered empowerment and HIV prevention: Policy and programmatic pathways to success in the MENA region. *Journal Of Acquired Immune Deficiency Syndromes (1999), 51*(Suppl. 3), S111–S118.

Dworkin, S. L., Treves-Kagan, S., & Lippman, S. A. (2013). Gender-transformative interventions to reduce HIV risks and violence with heterosexually-active men: A review of the global evidence. *AIDS and Behavior, 17*(9), 2845–2863. doi: 10.1007/s10461-013-0565-2

Ellsberg, M., Arango, D. J., Morton, M., Gennari, F., Kiplesund, S., Contreras, M., & Watts, C. (2015). Prevention of violence against women and girls: What does the evidence say? *The Lancet, 385*(9977), 1555–1566. doi: 10.1016/S0140-6736(14)61703-7

Enarson, E. (2008). *Gender mainstreaming in emergency management: Opportunities for building community resilience in Canada.* Ottawa: Public Health Agency of Canada, Centre for Emergency Preparedness and Response.

Fang, M. L., Gerbrandt, J., Liwander, A., & Pederson, A. (2014). Exploring promising gender-sensitive tobacco and alcohol use interventions: Results of a scoping review. *Substance Use & Misuse, 49*(11), 1400–1416. doi: 10.3109/10826084.2014.912225

Fulu, E., Kerr-Wilson, A., & Lang, J. (2014). *What works to prevent violence against women and girls? Evidence Review of interventions to prevent violence against women and girls.* Pretoria: Medical Research Council.

Gaillard, J. C., Sanz, K., Balgos, B. C., Dalisay, S. N. M., Gorman-Murray, A., Smith, F., & Toelupe, V. A. (2016). Beyond men and women: A critical perspective on gender and disaster. *Disasters.* doi: 10.1111/disa.12209

García-Moreno, C., Hegarty, K., d'Oliveira, A. F. L., Koziol-McLain, J., Colombini, M., & Feder, G. (2015). The health-systems response to violence against women. *Lancet (London, England), 385*(9977), 1567–1579. doi: 10.1016/S0140-6736(14)61837-7

Gladwell, M. (2000). *The tipping point: How little things can make a big difference.* New York, NY: Back Bay Books/Little, Brown and Company.

Government of Alberta. (2013). *Family violence hurts everyone: A framework to end family violence in Alberta.* Retrieved from www.humanservices.alberta.ca/documents/family-violence-hurts-everyone.pdf

Government of British Columbia. (2015). *A vision for a violence free BC: Addressing violence against women in British Columbia.* Retrieved from www2.gov.bc.ca/assets/gov/law-crime-and-justice/criminal-justice/bc-criminal-justice-system/if-victim/publications/violence-free-bc.pdf

Government of Ontario. (2015). It's never okay: An action plan to stop sexual violence and harassment. Toronto: Queen's Printer for Ontario.

Greaves, L., Pederson, A., & Poole, N. (Eds.). (2014). *Making it better: Gender-transformative health promotion*. Toronto: Canadian Scholars' Press.

Gupta, G. R. (2000). *Gender, sexuality and HIV/AIDS: The what, the why and the how. Plenary address at the XIII International AIDS Conference*. Paper presented at the XIII International AIDS Conference, Durban, SA. Retrieved from www.un.org/womenwatch/daw/csw/hivaids/Gupta.html

Guruge, S., & Khanlou, N. (2004). Intersectionalities of influence: Researching the health of immigrant and refugee women. *Canadian Journal of Nursing Research, 36*(3), 33–47.

Hankivsky, O., Reid, C., Cormier, R., Varcoe, C., Clark, N., Benoit, C., & Brotman, S. (2010). Exploring the promises of intersectionality for advancing women's health research. *International Journal for Equity in Health, 9*(1), 1.

Ha-Redeye, O. (2009). "Engendering" change in disaster response: Increasing women in leadership roles. In M. Provost & D. Griffiths (Eds.), *Gender and disaster in Canada: New thinking, new direction (Workshop report)* (pp. 53–60). Sydney, Nova Scotia: Cape Breton University.

Hunt, K., McCann, C., Gray, C. M., Mutrie, N., & Wyke, S. (2013). You've got to walk before you run: Positive evaluations of a walking program as part of a gender-sensitized, weight-management program delivered to men through professional football clubs. *Health Psychology, 32*(1), 57–65. doi: 10.1037/a0029537

Jack, S. M., Busser, L. D., Sheehan, D., Gonzalez, A., Zwygers, E. J., & MacMillan, H. L. (2012). Adaptation and implementation of the nurse-family partnership in Canada. *Canadian Journal of Public Health/Revue Canadienne de Sante'e Publique, 103*, S42–S48.

Jack, S. M., Sheehan, D., Gonzalez, A., MacMillan, H. L., Catherine, N., & Waddell, C. (2015). British Columbia Healthy Connections Project process evaluation: A mixed methods protocol to describe the implementation and delivery of the Nurse-Family Partnership in Canada. *BMC Nursing, 14*, 47.

Jewkes, R., Rachel, J., Michael, F., & James, L. (2015). From work with men and boys to changes of social norms and reduction of inequities in gender relations: A conceptual shift in prevention of violence against women and girls. *The Lancet (British edition), 385*(9977), 1580–1589. doi: 10.1016/S0140-6736(14)61683-4

Johnson, J. L., Greaves, L., & Repta, R. (2009). Better science with sex and gender: Facilitating the use of a sex- and gender-based analysis in health research. *International Journal for Equity in Health, 8*(14).

MacMillan, H. (2010). *Research brief: Interventions to prevent child maltreatment*. London, ON: Preventing Violence Across the Lifespan Research Network.

Metcalfe-Chenai, D. (Ed.). (2016). *In this together: Fifteen stories of truth & reconciliation*. Victoria, BC: Brindle & Glass.

Morrow, M. H., & Varcoe, C. (2000). *Violence against women: Improving the health care response: A guide for health authorities, health care managers, providers and planners*. Victoria: British Columbia Women's Health Bureau.

Mullings, L., & Schulz, A. (2006). Intersectionality and health: An introduction. In A. Schulz & L. Mullings (Eds.), *Gender, race, class, and health: Intersectional approaches* (pp. 3–17). New York, NY: Jossey-Bass.

Native Women's Association of Canada. (2010). *Fact sheet: Missing and murdered Aboriginal women and girls in British Columbia.* Ottawa, ON: Author.

Pearce, M. E., Blair, A. H., Teegee, M., Pan, S. W., Thomas, V., Zhang, H., … Spittal, P. M. (2015). The Cedar Project: Historical trauma and vulnerability to sexual assault among young Aboriginal women who use illicit drugs in two Canadian cities. *Violence Against Women, 21*(3), 313–329.

Pederson, A., Greaves, L., & Poole, N. (2014). Gender-transformative health promotion for women: A framework for action. *Health Promotion International.* doi: 10.1093/heapro/dau083

Perreault, S. (2009). *Criminal Victimization and health: A profile of victimization among persons with activity limitations or other health problems.* Statistics Canada. Canadian Centre for Justice Statistics. Catalogue no. 85F0033M—No. 21. Retrieved from www.statcan.gc.ca/pub/85f0033m/85f0033m2009021-eng.pdf

Poole, N., Bopp, J., & Greaves, L. (2014). Provoking gender-transformative health promotion. In L. Greaves, A. Pederson, & N. Poole (Eds.), *Making it better: Gender-transformative health promotion* (pp. 195–211). Toronto: Canadian Scholars' Press.

Province of Québec. (2012). *Preventing, detecting, ending: 2012–2017 government action plan on domestic violence.* Québec City, Québec: Author.

Provincial Health Officer. (2011). *The health and well-being of women in British Columbia: Provincial Health Officer's 2008 annual report.* Victoria, BC: Office of the Provincial Health Officer.

Public Health Agency of Canada. (2016). *The Chief Public Health Officer's report on the state of public health in Canada 2016. A Focus on Family Violence in Canada.* Ottawa: Author.

Reid, C., Pederson, A., & Dupéré, S. (2012). Addressing diversity and inequities in health promotion: The implications of intersectional theory. In I. Rootman, S. Dupéré, A. Pederson, & M. O'Neill (Eds.), *Health promotion in Canada: Critical perspectives on practice* (pp. 54–66). Toronto, ON: Canadian Scholar' Press.

Rezaeian, M. (2013). The association between natural disasters and violence: A systematic review of the literature and a call for more epidemiological studies. *Journal of Research in Medical Sciences: The Official Journal of Isfahan University of Medical Sciences, 18*(12), 1103–1107.

Royal Canadian Mounted Police. (2014). Missing and murdered Aboriginal women: A national operational overview. Ottawa: Author.

Sen, G., & Ostlin, P. (2010). Gender as a social determinant of health: Evidence, policies, and innovations. In G. Sen & P. Ostlin (Eds.), *Gender equity in health: The shifting frontiers of evidence and action* (pp. 1–46). New York and London: Routledge.

Sinha, M. (2013). *Measuring violence against women: Statistical trends.* Ottawa: Statistics Canada.

Statistics Canada. (2016). *Family violence in Canada: A statistical profile, 2014.* Ottawa: Author.

Status of Women Canada. (2017). *About the federal strategy on gender-based violence.* Ottawa: Government of Canada. Retrieved from www.swc-cfc.gc.ca/violence/strategy-strategie/index-en.html

United Nations Office on Drugs and Crime. (2014). *Global study on homicide, 2013: Trends, contexts, data.* Vienna: Author.

UN Women. (2015). *A framework to underpin action to prevent violence against women.* New York, NY: Author.

Wathen, N. (2013). *Health impacts of violent victimization on women and their children.* Ottawa: Research and Statistics Division, Department of Justice Canada.

Wathen, N., & MacMillan, H. (2014). *Research brief: Identifying and responding to intimate partner violence against women.* London: PreVAiL.

Wilkinson, A. (2013). Violence against women. *CMAJ: Canadian Medical Association Journal, 185*(12), E580. doi: 10.1503/cmaj.109-4567

World Health Organization (WHO). (1986). Ottawa Charter for Health Promotion. *Can J Public Health, 77*(6), 425–430.

World Health Organization (WHO). (1997). *Violence against women: Definition and scope of the problem.* Geneva: Author.

World Health Organization (WHO). (2009). *Integrating gender into HIV/AIDS programmes in the health sector: Tool to improve responsiveness to women's needs.* Geneva: Author.

World Health Organization (WHO). (2011a). *Evidence for gender responsive actions to prevent and manage chronic conditions: Young people's health as a whole-of-society response.* Copenhagen: Author.

World Health Organization (WHO). (2011b). *Evidence for gender responsive actions to promote mental health: Young people's health as a whole-of-society response.* Copenhagen: Author.

World Health Organization (WHO). (2013). *Global and regional estimates of violence against women: Prevalence and health effects of intimate partner violence and non-partner sexual violence.* Geneva: Author.

CHAPTER 8

Implications of Inequities in Health for Health Promotion Practice

Dennis Raphael

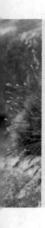

LEARNING OBJECTIVES

1. Appreciate the magnitude of health inequities in Canada
2. Identify the public policy antecedents of these health inequities
3. Gain knowledge of the different ways that health inequities can be addressed by health promoters
4. Come to understand how effecting societal change may be the most effective means of reducing health inequities

INTRODUCTION

Health promotion has the goal of improving the health of populations. It is becoming increasingly clear that in wealthy developed nations such as Canada, the primary component of this effort involves reducing health inequities. One way to think about this is that the average health of the top 20 percent of Canadians represents the best that can be reasonably expected of the entire population. The primary health promotion task is to "level up" the health of the remaining 80 percent of the population, which falls below this 20 percent benchmark (Dahlgren & Whitehead, 2006; Whitehead & Dahlgren, 2006). While there is disagreement regarding how this levelling up may be accomplished, it is generally agreed that these differences or inequalities in health are unjust and unfair.[1] They are therefore health inequities (Braveman & Gruskin, 2003).

Health promoters should not forget about improving the health of the top 20 percent, but must recognize that their health issues are rather minor in the overall health situation. Actually, levelling up the health of the lower 80 percent may improve the health of the top 20 percent by improving the overall quality of societal functioning. That is, as measures are taken to reduce the health gap between the rich and everybody else, the increases in social cohesion and solidarity and reductions in class-related conflicts will promote the health of all (Wilkinson & Pickett, 2009).

How can the health of this 80 percent be levelled up? This question exposes a range of contentious issues concerning the definition of health promotion, means of intervention, and barriers to action. I argue that the most effective health promotion approach for reducing health inequities is contained in the *Ottawa Charter for Health Promotion* (WHO, 1986) and reiterated by the Commission on Social Determinants of Health (CSDH, 2008): Create public policy that strengthens the prerequisites or social determinants of health. I also recognize that this is not a value-free exercise uninfluenced by politics. Indeed, the World Health Organization states, "These circumstances are shaped by the distribution of money, power and resources at global, national and local levels" (WHO, 2013).

STATUS OF HEALTH INEQUITIES IN CANADA

Health inequities in Canada are widespread and manifest in numerous indicators of health status at every stage of the life-course. The primary category for identifying health inequities in Canada is family or individual income: those of differing incomes experience differing health outcomes (Auger & Alix, 2016). There are three explanations as to why income differences are a driver of health inequities:

> First, income inequality places people in material life circumstances that lead to different health outcomes. Second, income inequality may be an intrinsic driver of health-related inequality as individuals experience health-threatening psychosocial distress by comparing their own situations to those who are better off. Third, income inequality may serve as a marker for a collection of societal structures and processes related to employment and working conditions, state provision of economic and social security, and the distribution of power and influence—all of which are important social determinants of health. (Bryant, 2015, pp. S10–S11)

Two main methodological approaches identify health inequities related to income (Raphael, 2011). One approach identifies the average income received within a specific geographic area—such as a census tract, neighbourhood, or health care service area—and then details the health situations of those residing in these areas. These geographic areas are placed into equal population-sized groups, from the wealthiest to the poorest, such as quartiles (four groups), quintiles (five groups), or deciles (ten groups), and the health situation among groups is then compared. Health differences between these areas are then compared.

The other approach categorizes individuals and families as a function of their income (e.g., high, upper-middle, middle, lower-middle, low) and then examines their health outcomes. This latter approach is more accurate as the former tends to be more conservative in its explication of health inequalities as it involves averages rather than individual scores.

Overviews of the extent of income-related health equalities in Canada acquired through both methods are available (Auger and Alix, 2016; Tjepkema, Wilkins, & Long, 2013). A few examples illustrate their extent in Canada.

Inequities in Death Rates or Mortality among Canadians

A 2013 report by Statistics Canada highlights how income is related to health inequities. The study shows that income differences are associated with the excess deaths of 40,000 Canadians a year (Tjepkema et al., 2013). That is equal to 110 Canadians dying prematurely each day. How does this report arrive at this conclusion? Researchers followed 2.7 million Canadians over a 16-year period and calculated death rates from a wide range of diseases and injuries as a function of individuals' income. Canadians in the study were divided into five quintiles of approximately equal numbers from poorest to wealthiest.

The study then compared the number of deaths each year among the wealthiest 20 percent of Canadians to the other 80 percent of Canadians. It came to the conclusion that if all Canadians were as healthy as the top 20 percent of Canadian income earners, there would be approximately 40,000 fewer deaths each year. Of these, 25,000 fewer deaths would be among Canadian men and 15,000 among Canadian women. *These numbers are comparable to eliminating all deaths from a major killer of Canadians, coronary artery disease.*

The report also calculates the relative rate of mortality, comparing the likelihood of death of someone in the poorest 20 percent of Canadians to one of the wealthiest 20 percent of Canadians. Overall, this figure is 1.67 for men and 1.52 for women, indicating that a poor male has a 67 percent greater chance of dying each year and a poor woman has

Table 8.1: Greater Risk of Dying Associated with Being Poor as Compared to Wealthy (RR) and Excess Deaths Associated with Income Inequality for Various Diseases and Injuries among Canadians

Disease	RR[1]		Excess Deaths[2]	
	Men	Women	Men	Women
Cardiovascular disease	1.67	1.53	19%	18%
Cancers	1.46	1.30	16%	11%
Diabetes	2.49	2.64	36%	38%
Respiratory disease	2.31	2.11	37%	30%
HIV/AIDS	3.57	11.1	39%	69%
Injuries	1.88	1.83	18%	17%

1 Inter-quintile rate ratio between poorest and wealthiest = (Q1—Poorest/Q5—Wealthiest)
2 Percentage of excess deaths due to differences between wealthy and all other Canadians = [100*(Total–Q5)/ Total]

Source: Adapted from Tjepkema, M., Wilkins, R. & Long, A. (2013). Cause-specific mortality by income adequacy in Canada: A 16-year follow-up study. *Health Reports, 24*(7), 14–22, tables 2 and 3, pp. 17–18.

a 52 percent greater chance of dying each year than their wealthy counterparts. That's an overall excess death rate of 19.4 percent for men and 16.6 percent for women.

The study goes into further detail, outlining income-related statistics for specific diseases. Table 8.1 shows the greater risk associated with being poor as compared to wealthy, and excess mortality associated with income differences between the wealthy and all other Canadians for various diseases and injuries. Poor Canadian males have a 67 percent greater chance of dying each year from heart disease than their wealthy counterparts. For women, it's a difference of 53 percent. The excess cardiovascular deaths each year associated with not being as healthy as the wealthy are 19 percent for men and 18 percent for women.

In relation to mortality from diabetes, the figures are even more striking. Poor Canadian men have a 150 percent greater chance and poor women a 160 percent greater chance of dying from diabetes each year than wealthy Canadians. This means that if all Canadians were as healthy as wealthy Canadians, there would be nearly 40 percent fewer deaths from diabetes and nearly 20 percent fewer deaths from cardiovascular disease every year. Similar numbers showing a profound difference between wealthy and poor Canadians and between wealthy and all other Canadians appear for virtually every known disease that can kill Canadians, including cancer, respiratory disease, injuries, and HIV/AIDS.

The Statistics Canada report also makes clear that these differences in health outcomes are primarily due to the material living circumstances and the associated psychosocial stresses associated with not being as well-off as the wealthiest 20 percent of Canadians, not differences in health-related behaviours: "Income influences health most directly through access to material resources such as better quality food and shelter" (Tjepkema et al., 2013, p. 14).

Similar findings are seen for infant mortality rates, an especially sensitive indicator of overall societal health. Rates in the poorest 20 percent of urban neighbourhoods across Canada (7.1/1,000) are 40 percent higher than in the wealthiest 20 percent (5.0/1,000) (Wilkins, 2007). In Québec, as a provincial example, during the period from 2009 to 2011, infant mortality rates in the poorest 20 percent of neighbourhoods (6.0/1,000) were 30 percent higher than in the wealthiest 20 percent (4.6/1,000) of neighbourhoods (Auger & Alix, 2016).

Inequities in Illness and Injuries or Morbidity

Incidence of low birth weight differs as a function of average neighbourhood income (Wilkins, Houle, Berthelot, & Ross, 2000). Rates are 40 percent higher in the poorest 20 percent of neighbourhoods (7.0/100) as compared to what occurs in the wealthiest 20 percent (4.9/100). In Québec, rates are 26 percent higher in the poorest 20 percent of neighbourhoods (10/100) as compared to what occurs in the wealthiest 20 percent (7.9/100) (Auger & Alix, 2016).

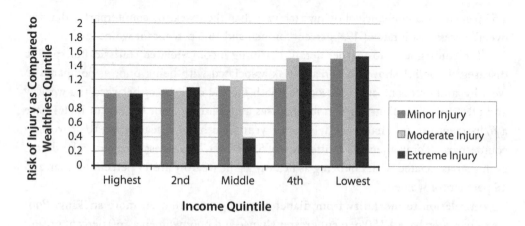

Figure 8.1: Association between Socio-economic Status and Childhood Injury, by Severity of Injury, Ontario 1996

Source: Data adapted from Faelker, T., Pickett, W., & Brison, R. J. (2000). Socioeconomic differences in childhood injury: A population-based epidemiologic study in Ontario, Canada. *Injury Prevention, 6* (3), 203–208, table 4, p. 206.

Figure 8.1 shows that children in the poorest Ontario neighbourhoods have injury rates 67 percent higher than children in the wealthiest neighbourhoods (Faelker, Pickett, & Brison, 2000). These differences are apparent for minor, moderate, and extreme injuries. The City of Toronto provides an analysis that shows neighbourhood income to be related to cardiovascular disease, type 2 diabetes, youth chlamydia, youth gonorrhea, teen pregnancy, and readiness to learn upon entry to school (Toronto Public Health, 2015).

SOURCES OF HEALTH INEQUITIES

Health inequities are primarily a result of exposures to varying qualities of living and working conditions, which have come to be known as the social determinants of health (see box 8.1) (Raphael, 2016). Wealthy, high-income Canadians enjoy the best health because their living and working conditions are superior to those experienced by other Canadians. These conditions affect health through pathways associated with material advantage and disadvantage; psychosocial stress and amount of control; and adoption of coping behaviours. These differences in living and working conditions and their manifestation in unequal health outcomes occur all the way from the top to the bottom of the Canadian socio-economic ladder.

Many Canadian health promoters' programs of practice say little, if anything, about living and working conditions and the importance of attempting to influence the public policies that create them (Raphael, 2008a). They work to improve health care systems' capacity to deal with health inequities or believe they can prevent health inequities by promoting "healthy lifestyle choices," "social capital," or "resiliency."

The belief is that reducing risk behaviours (i.e., adopting healthy lifestyle choices), building connections and networks among individuals and communities (i.e., building

---

Box 8.1: Social Determinants of Health with Particular Relevance to Health Inequities in Canada

---

- Disability
- Early life
- Education
- Employment and working conditions
- Food security
- Gender
- Geography
- Health care services
- Housing
- Immigration status
- Income and its distribution
- Indigenous ancestry
- Race
- Social safety net
- Social exclusion
- Unemployment and employment security

Source: Raphael, D. (2016). *Social determinants of health: Canadian perspectives* (3rd ed.). Toronto: Canadian Scholars' Press.

---

social capital), and enhancing individual coping strategies (i.e., promoting resiliency) can improve health and reduce inequities without addressing the upstream determinants of both these mediating processes and their resultant health inequities. Critiques of these approaches are available (Muntaner, Lynch, & Davey Smith, 2000; Smith & Scott-Samuel, 2015).

It may be more useful to adopt a structural analysis of how health inequities come about. Here, health inequities—as well as the mediating outcomes of lifestyle choices, social capital, and resiliency—are due to the workings of the economic system, a governmental apparatus that maintains or reinforces these inequities, and a public discourse that justifies them (Grabb, 2007). It can be reasoned, then, that health inequities can best be reduced by changing or modifying the economic system, adjusting how governments operate, and shifting how these issues are understood by policy makers and the public (Raphael, 2015a).

HEALTH INEQUITIES AND HEALTH PROMOTION PRACTICE

While health inequities result primarily from differences in Canadians' living and working conditions, there are at least seven different ways in which "health promoters"—broadly defined—have interpreted this reality. These interpretations lead to different ways of taking on the task of reducing health inequities. Table 8.2 outlines these different approaches.

Approach 1: Health Inequities and Access to and Quality of Health Care and Social Services

In this approach health inequities are seen as resulting from health care and social service issues. Particular individuals have less access to necessary services, or these services may be of less than optimal quality. Health promoters strive to reduce barriers to care and improve the quality of these services. "Health promoting" hospitals are part of this approach.

Some examples include addressing the health needs of homeless individuals, managing chronic diseases among vulnerable communities, and providing primary health care to immigrant groups, among others. Public health agencies provide preventive health services, and social service agencies support at-risk individuals and communities.

These activities are important, but do rather little to reduce health inequities. Moreover, limiting research and activity to these issues neglects the sources of health inequities. It can reinforce already dominant care emphases, obscuring the role that living and working conditions play in creating health inequities.

Approach 2: Health Inequities and Modifiable Medical and Behavioural Risk Factors

Modifying individual risk factors has been a primary concern of health promoters. Although, as noted in chapter 1, the 1974 Lalonde Report identified risk behaviours as only one of four health fields, the healthy lifestyles approach came to dominate health promotion activity in Canada (Legowski & McKay, 2000).

The medical and public health concern with medical (e.g., high blood sugar and "bad" cholesterol levels) and behavioural (e.g., poor diet, lack of physical activity, and tobacco and excessive alcohol use) risk factors is so prevalent as to dominate professional thinking, media coverage (Hayes et al., 2007), and public understandings about the mainsprings of health and the causes of illness (Canadian Population Health Initiative, 2004). Many government and health agency documents discuss broader approaches to reducing health inequities, but these have had little penetration into medical and public health activity and media and public awareness (Raphael, 2008b).

Unlike Approach 1, which stresses provision and improvement of services, this approach has many negative aspects. First, medical and behavioural risk factors account for relatively little of the health inequities that exist in Canada. Second, this approach assumes that individuals are capable of "making healthy lifestyle choices" such that individuals who fail to do so are responsible for their own adverse health outcomes (Labonté & Penfold, 1981). Third, programs show rather little evidence of effectiveness among the most vulnerable and may increase health inequities as "healthy living" messaging is more likely to be taken up by the already advantaged (Jarvis & Wardle, 2003). Investing in the approach may further disenable vulnerable populations and the health promoters administering these programs as these approaches show little for their efforts.

Table 8.2: Health Promotion Approaches Directed toward Reducing Health Inequities

Health Inequities Interpretation	Key Health Promotion Concept	Health Promotion Practice Approach	Practical Implications of the Approach
1. Health inequities result from differences in access and quality of health and social services.	Health inequities can be reduced by strengthening health care and social services.	Create "health promoting" hospitals, clinics, and social service agencies.	Focus is limited to promoting the health of those already experiencing health inequities.
2. Health inequities result from differences in important modifiable medical and behavioural risk factors.	Health inequities can be reduced by enabling people to make "healthy choices" and adopt "healthy lifestyles."	Develop and evaluate healthy living and behaviour modification programs and protocols.	Healthy lifestyle programming may ignore the material basis of health inequities and widen existing health inequities.
3. Health inequities result from differences in material living conditions.	Health inequities can be reduced by improving material living conditions.	Ensure that community development and participatory research enable people to gain control over their health.	There is the assumption that governmental authorities are receptive to and will act upon community voices and research findings.
4. Health inequities result from differences in material living conditions that are a function of group membership.	Health inequities can be reduced by improving the material living conditions of particular disadvantaged groups.	Targeted development and research activities among disadvantaged groups improve their material living conditions.	There is the assumption that governmental authorities are receptive to such activities and anticipated outcomes.
5. Health inequities result from differences in material living conditions shaped by public policy.	Health inequities can be reduced by advocating for healthy public policy that reduces disadvantage.	Analyze how public policy decisions impact health (i.e., health impact analysis).	There is the assumption that governments will create public policy on the basis of its effects upon health.
6. Health inequities result from differences in material living conditions that are shaped by economic and political structures and their justifying ideologies.	Health inequities can be reduced by influencing the societal structures that create and justify health inequities.	Analyzing how the political economy of a nation creates inequities identifies avenues for social and political action.	Requires health promotion to engage in building social and political movements that will reduce health inequities.
7. Health inequities result from the power and influence of those who create and benefit from health and social inequities.	Health inequities can be reduced by increasing the power and influence of those who experience these inequities.	Critical analysis empowers the disadvantaged to gain an understanding of, and a means of increasing, their influence and power.	Requires health promotion to engage in building social and political movements that increase the power of the disadvantaged.

Approach 3: Health Inequities and Differences in Material Living Conditions

Living conditions operate through material, psychological, and behavioural pathways to "get under the skin" to shape health. Society's structures, such as employment and working conditions, and neighbourhood characteristics produce health inequities across the lifespan. In this view, health inequities can be reduced by levelling up the living conditions experienced by the less well-off.

How do health promoters implement this approach? In Canada, it frequently involves community development, and participatory or action research (Minkler, 2005). The idea is that when community members uncover the factors that shape their health—and, in the case of disadvantaged communities, cause health inequities—governmental and other societal authorities will act upon this knowledge to improve the situation (Raphael, Steinmetz, & Renwick, 1999).

All of this assumes that governmental and other authorities are receptive to the information that comes from such activities. This has become increasingly questionable over the past three decades as Canadian governments have (1) reduced provision of supports and services to the population; and (2) demonstrated less willingness to create public policy to reduce health inequities (Bryant, Raphael, Schrecker, & Labonté, 2011).

Approach 4: Health Inequities, Material Living Conditions, and Group Membership

Health promoters recognize that health inequities are frequently a function of class, gender, and race. Therefore, community development, and participatory and action research become focused on disadvantaged or marginalized individuals. Again, the key idea is that uncovering factors that shape health and cause health inequities will lead authorities to act upon this knowledge.

Approach 5: Health Inequities Result from Differences in Material Living Conditions Shaped by Public Policy

This analysis considers that the primary means of reducing health inequities is through public policy action. This approach is clearly endorsed by the World Health Organization's recent social determinants report (CSDH, 2008).

As an illustration of this approach, the presence of health inequities is shaped by access (or lack thereof) to material resources such as income, housing, food, and educational and employment opportunities, among others. These resources are related to parents' employment security, wages, and the quality of their working conditions and availability of quality, regulated child care, all of which are shaped by public policy decisions (Raphael, 2015a).

Raising these issues is uncommon among health promoters. The health promotion activity most consistent with this approach is health impact assessment (HIA) (Scott-Samuel, Birley, & Ardern, 2001). The health promotion organization analyzes the effects a proposed public policy will have on existing health inequities. This process is similar to that of environmental assessment. Prior to the construction of a bridge or tunnel, an environmental assessment is done to identify the impacts—both positive and negative—on local flora and fauna. A health impact assessment would determine the probable impacts of, say, the reduction of affordable recreational services upon the health of local residents. Opportunities to do just this arise rather often in Canada.

Hardly a day goes by without a public policy issue arising at either the municipal/regional, provincial, or federal level that has health inequities implications: minimum wages, social assistance rates, recreation fees, labour laws, public transportation, education, child care, and just about every other social determinant of health. HIA is rarely, if ever, seen in Canada. Why this is so is considered in the following section.

Approach 6: Health Inequities Are Shaped by Economic and Political Structures and Their Justifying Ideologies

It seems reasonable that health promoters would carry out HIA of proposed policies to inform public policy-making. This view is consistent with the belief (pluralism) that public policy decisions are made on the basis of evidence (Brooks & Miljan, 2003). Pluralism is the belief that public policy decisions are made by weighing the pros and cons of policy advice contributed by a wide range of societal sectors (e.g., business, labour, and civil society). In this model, information of all kinds is valued and policy options are informed by such data. Health promotion knowledge production, dissemination, transfer, and exchange in the service of reducing health inequities is part of this approach (Bryant, 2015).

How, then, can we explain the last two decades of government policy-making in Canada, which have widened the social inequalities that create health inequities, as well as the lack of any significant health impact assessment of public policies on the part of health promoters, their agencies, and institutions? The alternative explanation (the materialist) is that governments make decisions on the basis of existing economic and political structures of influence and power (Brooks & Miljan, 2003). In this model, policy-making is seen as being made in the interests of the wealthy and powerful rather than in the interests of all. These decisions are then justified on the basis of particular ideologies and positions, such as what is good for business is good for society. If there are resulting health inequities from such decisions, they are justified on the basis that people bring their own health problems on themselves by making poor lifestyle decisions.

This analysis goes far in explaining why Canada, which is seen as a leader in creating health promotion and population concepts that have been applied in the service of reducing health inequities elsewhere, has always been somewhat of a health equity laggard. Public policy, it is argued, is not being made in the interests of the majority of Canadians but in the interests of those with more influence and power (Raphael, 2015a).

These economic and political approaches to creating public policy that either creates or reduces health inequities differ from one jurisdiction to another. Sweden, Norway, and Finland have placed the reduction of health inequities high on their public policy agenda; nations such as Canada and the US, rather less so (Raphael, 2012). Health promoters and their agencies are embedded within these differing economic and political structures.

Three distinct types of welfare states have been identified: social democratic (e.g., Sweden, Norway, Denmark, and Finland); liberal (e.g., the US, the UK, Canada, and Ireland); and conservative (e.g., France, Germany, Netherlands, and Belgium) (Esping-Andersen, 1990). Canadian sociologists add a fourth Latin welfare state that includes Greece, Italy, Portugal, and Spain (Saint-Arnaud & Bernard, 2003).

The approach suggests that differences in political and economic structures and processes (political economy)—themselves a result of historical traditions and governance by specific political parties over time—determine the living conditions Canadians experience. Two important examples of factors shown to create health inequities—income inequality and poverty rates—illustrate the power of such an analysis (see figures 8.2 and 8.3).

The liberal political economies (shaded dark) tend towards the highest income inequality and poverty rates, while the social democratic nations (unshaded) tend towards the lowest. The Latin undeveloped welfare states (dotted) show many similarities with the liberal states. Even the conservative welfare states (lightly shaded) deal better with these important determinants of health inequities than Canada does. Since the dominant inspiration of liberal political economies is to minimize governmental intervention in the operation of its central institution—the market—it should not be surprising that Canada and its liberal partners fall well behind other nations in addressing health inequities (Raphael & Bryant, 2015). Instead, emphasis is on facilitating the operation of the economic system, which tends to benefit the wealthy and powerful. This health promotion analysis broadens the health promotion role beyond simply identifying public policy implications to one of attempting to influence the political and economic structures that shape such policy.

Health promoters must recognize that the implementation of health-promoting public policies that strengthen the social determinants of health will require shifts in existing economic and political structures. This will require the building of social and political movements that will increase the influence of those whose health is threatened by existing public policies. The means of doing so involves educating and engaging the public in the political process to force fundamental changes in how society works and resources are distributed.

The institution of new public policies that support health will gradually change these existing structures. As citizens come to appreciate how these public policies are supporting their health and wellbeing, there will be fundamental changes in the operation of society (i.e., economic and political structures) that will institutionalize these changes. Indeed, such transformation through public policy change is at the heart of every credible analysis of the means by which health inequities can be reduced (see Bryant, 2015; Raphael, 2015b).

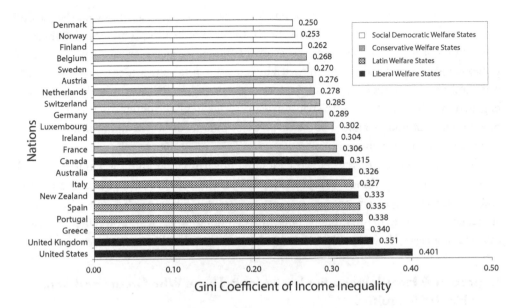

Figure 8.2: Income Inequality Rates, Selected OECD Nations, 2013

Source: Data adapted from Organisation for Economic Co-operation and Development. (2016). *Income inequality.* Available at www.oecd.org/els/soc/income-distribution-database.htm.

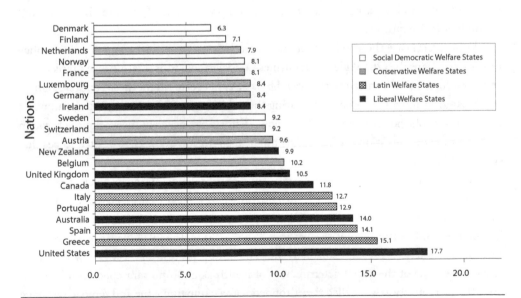

Figure 8.3: Poverty Rates, Selected OECD Nations, 2013

Source: Data adapted from Organisation for Economic Co-operation and Development. (2016). *Income inequality.* Available at www.oecd.org/els/soc/income-distribution-database.htm.

Why, then, is there such a lack of public policy analysis and advocacy on the part of health promoters in Canada? I suggest that in the case of health promoters who are government employees or who work for government-funded agencies, there is a perception of professional and personal danger in criticizing governmental authorities that pay their salaries and determine their opportunities for advancement. In the case of health promoters engaged by other institutions, the reluctance to engage in public policy discussions may be based on lack of understanding of the social determinants of health and health inequities or a perception that such activities are not part of their mandate or role.

The fear of governmental blowback among governmental and government-funded agencies is rather disturbing as it suggests we really do not live in such a democratic society, and that earnest, sincere people can get into real trouble for doing their jobs. The lack of appreciation for the role that public policy plays among other health promoters is also a cause for concern. How to deal with these barriers is discussed in later sections.

Approach 7: Health Inequities Result from Those Who Create and Benefit from Health Inequities

In this final approach the individuals and groups who—through their undue influence upon governments—create and benefit from health inequities are identified. These individuals and groups lobby for shifting the tax structures to favour the corporate sector and the wealthy, reducing public expenditures, controlling wages and employment benefits, and relaxing labour standards and protections. These are all factors that create health inequities.

Who exactly are these villains and how can their undue influence upon public policy be resisted? Langille (2016) identifies business associations, conservative think tanks, citizen front institutions, and conservative lobbyists. What form might these counterbalances take? Langille and others propose educating the public and using their strength in numbers to promote public policy to oppose this agenda. Efforts can occur in the workplace through greater union organization and increasing public recognition of the class-related forces that shape public policy.

Activities can also occur in the electoral and parliamentary arena by electing political parties that favour action to reduce health inequities. It is clear that social democratic parties are more receptive to and successful at implementing public policies that reduce social inequalities and health inequities (Navarro & Shi, 2002). The 2011 elevation of the New Democratic Party (NDP) in Canada to the Official Opposition in Ottawa saw the NDP raising the issue of the social determinants of health as an important concern. However, once the 2015 election was called they dropped it as a campaign issue and removed its page from their website. The newly appointed Federal Minister of Aboriginal Affairs is quoted as saying that the social determinants of health—and apparently health equity—will be an important governmental concern (Duggan, 2015).

HEALTH PROMOTION DILEMMAS

If health inequities are a result of political and economic structures and the public policies that flow from such structures, generating knowledge and disseminating information about the sources of health inequities and the means of reducing them are a necessary but not sufficient condition for reducing them.

There are three ways health promoters can help reduce health inequities, and these are focused on education and knowledge transmission (Raphael, 2008b). These will not by themselves lead to public policy to reduce health inequities, but will assist others engaged in public policy advocacy.

Education and Knowledge Transmission

The Canadian public remains woefully uninformed about health inequities and their sources. In addition to the constant barrage of "healthy living" messages, Canadians are subject to continual messaging as to the benefits of a business-oriented, laissez-faire approach to governance. What this messaging has not included are the societal effects of this approach: increasing income and wealth inequality, persistent poverty, and growing health inequities.

Telling the Solid Facts

At a minimum, health promoters can carry out and publicize the findings from analyses of the causes of health inequities. A public-oriented document, *Social Determinants of Health: The Canadian Facts* (thecanadianfacts.org) can assist in this task (Mikkonen & Raphael, 2010).

There are numerous health inequity–related policy areas in which health promoters could engage in public education and their importance in promoting health: reducing poverty and housing and food insecurity, improving employment and working conditions, and fostering early child development and others. My short list of afflictions where significant health inequities are related to these living conditions include coronary heart disease, type 2 diabetes, arthritis, stroke, many forms of cancer, respiratory disease including asthma, HIV/AIDS, death from injuries, mental illness, suicide, emergency room visits, school dropout, delinquency and crime, unemployment, alienation, distress, and depression.

Telling Stories

Health promoters can shift public, professional, and policy makers' focus from the dominant biomedical and lifestyle health paradigms to a broader public policy perspective by collecting and presenting stories about the impact that living conditions—and the public policy decisions that influence these—have on people's lives. Ethnographic and qualitative approaches to individual and community health produce vivid illustrations of the importance of these issues for people's health and wellbeing (Popay & Williams, 1994). There is some indication that policy makers—and certainly the media—may be responsive to such forms of evidence.

There is increasing recognition of the importance of community-based action, such as community needs assessment, that applies these approaches. Such activities can be a rich source of insights about the mainsprings of health inequities and the means of influencing public policy. Such a perspective allows community members to provide their own critical reflections on society, power, and inequality. At a minimum, these approaches allow the voices of those most influenced by the public policy decisions that create health inequities to be heard and hold out the possibility of their concerns being translated into political activity on their part, and policy action on the part of health and government officials.

Providing Support for Policy Action

The final role is the most important, but potentially the most difficult: supporting policy action in support of health. And implicit in such a course of action is recognizing the important role that politics play in these activities.

Numerous public health units and health-promotion agencies have taken up the task of speaking out about public policy choices and their effects upon health inequities. Sometimes these units and agencies work in partnership with community organizations to raise these important health equity issues. The Sudbury and District Health Unit's video animation *Let's Start a Conversation about Health and Not Talk about Health Care at All* (Sudbury and District Health Unit, 2011) has been adapted for use—including public education—by no less than 19 other public health units in Ontario (out of the total of 36), numerous others across Canada, and jurisdictions in the US and Australia. These examples should spur other agencies to take up this task.

Professional Association and Agency Network Action

For health promoters and their agencies that feel vulnerable about raising these issues in their workplace, avenues of action are possible through professional associations and agency networks. Professional associations, such as the Canadian Public Health Association and provincial/territorial health associations, can raise the profile of health inequities and their impact on Canadian society. The Canadian Medical Association, Registered Nurses' Association of Ontario, the Canadian Nurses Association, the Association of Ontario Health Centres, and the British Columbia Healthy Living Alliance have all produced clearly stated policy documents that raise the issue of health inequities and the importance of applying public policy analysis and action to reduce them (Raphael, 2016).

Political Engagement

Health promoters are also citizens who can vote and support particular political parties between and during political campaigns. Canadians are not a particularly politicized people, and there is no reason to think that health promoters are much different from the average Canadian (Schellenberg, 2004). The relevance of addressing health inequities to their employment goals—better health for all—should serve as a spur to increase such participation among health promoters.

CONCLUSION

Health promotion approaches that acknowledge the importance of public policy activity for reducing health inequities may be the best means of accomplishing this goal. There are significant barriers to such action in Canada. It may be necessary to elect specific political parties and modify economic and political structures to effect the reduction of health inequities (Raphael, 2015a).

Such transformations will result in more equitable distribution of income and wealth, which will reduce the profound social inequalities that spawn health inequities. Strong programs that support children, families, and women, and economies that support full employment are required (Raphael, 2016).

My analysis indicates that health promotion activities operate within the confines of the dominant political and economic discourses of Canadian society. In Canada, governmental withdrawal from intervening in the operation of the economic marketplace has made concern with reducing health inequities not only unpopular among governing circles, but actually threatening to agency funding and individual health promoters' career prospects.

Despite the barriers to addressing health inequities in Canada, the best means of reducing health inequities involve health promoters and their agencies and organizations navigating the difficult task of informing citizens about the political and economic forces that shape the health of a society.

Establishing an environment in which health promoters can do this would be an important first step in reducing health inequities in Canada. This would provide a solid base for public policy activity in reducing health inequities. Without this base and the public policy activity that would flow from it, significant reduction in health inequities in Canada seems unlikely.

CRITICAL THINKING QUESTIONS

1. Review the health-related stories in your local newspaper over the next few weeks. If you based your understanding of health inequities on these stories, what would be your views of what makes some people healthy and others ill?
2. What evidence is available concerning the extent of health inequities in your jurisdiction? What are the current indicators of the incidence of poverty, homelessness, and food bank use in your area? Have conditions been improving or declining?
3. To what extent have other health-related courses you have taken addressed issues of health inequities? What could be done to increase your discipline's emphasis on health inequities?

4.   What could be done to improve the public's understanding of the importance of tackling health inequities? What should be the role of your local public health unit or health care agencies?

5.   What are some of the personal and professional dilemmas health promoters face in applying the more sophisticated approaches described in this chapter? How can these problems be overcome?

RESOURCES

Further Readings

Bryant, T., Raphael, D., & Rioux, M. (Eds.). (2010). *Staying alive: Critical perspectives on health, illness, and health care* (2nd ed.). Toronto: Canadian Scholars' Press.
This volume emphasizes the political economy of health and contains chapters on the social determinants of health and health inequities associated with social class, gender, and race.

Graham, H. (2007). *Unequal lives: Health and socioeconomic inequalities*. New York: Open University Press.
This is an excellent overview of how public policy comes to shape the living conditions that lead to health inequities. By reviewing the various approaches to addressing health inequities, it identifies strengths of a public policy approach.

Raphael, D. (2016). *Social determinants of health: Canadian perspectives* (3rd ed.). Toronto: Canadian Scholars' Press.
This book summarizes how socio-economic factors affect the health of Canadians, surveys the current state of the social determinants of health across Canada, and provides an analysis of how these determinants affect Canadians' health.

Smith, K., Bambra, C., & Hill, S. (Eds.). (2015). *Health inequalities: Critical perspectives*. Oxford: Oxford University Press.
This book examines a variety of research and policy topics concerned with identifying and addressing health inequities. It considers ways of improving the links between health inequalities research, policy, and practice, including the role of advocacy by researchers and practitioners.

Whitehead, M. (2007). A typology of actions to tackle social inequalities in health. *Journal of Epidemiology and Community Health, 61*, 473–478.
This article outlines some of the ways by which health inequities can be remedied. More extensive presentations are provided by Whitehead and Dahlgren (2006) and Dahlgren and Whitehead (2006).

Relevant Websites

Canadian Public Health Association, CPHA Policy Statements

www.cpha.ca/en/programs.aspx

These reports and statements situate the CPHA as having been in the forefront of identifying the sources of health inequities and outlining the means of reducing them.

Chief Public Health Officer's Reports on the State of Public Health in Canada

www.phac-aspc.gc.ca/publicat/cpho-acsp/index-eng.php

These reports provide the evidence concerning the profound health inequities among the Canadian population.

National Collaborating Centre for Determinants of Health (NCCDH)

www.nccdh.ca

The NCCDH focuses on the social and economic factors that influence the health of Canadians. It translates and shares evidence with public health organizations and practitioners to influence interrelated determinants and advance health equity. Through various products and services, it works to advance knowledge, foster knowledge use, and accelerate network development.

Wellesley Institute

www.wellesleyinstitute.com/

The Wellesley Institute focuses on developing research and community-based policy solutions to problems of urban health and health inequities.

World Health Organization: Social Determinants of Health

www.who.int/social_determinants/en

The WHO established the Commission on Social Determinants of Health to provide advice on how to reduce persisting and widening inequities in health. See especially its final report, *Closing the Gap in a Generation: Health Equity through Action on the Social Determinants of Health.*

NOTE

1.   An inequality in health is simply a recognition that some measurable difference in health exists. An inequity in health is a moral statement that this difference is unfair and unjust and needs to be addressed.

REFERENCES

Auger, N., & Alix, C. (2016). Income, income distribution, and health in Canada. In D. Raphael (Ed.), *Social determinants of health: Canadian perspectives* (3rd ed.) (pp. 90–109). Toronto: Canadian Scholars' Press.

Braveman, P., & Gruskin, S. (2003). Defining equity in health. *Journal of Epidemiology and Community Health, 57*, 254–258.

Brooks, S., & Miljan, L. (2003). Theories of public policy. In S. Brooks & L. Miljan (Eds.), *Public policy in Canada: An introduction* (pp. 22–49). Toronto: Oxford University Press.

Bryant, T. (2015). Implications of public policy change models for addressing income-related health inequalities. *Canadian Public Policy, 41*(Suppl. 2), S10–S16.

Bryant, T., Raphael, D., Schrecker, T., & Labonté, R. (2011). Canada: A land of missed opportunity for addressing the social determinants of health. *Health Policy, 101*(1), 44–58.

Canadian Population Health Initiative. (2004). *Select highlights on public views of the determinants of health*. Ottawa: CPHI.

Commission on Social Determinants of Health (CSDH). (2008). *Closing the gap in a generation: Health equity through action on the social determinants of health*. Geneva: World Health Organization.

Dahlgren, G., & Whitehead, M. (2006). *Leveling up (Part 2): A discussion paper on European strategies for tackling social inequities in health*. Copenhagen: WHO Regional Office for Europe.

Duggan, K. (2015). Bennett says new government will tackle social determinants of health. *iPolitics*, November 30. Available at ipolitics.ca/2015/11/30/bennett-says-new-government-will-tackle-social-determinants-of-health/

Esping-Andersen, G. (1990). *The three worlds of welfare capitalism*. Princeton: Princeton University Press.

Faelker, T., Pickett, W., & Brison, R. J. (2000). Socioeconomic differences in childhood injury: A population-based epidemiologic study in Ontario, Canada. *Injury Prevention, 6*, 203–208.

Grabb, E. (2007). *Theories of social inequality* (5th ed.). Toronto: Harcourt Canada.

Hayes, M., Ross, I., Gasherc, M., Gutstein, D., Dunn, J., & Hackett, R. (2007). Telling stories: News media, health literacy, and public policy in Canada. *Social Science and Medicine, 54*, 445–457.

Jarvis, M. J., & Wardle, J. (2003). Social patterning of individual health behaviours: The case of cigarette smoking. In M. G. Marmot & R. G. Wilkinson (Eds.), *Social determinants of health* (2nd ed.) (pp. 224–237). Oxford: Oxford University Press.

Labonté, R., & Penfold, S. (1981). Canadian perspectives in health promotion: A critique. *Health Education, 19*, 4–9.

Lalonde, M. (1974). *A new perspective on the health of Canadians*. Ottawa: Government of Canada.

Langille, D. (2016). Follow the money: How business and politics shape our health. In D. Raphael (Ed.), *Social determinants of health: Canadian perspectives* (3rd ed.) (pp. 470–490). Toronto: Canadian Scholars' Press.

Legowski, B., & McKay, L. (2000). *Health beyond health care: Twenty-five years of federal health policy development*. CPRN Discussion Paper no. H04. Ottawa: Canadian Policy Research Networks.

Mikkonen, J., & Raphael, D. (2010). *Social determinants of health: The Canadian facts*. Toronto: York University School of Health Policy and Management. Available at thecanadianfacts.org/

Minkler, M. (2005). Community-based research partnerships: Challenges and opportunities. *Journal of Urban Health, 82*(Suppl. 2), ii3–ii12.

Muntaner, C., Lynch, J., & Davey Smith, G. (2000). Social capital and the third way in public health. *Critical Public Health, 10*(2), 107–124.

Navarro, V., & Shi, L. (2002). The political context of social inequalities and health. In V. Navarro (Ed.), *The political economy of social inequalities: Consequences for health and quality of life* (pp. 403–418). Amityville: Baywood.

Popay, J., & Williams, G. H. (Eds.). (1994). *Researching the people's health*. London: Routledge.

Raphael, D. (2008a). Grasping at straws: A recent history of health promotion in Canada. *Critical Public Health, 18*(4), 483–495.

Raphael, D. (2008b). Getting serious about health: New directions for Canadian public health researchers and workers. *Promotion and Education, 15*, 15–20.

Raphael, D. (2011). Who is poor in Canada? In D. Raphael (Ed.), *Poverty in Canada: Implications for health and quality of life* (2nd ed.) (pp. 62–89). Toronto: Canadian Scholars' Press.

Raphael, D. (Ed.). (2012). *Tackling health inequalities: Lessons from international experiences*. Toronto: Canadian Scholars' Press.

Raphael, D. (2015a). Beyond policy analysis: The raw politics behind opposition to healthy public policy. *Health Promotion International, 30*, 380–396.

Raphael, D. (2015b). The political economy of health: A research agenda into means of addressing health inequalities in Canada. *Canadian Public Policy, 41*(Suppl. 2), S17–S25.

Raphael, D. (Ed.). (2016). *Social determinants of health: Canadian perspectives* (3rd ed.). Toronto: Canadian Scholars' Press.

Raphael, D., & Bryant, T. (2015). Power, intersectionality and the lifecourse: Identifying the political and economic structures of welfare states that support or threaten health. *Social Theory and Health, 13*, 245–266.

Raphael, D., Steinmetz, B., & Renwick, R. (1999). The community quality of life project: A health promotion approach to understanding communities. *Health Promotion International, 14*, 197–210.

Saint-Arnaud, S., & Bernard, P. (2003). Convergence or resilience? A hierarchical cluster analysis of the welfare regimes in advanced countries. *Current Sociology, 51*(5), 499–527.

Schellenberg, G. (2004). *2003 General Social Survey on Social Engagement, cycle 17: An overview of findings*. Ottawa: Statistics Canada.

Scott-Samuel, A., Birley, M., & Ardern, K. (2001). *The Merseyside guidelines for health impact assessment*. Liverpool: International Health Impact Assessment Consortium.

Smith, K., & Scott-Samuel, A. (2015). Fantasy paradigms of health inequalities: Utopian thinking? *Social Theory & Health, 13*, 418–436.

Sudbury and District Health Unit. (2011). *Let's start a conversation about health ... and not talk about health care at all*. Retrieved from www.sdhu.com/wp-content/uploads/2015/03/LSAC_User_Guide_ENG-3.pdf

Tjepkema, M., Wilkins, R., & Long, A. (2013). Cause-specific mortality by income adequacy in Canada: A 16-year follow-up study. *Health Reports, 24*(7), 14–22.

Toronto Public Health. (2015). *The unequal city 2015: Income and health inequities in Toronto*. Toronto: Author.

Whitehead, M., & Dahlgren, G. (2006). *Concepts and principles for tackling social inequities in health: Leveling up, part 1*. Copenhagen: WHO Regional Office for Europe.

Wilkins, R. (2007). *Mortality by neighbourhood income in urban Canada from 1971 to 2001*. Ottawa: Statistics Canada, Health Analysis and Measurement Group.

Wilkins, R., Houle, C., Berthelot, J.-M., & Ross, D. P. (2000). The changing health status of Canada's children. *ISUMA, 1*(2), 57–63.

Wilkinson, R. G., & Pickett, K. (2009). *The spirit level: Why more equal societies almost always do better*. London: Allen Lane.

World Health Organization (WHO). (1986). *Ottawa Charter for Health Promotion*. Geneva: World Health Organization European Office.

World Health Organization (WHO). (2013). Social determinants of health. Retrieved from www.who.int/social_determinants/en/

CHAPTER 9

A Culture Shift towards Promoting Mental Health and Wellbeing in Canada

Paola Ardiles

LEARNING OBJECTIVES

1. Understand the context of mental health promotion in Canada
2. Identify promising practices, key barriers, and enablers in mental health promotion in Canada
3. Explore how to integrate mental health promotion into health promotion practice in Canada

There is no health without mental health.
There is no health promotion without mental health promotion.

INTRODUCTION

Mental Health Promotion is the process of enhancing the capacity of individuals and communities to take control over their lives and improve their mental health. By working to increase self-esteem, coping skills, social support and well-being in all individuals and communities, MHP empowers people and communities to interact with their environments in ways that enhance emotional and spiritual strength. It is an approach that fosters individual resilience and promotes socially supportive environments.

—Centre for Health Promotion, 1997

Everyone has a role to play in promoting mental health. This chapter aims to support the health promotion practitioners in Canada to enhance their understanding of their role in mental health promotion (MHP) and facilitate a culture shift towards the promotion of mental health and wellbeing.

A NATIONAL COMMITMENT TO PROMOTING MENTAL HEALTH

Even though the concept of mental health promotion has been alive in Canada since 1997, it has remained in the shadows of health promotion. This is surprising given that every week, if not every day, in the mainstream and social media we hear about the overwhelming demand for upstream and comprehensive approaches to deal with the growing burden of mental health and substance use issues affecting urban and rural communities. However, over the last six years, all levels of government in Canada, regardless of their geography or political affiliation, have come to agree that promoting mental health at a population level is a key social and economic investment for all Canadians.

In 2012, the Mental Health Commission of Canada (MHCC)[1] released Canada's first national mental health strategy, entitled *Changing Directions, Changing Lives*, to address the need for service-delivery efforts as well as MHP and mental illness prevention[2] efforts, as both are critical elements to implement mental health policies for the Canadian population. Its purpose is to help improve mental health and wellbeing and to create a mental health system that can meet the needs of people of all ages living with mental health problems and illnesses and their families[3] (MHCC, 2012). The strategy mentions the social determinants of mental health and has a specific strategic direction to reduce disparities and address diversity. In addition, the strategy prioritizes the mental health needs of First Nations, Inuit, and Métis in urban and rural areas, and the complex social issues that have an impact on Aboriginal people's mental health across Canada.

Since the release of the national mental health strategy, nearly all provinces and territories have released new strategies and action plans specifically addressing mental health and substance use[4] (NCCHPP, 2014). The majority of the provincial/territorial plans recognize the importance of the downstream (service-delivery) and upstream (prevention and promotion) elements that are necessary to effectively promote population mental health. Similarly, all of the provincial/territorial plans focus on reducing risk factors and promoting protective factors for people living with mental health and substance use issues.

One of the most transformative policy examples in Canada was the creation of *A Path Forward: BC First Nations and Aboriginal People's Mental Wellness and Substance Use—Ten Year Plan*[5] in early 2013 by British Columbia's First Nations Health Authority. This plan acknowledges the social, historical, and structural determinants that impact Aboriginal people and their mental wellness, such as the effects of colonization, residential schools, First Nations and Métis land appropriation, Indian hospitals and child welfare, and the impact of learned violence, loss of language, loss of emotional security and family connections, and a loss of respect for First Nations and Aboriginal culture (FNHA, 2013). Various action areas of the plan address social determinants of mental health including social support, housing, early childhood education, discrimination, and cultural safety.

The success of these policy initiatives will largely be determined by the extent that these efforts can be implemented, and how effective they will be in actively engaging communities and other policy sectors. Given national and provincial economic trends to lower public social and health expenditure in order to meet fiscal budget needs, what is critical now is the sustainability of these policy efforts. Strategies are only realized with implementation plans that are well managed with appropriate resources, meaningful indicators, and performance systems in place.

Health promotion practitioners can advocate for interventions across the five action areas of the *Ottawa Charter* in order to promote mental health and wellbeing of individuals, families, and communities at large. A comprehensive MHP approach requires a focus on reducing risk factors and promoting protective factors, as well as addressing the determinants of mental health. Given the complexity of mental health and its broader structural determinants—which lie outside of the "mental health," "public health," and "health service" sector—almost every public policy (e.g., housing, employment, justice, education, economic development, and environmental) can be considered a determinant of mental health. Health promotion practitioners need to have the skills to communicate the evidence-base across disciplines and make a strong case for public investments in various policies in other sectors.

BARRIERS AND FACILITATORS TO INTEGRATING MENTAL HEALTH INTO HEALTH PROMOTION

While approaches may vary across different provinces, regions, and settings, several key interrelated principles guide MHP initiatives, such as (1) a positive conceptualization of mental health; (2) an emphasis on meaningful engagement, participatory and empowerment-oriented approaches that enable individuals, groups, and communities to achieve and maintain their health; (3) a special focus on building upon existing strengths, assets, and capacities rather than a focus on problems and/or deficits; (4) collaborative action on the determinants of mental health; (5) multiple interventions across a wide range of sectors, policies, programs, settings, and environments; (6) approaches that are tailored and culturally appropriate; and (7) actions informed by evidence and practice (GermAnn & Ardiles, 2009).

Misconceptions that mental health is only relevant to the segment of the population experiencing (or at high risk of) mental illness, or that mental health and physical health issues exist in isolation of each other, act as barriers in MHP. Raising awareness about the importance of mental health in health promotion practice and building consensus around a common understanding is critical for successful MHP initiatives. However, a study in 2010 of health providers in BC showed that participants had difficulty defining and identifying MHP goals and outcomes, alongside the social determinants of mental health; instead, there was a greater focus on poor mental health and illness (Rauscher, Ardiles, & Griffin, 2013). Furthermore, MHP was mostly defined within a healthy lifestyle approach and there was no mention of health-promoting activities extending beyond health education (Rauscher et al., 2013). As a result of these findings, the Provincial Health Service Authority in BC launched a participatory capacity-building project to enhance the MHP skills and knowledge of health and community service providers (PHSA, 2014).

In July 2013, the Provincial System Support Program at the Centre for Addiction and Mental Health (CAMH) released its *Connecting the Dots* report, aimed to better understand how Ontario public health units are addressing child and youth mental health. They noted that historically in Canada, the role of public health in mental health has not been well described, and that MHP is a field that is not well understood in the context of public health's core business of illness prevention and health promotion. Nonetheless, the public health workforce across Canada is mandated to respond to local health issues, which include mental health needs as well (CAMH, Public Health Ontario, & Toronto Public Health, 2013). This report identified key enablers for public health, including partnerships, strong leadership, and commitment within public health; fundamental public health approaches, principles, and frameworks; and staff expertise. Common barriers were also reported that related to a lack of a provincial mandate contributing to unclear roles in public health; a lack of dedicated resources; coordination challenges among community partners; a lack of focus on MHP and mental illness prevention; stigma; and gaps in mental health services (CAMH et al., 2013). In 2015, CAMH released a survey of public health units in Ontario revealing that 39 percent of them mentioned MHP explicitly in their organizational strategic planning and other accountability documents, 31 percent had staff exclusively dedicated to MHP, and 58 percent reported having staff with MHP as a primary function of their work (CAMH, 2015).

In 2014, the National Collaborating Centre for Healthy Public Policy (NCCHPP) released a framework for a population health approach to mental health in Canada that includes an exploration of public policy approaches, social determinants of mental health, and pathways to mental health inequities (Mantoura, 2014). The following year, the NCCHPP conducted a survey of more than 450 public health practitioners to assess their needs in the area of population mental health. The participants revealed that they understood the link between mental health, physical health, and the social determinants of health, and used this understanding to explain how their public health practice is associated with mental health in various settings, such as perinatal activities, early childhood and parenting, schools, or work in clinical prevention and MHP specifically. However, participants also identified the lack of a clear mandate and, importantly, a lack of understanding of public health's role in mental health and in addressing the determinants of health, and a lack of resources to promote mental health. The report outlined the need for clear and fully supported guidelines for public health practice in mental health, which include clear mandates, institutional/organizational support (human and financial resources), and clear roles for practitioners at different levels, as well as support for ongoing collaboration (Mantoura, 2016).

Lack of Common Agenda

Health promotion practitioners across Canada use various terminologies in MHP including: positive mental health, mental wellness, population mental health, public mental health, mental fitness, and mental wellbeing. Ideally, the language used for promoting mental health is reflective of cultural, social, and political context in order to capture the attention of stakeholders (GermAnn, McKean, & Ardiles, 2011). Yet there are numerous untapped opportunities to embed mental health messaging into other existing health promotion initiatives, such as child/maternal/paternal health, healthy living programs, disaster preparedness, and health literacy. Further, it is imperative to bring those working in public health and MHP together, while also broadening the agenda to other sectors. As is the case with health promotion, it is important to consider how to embed mental health promotion into other fields of practice such as social work, health care, mental health, human resources, and veterans' affairs.

Interestingly, the lack of consensus around language may have an unintentional benefit. It can allow MHP to be integrated into diverse policy and programs, with a focus on promoting mental health for everyday life, as part of a broader lifespan approach that facilitates shared ownership across sectors. For instance, several provinces are implementing the Nurse-Family Partnership model that encourages nurse home visits during pregnancy and/ or postpartum, using a strength-based approach. These types of initiatives have multiple outcomes (e.g., improved maternal, infant, and child mental health; improved parenting skills; healthier relationships; higher employment rates; social connectedness; increased high-school completion rates) across what have traditionally been considered distinct policy sectors or domains (e.g., education, employment, health and social services). Moreover, policies and programs promoting mental health are now being evaluated across the country (e.g., Public Health Agency of Canada's Innovation Strategy), making it easier to position MHP as a key area of future investment in Canada.

Perhaps what is more essential than consensus on language is a common agenda and a shared responsibility to promote mental health. The Council of the Federation, which brings together premiers from across Canada, organized a Mental Health Summit in 2012 that laid the foundation for a intersectoral approach to promote mental health, as "it is important that we find ways to communicate the connection between mental wellbeing and economic prosperity, school performance, and physical health and wellbeing, so that mental health can be promoted in policies and practices in all areas of social and economic life" (Mental Health Summit Steering Committee, 2013, p. 7).

Ultimately, a common agenda is one that improves mental health for all Canadians. The health promotion workforce is diverse across disciplines, sectors, and even geography in Canada. Given this, how can we best integrate the promotion of mental health into our current roles? Below is a framework that proposes five key roles that support a mental health promotion practice, across the lifespan and the continuum of care, including MHP, mental illness prevention, along with mental health services and supports. The following framework highlights five roles to champion the promotion of mental health:

1. Monitoring and assessing the mental health of the population or sub-populations to identify mental health problems across the lifespan

2. Ensuring early identification and culturally safe interventions to promote mental health at the individual, family, and societal levels

3. Using collaborative approaches, developing policies, and designing programs and services to address the mental health and mental wellbeing of communities

4. Delivering services directly with stakeholders within and beyond the health system to help promote protective factors or mitigate risk factors related to mental health problems, and reduce mental health inequities

5. Engaging communities and enabling policy makers and professionals in other sectors to better understand the scale and impact of population mental health issues so they can take appropriate strategic or remedial action (Adapted from British Columbia Ministry of Health, *Promote, Protect, Prevent: Our Health Begins Here: BC's Guiding Framework for Public Health*, 2013; Government of Ontario, *Open Minds, Healthy Minds Progress Report*, 2014; and Public Health England's *Public Mental Health Leadership and Workforce Development Framework*, 2015)

PROMISING PRACTICES IN MENTAL HEALTH PROMOTION IN CANADA

This section will showcase three promising practices as examples of how MHP work is being shared with various partners and sectors across Canada, and across practice, research, and policy areas. They were chosen on the basis of demonstrating various interventions and leadership across different geographical regions of Canada, as well as demonstrating different levels of intervention, such as community versus provincial, and across the lifespan. The examples also take place in different settings: one specifically addresses the issues of cultural competency, and two specifically address the issue of mental health inequities. These three examples will include efforts along the continuum, from MHP to mental health services and supports. Barriers and enablers faced in promoting mental health are also outlined below.

BC Healthy Connections Research Project: Creating Supportive Environments at Home

Public health in British Columbia is demonstrating leadership in this area by participating in a randomized controlled trial (RCT) called the BC Healthy Connections Project (BCHCP) to study the effectiveness of an intensive home-visiting program called the Nurse-Family Partnership (NFP) program. NFP is designed to help disadvantaged young first-time mothers and their children using a strength-based approach.

Public health prenatal services complement the multidisciplinary reproductive health care services to support pregnant women with screening, health promotion, education, and referral to other needed health or community services. Public health can offer underserved women more intensive follow-up and enhanced services, supporting them to make the healthiest choices possible during pregnancy, including accessing community resources that would be of benefit. The goals are to improve children's mental health and early development, while also improving mothers' life situations. Public health nurses (PHN) play an important role in supporting women throughout the pregnancy and into children's early years in the women's own homes, in order to enhance their coping skills and strengthen their emotional wellbeing. The home setting enables PHNs to gain a genuine understanding of each woman's unique living situation, to help enable mothers to gain control over their own social and built environment. Every health authority in BC has set up a prenatal registry to connect families to public health nurses and community supports. While NFP was tested in a pilot study at McMaster University, it has never been fully evaluated in Canada before. Over the next five years an evaluation will determine how well this program works in BC communities.

Enablers

Stable funding and multi-level partnerships are key enablers of this program.[6] In addition, as a research collaborative, the NFP program is being evaluated in two parts: (1) an RCT of the program's effectiveness compared with existing services, and (2) a process evaluation of nurses' experiences and the program adaptations needed in BC. In October 2013, the RCT was launched, and over three years more than 700 families were recruited to participate (Children's Health Policy Centre, 2016). Child and maternal outcomes will be evaluated throughout pregnancy and until children reach their second birthday. The process evaluation studies how the program is being implemented in the five regional Health Authorities to meet the needs of families across the province and will also help understand BC's (and Canada's) unique context, including the situations faced by PHNs, their supervisors, and the families they visit, alongside the solutions developed by the NFP teams to resolve any emergent challenges.

Barriers

Coordination across BC's primary care and public health prenatal services is challenged in reaching *all* pregnant mothers who may benefit from public health services, especially if they are vulnerable. A growing number of women are registering in the project through prenatal registries and/or are being referred by their care providers as early in pregnancy as possible. However, these young women are often hard to reach because they may not have stable housing, reliable work, or supportive extended families. PHNs may find it challenging to locate young mothers who may be highly mobile, and financial difficulties may also lead to some women having limited access to telephones or cellphones.

Another challenge is that many of these young women may not have had good role models to help them learn what a trusting relationship looks like or how to maintain healthy relationships. The trusting relationship that is built with the NFP PHN is sometimes the first positive, supportive relationship in a woman's life. PHNs are trained with specialized skills to support effective communication with young women, as well as the families they serve. The process evaluation will involve collecting comprehensive data on some of the enablers and barriers PHNs (and other care providers) are facing in the implementation of BCHCP, in order to better support families to promote health and wellbeing (Children's Health Policy Centre, 2017).

White Raven Healing Centre Team: Enhancing Emotional Health and Spiritual Strength

Mental health wellness teams are multidisciplinary teams developed and driven by communities. Through community engagement and partnerships, the teams provide a variety of cultural, clinical, and community-as-a-whole services and supports for mental health and addictions to a small cluster of First Nations communities on an ongoing basis. To enhance the capacity of individuals and community, the services provided vary depending on the community needs, approaches, local infrastructure, and availability of cultural, clinical, and community expertise. The Mental Wellness Teams (MWTs) concept has been demonstrated as an effective model for developing relationships that support service delivery collaborations both with provinces and territories and between community, cultural, and clinical service providers (Health Canada, 2015).

The White Raven Healing Centre (WRHC) is a program of the File Hills Qu'Appelle Tribal Council, which has 11 member First Nations. The Centre was established in 2003 and became designated as an MWT in 2008. WRHC provides mental health services, addictions counselling, Indian Residential School IAP Support, and cultural and spiritual services to First Nations within the File Hills Qu'Appelle Tribal Council area. WRHC is located at the All Nations' Healing Hospital in Fort Qu'Appelle, Saskatchewan (approximately 74 kilometres northeast of Regina), and all the services of WRHC are housed in one facility. WRHC has an open door policy in which First Nations people are welcome to visit at any time. They offer afterhours and/or crisis services, and outreach in-community services are also available on request by FHQ Tribal Council First Nations. WRHC has an interdisciplinary MWT composed of First Nations and Inuit Health Branch[7]–approved therapists, certified addictions counsellors, Indian Residential School support workers, and Elders. They provide a range of services for holistic counselling programs in a safe, culturally sensitive environment to assist individuals, families, and communities in healing past trauma and to maintain emotional wellness (FHQ Tribal Council, 2016).

Enablers
WRHC has a strong team of qualified personnel whose background, training, and experience equip them uniquely to enhance peoples' emotional health and spiritual strength and demonstrate sensitivity to their communities' values and traditions. One of the key enablers of WRHC is that it operates within a First Nation culturally appropriate, community specific framework, using the principle of empowerment to promote and facilitate individual resiliency and collective development.

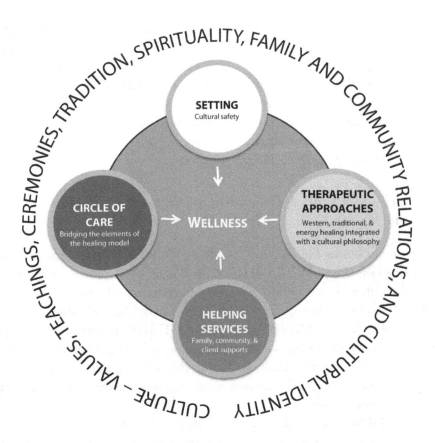

Figure 9.1: White Raven Healing Model

Source: Adapted from the White Raven Healing Centre, File Hills Qu'Appelle Tribal Council website. *White Raven Healing Centre.* Retrieved from http://fhqtc.com/entities/white-raven-healing-centre/

This framework allows for team members to collaborate and effectively communicate their philosophy of "traditional healing," in service of using culture as healing. The vision of WRHC Elders and leadership has been to provide client-centred mental health programming that integrates the best of mainstream therapeutic techniques with traditional First Nations healing practices to provide a holistic approach to heal from past traumatic experiences and current psychological issues (FHQ Tribal Council, 2016.).

Barriers
Instability of funding has been recognized by WRHC as the single most important barrier to their work in mental wellness. Over the course of nearly a decade of operations, WRHC has been able to count on only a few stable sources of funding. They receive some mental health funding from the federal government through the MWTs; however, the needs of the community are complex and require funding for services to address issues of trauma, violence, and substance use. WRHC had a mandate to provide gambling addictions

services as per an agreement with the Federation of Saskatchewan Indians, although they provide in-kind alcohol and drug addiction services for which they receive no funding. Insecure funding from multiple sources under "sunset" provisions leaves the WRHC vulnerable, making it difficult to plan effectively for the long-term, especially when it comes to maintaining the staff who serve the needs of more than 20,000 in the community (FHQ Tribal Council, 2016). A truly sustainable model for Indigenous wellness requires the enablement of self-governance and community-building initiatives that acknowledge Indigenous knowledge, Elders, and community values.

Provincial System Support Program at the Centre for Addiction and Mental Health, Ontario: Healthy Public Policy

Based within the Centre for Addiction and Mental Health's (CAMH) Provincial System Support Program (PSSP), the CAMH Health Promotion Resource Centre (CAMH HPRC) strengthens public health leadership and provides system-level support in the area of MHP and substance misuse prevention. Funded by Ontario's Ministry of Health and Long-Term Care, CAMH HPRC works to build MHP capacity in Ontario's public health workforce by supporting system-level capacity-building and knowledge exchange; investing in partnerships that are strategic, outcome-oriented, and contribute to system improvement; and making evidence-based tools and resources relevant and applicable for public health professionals.

CAMH HPRC works with CAMH researchers, clinicians, and public health partners to share evidence through webinars, conferences, and other tools to inform program planning, practice, and policy in public health. For example, during the first three years of Ontario's comprehensive ten-year mental health and addictions strategy, Open Minds, Healthy Minds (Government of Ontario, 2011), CAMH HPRC helped to share research such as CAMH's Ontario Student Drug Use and Health Survey, Canada's longest ongoing school survey regarding student mental health and addictions. In addition, CAMH HPRC worked to promote access and use of evidence-based resources like CAMH's *Best Practice Guidelines for MHP Programs: Children and Youth* (2014), a resource developed in partnership with University of Toronto's Dalla Lana School of Public Health and Toronto Public Health to inform public health practice in MHP.

Enablers

CAMH HPRC invests in partnerships that are strategic, outcome-oriented, and contribute to system improvement. For example, partnering with key provincial public health system partners and local partners, CAMH HPRC worked with Public Health Ontario and Toronto Public Health on a provincial public health survey to understand the range of activities, initiatives, services, and programming undertaken by public health units to address and promote mental health in children and youth. The research also aimed to describe the enablers and barriers that public health units experience when implementing activities to promote mental health and prevent mental illness in children and youth. The resulting report, *Connecting the Dots: How Ontario Public Health Units are Addressing Child and Youth Mental Health* (CAMH, Public Health Ontario, & Toronto Public Health, 2013), found that public health units were involved in a wide range of activities and initiatives and that these activities were often driven by local need. Findings from the report identified that key enablers included partnerships, strong leadership and commitment from within public health units, staff expertise, and embedded approaches to addressing child and youth mental health.

Barriers

Barriers identified included limited resources, such as evidence and expertise, a lack of a specific provincial mandate to guide public health activity related to MHP, coordination challenges with local partners, public perceptions regarding stigma and conceptualizations of mental health and mental illness, and unmet needs/gaps within the mental health service system. Findings also demonstrated a need for system-level discussions to clarify the role of public health in MHP for children and youth.

Summary

All three of these examples demonstrate that integrating mental health into health promotion research, policy, and practice is possible. As was noted above, funding constraints, lack of capacity or resources, and the multiplicity of stakeholders are often common challenges. Nevertheless, the above examples demonstrate that clear roles and mandates, as well as program and policy support and engagement, are key enablers to make this work effective and impactful. Taking a leadership role in MHP requires attention to setting common goals, stable funding, the building of strategic partnerships, and collaboration within health promotion and beyond. However, to date there has been a lack of recognition as to how mental health is an essential aspect of everyday health promotion practice, as well as how these initiatives are related to core health promotion principles such as empowerment and participation.

As is evidenced in this section above, promotion of mental health is happening in various settings, with multiple partnerships and across various policy areas. Given the wider range of approaches outlined above, as well as some common barriers and enablers identified in the promising practices, how can we best promote partnerships and networks, and coordinate mental health efforts across Canada?

A CULTURAL SHIFT IN HEALTH PROMOTION: LEADERSHIP SKILLS TO PROMOTE MENTAL HEALTH AND WELLBEING

In addition to gathering more evidence about MHP, it is also necessary to equip the health promotion workforce with leadership skills to support a culture shift that promotes mental health. Why? *Knowledge is not enough.* In order to create change towards a common agenda and a shared responsibility for promoting mental health, health promotion practitioners require dedicated resources and leadership skills to build and support partnerships and networks, and coordinate efforts across Canada.

Leadership can refer to the ability of an individual to influence, motivate, and enable others to contribute towards the effectiveness and success of the community/organization in which they work. It involves inspiring people to craft and achieve a shared vision and goals. Leaders provide mentoring, coaching, and recognition; they encourage empowerment, allowing other leaders to emerge (PHAC, 2008).

Leadership is key to shifting the health promotion workforce culture to promote mental health and involves individual, team, and organizational levels. Workforce culture here refers to shared values, beliefs, assumptions, perceptions, and norms that lead to patterns of behaviour within the workforce; it shapes how things get done, what people think, how

Table 9.1: A Cultural Shift in Health Promotion: Leadership Skills to Promote Mental Health and Wellbeing

	Individual Practitioner	Team	Organizations
Skills	- Self-reflection - Self-awareness	- Communication - Collaboration - Partnership building	- Leadership skills - Management skills
Key reflective questions	1. How does your workplace demonstrate that you are a champion promoting mental health and wellbeing (e.g., what things do you do to explicitly build your own resiliency at work)? 2. How are your attitudes, beliefs, and values about mental health impacting those around you (e.g., how do you convey your priorities)? 3. What can you continue to do (or change) in order to engage your staff, management, colleagues, and community partners in the work to promote mental health and wellbeing?	1. How does your team establish reflective and effective communication to promote mental health and wellbeing? 2. What are the structures and processes in place to support regular team reflection and evaluation of work related to mental health and wellbeing? 3. What are the processes in place that can support your team to collaborate and partner with key stakeholders in order to promote positive mental health and wellbeing?	1. What are some of the policies and processes in place in your setting that support the health promotion workforce to effectively deliver service to promote mental health and wellbeing? 2. What kind of resources, technologies, and capacities does your management support in order to deliver effective services to promote mental health and wellbeing? 3. How can your management influence the organization's strategic priorities and/or mission to promote mental health and wellbeing?

people feel, and the actions people take. Leadership skills can be used at the individual, team, or management level, regardless of job title or position.

Table 9.1 shows how leadership skills can support this culture shift so that everyone in health promotion understands their role and their responsibility in promoting mental health and wellbeing. This section has been adapted from *Health Compass: Transformative Practices, Embracing Mental Wellbeing* (PHSA, 2014), an innovative, collaborative capacity-building project aimed to enhance the capacity of health care providers in the area of MHP.

In championing mental health and wellbeing, it is important to lead by example so that others can see opportunities for themselves, too. While acknowledging that everyone has a role to play in promoting mental health, it is often challenging to see what the first step is in creating a culture shift. Ultimately, it starts with one step, big or small—that one step can be as simple as beginning a conversation. The critical element that will support mental health promotion leadership is to ensure you set up metrics to be able to find meaningful indicators of success, and systems to support implementation and sustainability of these efforts.

CONCLUSION

In July 2013, the Council of the Federation, which brings together premiers from across Canada, made a commitment to a fair and inclusive society where citizens have access to public services that support their wellbeing and help them contribute to the social and economic fabric of society. The premiers directed their ministers to continue to develop best practices for MHP and mental illness prevention and identify how approaches, treatments, and supports can be shared across jurisdictions to reach all individuals and communities, including in Aboriginal and remote regions (Council of the Federation, 2013).

As health promotion advocates, we need to understand that inequities that arise from a lack of availability, accessibility, and acceptability of services cannot be addressed through one isolated policy, program, or educational initiative. Dedicated resources and infrastructure at all levels are essential to ensure that MHP is prioritized and that health promotion can continue to serve as a catalyst, convener, and leader towards a flourishing Canada.

ACKNOWLEDGEMENTS

Many thanks to all those who contributed case studies and materials to this chapter, including Elaine Lavallee, Tamar Meyer, Donna Jepsen, Pascale Mantoura and the members of the Pan Canadian Mental Health working group, as well as the Public Health Agency of Canada, who commissioned a report that served as a foundation for this chapter. A special thank you to Crystal Hutchinson, Jim Frankish, Irving Rootman, Michelle Aslan, and Zainah Merani for reviewing earlier drafts and providing thoughtful feedback. This chapter is dedicated to Dr. Elliot Goldner, who we lost at the end of 2016 when I was finishing this chapter. Elliot was a champion for mental health, both in Canada and globally, and I had the good fortune to work with him at Simon Fraser University. He will be remembered as a very generous, creative, caring, and humble person who mentored and supported many of us in our professional development.

CRITICAL THINKING QUESTIONS

1. What are some key principles and features of mental health promotion?
2. What are some of the key enablers and barriers experienced by health promotion practitioners in addressing mental health and wellbeing?
3. How can health promotion practitioners, researchers, and policy makers embed mental health promotion principles into their daily practice?
4. Why is it important to embed mental health promotion across disciplines and across sectors? Give examples.
5. What are some of the key leadership skills needed to promote mental health and wellbeing?

RESOURCES

Further Readings

Centre for Addiction and Mental Health (CAMH). (2012). *Mental health promotion for youth in Canada.* Toronto: CAMH.
This review discusses significant topics in the area of youth mental health. An overview of key terms, issues, and interventions is presented, as well as promising practices and recommendations in youth mental health promotion.

Centre for Addiction and Mental Health (CAMH). (2014). *Best practice guidelines for mental health promotion programs: Children (7–12) and youth (13–19).* Toronto: CAMH.
This resource presents current concepts, principles, evidence-based approaches, and best practice guidelines for mental health promotion initiatives and programs targeting children and youth.

Watson, S., & McDonald, K. (2016). *Mental health promotion: Let's start speaking the same language.* Waterloo: Region of Waterloo Public Health & Emergency Services.
The authors define mental health, review key concepts and theories, and highlight effective interventions related to mental health promotion.

Relevant Websites

CAMH Health Promotion Resource Centre (CAMH HPRC)
www.porticonetwork.ca/web/camh-hprc

CAMH HPRC is Ontario's source for health promotion evidence regarding mental health and substance use, and it builds related capacity in health promotion, public health, and allied health professionals. Other primary activities include partnership development and knowledge exchange to impact local and system-level practice, planning, and policy.

Canadian Best Practices Portal: Mental Health and Wellness
cbpp-pcpe.phac-aspc.gc.ca/public-health-topics/mental-health-and-wellness/
The Public Health Agency of Canada has compiled these relevant and evidence-based resources to provide information to help you plan programs that promote mental health and wellness.

Health Compass: Transformative Practices, Embracing Mental Wellbeing
www.bcmhsus.ca/health-compass
Health Compass was developed by the Provincial Health Service Authority, in collaboration with local and global experts, as well as health care providers. Health Compass is an online course and electronic information guide aimed to provide education and training to health care providers and non-clinical staff to deepen their knowledge of, and strengthen their skills to promote, patient and family mental health and wellbeing.

NOTES

1. Mental Health Commission of Canada, funded by the federal government.
2. Mental illness prevention focuses on reducing risk factors and enhancing protective factors associated with mental ill-health. This involves reducing the risk, incidence, prevalence, and recurrence of mental disorders, as well as the time spent with symptoms or the risk condition of a mental illness. Focus is also on preventing or delaying recurrences and decreasing the impact of illness on the affected persons, their families, and society (Jané-Llopis & Anderson, 2006, p. 7).
3. The national strategy serves as a guideline for stakeholders across the country, as the MHCC does not have the jurisdictional authority or the resources necessary to implement a plan across Canada.
4. In 2014 NCCHPP conducted an environmental scan.
5. *A Path Forward: BC First Nations and Aboriginal People's Mental Wellness and Substance Use—Ten Year Plan* was released in early 2013 by British Columbia's First Nations Health Authority.
6. BCHCP is being funded by the BC Ministry of Health, with support from the BC Ministry of Children and Family Development and the five regional BC Health Authorities (Fraser Health, Interior Health, Island Health, Northern Health, and Vancouver Coastal Health).
7. At a federal level, the First Nations and Inuit Health Branch (FNIHB) of Health Canada has taken a leadership role in terms of policy and program development, specifically through the FNIHB's mental wellness initiatives. One of these initiatives has been the funding of Mental Wellness Teams across Canada.

REFERENCES

British Columbia Ministry of Health. (2013). *Promote, protect, prevent: Our health begins Here: BC's guiding framework for public health*. Victoria: British Columbia Ministry of Health.

Centre for Addiction and Mental Health (CAMH). (2014). *Best practice guidelines for mental health promotion programs: Children (7–12) and youth (13–19)*. Toronto: CAMH.

Centre for Addiction and Mental Health (CAMH). (2015). *Pathways to promoting mental health: A 2015 survey of Ontario Public Health units*. Toronto: CAMH Health Promotion Resource Centre.

Centre for Addiction and Mental Health (CAMH), Ontario Agency for Health Protection and Promotion (Public Health Ontario), & Toronto Public Health. (2013). *Connecting the dots: How Ontario public health units are addressing child and youth mental health*. Toronto: CAMH.

Centre for Health Promotion. (1997). *Proceedings from the International Workshop on Mental Health Promotion*. Toronto: University of Toronto. Cited on p. 16 in Joubert, N., & Raeburn, J. (1999). Mental health promotion: People, power and passion. *International Journal of Mental Health Promotion, 1*, 15–22.

Children's Health Policy Centre. (2016). *Study Milestone Reached: BC Healthy Connections recruitment closing as planned*. Vancouver: Simon Fraser University. Retrieved from childhealthpolicy.ca/nfp-in-bc/

Children's Health Policy Centre. (2017). *BC Healthy Connections Project*. Vancouver: Simon Fraser University. Retrieved from childhealthpolicy.ca/bc-healthy-connections-project/

Council of the Federation. (2013). *Council of the Federation Communiqué: Canada's premiers are committed to a fair and inclusive society*. Ottawa: Council of the Federation. Retrieved from www.canadaspremiers.ca/en/latest-news/13-2013/340-canada-s-premiers-are-committed-to-a-fair-and-inclusive-society

File Hills Qu'Appelle (FHQ) Tribal Council. (2016). *White Raven Healing Centre*. Retrieved from fhqtc.com/entities/white-raven-healing-centre/

First Nations Health Authority (FNHA), British Columbia Ministry of Health, & Health Canada. (2013). *A path forward: BC First Nations and Aboriginal people's mental wellness and substance use ten-year plan*. British Columbia: FNHA, BC Ministry of Health, & Health Canada. Retrieved from www.fnha.ca/Documents/FNHA_MWSU.pdf

GermAnn, K., & Ardiles, P. (2009). *Toward flourishing for all*. Mental Health Promotion and Mental Illness Prevention Policy Background Paper and Companion Document. Pan-Canadian Steering Committee for Mental Health Promotion and Mental Illness Prevention. Retrieved from www.bcmhsus.ca/toward-flourishing-for-all-

GermAnn, K., McKean, G., & Ardiles, P. (2011). *Trends in international mental health promotion policy and action*. A Background Paper for the Public Health Agency of Canada. Unpublished Manuscript.

Government of Ontario. (2011). *Open minds, healthy minds: Ontario's comprehensive mental health and addictions strategy*. Ontario: Queen's Printer for Ontario.

Government of Ontario. (2014). *Open minds, healthy minds: Ontario's comprehensive mental health and addictions strategy. Progress Report*. Ontario: Queen's Printer for Ontario.

Health Canada. (2015). *First Nations mental wellness continuum framework.* Ottawa: Health Canada. Retrieved from www.hc-sc.gc.ca/fniah-spnia/alt_formats/pdf/pubs/promotion/mental/2014-sum-rpt-continuum/2014-sum-rpt-continuum-eng.pdf

Jané-Llopis, E., & Anderson, P. (Eds). (2006). *Mental health promotion and mental disorder prevention across European Member States: A collection of country stories.* Luxembourg: European Communities. Retrieved from ec.europa.eu/health/ph_projects/2004/action1/docs/action1_2004_a02_30_en.pdf

Mantoura, P. (2014). *Defining a population mental health framework for public health.* Montréal: National Collaborating Centre for Healthy Public Policy.

Mantoura, P. (2016). *Main types of needs of the public health workforce for population mental health.* Montréal: National Collaborating Centre for Healthy Public Policy.

Mental Health Commission of Canada (MHCC). (2012). *Changing directions, changing lives: The mental health strategy for Canada.* Calgary: MHCC.

Mental Health Summit Steering Committee. (2013). *Background: Mental Health Summit 2012.* Unpublished Manuscript.

National Collaborating Centre for Healthy Public Policy (NCCHPP). (2014). *Scan of mental health strategies across Canada.* Montréal: NCCHPP.

Provincial Health Service Authority (PHSA). (2014). *Health compass: Transformative practices, embracing mental wellbeing.* Retrieved from www.bcmhsus.ca/health-compass

Public Health Agency of Canada (PHAC). (2007). *Public Health Agency of Canada's Innovation Strategy: A closer look at the Innovation Strategy.* Ottawa: PHAC.

Public Health Agency of Canada (PHAC). (2008). *Core competencies for public health in Canada regional consultations: Final report.* Ottawa: PHAC.

Public Health England. (2015). *Public mental health leadership and workforce development framework: Confidence, competence and commitment.* London: Public Health England. Retrieved from www.gov.uk/government/publications/public-mental-health-leadership-and-workforce-development-framework

Rauscher, A., Ardiles, P., & Griffin, S. (2013). Building mental health promotion in health care: Results from Phase I of a workforce development project. *International Journal of Mental Health Promotion, 15*(2), 76–92.

CHAPTER 10

Promising Practices in Indigenous Community Health Promotion

Charlotte Loppie

LEARNING OBJECTIVES

1. Understand the historical, cultural, political, social, and economic contexts that shape Indigenous peoples' health
2. Understand the diversity of Indigenous cultures and the importance of culturally grounded and safe Indigenous health promotion
3. Understand the value and implications of community-led and engaged Indigenous health promotion

INTRODUCTION

The World Health Organization defines health promotion as "the process of enabling people to increase control over their health and its determinants, and thereby improve their health" (WHO, 2007, p. 10). Similarly, within Indigenous contexts, health promotion is considered most promising when it involves shared decision-making and collaborative processes that maximize self-determination (i.e., control) over health determinants such as self-governance, environmental stewardship, community development, food security, education, and many others (Chandler & Lalonde, 1998; Loppie Reading & Wien, 2009; NAHO, 2002).

POLITICAL CONTEXTS

The United Nations estimates that there are more than 370 million Indigenous people worldwide, including those in North, Central, and South America, northern Europe, Australia, and New Zealand (United Nations, 2016). While no definitive description of

Indigeneity exists, a distinction has been made between European settler societies and peoples with ancestral connections to colonized lands, languages, and cultural traditions.

In 1982, in the absence of consultation with Indigenous peoples, the Constitution Act of Canada (Section 35, 2) established the term *Aboriginal* to denote Inuit, Métis, and First Nations peoples. Although each of these federally designated groups has a unique relationship with the Crown (Government of Canada, 2016), there are several important political distinctions between them, which can substantially influence the processes and outcomes of health promotion policies and programs. Within the Canadian context, the term *Indigenous* is beginning to replace *Aboriginal* as a more appropriate representation of First Peoples and is therefore used whenever possible and appropriate in this chapter.

The homeland of the Inuit is known as Inuit Nunangat, which encompasses the land, water, and ice of the Arctic region. In 1999, the largest Aboriginal land claims agreement occurred between the Canadian government and the Inuit people, resulting in the formation of Nunavut, which was formerly part of the Northwest Territories (Dewar, 2009). During that year, the Nunavut government was officially formed and, like other jurisdictions, receives transfers from the federal government under the Canada Health Transfer, Canada Social Transfer, and the Territorial Financing Formula (Government of Nunavut, n.d.). The Inuit now live in the territory of Nunavut (Canadian Arctic and Subarctic), Nunavik (northern Québec), Nunatsiavut and NunatuKavut (Labrador), as well as parts of the Northwest Territories, in addition to urban, rural, and remote locations across the country.

First Nations people (formerly referred to as "Indians" or "Natives") make up approximately 60 percent of the Indigenous peoples of the land known as Canada. First Nations people live on lands reserved for their use by the colonial government (known as reserves) as well as in urban, rural, and remote locations across the country. In 1876, the recently formed Canadian government passed the Indian Act, a piece of legislation that exerted control over almost every aspect of First Nations' identity, lands, languages, and cultural practices (Department of Justice Canada, 2013). Shortly after, the Department of Indian Affairs (DIA) was established to oversee this and other colonial policies. During the ensuing years, both the Indian Act and the DIA have undergone a series of revisions, yet both continue to regulate the economic, social, and political lives of First Nations people (Makarenko, 2008).

Métis people have both European and Indigenous ancestry but were not historically considered "Indians" under the Canadian Constitution and therefore did not fall under federal jurisdiction. In April 2016, the Supreme Court of Canada ruled that non-status Indians (those not recognized under the Indian Act) and Métis should be classified as "Indians" under section 91(24) of the Constitution. This clarifies that both groups are a constitutional responsibility of the federal government and not the provinces (CBC News, 2016). However, the federal government's role in providing these groups with health and social programs as well as benefits similar to status First Nations people remains undecided.

CULTURAL CONTEXT

Within the Americas and elsewhere, Indigenous cultures and languages are as diverse as any within Europe (e.g., Italian, German, Spanish). Yet one of the most widespread misconceptions held by non-Indigenous people is that a single Indigenous worldview and culture exists. In fact, there is vast national and regional diversity with respect to Indigenous cultures, languages, traditions, and practices. In Canada alone there are more than 60 Indigenous languages (Statistics Canada, 2011).

Indigenous cultures are best understood as locally situated. Even language groups, which may span entire provinces or regions, often have distinct local dialects that may construct concepts differently. Health promotion professionals who have established respectful relationships with Indigenous partners take the time to learn about local, regional, and national distinctions and similarities. In this way, health promotion processes and, more importantly, supports[1] are designed, implemented, and assessed within the most appropriate cultural contexts.

A number of similar historical circumstances have shaped the health and wellbeing of all Indigenous peoples living in Canada. Most notably, all three Indigenous groups have undergone a process of colonization[2] that included the dispossession of ancestral lands, the imposition of colonial institutions, and the disruption of traditional lifestyles (RCAP, 1996). It is critical that health professionals and policy makers gain a comprehensive appreciation of how historical and current political intrusions have shaped social inequities as well as the health promotion needs of Indigenous communities. Otherwise, health promotion programs might duplicate disrespectful practices and represent a form of colonial oppression.

INDIGENOUS HEALTH INEQUITIES

Indigenous peoples in Canada, and indeed globally, experience substantial health inequities relative to people of European settler ancestry. A critical mass of literature, accumulated by governments and researchers since the early days of colonization, describes a rapid decline in the overall health of Indigenous children, youth, adults, and elders (Adelson, 2005; Loppie Reading & Wien, 2009; RCAP, 1996; TRC, 2015; United Nations, 2008). Although there is now substantial evidence that geographic colonization, political domination, economic disadvantage, and social discrimination are key determinants of Indigenous health, both Indigenous and allied[3] researchers are becoming reluctant to focus too much attention on the health disparities facing Indigenous peoples, as those very statistics have been repeatedly used to pathologize and further stereotype them. Nevertheless, it is critical that we acknowledge these disparities so we can accurately trace their origins and move forward in our collective attempt to assist in the most appropriate places, using the most suitable and relevant approaches.

SOCIAL DETERMINANTS OF INDIGENOUS HEALTH

The foundational premise of health promotion is that health and/or illness occurs within specific contexts. According to the Commission on Social Determinants of Health

> the social determinants of health are the conditions in which people are born, grow, live, work and age, including the health system. These circumstances are shaped by the distribution of money, power and resources at global, national and local levels, which are themselves influenced by policy choices. The social determinants of health are mostly responsible for health inequities—the unfair and avoidable differences in health status seen within and between countries. (WHO, 2016, para. 1)

Despite this globally recognized definition, Indigenous ancestry remains listed among the social determinants of health, as though simply being Indigenous causes one to get sick more often and to die prematurely. In fact, being Indigenous—or a member of any other racialized[4] group, does not inherently predispose one to good or ill health. It is the social, political, and economic marginalization and discrimination of Indigenous peoples, by those in racialized positions of power, that leads to health inequities. So, in addition to the other social determinants of health, racism, colonization, and colonialism are among the most critical determinants of Indigenous peoples' health (Loppie Reading & Wien, 2009; Reading, 2014).

Colonization, Racism, and Colonialism

Indigenous peoples across the globe have experienced centuries of European colonization and colonialism[5] resulting in the loss of territories, languages, and traditions as well as an increasingly disproportionate burden of disease, injury, and early death (Loppie Reading & Wien, 2009). Indigenous peoples have also been the subjects of European "intervention" since first contact. Unfortunately, racist beliefs as well as political, social, and economic domination shape much of the practice, which often pathologizes and sometimes harms Indigenous peoples. An example can be found in government-sanctioned experiments that withheld nutrition from Indigenous children in residential schools during the 1940s and 1950s (Mosby, 2013).

Fortunately, the emergence of social justice philosophies during the late twentieth century led to a rise in health promotion that considers ethno-cultural inequities, which continue to shape Indigenous health. Nevertheless, historical traumas have created a justifiable distrust in colonial structures, including institutions of health. Trust is slowly being established but far too many health professionals continue to unwittingly or intentionally ignore cultural and other critical contexts, thus perpetuating a colonial relationship with

Indigenous peoples and negatively affecting their health and wellbeing. The relevance and practice of cultural safety is discussed in the section on decolonizing health promotion.

INDIGENOUS CONSTRUCTIONS OF HEALTH

Despite diversity in geography, language, and cultural practice, Indigenous peoples share certain metaphysical and philosophical beliefs. Indigenous knowledge systems are predicated on the belief that many truths exist and are manifest in subjective life experiences. Humility is emphasized in belief systems that not only acknowledge all life as equal and related but that do not necessarily recognize humans as the most important beings in the cosmos (Oakes, Riewe, Koolage, Simpson, & Schuster, 2000).

Many Indigenous cultures embrace a gestalt paradigm, often reflected in value themes of holism, which emphasizes the complete person in the entirety of their life; personalism, which places value on individual autonomy and freedom; relationality, which acknowledges responsibility for the self, community, environment, and cosmos; as well as balance and harmony, which acknowledge the sacredness of all existence and unconditional respect for humans and non-humans alike (Gunn Allen, 1986; Klein & Ackerman, 1995; McMillan, 1995). Biomimicry[6] is also typically used in Indigenous models, as the natural environment is helpful in representing complex concepts such as wellness.

Holism

Indigenous peoples often conceptualize health (or wellness) within multiple domains (physical, emotional, mental, and spiritual), which are bound together and reciprocally shaped. In general, Indigenous cultures reflect a philosophical structure that positions the life of an individual within a network of family, community, and nation. Within this context, each individual is a vital thread in the social fabric (Paul, 2000). Holistic health is achieved when there is balance within and between health domains, as well as families, communities, nations, and the natural environment (Kelm, 1998).

Indigenous metaphysics often situate the human body where physical and spiritual realms intersect (Paul, 2000; Tagalik, 2015). Hence, we are individually and collectively shaped by activities in both realms that sometimes require healing that is "possessed of the ability to move between and among these states" (Kelm, 1998, p. 84). Complete wellness is thought to be achieved through harmony with the Creator, family, community, and nature (Long & Fox, 1996). This harmony extends temporally, thus symbolizing respect for ancient wisdom as well as connection and concern for future generations. This paradigm, based on unity, interrelatedness, and balance, differs considerably from Western Cartesian-based notions of health, which often deconstruct the physical body in isolation of the spiritual realm.[7]

Within many Indigenous cultures, a circle is used to represent the cyclical and dynamic nature of human life, consisting of many stages—birth, growth, death, and renewal (Leavitt, 1995). The circle also symbolizes an intimate connection between beliefs, knowledge, feelings, and actions, as well as among the individual, family, community, culture, and cosmos. The medicine wheel has been used traditionally by Indigenous peoples of the central regions of North America but has recently been adopted by others as a symbol of this holistic model (Canadian Encyclopedia, 2016). However, it is important to note that this symbol does not hold meaning for all Indigenous peoples.

Pluralism

Pluralism refers to the value of diversity and the practice of ensuring that people within a society are not excluded or humiliated for possessing different beliefs, spiritualities, cultures, languages, social practices, and so on (Pluralism, n.d.). Indigenous knowledge is pluralistic; it "overcomes [binaries] and oppositional logic that demands adherence to one absolute and rejection of its opposite" (Yunkaporta, 2007). In this way, Indigenous rationality allows for conflicting ideas to coexist simultaneously. Indeed, tension and balance between opposites is often the source of both new creation and social cohesion (Yunkaporta, 2007). An example of this can be found in the Haudenosaunee (Iroquois) Confederacy, formed during the seventeenth and eighteenth centuries, in which the Mohawk, Oneida, Onondaga, Cayuga, Seneca, and Tuscarora united to form a common council to oversee affairs at the intertribal level (Haudenosaunee Confederacy, 2016).

Conceptualized by Elder Albert Marshall (Eskasoni Mi'kmaq First Nation, Cape Breton, NS), "two-eyed seeing" reflects the concept of pluralism and offers an alternative to the existing divisiveness between Indigenous and Western approaches to health promotion. Rather than viewing these culturally distinct approaches as incommensurate with one another, Elder Marshall advises that we view health from "one eye with the strengths of Indigenous knowledges and ways of knowing, and from the other eye with the strengths of Western (or Eurocentric, conventional, or mainstream) knowledges and ways of knowing … and to use both these eyes together, for the benefit of all" (Marshall, Marshall, & Bartlett, 2015, pp. 17–18). In this way, health promotion strategies can draw from the perspectives of both Indigenous and Western thought, rather than the domination or assimilation of either. Willie Ermine conceptualizes the site of this plurality as "the ethical space," which "is formed when two societies, with disparate worldviews, are poised to engage each other. It is the thought about diverse societies and the space in between them that contributes to the development of a framework for dialogue between human communities" (Ermine, 2007, p. 193).

HEALTH PROMOTION AND INDIGENOUS PEOPLES IN CANADA

Decolonizing Health Promotion

Article 23 of the *United Nations Declaration on the Rights of Indigenous Peoples* (UNDRIP) states that "Indigenous peoples have the right to … be actively involved in developing and determining health, housing and other economic and social programmes affecting them and, as far as possible, to administer such programmes through their own institutions" (United Nations, 2008, p. 9). This appeal to decolonize Indigenous health systems and structures is likewise found in Articles 21 to 24 of Canada's *Truth and Reconciliation Commission: Calls to Action*, which recommend changes to the funding, implementation, and staffing of Indigenous health services, programs, and promotion as well as cultural safety training for all health professionals working in the area of Indigenous health (TRC, 2015).

Cultural safety refers to relationships and environments that are perceived by Indigenous peoples to be inoffensive, respectful, and non-violent (Wilson et al., 2013). Creating those relationships and environments requires a lifelong commitment, on the part of health professionals, to self-reflection of one's own culture and belief system. As well, we must critique the underlying assumptions and power imbalances that come with our social position, which subsequently guide our practice, and finally, be aware of "blindspots" that can unintentionally cause one to come across as paternalistic or domineering (Wilson et al., 2013). Wiebe, van Gaalen, Langlois, and Costen (2013) claim that it is "essential that service providers and administrators [including those working in health promotion] understand the impacts of history, traditions, values and forces on families and communities and those of their own social position, on the development and delivery of programs and services" (pp. 19–20).

Decolonizing Processes

Community Control

To some degree, Indigenous health promotion continues to be undertaken by "outsiders" who rarely consult with or engage community members. This form of "colonizing health promotion" occurs when practitioners develop "supports" based on their own socio-political and cultural contexts, then enter Indigenous communities uninvited to implement and evaluate the extent to which the programs are "successful" using criteria that are often not relevant to community members.

Evolving within the context of decolonizing health research, Indigenous communities have affirmed the right to *control* the process of programs and practices undertaken about, with, and for them. In this case, *control* refers to "the aspirations and rights of First Nations [and other Indigenous] Peoples to maintain and regain control of all aspects of their lives and institutions" (First Nations Information Governance Centre, 2005, p. 5).

Community Engagement

Indigenous community engagement represents a process by which members take meaningful actions aimed at benefiting the entire community. Indigenous values of relationship, reciprocity, and collective vision underpin this process, whereby community members collaborate, with one another and/or people from outside the community, to move the community towards positive change. As in other contexts, community engagement in health promotion reflects a critical component of self-determination.

When political and professional stakeholders collaborate with Indigenous communities in the development and implementation of health promotion activities, true partnerships can emerge in an atmosphere of mutual trust. Collaborative partnerships also enhance the degree to which Indigenous communities share decision-making power, as well as help to ensure that health promotion is undertaken in a respectful, relevant, reciprocal, and culturally appropriate manner, with benefits shared among all partners.

Cultural Relevance

When Indigenous communities initiate, develop, and control the processes and products of health promotion, cultural relevance is enhanced. However, the cultural diversity of Indigenous peoples across Canada requires the engagement of local perspectives in order to adequately acknowledge and address the diversity of contexts in which health promotion occurs. For instance, a "pan-Indigenous" approach to health promotion might erroneously posit that all Indigenous peoples view tobacco as culturally significant, and that promoting respect for the sacredness of tobacco might be a means of reducing its non-traditional or recreational use. While this approach is convenient for a national-level campaign, it lacks sensitivity to culturally specific contexts. In this case, Indigenous peoples from the west coast do not often use tobacco in their ceremonies, which traditionally involve the sacred use of cedar (Aboriginal Health Practice Council, n.d.).

PROMISING PRACTICES

In any given year, there are myriad innovative, community-based, and collaborative health promotion programs and activities addressing the health and wellness of Indigenous populations across Canada. What follows is a description of four such programs, situated in urban and reserve contexts and serving First Nations, Métis, and Inuit peoples.

The Tu'wusht Project

Initiated in 2005, and formerly known as the Urban Aboriginal Community Kitchen/ Garden Project, the Tu'wusht (Tla'amin Coast Salish for "we belong") Project, located on the UBC Farm, on Musqueam territory in British Columbia, provides opportunities for urban Indigenous people to access the natural enviornment as well as nutritional traditional foods (Vancouver Native Health Society, 2016). The Tu'wusht Project is guided by several Indigenous cultural teachings including the medicine wheel and involves the sharing of Indigenous knowledge. Its mission is "to provide the support and opportunity for Aboriginal people living in east Vancouver to improve their health and capacity [and to] create a safe space for Elders and youth to interact, to promote healing through gardening" (University of British Columbia, 2016, para. 3). The project hosts a weekly community kitchen activity in which Indigenous Elders and community participants, including several Indigenous youth organizations, share in growing, gathering, preparing, and eating healthy food from the garden. In addition to sharing knowledge and skills (e.g., smoking fish in a cedar smokehouse) during the project's activities, Indigenous ceremonies (e.g., harvest feast) are used to mark seasonal changes.

In an evaluation of this project, Mundel and Chapman (2010) interviewed resident project Elders as well as participants, who reported that the project encourages relationship building in which participants become like family, providing practical knowledge and emotional support within and beyond the project. One participant claimed, "it's community, it's love, it's family, it's belonging." In addition to improving their physical health through increased activity and consumption of healthy foods like vegetables from the garden, community participants also described how the informal learning environment helped them to feel inspired and to develop several health-promoting skills.

The Tu'wusht Project promotes more than just individual health, including a focus on the health of the community, the ecosystem, and the universe. Participants reported that the project helped them connect with their culture through time spent on the land and engaging in Tu'wusht Project activities. Some participants also viewed the project activities as decolonizing. For example, one participant suggested that the project represents a form of "decolonization because part of colonization is that we live in dependency."

By providing a space for Indigenous people to come together on the land and learn from Elders, the Tu'wusht Project serves as an excellent example of how decolonizing health promotion can facilitate Indigenous healing and self-determination in an urban context.

Kahnawake Schools Diabetes Prevention Project

In response to advice from community Elders to address the epidemic of diabetes within the Mohawk community of Kahnawake, in 1993, community members collaborated with physicians, dietitians, researchers, and school officials to develop the Kahnawake Schools Diabetes Prevention Project (KSDPP). Since that time and with active participation of a local advisory board, the KSDPP continues to provide a holistic and culturally appropriate, classroom-based health education program that includes nutrition, fitness, diabetes, understanding the human body, and healthy lifestyles, as well as a home support program for parents and caregivers on nutrition, physical activity, and healthy lifestyles (Macaulay et al., 1997).

Although initially developed as a three-year pilot project to increase healthy eating and physical activity among elementary school students (grades 1–6), the KSDPP has since expanded to serve all community schoolchildren. Collaborations now also include mutually beneficial research partnerships with local universities, as well as capacity-building through training for service providers from other communities (Macaulay et al., 1997).

This community-controlled program embraces a pluralistic model of health promotion through the incorporation of Indigenous and Western theories, including social learning theory, the PRECEDE-PROCEED model, the *Ottawa Charter for Health Promotion*, and traditional Indigenous teachings. In addition to the physical health–related objectives, KSDPP strives to maximize community engagement through information-sharing, capacity-building, and collective decision-making.

The Sprouts Day Camp Program

Early childhood development is recognized as an important determinant of health (Mikkonene & Raphael, 2010); this is equally true for Indigenous families. Since 2001, the Sprouts Day Camp Program has been providing children and youth in Iqaluit, Nunavut, (and elsewhere) with opportunities for learning that promotes culture, health, and education utilizing traditional Inuit knowledge and practices. Every summer Inuit children aged 7 to 15 attend a series of week-long summer day camps offered through a partnership between the Qikiqtani Inuit Association and Actua Canada's Aboriginal Outreach Program (Indspire, 2014).

The Sprouts Day Camp curriculum incorporates science and technology so Inuit can pursue career opportunities in the growing mineral, oil, and gas potential of Nunavut. For example, learning includes hands-on activities such as making blubber mitts from lard and immersing hands in cold water to understand how arctic mammals keep warm through the insulating properties of blubber; using traditional Inuit throat singing as a way to explore how Beluga whales hear; engaging in scavenger hunts and hikes using GPS technology to discuss how the Inuksuk was used as guidance (Indspire, 2014).

Indigenous Elders and community members volunteer their time to lead activities and provide students with important connections to the local culture and traditional knowledge. Elders conduct opening and closing ceremonies and share culturally relevant teachings, while community volunteers take students on field trips (sometimes overnight) to places of cultural significance (Indspire, 2014).

The Day Camp employs graduates of Nunavut Sivuniksavut as instructors. For 30 years, this Ottawa-based college program has been facilitating Inuit youths' transition from high school to post-secondary education and/or the workforce. The Sivuniksavut-prepared instructors are also seen as role models for the children in terms of academic achievement, community involvement, and volunteering, as well as for encouraging Inuit children to be proud of their heritage and make positive choices for their futures (Indspire, 2014).

Hulitan Family and Community Services Society

Indigenous models of wellness emphasize relationships as key (Loppie Reading & Wien, 2009), with the majority of Indigenous people identifying their family as a major source of strength (First Nations Information Governance Centre, 2010). The most important preface to any discussion of Indigenous family wellness is that the majority of Indigenous families are happy and well balanced (Canadian Institute for Health Information, 2009).

In fact, between 60 and 75 percent of First Nation youth report feeling physically, emotionally, mentally, and spiritually balanced most or all of the time as well as feeling loved and supported by their parents (First Nations Information Governance Centre, 2010).

Unfortunately, poverty is a key determinant of Indigenous peoples' health, resulting from a colonial history and continued social and political oppression (Battiste & Youngblood Henderson, 2012; Loppie Reading & Wien, 2009). Substance use has also been identified as a challenge to Indigenous health and wellbeing and is likewise linked to deleterious social conditions, residential school, and a legacy of colonization (Assembly of First Nations & Native Addictions Partnership Foundation, 2011). Substance use and poverty are both strongly associated with higher risk of child apprehension (Denison, Varcoe, & Browne, 2014). According to Blackstock, Trocme, and Bennett (2004), "cases of substantiated or suspected maltreatment involving Aboriginal children were more likely to involve neglect and, in particular, supervision issues, rather than physical or sexual abuse" (p. 12).

Located in Victoria, BC, Hulitan Family and Community Services Society is an urban Indigenous agency providing culturally relevant and safe programs and services to support the wellbeing of Indigenous children, youth, and families living in Victoria.

The primary goal of the Journeys of the Heart Cultural Learning Program is to facilitate the physical, intellectual, emotional, and spiritual development of Indigenous children. The ten-month program is designed to nurture the cultural identity of Indigenous children aged two to five, while preparing them to make a positive transition into the public school system. Program activities include culturally relevant curriculum for kindergarten preparation; role modelling, parenting, and socialization techniques for parents; family-based physical activity; and connecting urban Indigenous families with community resources and organizations. Although Hulitan recognizes parents as primary teachers, they also embrace traditional Indigenous values related to the important role of extended family members in the upbringing of children. Therefore, the Journeys of the Heart program works closely with and has the support of family networks as well as local Indigenous community programs.

The L, KI, L (meaning confidence) Child and Youth Mental Health Program facilitates improved mental health and wellbeing among Indigenous children and youth (aged 0–18) and their families through activities tailored to their specific needs and interests. The program employs a number of traditional Western and Indigenous modalities including, but not limited to, one-on-one and family counselling, healing circles, art therapy, cultural supports (smudging, seven teachings, drumming, medicine wheel, storytelling, and music), and land-based activities. The program also involves knowledge-sharing (with youth and adults) about the intergenerational impacts of colonization and residential schools on Indigenous families and parenting. Although the program's primary focus is mental wellness, a holistic approach, which embraces the teachings of the medicine wheel, also acknowledges and supports the emotional, physical, and spiritual needs of Indigenous children, youth, and families.

The *Kwen'an'latel* Intensive Parenting Program is a parenting program for urban Indigenous parents who have had their children removed by the Ministry of Children and Family Development (MCFD). This locally designed and culturally appropriate program employs holistic approaches that are relevant to the social realities and cultural values of Indigenous peoples living on Vancouver Island (Hulitan, n.d.).

The goals of *Kwen'an'latel* are to increase parenting knowledge and skills among Indigenous families; increase parents' understanding of the risks/behaviours that impact child safety; and increase parents' connection to cultural and community resources. In this six- to nine-month, three-stage program, parents have opportunities to incorporate Western and traditional Indigenous parenting knowledge and skills into their own parenting practice and receive support from culturally sensitive Hulitan Family Development Workers if they encounter challenges. Upon completion of the program, Hulitan holds a graduation celebration for parents, family, and friends (Hulitan, n.d.).

CONCLUSION

Indigenous peoples in Canada, including First Nations, Inuit, and Métis, are culturally diverse, geographically dispersed, and undergoing rapid social, cultural, and economic transitions. In the face of challenging obstacles, numerous inspirational, community-based programs demonstrate how to balance the development of community health promotion initiatives with broader socio-cultural public policy to create healthy environments for Indigenous peoples.

The success of these programs can be attributed, at least in part, to the appreciation and application of Indigenous concepts, contexts, and processes. Initially, incorporation of the distinct perspectives of Indigenous and Western paradigms reflects a more pluralistic alternative to the existing divisiveness between Indigenous and Western approaches to health promotion. Most notably, it is clear that, in developing and implementing these successful health promotion supports for Indigenous peoples and communities, policy makers as well as program planners and practitioners considered the distinct contexts that influence all dimensions of Indigenous health. Whether they were responding to food security, diabetes, child development, or family cohesion, all of these programs are premised on the belief that the solutions to the health and social challenges facing Indigenous people can be found in the teachings and traditions of their ancestors as well as those of their allies, thus demonstrating the principle of two-eyed seeing.

Over the past three decades, social theorists and researchers have established that control over one's life (i.e., self-determination) is key to improving health and wellbeing (Ermine & Hampton, 2007). Repressive colonial structures and systems have diminished opportunities for self-determination among Indigenous peoples, thereby deleteriously influencing all other determinants of health. However, in the case of health promotion, self-determination is evolving in that Indigenous communities are beginning to take control over and actively engage in all decisions and activities related to health supports.

The Truth and Reconciliation Commission's *Calls to Action* (2015) are clear that supports must be based on values of equity and justice and aimed at reducing the influence of colonial practice, programs, and policies. Priorities identified by community members, those most affected and who ultimately understand the context of their own lives best, must drive the development and implementation of health promotion supports.

According to Waziyatawin and Yellow Bird (2012), decolonization is a process of "engaging in the activities of creating, restoring, and birthing … new ideas, thinking, technologies, and lifestyles that contribute to the advancement and empowerment of Indigenous Peoples" (p. 3). This begins by organizing supports with the clear consent and guidance of an Indigenous community or group, building long-term relationships of accountability, and never assuming or taking for granted the personal and political trust that non-Indigenous people may earn from Indigenous peoples over time. It also requires that non-Indigenous health promotion professionals understand themselves as beneficiaries of the illegal settlement of Indigenous peoples' land and unjust appropriation of Indigenous peoples' resources and jurisdictions. When faced with this truth, it is common for activists to get stuck in feelings of guilt; yet, while guilt is often a sign of a much-needed shift in consciousness, in itself it does nothing to motivate the responsibility necessary to actively dismantle entrenched systems of oppression. "Solidarity is not the same as support; to experience solidarity, we must have a community of interests, shared beliefs and goals around which to unite" (hooks, 2014).

CRITICAL THINKING QUESTIONS

1. What are the fundamental elements of promising health promotion practice in Indigenous communities? Why are these elements important to consider when developing and implementing Indigenous health promotion?
2. In what ways might community engagement facilitate successful health promotion programs in Indigenous communities? What are some examples of promising Indigenous community engagement strategies?
3. What are the unique historical and cultural contexts within which social determinants influence the health of Indigenous peoples in Canada? Why is it important to consider these contexts when developing and implementing Indigenous health promotion?
4. In what ways might integration of concepts such as two-eyed seeing facilitate successful health promotion with Indigenous peoples?
5. In what ways might the health promotion programs described in this chapter also represent actions of self-determination?

RESOURCES

Further Readings

Bagelman, J., Deveraux, F., & Hartley, R. (2016). Feasting for change: Reconnecting with food, place & culture. *International Journal of Indigenous Health, 11*(1).

This paper explores the Feasting for Change project in BC, which aims to facilitate the revitalization of traditional food sovereignty. Through experiential and holistic methods, this research highlights the benefits of "intergenerational, land-based, and hands-on learning about the value of traditional food and cultural practices. It also demonstrates how resources (digital stories, plant knowledge cards, celebration cookbooks, and language videos) can be successfully developed with and used by community to ensure the ongoing process of healthful revitalization."

Monchalin, R., Flicker, S., Wilson, C., Prentice, P., Oliver, V. Jackson, R., Larkin, J., Mitchell, C., Restoule, J-P., & Native Youth Sexual Health Network. (2016). "When you follow your heart, you provide that path for others": Indigenous models of youth leadership in HIV prevention. *International Journal of Indigenous Health, 11*(1).

This study explored "how a group of Indigenous youth leaders took up the notion of leadership in the context of HIV prevention." Through individual interviews, 18 Indigenous youth leaders from across Canada shared narratives about their passion for HIV prevention through digital storytelling. Thematic analysis identified the "qualities of an Indigenous youth leader as being confident, trustworthy, willing to listen, humble, patient, dedicated, resilient, and healthy. In contrast to individualized mainstream ideals, Indigenous youth in our study viewed leadership as deeply connected to relationships with family, community, history, legacies, and communal health."

Oster, R., Grier, A., Lightning, R., Mayan, M., & Toth, E. (2014). Cultural continuity, traditional Indigenous language, and diabetes in Alberta First Nations: A mixed-methods study. *International Journal for Equity in Health, 13*(1), 92–103.

This exploratory sequential mixed-methods study explores the association between "cultural continuity ('being who we are'), self-determination, and diabetes prevalence in First Nations in Alberta, Canada. Interviews with 10 Cree and Blackfoot leaders (members of Chief and Council) from across the province reveals understandings of cultural continuity, self-determination, and their relationship to health and diabetes, in the Alberta First Nations context." Based on a cross-sectional analysis of provincial administrative data and publically available data for 31 First Nations communities, the authors seek relationships between cultural continuity and diabetes prevalence. Results indicate that First Nations with higher levels of cultural continuity had lower diabetes prevalence.

Petrucka, P., Bickford, D., Bassendowski, S., Goodwill, W., Wajunta, C., Yuzicappi, B., ... Rauliuk, M. (2016). Positive leadership, legacy, lifestyles, attitudes, and activities for Aboriginal youth: A wise practices approach for positive Aboriginal youth futures. *International Journal of Indigenous Health, 11*(1).

This community-based participatory research project, entitled *Positive Leadership, Legacy, Lifestyles, Attitudes, and Activities for Aboriginal Youth*, involved Elder-youth dyads to explore cultural practices that might inform the youth's wellness. The Elder-youth dyads developed and delivered five cultural wellness modules to students at a local elementary school. This teaching method was found to be highly effective in strengthening the youth's ability to achieve holistic personal and community wellness.

Relevant Websites

Canadian Aboriginal AIDS Network
www.caan.ca

CAAN is a national organization committed to addressing issues related to HIV and AIDS among Indigenous peoples in Canada. CAAN engages closely with Indigenous peoples and agencies to create national forums for Indigenous peoples to address sexually transmitted and blood-borne infections, as well as co-morbidities and related mental health and aging issues.

First Nations Health Authority
www.fnha.ca

In 2013, the first provincial health authority of its kind in Canada, the First Nations Health Authority (FNHA), assumed responsibilities formerly held by Health Canada's First Nations Inuit Health Branch—Pacific Region. In partnership with First Nations communities in BC, the FNHA is now responsible for planning, management, service delivery, and funding of health programs for First Nations in BC.

NOTES

1. I have intentionally used the term *support* rather than *intervention* as *intervention* is not always a benign word for Indigenous people, whose lives have been intervened (imposed) upon for centuries.

2. To create a colony in or on (a place): to take control of (an area) and send people to live there (Colonize, n.d.).

3. Allies are defined here as non-Indigenous people working in solidarity with Indigenous people.

4. *Racialize* refers to the practice of assigning a racial identity to a person or group of people (Racialize, n.d.).

5. The imposition of control or governance of one nation over another (Colonialism, n.d.).

6. Biomimicry is the imitation of models, systems, and elements of nature (Vincent, Bogatyreva, Bogatyrev, Bowyer, & Anja-Karina Pahl, 2006).

7. See the works of Rene Descartes at plato.stanford.edu/entries/descartes-works/

REFERENCES

Aboriginal Affairs and Northern Development Canada. (2017). *Nutrition north Canada*. Retrieved from nutritionnorthcanada.ca/index-eng.asp

Aboriginal Health Practice Council. (n.d.). *Aboriginal traditional medicines*. Retrieved from www.sanyas.ca/downloads/aboriginal-traditional-medicine.pdf

Adelson, N. (2005). The embodiment of inequity: Health disparities in Aboriginal Canada. *Canadian Journal of Public Health, 96*(Suppl. 2), S45.

Assembly of First Nations & Native Addictions Partnership Foundation. (2011). *Honouring our strengths: A renewed framework to address substance use issues among First Nations people in Canada*. Ottawa, ON: Health Canada. Retrieved from nnadaprenewal.ca/wp-content/uploads/2012/01/Honouring-Our-Strengths-2011_Eng1.pdf

Battiste, M., & Youngblood Henderson, S. (2012). Oppression and the health of Indigenous peoples. In E. McGibbon (Ed.), *Oppression: A social determinant of health* (pp. 89–96). Halifax: Fernwood.

Blackstock, C., Trocme, N., & Bennett, M. (2004). Child maltreatment investigations among Aboriginal and non-Aboriginal families in Canada. *Violence Against Women, 10*(8), 901–916.

Canadian Encyclopedia. (2016). *Medicine wheels*. Retrieved from www.thecanadianencyclopedia.ca/en/article/medicine-wheels/

Canadian Institute for Health Information. (2009). *Mentally healthy communities: Aboriginal perspectives*. Ottawa: Author.

CBC News. (2016, April). *What a landmark ruling means—and doesn't—for Métis, non-staus Indians*. Retrieved from www.cbc.ca/news/indigenous/landmark-supreme-court-decision-metis-non-status-indians-1.3537419

Chandler, M., & Lalonde, C. (1998). Cultural continuity as a hedge against suicide in Canada's First Nations. *Transcultural Psychiatry, .352*, 191–219.

Colonialism. (n.d.). *Merriam-Webster Online*. In Merriam-Webster. Retrieved from www.merriam-webster.com/dictionary/colonialism

Colonize. (n.d.). *Merriam-Webster Online*. In Merriam-Webster. Retrieved from www.merriam-webster.com/dictionary/colonize

Denison, J., Varcoe, C., & Browne, A. (2014). Aboriginal women's experiences of accessing health care when state apprehension of children is being threatened. *Journal of Advanced Nursing, 70*(5), 1105–1116.

Department of Justice Canada. (2013). *The Constitution Acts 1867–1982*. Ottawa, ON: Minister of Public Works and Government Services.

Dewar, B. (2009, July–August). Nunavut and the Nunavut land claims agreement—An unresolved relationship. *Policy Options*, 74–79.

Ermine, W. (2007). The ethical space of engagement. *Indigenous Law Journal, 6*(1), 193–203.

Ermine, W., & Hampton, E. (2007). Miyo-mahcihowin: Self-determination, social determinants, and Indigenous health. In B. Campbell & G. Marchildon (Eds.), *Medicare: Facts, myths, problems, and promise* (pp. 342–348). Toronto: James Lorimer and Company.

First Nations Information Governance Centre. (2005). *Ownership, control, access, and possession (OCAP) or self-determination applied to research: A critical analysis of contemporary First Nations research and some options for First Nations communities.* Ottawa: National Aboriginal Health Organization.

First Nations Information Governance Centre. (2010). *RHS—Regional Health Survey.* Retrieved from fnigc.ca/our-work/regional-health-survey/about-rhs.html

Government of Canada. (2016). *Constitution Act 1867.* Retrieved from laws-lois.justice.gc.ca/eng/const/

Government of Nunavut. (n.d.). *Facts about Nunavut. Government of Nunavut.* Retrieved from www.gov.nu.ca

Gunn Allen, P. (1986). *The sacred hoop: Recovering the feminine in American Indian traditions.* Boston, MA: Beacon Press.

Haudenosaunee Confederacy. (2016). *Haudenosaunee Confederacy, OSWE: GE Grand River.* Retrieved from www.haudenosauneeconfederacy.com

hooks, b. (2014). *Feminist theory: From margins to center.* New York: Routledge.

Hulitan Family & Community Services Society. (n.d.). Our services. Retrieved from www.hulitan.ca/kwenanlatel_intensive_parent_support_program.html

Indspire. (2014). *Case studies on Actua's national Aboriginal outreach program.* Ottawa: Author.

Kelm, M. (1998). *Colonizing bodies: Aboriginal health and healing in British Columbia.* Vancouver: UBC Press.

Klein, L., & Ackerman, L. (Eds.). (1995). *Women and power in Native North America.* Norman: University of Oklahoma Press.

Leavitt, R. (1995). *Malliseet and Micmac: First Nations of the Maritimes.* Fredericton: New Ireland Press.

Long, D., & Fox, T. (1996). Circles of healing: Illness, healing, and health among Aboriginal people in Canada. In D. Long & O. Dickason (Eds.), *Visions of the heart: Canadian Aboriginal issues* (pp. 239–269). Toronto: Harcourt Brace.

Loppie Reading, C., & Wien, F. (2009). *Health inequalities, social determinants, and life course health issues among Aboriginal peoples in Canada.* Prince George, BC: National Collaborating Centre for Aboriginal Health.

Macaulay, A., Paradis, G., Potvin, L., Cross, E., Saad-Haddad, C., McComber, A., Desrosier, S., Kirby, R., Montour, L., Lamping, D., Leduc, N., & Rivard, M. (1997). The Kahnawake Schools Diabetes Prevention project: Intervention, evaluation, and baseline results of a diabetes primary prevention program with a Native community in Canada. *Preventive Medicine, 26*(6), 779–790.

Makarenko, J. (2008, June 2). *The Indian Act: Historical overview.* Retrieved from www.mapleleafweb.com/features/the-indian-act-historical-overview

Marshall, M., Marshall, A., & Bartlett, C. (2015). Two-eyed seeing in medicine. In M. Greenwood, S. de Leeuw, L. M. Lindsay, and C. Reading (Eds.), *Determinants of Aboriginal peoples' health: Beyond the social* (pp. 16–24). Toronto: Canadian Scholars' Press.

McMillan, A. (1995). *Native peoples and cultures of Canada: An anthropological overview* (2nd ed.). Vancouver: Douglas & McIntyre.

Mikkonene, J., & Raphael, D. (2010). *Social determinants of health: The Canadian facts.* Toronto: University School of Health Policy and Management.

Mosby, I. (2013). Administering colonial science: Nutrition research and human biomedical experimentation in aboriginal communities and residential schools, 1942–1952. *Histoire Sociale/ Social History, 46*(91), 145–172.

Mundel, E., & Chapman, G. (2010). A decolonizing approach to health promotion in Canada: The case of the urban Aboriginal community kitchen garden project. *Health Promotion International, 25*(2), 166–173.

National Aboriginal Health Organization (NAHO). (2002). *Improving population health, health promotion, disease prevention, and health protection services and programs for Aboriginal people.* Ottawa: Author.

Oakes, J., Riewe, R., Koolage, S., Simpson, L., & Schuster, N. (Eds.). (2000). *Aboriginal health, identity, and resources.* Winnipeg: Departments of Native Studies and Zoology and Faculty of Graduate Studies, University of Manitoba.

Paul, D. (2000). *We were not the savages: A Mi'kmaq perspective on the collision between European and Native American civilizations.* Halifax: Fernwood.

Pluralism. (n.d.). *Merriam-Webster Online.* In Merriam-Webster. Retrieved from www.merriam-webster.com/dictionary/pluralism

Racialize. (n.d.). *Merriam-Webster Online.* In Merriam-Webster. Retrieved from www.merriam-webster.com/dictionary/racialize

Reading, C. (2014). *Policies, programs and strategies to address Aboriginal racism.* Prince George, BC: National Collaborating Centre For Aboriginal Health.

Royal Commission on Aboriginal Peoples (RCAP). (1996). *Royal Commission report on Aboriginal Peoples.* Retrieved from www.aadnc-aandc.gc.ca/eng/1100100014597/1100100014637 Document 14

Statistics Canada. (2011). *Aboriginal languages in Canada.* Retrieved from www12.statcan.gc.ca/census-recensement/2011/as-sa/98-314-x/98-314-x2011003_3-eng.cfm

Tagalik, S. (2015). Inuit knowledge systems, Elders, and determinants of health: Harmony, balance, and the role of holistic thinking. In M. Greenwood, S. de Leeuw, L. M. Lindsay, & C. Reading (Eds.), *Determinants of Aboriginal peoples' health: Beyond the social* (pp. 25–32). Toronto: Canadian Scholars' Press.

The Truth and Reconciliation Commission of Canada (TRC). (2015). *Truth and Reconciliation Commission of Canada: Calls to Action.* Retrieved from www.trc.ca/websites/trcinstitution/File/2015/Findings/Calls_to_Action_English2.pdf

United Nations. (2008). *United Nations Declaration on the Rights of Indigenous Peoples.* Retrieved from www.un.org/esa/socdev/unpfii/documents/DRIPS_en.pdf

United Nations. (2016). *Permanent forum on Indigenous issues: Report on the fifteenth session.* Retrieved from www.un.org/esa/socdev/unpfii/documents/2016/15th-session/Report_of_the_Permanent_Forum_15th_Session_unedited.pdf

University of British Columbia. (2016). *Indigenous initiatives: Tu'wusht pen Project.* Retrieved from ubcfarm.ubc.ca/community/indigenous-initiatives/

Vancouver Native Health Society. (2016). *The Tu'wusht Project.* Retrieved from www.vnhs.net/programs-services/tuwusht-project/about

Vincent, J., Bogatyreva, O., Bogatyrev, N., Bowyer, A., & Anja-Karina Pahl, A. (2006). Biomimetics: Its practice and theory. *Journal of the Royal Society Interface.* doi: 10.1098/rsif.2006.0127

Waziyatawin & Yellow Bird, M. (2012). Introduction: Decolonizing our minds and actions. In Waziyatawin & M. Yellow Bird (Eds.), *For Indigenous minds only: A decolonization handbook* (pp. 57–83). Santa Fe, NM: School for Advanced Research Press.

Wiebe, P., van Gaalen, R., Langlois, K., & Costen, E. (2013). Toward culturally safe evidence-informed decision-making for First Nation and Inuit community health policies and programs. *Pimatisiwin: A Journal of Aboriginal and Indigenous Community Health, 11*(1), 17–26.

Wilson, D., Ronde, S., Brascoupé, S., Nicole Apale, A., Barney, L., Guthrie, B., ... Wolfe, S. (2013). Health professionals working with First Nations, Inuit, and Métis—Consensus guidelines. *Journal of Obstetrics and Gynaecology Canada, 35*(6), 550–553.

World Health Organization (WHO). (2007). The Bangkok Charter for Health Promotion in a globalized world. *Health Promotion International, 21*(S1), 10–14.

World Health Organization (WHO). (2016). *Social determinants of health.* Retrieved from www.who.int/social_determinants/en/

Yunkaporta, T. (2007). *Indigenous knowledge systems: Comparing Aboriginal and Western ways of knowing* (Doctoral dissertation). Retrieved from researchonline.jcu.edu.au/10974/4/04Bookchapter.pdf

CHAPTER 11

No One Should Be Left Behind: Identifying Appropriate Health Promotion Practices for Immigrants

Mushira Mohsin Khan and Karen Kobayashi

LEARNING OBJECTIVES

1. Develop an understanding of the health status of immigrants in Canada
2. Identify the salient barriers that challenge the uptake of health promotion practices among immigrants
3. Identify and critically analyze "promising practices" for health promotion among immigrants in Canada

INTRODUCTION

Currently in Canada, almost two-thirds of population expansion can be attributed to immigration (Statistics Canada, 2013). Our immigrant population has grown and continues to grow rapidly to the point that we now have the highest proportion of foreign-born citizens (nearly 21 percent) among the G8 countries (Statistics Canada, 2013). The country of birth of Canadian immigrants, however, has changed significantly. Up until the 1950s, most immigrants to Canada were of European origin; however, this trend has shifted to visible minorities[1] since the late 1990s (Hyman, 2001). In particular, findings from the 2011 National Household Survey indicate that Asia (including the Middle East) is the region from which the largest proportion of individuals have emmigrated. The share of immigrants from Africa, the Caribbean, and Central and South America has also increased slightly. And, according to the most recent report from Statistics Canada (2013), nearly 70 percent of the visible minority population in Canada is now foreign-born.

The increasing diversity of Canada's immigrant population raises important concerns regarding the health-related needs of immigrants, particularly in the context of the challenges posed by the social, economic, geographical, cultural, and environmental exigencies that accompany the process of migration. The health of immigrants and their families then has important implications for the future health profile of the nation. Of significant importance is the need for policy makers and other key stakeholders to address complex and intricate questions on immigrant health, such as, What are the determinants of immigrant health? What are the barriers to the uptake of health promotion practices among immigrants? How can we optimize the uptake of health promotion practices among immigrants?

In this chapter, we use the social determinants of health approach to respond to these questions. First, we provide a brief overview of the health status of immigrants.[2] We then identify the salient barriers that may challenge the successful uptake and implementation of health promotion practices among this population. Finally, we conclude with a discussion on "promising practices" in health promotion and provide insights into how discourses and techniques such as social marketing, working with the mass and social media, and collaborative processes such as community capacity-building may be effectively used to optimize the uptake of health promotion practices among immigrants, and, ideally, ensure better health for all.

IMMIGRANT HEALTH: AN OVERVIEW

Research has suggested that upon arrival, immigrants typically have better health as measured by age-standardized mortality rates (ASMRs) than their Canadian-born counterparts, a phenomenon that has been referred to in the literature as the "healthy immigrant effect" (HIE) (Ng, 2011).

This can largely be attributed to the selective nature of international migration. The selective migration hypothesis, for example, suggests that healthy individuals may consider themselves better positioned to successfully negotiate the challenges of settlement and adapting to an unfamiliar environment (Jasso, 2003), and, therefore, self-select themselves for migration. Immigration policies of the receiving country, such as the mandatory "health exam" for Canadian immigrants, may also act as a "second filter" for these individuals, thereby ensuring that only the healthiest immigrants are admitted into the country (Urquia, Vang, & Bolumar, 2015). The health advantage of new immigrants, however, tends to lessen over time (Ng, 2011), and those who immigrate in later life (65 years and older) tend to report poorer overall health in comparison to Canadian-born older adults (Gee, Kobayashi, & Prus, 2004).

More recently, Vang, Sigouin, Flenon, and Gagnon (2015) found that the healthy immigrant advantage varies across and within each stage of the life-course and according to different health outcomes. The healthy immigrant effect appears to be strongest during adulthood and less so during childhood/adolescence and late life. But even in adulthood, some discrepancies between different immigrant subgroups persist, depending on the type of health measure used, including greater variation for self-rated health but less variation for mental health, disability/functional limitations, risk behaviours, and chronic conditions.

In a scoping review of the available literature on the health of visible minorities, 70 percent of whom are foreign-born, Khan, Kobayashi, Vang, and Lee (2017) found that while national-level estimates seem to suggest a lower prevalence of diabetes, hypertension, smoking, and obesity among visible minorities as a whole, at the provincial level, they are actually at greater *risk* for chronic diseases such as diabetes (Alangh, Chiu, & Shah, 2013), hypertension (Leenen et al., 2008) and stroke (Chiu, Austin, Manuel, & Tu, 2010) than their white counterparts. And while mental health appears to be better among visible minorities overall (Pahwa, Karunanayake, McCrosky, & Thorpe, 2012), they are less likely to report, seek help, and receive a proper diagnosis for mental health issues (McCleary & Blain, 2013).

In addition, the mortality rate from ischemic heart disease is highest among South Asians, the fastest growing visible minority group in Canada (Arasaratnam, Ayoub, & Ruddy, 2015). Compared to the white population, South Asians also have a higher prevalence of hypertension, nearly double the prevalence of type 2 diabetes, a higher percentage of body fat, lower levels of physical activity, and higher carbohydrate intake. All of these factors contribute to the unique cardiovascular disease (CVD) profile of this group (Rana, De Souza, Kandaswamy, Lear, & Anand, 2014). South Asian Canadian adolescents also have higher triglyceride and lower HDL cholesterol levels than white adolescents (Rana et al., 2014).

Given such epidemiological evidence, the health-related needs of Canada's rapidly growing immigrant population require focused attention in order to ensure optimal health for current and future generations of Canadians. A social determinants of health approach provides us with a relevant framework with which to address some of these concerns. According to the World Health Organization (WHO), "the social determinants of health (SDH) are the conditions in which people are born, grow, work, live, and age, and the wider set of forces and systems shaping the conditions of daily life" (WHO, 2015). Key social determinants of health include income, education, employment and working conditions, early childhood development, Aboriginal status, immigrant status, cultural beliefs and practices, social isolation, visible minority status, age, housing, and gender (Mikkonen & Raphael, 2010).

A social determinants of health approach is particularly useful in that it provides insights into how the status of "foreign-born" and markers of identity as related to ethnicity, language, culture, age, and gender may preclude immigrants from accessing and effectively using health promotion resources. Indeed, these may intersect to produce conditions of "multiple jeopardy" (Khan et al., 2017), thereby limiting the uptake of health promotion practices within this group.

BARRIERS TO THE UPTAKE OF HEALTH PROMOTION PRACTICES AMONG IMMIGRANTS

We undertook a critical literature review to identify barriers to the uptake of health promotion practices among immigrants in Canada. A number of factors were then identified as hindering the uptake and use of such practices. These are identified and discussed below.

Migration

One of the most important determinants of health, life-course transitions such as immigration and the stressors associated with settling down in an unfamiliar country, may preclude immigrants from taking up health promotion practices. In particular, recent immigrants may find it difficult to access health-related information due to (1) a lack of knowledge about the formal health care system; (2) a history of reliance on informal means of health information gathering in their countries of origin; and (3) limited knowledge on disease prevention measures such as healthy eating and nutritional awareness (Rosenmoller et al., 2011). And while the increased availability of nutritional knowledge in the host country may result in a change in dietary habits based upon length of residence, the consumption of red meat, convenience foods, sugar-sweetened beverages, and desserts and candy may increase due to their easy access and low cost (Varghese & Moore-Orr, 2002, as cited in Lesser, Gasevic, & Lear, 2014). In addition, sponsored older adults, such as parents and grandparents, may not seek out preventive services due to a desire not to burden adult children with health-related concerns (Koehn, 2009).

Socio-economic Status or Class

Socio-economic status (SES) or class is a key social determinant of health (Mikkonen & Raphael, 2010). Research on immigrant populations suggests that they are generally more educated than "mainstream" populations, and yet they tend to be underemployed; when they are employed, they tend to earn less, and are less likely to hold managerial positions (Saraswati, 2000). In addition, a troubling over-representation of visible minority women in low-paying jobs is reflective of the continued racialization and gendered nature of the labour market (Saraswati, 2000). The immigrant experience, therefore, is often characterized by unemployment, underemployment, and even poverty (Zuberi & Ptashnick, 2012). Indeed, immigrants who live in poverty may encounter specific economic barriers to adopting health promotion practices, such as those related to good nutrition and physical activity (Rusch, Frazier, & Atkins, 2015). And, in mid-life, recently landed immigrant women may be caught between managing the stressors of a competitive labour market with the demands of care provision for their older relatives at home (Khan & Kobayashi, 2017), constraints that may result in even greater difficulties in taking up health promotion practices.

Language Proficiency and Health Literacy

Language proficiency is perhaps the most salient barrier to the uptake of health promotion practices among immigrants. The lack of charter language skills, limited availability of translator services in Canada, little acknowledgement of the importance of cultural interpretation as well as the expertise required in translator services, and the poor quality of clinical interactions due to language barriers may result in low levels of resource use (Koehn, Jarvis, Sandhra, Bains, & Addison, 2014). This may particularly be the case for foreign-born older adults who prefer to seek out informal sources for health information such as traditional and complementary medicine practitioners (Zhang & Verhoef, 2002).

Similarly, the inability to access and process health-related information that is typically delivered in one of the charter languages may prevent the effective uptake of health promotion practices. The limited availability of health promotion resources such as pamphlets and brochures in vernacular languages may also adversely impact the uptake of interventions. Linguistic capacity is also an important determinant of the ability of immigrants to effectively advocate for themselves in the health care domain.

In addition, with regard to health literacy, or the capacity to make informed and appropriate decisions about their health, immigrants in general score significantly below the national average (Canadian Council on Learning, 2008, as cited in Omariba & Ng, 2011). Thus, low levels of health literacy may compound the issues related to linguistic capability, resulting in a limited uptake of health promotion practices.

Visible Minority Status

Between 2006 and 2011, Asia (including the Middle East) remained Canada's largest source of immigrants, with approximately 57 percent of immigrants migrating from this region compared to only 14 percent from Europe (Statistics Canada, 2013). In terms of proportion, visible minorities account for 70 percent of the immigrant population. Veenstra (2009), in his analysis of survey data from the 2003 Canadian Community Health Survey, found that visible minority status comes with its share of challenges, particularly those rooted in racialization and discrimination. Visible minorities are also less likely to use cancer-screening services (Quan et al., 2006); specifically, recently immigrated visible minority women are more likely to have never had a Pap test, partly due to the limited availability of culturally competent physicians (Amankwah, Ngwakongnwi, & Quan, 2009).

Gender

Research suggests that often, the burden of caring for young children as well as older adults falls disproportionately on women in immigrant families (Spitzer, Neufeld, Harrison, Hughes, & Stewart, 2003). Further, immigrant women often disregard their health-related needs due to traditional and cultural practices, thereby making gender a significant barrier to the uptake of health promotion practices, particularly those related to preventive health screening (Ahmad et al., 2004). In addition, transportation issues may be gender-related, in that they can be perceived as being linked to an adherence to traditional patriarchal norms and dependence on men, values and behaviours that preclude immigrant women from participating in health promotion programs and/or accessing important health care resources.

The FAB 55+ or the Forever Active Bodies incentive program offered by the BC Ministry of Health provides an example of an initiative that is designed to encourage non-active women over the age of 55 to participate in sports. However, adherence to traditional norms, values, and beliefs around modesty and propriety may discourage immigrant women from participating in such a program. Further, lack of same-gender instructors for exercise and fitness classes such as those offered in local recreation centres may make access to these programs difficult for many.

Cultural Perceptions around Health and Disease Prevention

Cultural perceptions around health and illness can also be a significant barrier to the uptake of health promotion practices. A fatalistic approach towards health and illness grounded in the idea that illness is beyond an individual's control, for example, is a predominant theme in the literature on the health-seeking behaviours of South Asians. In a comprehensive review of the literature on the barriers and facilitators to exercise and physical activity uptake among South Asian older adults, Horne and Tierney (2012, as cited in Khan & Kobayashi, 2015) report that becoming less active is often depicted as a normal part of aging. Conversely, others view a decline in health as a warning sign from God that they need to modify their lifestyle (Khan & Kobayashi, 2015).

Further, the idea of "mastery," or an individual's belief that his or her choices and actions influence outcomes later in life as well as in the hereafter (Collins & Benedict, 2006, p. 45), is an important construct that is positively related to self-efficacy and the self-evaluation of health. In Weerasinghe and Numer's (2011) study on the physical and emotional behaviours of widowed South Asian women in Canada, for example, the authors indicate that women's ambivalence towards leisure activities is (1) largely determined by culture and tradition-driven prescriptions, such as a stoic approach towards health and illness; and (2) guided by strict gender-based normative ideals constructed during the earlier stages of their lives in their country of birth. The ability to make choices based upon internalized and culture-specific values, therefore, is an important determinant of access to, and uptake of, health promotion practices.

Age

Migration in later life brings with it a host of challenges as older immigrants struggle with settling down in an unfamiliar land (Koehn, 2009). Canada's older adults are increasingly lonely and isolated, so much so that health and social researchers have recently referred to loneliness among older adults as a "public epidemic" that may lead to depression, hypertension, sleep disturbances, and dementia (De Jong Gierveld, Keating, & Fast, 2015). And Canadians who have immigrated later in life are at an even greater risk of loneliness and isolation. Older immigrants of non-European descent, in particular, are more likely to be lonely compared to their European counterparts for a number of reasons, including (1) language and cultural barriers that may make forging new connections more difficult in the host country; and (2) the fact that the immigration experience oftentimes separates people from lifelong networks of family and friends (De Jong Gierveld, 2015). These factors may hinder effective engagement with health promotion practices among immigrant older adults.

Further, embarrassment and fear of bringing shame to their children due to limited linguistic ability in mainstream languages may inhibit immigrant older adults from participating in health promotion programs (Ahmad et al., 2004). As mentioned earlier vis-à-vis gender, transportation and mobility also play a key role in access to health promotion resources for immigrant older adults. For those who immigrated later in life and are dependent upon their adult children for transportation, mobility issues may impact their ability to participate in health promotion programs. The cold Canadian weather may also hamper their ability to exercise outside the home.

The factors identified and discussed are by no means exhaustive; yet clearly, they are salient and complex and often intersect with one another, thereby significantly reducing the uptake of health promotion practices among immigrants. There is a need, therefore, to develop health promotion practices and programs that are not only "targeted," that is, specifically designed for and delivered to a particular immigrant population subgroup such as older immigrants, immigrant women, or visible minority immigrants, but also "tailored" for them in culturally relevant ways. In the following section, we critically examine a broad health promotion initiative in the province of BC, the Healthy Families BC program. We then highlight two "promising practices"—programs specifically *targeted* and *tailored* towards optimizing engagement with health promotion practices among visible minority immigrants. These are (1) the South Asian Exercise Trial (SAET) program run by CoHeaRT in Surrey, BC; and (2) the REACH Multicultural Family Centre's Creating a Sense of Belonging: Mental Health Promotion within Immigrant and Refugee Communities program.

Box 11.1: Key Barriers to Accessing Health Promotion Interventions among Immigrants

---

- Migration
- Socio-economic status or class
- Language proficiency and health literacy
- Visible minority status
- Gender
- Cultural perceptions around health and disease prevention
- Age

HEALTH PROMOTION PRACTICES

Healthy Families BC

Healthy Families BC is a province-wide initiative to promote an active lifestyle and encourage residents to better manage their own health and reduce chronic disease (Healthy
Families BC, 2016). Some commendable health promotion initiatives introduced by
the provincial government include the 2011 Healthy Families BC Walking Challenge;
Informed Dining, a program that promotes access to nutritional information before making menu choices when dining out; Shopping Sense, which, in partnership with five major
grocery chains, assists families in planning and preparing healthy, affordable meals; and
BC's Sodium Reduction Plan. And, more recently, the BC government has launched
"Carrot Rewards," an innovative rewards program app that promotes healthy lifestyle
choices among its users.

These health promotion programs, although commendable for their population health
objectives, may not, however, be suitable for immigrant groups. There are a number of
reasons for this. Health and nutrition programs like Informed Dining and BC's Sodium
Reduction Plan, for example, primarily cater to "Westernized" notions around meal
planning and cooking. A quick review of the website of BC's Informed Dining initiative
suggests that of the several dozen restaurants participating in the program, only a few
"ethnic" restaurants have signed up to participate. The low level of engagement by "ethnic"
proprietors may be attributed, in part, to the practical difficulties around tailoring and
modifying non-Western cuisine to standard Canadian nutritional guidelines. And, while
the BC government's handbook for older adults, *Healthy Eating for Seniors*, is available
in Chinese and Punjabi, the initiative fails to acknowledge the heterogeneity among the
foreign-born population according to (first) language and literacy levels. Further, related
to technology, older immigrants, particularly those sponsored by and dependent on their
adult children for support, may not have access to and/or an understanding of smartphones
or electronic notepad devices, thereby creating issues with the Carrot Rewards program
for a large and growing number of family-sponsored older adults.

These shortcomings notwithstanding, there are several ways in which the initiatives
under the Healthy Families program could be both targeted and tailored towards an increasingly diverse immigrant population. The *Healthy Eating Guide*, for example, could
be translated into vernacular languages such as Tamil, Urdu, Filipino, Bengali, Hindi,
Arabic, and Persian, and be made available in audio format (to address literacy issues) in
order to reach a larger proportion of the visible minority immigrant population. The preparation of healthy ethnic food requires specific ingredients and cooking equipment, thus, an
increased availability of these items in local markets and stores may facilitate the cultural
adaptation of "healthy recipes" included in the guide. To this end, the BC government
could partner with ethnic grocery stores under its Shopping Sense program. Similarly, exercise and fitness programs like FAB 55+ could be tailored in culturally appropriate ways to

address traditional notions around modesty among immigrant women. An example of such a program is the South Asian Exercise Trial (SAET), the first of two "promising practices" identified here, run by CoHeaRT, a team of community health researchers in Surrey, BC.

Promising Practice #1: The South Asian Exercise Trial (SAET)

The South Asian Exercise Trial (SAET) program was designed to test the efficacy of cardiovascular exercise on body fat distribution in post-menopausal South Asian women. This free program uses culturally appropriate bhangra dance-based exercises in combination with standard aerobic exercise (e.g., stationary biking and treadmill) to address the risks of CVD in South Asian women. In a 12-week randomized trial, 75 post-menopausal women with a waist circumference greater than 80 centimetres participated in the program. The exercise intervention group was asked to attend one-hour exercise classes three times a week during the 12-week period. Baseline and post-intervention inner abdominal fat, lean and fat mass, cardiovascular risk, and physical activity measures were recorded. Preliminary results from the trial indicate that attendance in the exercise program remained high throughout the 12-week period, visceral adipose tissue (VAT) was significantly reduced among women who adhered to the program, and several women reported an improvement in their sense of wellbeing (Lesser et al., 2016).

Appropriately targeted and culturally tailored health promotion programs such as SAET are important for several reasons:

- The program was offered at a community centre in Surrey, which has a large South Asian population; geographic proximity to the target population facilitated both the recruitment and participation of older women in this study.
- A culturally appropriate exercise program such as bhangra encourages older women who may be feeling ambivalent about such programs to overcome some of their inhibitions around community exercise and fitness initiatives. Indeed, Koehn et al. (2016) have found that for Indian and Pakistani women, the ability to wear comfortable ethnic clothing such as the salwar kameez greatly improves the chances of their participation in fitness programs.
- Given the active involvement of women in the study, as evidenced by the high participation rate in the program, it is likely that they were more receptive to onsite health promotion practices and messages on active living and healthy lifestyle choices (Jepson et al., 2012).

Along with diet and nutrition interventions such as the province of BC's *Healthy Eating Guide* and exercise and fitness programs like SAET, there is also a need to tailor health promotion strategies to address the mental health and wellbeing of immigrants, given, as previously discussed, their exposure to multiple cultural, economic, and social stressors associated with migration and settlement. The REACH Multicultural Family

Centre's Creating a Sense of Belonging: Mental Health Promotion within Immigrant and Refugee Communities is an example of one such program.

Promising Practice #2: Mental Health Promotion within Immigrant Communities

Funded by the Community Action Initiative, East Vancouver's REACH Multicultural Family Centre partnered with immigrant-serving organizations, community centres, and community health and mental health agencies to promote the mental health and wellbeing of high-risk immigrant communities in Metro Vancouver (Blanco, Debiri, & Ramirez, 2014). The two-year program, which ran from April 2010 to March 2012, was unique in that it involved cross-cultural health promoters (CCHPs), also known as cross-cultural health brokers (CCHBs), trusted leaders of a cultural community, who not only served as language translators but also facilitated the effective transfer of information in culturally sensitive ways. In essence, these "brokers" acted as a bridge between the values and beliefs of "mainstream" Canadian culture and the traditions and values of the client's culture. The CCHP/Bs were either certified Canadian social work or counselling practitioners and/or they were foreign-trained health professionals. The program had two components: (1) social support groups; and (2) community capacity-building activities.

The Afghan Women's Social Circle is one example of such a social support group. The aim of the program was to reduce social isolation among Afghan women and to equip them with better coping and stress-management skills. Facilitated by a CCHB from the Afghan community, the group fostered a sense of belonging in the participants. The capacity-building module of the program involved several initiatives, as detailed below:

- In partnership with Vancouver Coastal Health's Cross-Cultural Mental Health Program, CCHBs participated in a cultural adaptation of the psychoeducational group therapy program, Changeways.
- CCHBs underwent training in Mental Health First Aid (MHFA), an international mental health program that familiarizes participants with a Western context on mental health and illness.
- CCHBs shared this knowledge with their communities, working to empower members with important mental health self-care skills.

Such measures facilitated the construction of an environment where respectful dialogue on mental health could be pursued, alleviating some of the stigma associated with mental illness in a number of ethno-cultural communities. Indeed, on-the-ground, slow-and-small-step approaches such as "awareness-building" initiatives are an important first step towards developing an understanding of, and thus a more empathetic response to, mental health issues in ethno-cultural communities.

The collaborative and community capacity-building focus of this program provides an excellent example of how health promotion can act as a mediating strategy between people and their environment by taking into account social, cultural, environmental, and historical factors that affect the health of individuals (Weber & Khademian, 2008). Such approaches, initiatives that encourage working with and supporting an immigrant community, building skills, and increasing opportunities tailored towards the unique needs of that community, have proven effective in addressing some of the barriers that community members may encounter in accessing health care services and the uptake of health promotion practices (Weber & Khademian, 2008). Indeed, for vulnerable immigrant groups like the Afghan women in this project, the recognition that "socio-environmental risk conditions" (Labonté, 1993, p. 5) are themselves important determinants of health is absolutely central to the development of effective health promotion strategies.

CONCLUSION: CREATING HEALTHY PUBLIC POLICIES

The rapid increase in Canada's immigrant population is a demographic shift that poses a unique set of challenges to the health care system. If we are to continue to be able to ensure that our collective goal of better health for all Canadians is being met, policy makers at multiple levels need to develop health promotion strategies that are both targeted as well as tailored to meet the unique needs of an increasingly diverse immigrant population. An important first step towards achieving this goal is to adopt an approach that addresses issues of inequity as well as inequality, both between immigrants and the Canadian-born population, as well as within immigrant groups. To this end, there is a need to confront political discourse that regards "immigrants as a burden on the health care system" by advocating for change. Advocacy initiatives that acknowledge the multiple axes of inequality that define the everyday lived experiences of immigrant groups are essential to the construction of socially just policy. In support of this call, Bacchi (2000) maintains the following:

> issues get represented in ways that mystify power relations and often create individuals responsible for their own "failures," drawing attention away from the structures that create unequal outcomes. The focus on "the ways issues get represented" produces a focus on language and on "discourse," meaning the conceptual frameworks available to describe social processes. (p. 46)

Second, we suggest that a social marketing approach that uses marketing principles to target population subgroups and one that facilitates the "acceptance, rejection, modification, abandonment, or maintenance of particular behaviors" (Grier & Bryant, 2005, p. 321) would effectively complement a policy-as-discourse approach. Here, the four Ps of commercial marketing—product, price, place, and promotion (Grier & Bryant, 2005, p. 321)—could be used to modify attitudes towards healthy eating, exercise, and preventive screening for chronic diseases among immigrants. For example, policy makers could collaborate with influential members of immigrant communities such as recognized celebrity chefs—Vancouver's Vikram Vij (Indian cuisine) and Toronto's Susur Lee (Chinese cuisine) come to mind—to produce and promote healthy, low-cost, and grocery store–available ethnic food.

Similarly, high-traffic areas such as religious venues, including local temples, mosques, and gurdwaras, could also be effectively utilized for the distribution of health promotion resources or as sites for free preventive screening for chronic diseases. Further, media outlets such as ethno-cultural newspapers and multi-cultural television channels, e.g., Vancouver Desi, ATN, AlphaPunjabi, Omni, Sher-e-Punjab Radio, Filipino TV (FTV), and CFMT-DT, could be used as informal and non-intimidating avenues to promote health literacy regarding healthy eating and preventive screening for chronic disease, particularly among immigrant women.

Third, from a cultural safety and cultural competency perspective, reflexive practice on the part of health care providers, an empathetic attitude, and the ability to consider the "context," be it cultural, social, religious, or geographical (McEldowney & Connor, 2011), are key to reaching out to immigrant populations. Targeted training and offering post-secondary–level courses and/or programs on cultural safety and competence would also be useful, particularly for health practitioners.

Fourth, it is also of critical importance to consider in the construction of health promotion strategies that the content be presented in culturally appropriate and simplified (if necessary) language and modes (audio and video in addition to text), in order to improve access to health promotion resources among immigrant groups.

Fifth, in our interactions with front-line workers at immigrant and settlement organizations, it has been suggested that the development of PSAs (public service announcements) would be an effective way of communicating with individuals and their families on challenging health-related topics (Kobayashi, 2016). Here, PSAs could be used to combat stigma and raise awareness of sensitive and difficult issues such as mental illness in immigrant communities.

Sixth, a facilitated amalgamation of health care professionals from ethno-cultural minority groups working as a collective to accelerate re-credentialization processes for immigrant health care professionals may help to ensure effective and efficient integration of this group into the existing health care system, resulting in improved patient-provider communication. Family members, trained volunteers, and outreach workers could also be used to facilitate dialogue and community engagement in the production and delivery of health promotion resources and interventions.

Along with these interventions, there is a need for evaluation studies that track the efficacy of health promotion initiatives in immigrant communities. The assessment report of the Seniors Support Services for South Asian Community Project in Surrey, BC, for example, found that the success of the active living program could be attributed to interventions such as reducing cultural and language barriers, providing child care for grandchildren, and offering programs where older adults naturally gather, such at parks and temples (Koehn et al., 2016).

Finally, it is important to acknowledge that with an almost exclusive focus on the importance of a healthy diet, regular physical activity, and tobacco cessation (Raphael, 2008), health promotion efforts today have created a neo-liberal anxiety among Canadians with regard to their health. Among immigrants this angst may be felt more acutely based on the extent to which interlocking markers of social location have affected and continue to affect their access to needed resources related to their health. Addressing this anxiety among immigrants, therefore, poses a unique set of challenges with regard to health promotion. We propose, by way of closing, that health promotion efforts for this population shift from a "one size fits all" focus on lifestyle and behaviour-modification vis-à-vis healthy eating, diet, exercise, and preventive screening, to the development of initiatives that acknowledge and reflect the social, economic, cultural, and historical *determinants* that may preclude immigrants from effectively using these interventions. Only then can we claim to be working towards ensuring that no one gets left behind in our health promotion and care system.

CRITICAL THINKING QUESTIONS

1. What are some key considerations in developing effective health promotion strategies for immigrants?
2. As compared to younger immigrants, what are some of the unique challenges to the uptake of health promotion practices for those who immigrate later in life?
3. Discuss the ways in which migration as a social determinant of health relates to the uptake and effective utilization of health promotion practices.

RESOURCES

Further Readings

Hyman, I., & Guruge, S. (2002). A review of theory and health promotion strategies for new immigrant women. *Canadian Journal of Public Health*, *93*(3), 183–187.
This article presents a thorough analysis of the major theoretical models of health promotion, discusses the characteristics of successful health promotion strategies for immigrant women, and highlights the salient barriers to accessing health promotion resources among new immigrant women in Canada.

Khanlou, N., & Gonsalves, T. (2011). An intersectional understanding of youth cultural identities and psychosocial integration: Why it matters to mental health promotion in immigrant-receiving pluralistic societies. In O. Hankivsky (Ed.), *Health inequities in Canada: Intersectional frameworks and practices* (pp. 166–179). Vancouver: UBC Press.
The authors examine the challenges of mental health promotion and the psychosocial integration of immigrant and second-generation youth in Canada. Drawing from two community-based mixed-method studies (including qualitative and quantitative methods),

they suggest that an intersectional approach, which accounts for life-stage, gender, ethnicity, immigrant status, and other identity markers, will provide for an in-depth understanding of positions of oppression and privilege for immigrants and their children.

Relevant Websites

Kids New to Canada
www.kidsnewtocanada.ca/care/parent-info
Provides evidence-based information on health promotion for those who care for immigrant and refugee children, youth, and families.

Migration as a Social Determinant of Health
www.migrationhealth.ca/new-immigrants-canada
Provides details on the Revisiting *Personal is Political*: Immigrant Women's Health Promotion project and discusses migration as a social determinant of health.

Multicultural Mental Health Resource Centre
www.multiculturalmentalhealth.ca
Provides resources to support the mental health needs of Canada's visible minority population.

NOTES

1. The Employment Equity Act defines visible minorities as "persons, other than Aboriginal peoples, who are non-Caucasian in race or non-white in colour." The visible minority population consists mainly of the following groups: Chinese, South Asian, Black, Arab, West Asian, Filipino, Southeast Asian, Latin American, Japanese and Korean (Statistics Canada, 2013).

2. Given space constraints, we unfortunately cannot explore the health experiences and health care needs of refugees in this chapter, an immigrant group that we acknowledge faces unique barriers to engagement with health promotion practices in Canada.

REFERENCES

Ahmad, F., Shik, A.,Vanza, R., Cheung, A., George, U., & Stewart, D. E. (2004). Popular health promotion strategies among Chinese and East Indian immigrant women. *Women and Health*, *40*(1), 21–40.

Alangh, A., Chiu, M., & Shah, B. R. (2013). Rapid increase in diabetes incidence among Chinese Canadians between 1996 and 2005. *Diabetes Care*, *36*(10), 3015–3017.

Amankwah, E., Ngwakongnwi, E., & Quan, H. (2009). Why many visible minority women in Canada do not participate in cervical cancer screening. *Ethnicity and Health*, *14*, 337–349.

Arasaratnam, P., Ayoub, C., & Ruddy, T. R. (2015). Canadian multiethnicity—Differences in coronary artery disease prevalence and progression and relevance to cardiac imaging. *Current Cardiovascular Imaging Reports, 8,* 9314. doi:10.1007/s12410-014-9314-9

Bacchi, C. (2000). Policy as discourse: What does it mean? Where does it get us? *Discourse: Studies in the Cultural Politics of Education, 21*(1), 45–57.

Blanco, G., Debiri, P., & Ramirez, P. (2014). Creating a sense of belonging: Mental health promotion within immigrant and refugee communities. *Visions, 9*(4), 33–35.

Canadian Council on Learning. (2008). *Health literacy in Canada: A healthy understanding.* Ottawa: Canadian Council on Learning.

Chiu, M., Austin, P. C., Manuel, D. G., & Tu, J. V. (2010). Comparison of cardiovascular risk profiles among ethnic groups using population health surveys between 1996 and 2007. *Canadian Medical Association Journal, 182,* E301–E310.

Collins, C. C., & Benedict, J. (2006). Evaluation of a community-based health promotion program for the elderly: Lessons from seniors CAN. *American Journal of Health Promotion, 21*(1), 45–48.

De Jong Gierveld, J. (2015). Intra-couple caregiving of older adults living apart together: Commitment and independence. *Canadian Journal on Aging, 34,* 356–365.

De Jong Gierveld, J., Keating, N., & Fast, J. (2015). Determinants of loneliness among older adults in Canada. *Canadian Journal on Aging, 34*(2), 125–136.

Gee, E. M., Kobayashi, K. M., & Prus, S. G. (2004). Examining the healthy immigrant effect in mid-to-later-life: Findings from the Canadian Community Health Survey. *Canadian Journal of Aging, 23,* S61–S69.

Grier, S., & Bryant, C. A. (2005). Social marketing in public health. *Annual Review of Public Health, 26,* 319–339.

Healthy Families BC. (2016). *Welcome to HealthyFamiles BC!* Retrieved from www.healthyfamiliesbc.ca/home/about-us

Horne, M., & Tierney, S. (2012). What are the barriers and facilitators to exercise and physical activity uptake and adherence among South Asian older adults: A systematic review of qualitative studies. *Preventive Medicine, 55*(4), 276–284.

Hyman, I. (2001). *Immigration and health* (No. 01–05). Health Policy Workshop Paper Series. Ottawa: Health Canada.

Jasso, G. (2003). Migration, human development, and the life course. In J. T. Mortimer & M. J. Shanahan (Eds.), *Handbook of the Life Course* (pp. 331–364). New York: Kluwer Academic/Plenum Publishers.

Jepson, R., Harris, F. M., Bowes, A., Robertson, R., Avan, G., & Sheikh, A. (2012). Physical activity in South Asians: An in-depth qualitative study to explore motivations and facilitators. *PLoS ONE, 7*(10), e45333. doi:10.1371/journal.pone.0045333

Khan, M. M., & Kobayashi, K. M. (2015). Optimizing health promotion among ethnocultural minority older adults (EMOA). *International Journal of Migration, Health and Social Care, 11*(4), 268–281.

Khan, M. M., & Kobayashi, K. M. (2017). Negotiating sacred values: Dharma, karma, and kin-work among migrant Hindu women. In P. Dossa & C. Coe (Eds.), *Transnational aging and reconfigurations of kin work* (pp. 102–119). New Brunswick: Rutgers University Press.

Khan, M. M., Kobayashi, K. M., Vang, Z., & Lee, S. M. (2017). Are visible minorities "invisible" in Canadian health data and research? A scoping review. *International Journal of Migration, Health and Social Care, 13*(1), 126–143.

Kobayashi, K. (2016). *"Working together to reduce elder abuse" capacity building grant: Final report.* Victoria: Institute of Aging and Lifelong Health, University of Victoria.

Koehn, S. (2009). Negotiating candidacy: Access to care for ethnic minority seniors. *Ageing and Society, 29*(4), 585–608.

Koehn, S., Habib, S., & Bukhari, S. (2016). S⁴AC case study: Enhancing underserved seniors' access to health promotion programs. *Canadian Journal on Aging, 35*(1), 89–102.

Koehn, S., Jarvis, P., Sandhra, S. K., Bains, S. K., & Addison, M. (2014). Promoting mental health of immigrant seniors in community. *Ethnicity and Inequalities in Health and Social Care, 7*(3), 146–156. doi: 10.1108/eihsc-11-2013-0048

Labonté, R. (1993). *Health promotion and empowerment: Practice frameworks.* Toronto: Centre for Health Promotion/ParticipACTION.

Leenen, F. H. H., Dumais, J., McInnis, N. H., Turton, P., Stratychuk, L., Nemeth, K., ... Fodor, G. (2008). Results of the Ontario survey on the prevalence and control of hypertension. *Canadian Medical Association Journal, 178*(11), 1441–1449.

Lesser, I. A., Gasevic, D., & Lear, S. A. (2014). The association between acculturation and dietary patterns of South Asian immigrants. *PLoS One, 9*(2), e88495. doi: 10.1371/journal.pone.0088495

Lesser, I. A., Guenette, J. A., Hoogbruin, A., Mackey, D. C., Singer, J., Gasevic, D., & Lear, S. A. (2016). Association between exercise-induced change in body composition and change in cardiometabolic risk factors in postmenopausal South Asian women. *Applied Physiology, Nutrition, and Metabolism, 41*(9), 931–937. doi: 10.1139/apnm-2016-0082

McCleary, L., & Blain, J. (2013). Cultural values and family caregiving for persons with dementia. *Indian Journal of Gerontology, 27*(1), 178–201.

McEldowney, R., & Connor, M. J. (2011). Cultural safety as an ethic of care: A praxiological process. *Journal of Transcultural Nursing, 22*(4), 342–349.

Mikkonen, J., & Raphael, D. (2010). *Social determinants of health: The Canadian facts.* Toronto: School of Health Policy and Management, York University.

Ng, E. (2011). The healthy immigrant effect and mortality rates. *Health Reports, 22*, 25–29.

Omariba, D. W., & Ng, E. (2011). Immigration, generation and self-rated health in Canada: On the role of health literacy. *Canadian Journal of Public Health, 102*(4), 281–285.

Pahwa, P., Karunanayake, C. P., McCrosky, J., & Thorpe, L. (2012). Longitudinal trends in mental health among ethnic groups in Canada. *Chronic Diseases and Injuries in Canada, 32*, 164–176.

Quan, H., Fong, A., De Coster, C., Wang, J., Musto, R., Noseworthy, T. W., & Ghali, W. A. (2006). Variation in health services utilization among ethnic populations. *Canadian Medical Association Journal, 174*, 787–791.

Rana, A., De Souza, R., Kandaswamy, S., Lear, S., & Anand, S. (2014). Cardiovascular risk among South Asians living in Canada: A systematic review and meta-analysis. *CMAJ Open, 2*(3), E183–E191.

Raphael, D. (2008). Grasping at straws: A recent history of health promotion in Canada. *Critical Public Health, 18*(4), 483–495.

Rootman, I., Dupéré, S., Pederson, A., & O'Neill, M. (2012). *Health promotion in Canada* (3rd ed.). Toronto: Canadian Scholars' Press.

Rosenmoller, D. L., Gasevic, D., Seidell, J., & Lear, S. A. (2011). Determinants of changes in dietary patterns among Chinese immigrants: A cross-sectional analysis. *International Journal of Behavioral Nutrition and Physical Activity, 18*(8), 42.

Rusch, D., Frazier, S., & Atkins, M. (2015). Building capacity within community-based organizations: New directions for mental health promotion for Latino immigrant families in urban poverty. *Administration and Policy in Mental Health and Mental Health Services Research, 42*(1), 1–5.

Saraswati, J. (2000). Poverty and visible minority women in Canada. *Canadian Woman Studies, 20*(3), 49–53.

Spitzer, D., Neufeld, A., Harrison, M., Hughes, K., & Stewart, M. (2003). Caregiving in a transnational context: "My wings have been cut; where can I fly?" *Gender and Society, 17*(2), 267–286.

Statistics Canada. (2013). *Immigration and ethnocultural diversity in Canada.* Retrieved from www12.statcan.gc.ca/nhs-enm/2011/as-sa/99-010-x/99-010-x2011001-eng.cfm

Urquia, M. L., Vang, Z. M., & Bolumar, F. (2015). *Birth outcomes of Latin Americans in two countries with contrasting immigration admission policies: Canada and Spain.* Retrieved from www.ncbi.nlm.nih.gov/pmc/articles/PMC4550416/pdf/pone.0136308.pdf

Vang, Z. M., Sigouin, J., Flenon, A., & Gagnon, A. (2015). The healthy immigrant effect in Canada: A systematic review. Population Change and Lifecourse Strategic Knowledge Cluster Discussion Paper Series 3(1), Article 4. Available at ir.lib.uwo.ca/pclc/vol3/iss1/4

Varghese, S., & Moore-Orr, R. (2002). Dietary acculturation and health-related issues of Indian immigrant families in Newfoundland. *Canadian Journal of Dietetic Practice and Research, 63*(2), 72–79.

Veenstra, G. (2009). Racialized identity and health in Canada: Results from a nationally representative survey. *Social Science and Medicine, 69,* 538–542.

Weber, E. P., & Khademian, A. (2008). Wicked problems, knowledge challenges, and collaborative capacity builders in network settings. *Public Administration Review, 68*(2), 334–349.

Weerasinghe, S., & Numer, M. (2011). A life-course exploration of the social, emotional and physical health behaviours of widowed South Asian immigrant women in Canada: Implications for health and social programme planning. *International Journal of Migration, Health and Social Care, 6*(4), 42–56.

World Health Organization (WHO). (2015). *Health Promotion.* Retrieved from www.who.int/topics/health_promotion/en/

Zhang, J., & Verhoef, M. J. (2002). Illness management strategies among Chinese immigrants living with arthritis. *Social Science and Medicine, 55*(10), 1795–1802.

Zuberi, D., & Ptashnick, M. (2012). In search of a better life: The experiences of working poor immigrants in Vancouver, Canada. *International Migration, 50*(S1), e60–e93.

CHAPTER 12

Healthy Cities and Communities: Urban Governance for Health and Wellbeing

Trevor Hancock

LEARNING OBJECTIVES

1. Understand the evolution of the Healthy Cities and Communities movement
2. Understand the broad focus of action of health promotion in urban settlements, especially the links to sustainable urban development
3. Understand what is meant by urban governance for health
4. Understand how improved urban governance can improve health

INTRODUCTION

We live in an urban world. Globally, 54 percent of the population lived in urban settlements in 2014, and that proportion is expected to increase to 66 percent by 2050. In Canada, we are 80 percent urbanized, as is the rest of North America, Latin America, and the Caribbean, while Europe is 73 percent urbanized. Asia is 48 percent urban, while Africa is 40 percent urban, and they are expected to be 64 percent and 56 percent urbanized, respectively, by 2050 (United Nations, Department of Economic and Social Affairs, Population Division, 2014). So health promotion is now largely an urban-based and urban-focused concern.[1]

Human settlements—cities, towns, villages, neighbourhoods, slums, and informal settlements—are not simply physical places ("a particular position, point, or area in space; a location" [Oxford Dictionaries]), they are also social spaces ("Space available or intended for social interaction; an area set aside for social interaction" [Oxford Dictionaries]), and they are always embedded within natural ecosystems. In fact, one important way to think of human settlements is that they are human-built eco-social systems, the settings within which most of us lead our lives.

But it is also important to recognize that these human-created urban ecosystems exist within a larger frame of reference—the bio-regional and ultimately planetary natural ecosystems. While much of humanity may spend much of its time indoors and in an urban setting, it is natural ecosystems, not urban ecosystems, that constitute the fundamental life support systems for humanity (see chapter 22).

What makes the urban ecosystem distinct from natural ecosystems, however, are the human aspects of the city; the fact that it is a human-built environment, and that it is a socio-cultural environment.

> Thus the urban settlement can be viewed as a human ecosystem—an ecosystem largely created by and inhabited by humans and consisting of both the built and human-modified physical environment and the social, economic, cultural and political environments that humans have created. Such an urban ecosystem is a dynamic complex of human, plant and animal communities situated within a given urban environment. (Hancock, 2000a)

This fits well with the long-established view that public health is a branch of the wider field of human ecology (Kartmann, 1967), which is "the inter-disciplinary study of the relationship between human society and nature" (Commonwealth Human Ecology Council [CHEC], 2017). In a much earlier pamphlet, CHEC added that human ecology is "concerned with the philosophy and quality of life in relation to the development of biological and geological resources, of urban and rural settlements, of industry and technology, and of education and culture" (Commonwealth Human Ecology Council, n.d.).

So, in seeking to create healthier cities and communities, we and all those with whom we work need to understand and adopt systems thinking, understanding and managing the city as a complex adaptive eco-social system. This has profound implications for urban governance and the work of health promoters. So how can this be done, and how is it being done? I see it in terms of the following questions:

- What business are we in?
- How do we measure our progress?
- What is governance for health in the twenty-first century?
- What are the new forms of governance we must develop?

But first, I begin with a brief introduction to the development of the Healthy Cities and Communities movement over the past 140 years, and especially the past 30 years.

THIRTY AND MORE YEARS OF HEALTHY CITIES AND COMMUNITIES

The concept of a healthy city is not new. As far back as 1875, Sir Benjamin Ward Richardson—a self-avowed disciple of Edwin Chadwick—described Hygeia as a City of Health in a speech to celebrate the "Great" Public Health Act of 1875 at the Social Science Congress in Brighton, England (Richardson, 1875). Many of the ideas he expressed are remarkably current—if understandably Victorian in their understanding and phrasing.

Richardson's work and that of another pioneering Victorian, Ebenezer Howard (1902), who created the concept of Garden Cities and stimulated their creation (influenced, I can't help but suspect, by Richardson's earlier ideas), was very influential in improving the health of urban dwellers in Britain and North America in the nineteenth and early twentieth centuries.

In 1914, those ideas were brought to Canada by Thomas Adams, a noted British planner and first Secretary of Letchworth Garden City. He was brought here by the Public Health Committee of the Commission on Conservation—what today we would call a commission on sustainable development—to help develop the town planning profession and legislation in Canada, which he did (Armstrong, 1959). At the same time, in Toronto, the Department of Public Health, under the leadership of Dr. Charles Hastings, was evolving into one of the best urban public health departments in the world (MacDougall, 1990), making Toronto the "healthiest of large cities" (Yorke, 1915).

The legacy of being the healthiest of large cities was a motivating factor 70 years later when we began to explore what it would take to make Toronto the healthiest city in North America, as our new mission statement declared. Our work there, as well as work in Britain and elsewhere, led Ilona Kickbusch to establish the WHO/Europe Healthy Cities Project in early 1986, as a way of taking the concepts of health promotion (then coalescing into the *Ottawa Charter*) out into the streets and making them concrete.

It turned out that she had established "the little idea that could" (Hancock, 2014) and the rest, as they say, is history (Hancock, 2017). Healthy Cities (in North America, Healthy Communities; in Latin America, Healthy Municipalities; in other parts of the world, variously Healthy Towns or Healthy Villages) has become a worldwide movement involving thousands of communities in countries all over the world. It is a prime—if somewhat neglected—vehicle for health promotion.

WHAT BUSINESS ARE WE IN?

Clearly, as health promoters, we are in the business of improving the health of the population while reducing inequalities in health. But that is not the business that cities are in, nor is it the business that many of our potential partners are in. So if we want to work with them, we need to find common ground and shared purpose, and not simply proceed as if health were all that mattered.

So what business are cities in? The good news is that they are not provincial or national governments, for whom the only thing that seems to matter is the economy, and especially the GDP. For these higher levels of government, the key objective seems to be to grow the economy, even though Simon Kuznets, the person who largely developed the national system of accounts that underlies the GDP, warned the US Congress that it should not be used as a measure of social welfare, noting that "the welfare of a nation can scarcely be inferred from a measure of national income" (Kuznets, 1934).

Instead, as discussed below, cities tend to focus on the wellbeing and quality of life of their citizens, which is understood in broad terms. Another area where municipalities and their citizens are leaders is in their focus on sustainable development, and especially on climate change and reduction of greenhouse gas emissions. They have also led on recycling and waste reduction, public transit, and a host of other sustainability initiatives. In general, they have been much more willing to come to grips with these issues than have national or provincial governments.

Taken together, it seems to me that municipalities are focused on five broad areas fundamental to quality of life and human wellbeing:

1. Human development
2. Sustainable development
3. Social and cultural development
4. Livable urban development
5. Economic development

Human-centred development is hardly a new concept; the 1986 UN *Declaration on the Right to Development* stated "the human person is the central focus of development." This was followed in 1990 by the creation of the Human Development Index (HDI) and its adoption by the UN Development Program.[2]

The admittedly utopian outcome of good human development would be that everyone achieves the highest level of human potential of which they are capable. It is important to recognize that while health is one part of human development, it is just one part. The concept encompasses much more, including the level of education, knowledge, and skills we achieve; our innovativeness and creativity; and our capacity for empathy and caring—not only for each other, but for the other species with whom we share the Earth, and for the Earth itself.

This, I believe, is where we can find common ground with many partners at the municipal level, not least municipal governments, urban planners, communities and community organizations, arts and culture organizations, local businesses, educators, and others who are focused on improving the quality of life of their community, maximizing the level of human development for all, and doing so in a manner that is ecologically sustainable. In fact, a 1992 Canadian Public Health Association report on human and ecosystem health suggested just such an approach when it redefined sustainable development:

> Human development and the achievement of human potential requires a form of economic activity that is environmentally and socially sustainable in this and future generations. (CPHA, 1992)

This is, or should be, the business we are in as health promoters, as communities, and as municipal, provincial, and national governments; it is a national tragedy that the latter two levels of government do not yet get it! But there is a real opportunity to make progress at the local level, while continuing to pressure the national and provincial governments to catch up.

A good recent summary of the business that cities should be in can be found in the Kuching Statement (International Institute for Global Health, 2016), the product of an Urban Thinkers Campus organized by the UN University's International Institute for Global Health (IIGH) in January 2016. This was one of a number of such events held in the lead-up to the third global conference on urban development organized by UN Habitat, but the only one focused on health and wellbeing.

Entitled *People, Planet and Participation*, the statement is focused on healthy, just, and sustainable urban development. The preamble states,

> In this rapidly urbanizing era, cities are key players in ensuring that humanity and all other species can live harmoniously and healthily on this one small planet. But this requires cities to adopt an eco-social approach, placing both the health of people and planet at the centre of urban planning and governance. The hallmark of successful 21st century cities will be an understanding of urban development in terms of the complex interconnections between the ecological, economic and social foundations of human development and health. (IIGH, 2016)

How Do We Measure Our Progress?

As noted above, cities do not measure their progress simply in economic terms. I do not know of a single municipality that is focused on the municipal equivalent of GDP—in fact I don't even think such a thing exists. Cities have a more holistic and human-centred, environmentally conscious approach, and they measure quality of life as revealed by the national set of indicators that has been developed and used in Canada for the past 20 years or so.

Led by the Federation of Canadian Municipalities (FCM), the Quality of Life Reporting System (QOLRS) "measures, monitors and reports on social, economic and environmental trends in Canada's largest cities and communities." The QOLRS is a member-based initiative. Starting with 16 municipalities in 1996, the QOLRS has grown to 24 communities in seven provinces (see www.fcm.ca/home/programs/quality-of-life-reporting-system.htm).

There are ten domains in the FCM's set of indicators, of which the economy is but one, as is health:

1. Demographic and background information
2. Affordable, appropriate housing
3. Civic engagement
4. Community and social infrastructure
5. Education

6. Employment and local economy
7. Natural environment
8. Personal and community health
9. Personal financial security
10. Personal safety

The FCM is not alone in this approach. Canada's Community Foundations have collaborated to create the Vital Signs indicators, and they have 11 somewhat similar domains (see box 12.1).[3]

Box 12.1: Vital Signs

Vital Signs is a community check-up conducted by community foundations across Canada that measures the vitality of our communities, identifies significant trends, and supports action on issues that are critical to our quality of life. The Toronto Community Foundation initially developed the Vital Signs concept and shared it, with Community Foundations of Canada supporting a coordinated national Vital Signs initiative.

The Vital Signs are based on the 11 categories created in the original Vital Signs report developed in Toronto, but local variants emerge. For example, a 12th category, sports and recreation, was added for the Victoria reports, based on local input.

The 12 categories for Victoria are

1. Arts and culture
2. Belonging and engagement
3. Economy
4. Environmental sustainability
5. Getting started in our community
6. Health and wellness
7. Housing
8. Learning
9. Safety
10. Sports and recreation
11. Standard of living
12. Transportation

On October 6, 2015, 28 community foundations across Canada released Vital Signs reports, while Community Foundations Canada released its third national Vital Signs report. For more information visit www.communityfoundations.ca/vitalsigns.

Source: Text adapted from *Victoria's Vital Signs 2015*, with permission.

Municipalities and community foundations are thus the national leaders in measuring what truly matters, and for them, what matters is quality of life measured across a wide range of environmental, social, and human dimensions. National and provincial governments need to learn from them and start measuring what matters. One new example of measuring what matters is the Happy Planet Index (HPI) (New Economics Foundation, 2016), which is discussed in the closing section of this chapter.

Defining and measuring what truly matters, and establishing public policies and community and corporate practices consistent with these aims, is one of the most important challenges we face in the twenty-first century. I believe that one of the key future roles for health promotion at the community level will be to work with the community and all the relevant local stakeholders to establish new forms of urban governance congruent with this understanding. This should begin by envisioning the community in the future where it is healthy, just, and sustainable. Then all the partners involved in governance must work together to figure out the path to this future.

WHAT IS GOVERNANCE FOR HEALTH IN THE TWENTY-FIRST CENTURY?

In its 2008 report, the WHO Commission on Social Determinants of Health (CSDH) noted that

> Within cities, new models of governance are required to plan cities that are designed in such a way that the physical, social, and natural environments prevent and ameliorate the new urban health risks, ensuring the equitable inclusion of all city dwellers in the processes by which urban policies are formed. (WHO Commission on Social Determinants of Health, 2008, p. 6)

Governance has been defined as "the management of the course of events in a social system" (Burris, Drahos, & Shearing, 2005), while urban governance has been defined as "the sum of the many ways individuals and institutions, public and private, plan and manage the common affairs of the city" (UN Habitat, 2002). It is important to recognize that governance is more than government (public institutions), including individual citizens, non-governmental and community organizations, and the private sector in the process.

Urban health promotion is rooted in the recognition that many of the main determinants of the health of urban populations lie within the domain of urban governments and other urban actors. Governance for health involves finding ways to establish collaboration and partnerships among all these stakeholders, around the common purpose of creating healthier, more just, and sustainable communities.

Governance for Health in the 21st Century is actually the title of a book published by WHO/Europe (Kickbusch and Gleicher, 2012). In it, they define governance for health as "the attempts of governments or other actors to steer communities, countries or groups of countries in the pursuit of health as integral to well-being through both whole-of-government and whole-of-society approaches" (pp. vii).

A couple of terms here are worth considering further:

- A *whole-of-government* approach requires the engagement of all municipal government departments—horizontal collaboration—and arguably, of all provincial and federal ministries whose activities affect the city—vertical collaboration. This calls for political leadership from the top (mayor or council), a coordinating structure and mechanism, and technical approaches such as health impact assessments and healthy public policy (see chapter 18).
- A *whole-of-society* (or at the municipal level, *whole-of-community*) approach has to extend beyond government to include all the other actors noted earlier. It requires broad civic leadership, with municipal-level leaders from many sectors working together to find common cause and take action. Here too, a coordinating structure and mechanism is needed (perhaps a civic leadership roundtable and a secretariat), and technical approaches would involve healthy *private* policy, community development, and capacity-building.

Indeed, right from the outset, the Healthy Cities and Communities approach has used four key approaches: political leadership, community engagement and capacity-building,

Box 12.2: Healthy City Examples: Toronto[4] and Vancouver

In late 1988, after a two-year process of research and consultation with the community and key stakeholders, the report "Healthy Toronto 2000" was approved by the Board of Health (1988). The report recognized the need to address the underlying determinants of health and laid out guidelines on how to create a healthier city, including the establishment of the Healthy City Office (HCO).

Importantly, the HCO was set up outside the Department of Public Health, and reported not to the Board of Health but, through the Committee of Departmental Heads, to City Council (and later to the mayor). It was given a two-pronged mandate: to work internally across departments within City Hall as a catalyst for change, and to work externally to build partnerships to help reach the goal of a Healthy City. The HCO was guided by a core group of champions from different departments who were key decision makers and acted as an advisory committee.

Underlying all the strategies was the idea of democratization: access to government processes and the importance of fostering the understanding of the Healthy City model. Healthy City staff used three main approaches: visioning, analysis, and action; the latter involved strengthening community engagement and capacity, building multi-sectoral partnerships, and developing healthy public policy.

continued

- Visioning: The Healthy City vision, which was encapsulated in the "Healthy Toronto 2000" report, identified future trends, detailed hopes and dreams, and recognized past successes. It was an important source of direction over the years.
- Analysis: *The State of the City* report was a way of organizing facts for public and political use. Led by the HCO, different departments collected and analyzed their pertinent data and helped prepare chapters for the report. The chapters covered economy, environment, community health, education, housing, transportation, and safety and identified areas for improvement and action.
- Strengthening community engagement and capacity was key to enabling community groups to work on solving issues, in part by ensuring access to decision makers and people with advocacy skills. Community grants were established, and groups were also recognized through The Healthy City Neighbourhood incentive awards (The Neighbourlies), which recognized groups that were helping make Toronto a better place to live. By the time of the HCO's demise (caused by the forced amalgamation of Toronto by the provincial government in 1998), there were approximately 200 Healthy City initiatives in Toronto.
- Intersectoral action and coalition-building: A wide range of initiatives such as urban gardening, homeless persons' self-help, and youth advocacy were strengthened by establishing partnerships between citizens and city government. For example, the Clean Air Partnership (CAP), hosted by the HCO, was an association of more than 50 businesses, community groups, and government agencies working on air quality issues for Toronto.
- Healthy public policy was key to the success of the HCO. By working across city departments and with internal and external partners, the HCO was able to recommend changes in policy. Many policy changes were implemented, such as the community safety strategy, clean air initiatives, youth employment initiative, and homeless initiatives, to name a few.

A more recent example of a comprehensive large-city Healthy City initiative can be found in Vancouver, where a partnership with the Vancouver Coastal Health Authority has been important right from the start. Beginning in 2010, an 18-month process of internal consultations in both organizations led to a joint agreement on a Healthy City framework, public consultations, and the creation of a Healthy City for All Leadership Table early in 2014. A ten-year Healthy City Strategy was approved by City Council in 2014 and the first four-year action plan was approved in mid-2015 (see vancouver.ca/people-programs/healthy-city-strategy.aspx).

The Strategy has three main themes—healthier people, healthier places, and a healthier planet—and "13 long-term goals for the well-being of the City and its people, including ambitious targets to reach by 2025" (City of Vancouver, 2014). Perhaps not surprisingly, the goals bear many similarities to the indicator categories identified by the FCM and the Community Foundations, as noted earlier.

intersectoral action, and the creation of healthy public policy (WHO/Europe, 1992); these are exemplified by the City of Toronto, which was, in many ways, the birthplace of the modern Healthy Cities movement (Hancock, 2017). It was one of the first large cities to adopt a comprehensive approach in its Healthy City Initiative, which ran from 1989 to 1999.

An Emerging International Agenda on Urban Governance for Health

Governance and health, especially urban governance and health, have been key areas of focus in several recent significant international statements:

- At the UN in 2015, the nations of the worlds adopted a set of 17 Sustainable Development Goals (SDGs) intended "to free the human race from the tyranny of poverty and want and to heal and secure our planet." Goal 3—"Ensure healthy lives and promote well-being for all ages"—and Goal 11—"Make cities and human settlements inclusive, safe, resilient and sustainable"—speak directly to the issue of healthy cities (see www.un.org/sustainabledevelopment/sustainable-development-goals/).
- The New Urban Agenda (UN Habitat, 2016), which was adopted at the Habitat III conference in Quito in October 2016, is "an action-oriented document which will set global standards of achievement in sustainable urban development." It includes a number of points that focus on strengthening urban governance and—unlike the Habitat II conference 20 years previously—has a number of references to the need to improve urban conditions to improve health and well-being. These include the provision of sustainable water, sanitation, and other key components of infrastructure; safe and green public spaces; "the generation and use of renewable and affordable energy and sustainable and efficient transport infrastructure and services"; access to public services and a clean environment; improved walkability and cyclability; improved housing and road safety; food security; and other issues very familiar to those working to create healthier cities and communities.
- In a report entitled "Health as the Pulse of the New Urban Agenda" prepared for Habitat III, the WHO (2016a) stated that in order for the ambitious New Urban Agenda to be realized, "the health of the nearly four billion people who dwell in cities today must be a central concern," and the report "provides a detailed vision for integrating health into urban planning and governance." The report stressed that healthy cities are environmentally sustainable, resilient, and socially inclusive and that "The good health of all its citizens is one of the most effective markers of any city's sustainable development"; one of its key recommendations was to "foster commitment to healthy cities as sustainable cities—recognizing the need for actions that involve all urban sectors" (see wcr. unhabitat.org/main-report/).

- Finally, the *Shanghai Declaration* (WHO, 2016b), the product of the 9th Global Conference on Health Promotion in November 2016, noted that

> We face a new global context for health promotion. People's health can no longer be separated from the health of the planet and economic growth alone does not guarantee improvement in a population's health.

The Declaration identified three priorities: good governance, local action through cities and communities, and people's empowerment by promoting health literacy. Under the heading "Cities and communities are critical settings for health" the Declaration noted that

> Health is created in the settings of everyday life—in the neighbourhoods and communities where people live, love, work, shop and play. Health is one of the most effective markers of any city's successful sustainable development and contributes to make cities inclusive, safe and resilient for the whole population.
>
> Together with city leaders we must address the toxic combination of rapid rural-to-urban migration, global population movements, economic stagnation, high unemployment and poverty as well as environmental deterioration and pollution. We will not accept that city residents in poor areas suffer ill-health disproportionately and have difficulty accessing health services.

This will require not only good governance but new forms of government that put people and the planet at the heart of governance, the topic to which I now turn.

WHAT ARE THE NEW FORMS OF GOVERNANCE WE MUST DEVELOP?

Informed by an understanding of their history, cities of the Anthropocene understand the journey ahead requires new tools and approaches. Past ways of working—characterized by simplistic, linear and siloed approaches that separate cultural, social, economic and ecological dimensions—do not work and indeed make things worse. We need an eco-social approach and sophisticated responses rooted in an understanding that cities are complex systems involving people/people, people/built environment and people/planet interactions. (The Kuching Statement, International Institute for Global Health, 2016)

The challenges we face in creating healthy, just, and sustainable communities in the twenty-first century are extraordinary—at least comparable to the challenges faced by nineteenth-century public health professionals and organizations in confronting the terrible living and working conditions of the slums and factories of the rapidly expanding and industrializing cities of those times. Yet we can take courage and inspiration from the fact that they succeeded to a large extent, and within only a few decades (remember, Rome was not built in a day!).

If we are to rise to the challenges of urban health in the age of the Anthropocene,[5] we will need new ways of working; this is not the nineteenth century, and we need approaches more suited to the twenty-first century. Three approaches worth considering are (1) the creation of a shared vision; (2) the creation of intersectoral partnerships, including with the planning sector and with the emerging sector of sustainable social entrepreneurship; and (3) the creation of a more engaged and participatory democracy using all the social media tools now available and yet to emerge.

The Power of a Shared Vision

The biggest challenge in establishing a whole-of-government and a whole-of-community approach is that each municipal department and each sector in the community has its own agenda and its own set of purposes and priorities. But as noted in the example of the City of Toronto, establishing a shared vision creates the common ground upon which people can converge. Particularly in smaller communities, creating a shared vision can be a powerful way of mobilizing volunteers to work with municipal governments and other partners doing this, and its impacts can last for years. Below are two examples of shared visions in communities in Canada that were established two or three decades ago and were a powerful motivating force for many years.

Rouyn-Noranda, Québec[6]

In 1986, the towns of Rouyn and Noranda, located at the heart of a gold and copper mining region and long one of the most polluted communities in Canada, were merged and new city council elections were held. One local councillor, inspired by Réal Lacombe, the "father" of healthy communities in Québec, ran on a healthy city ticket and came first in the election! Within months, the new city council launched its Healthy City project, the first in the Americas.

The project began with a widespread community consultation, including visioning, involving 6,000 of the 40,000 population, mainly children—on the grounds that it was their future that was being discussed. Out of this process, several clear visions emerged, one of which was to beautify and revitalize a small downtown lake that had been used as a dump, creating instead a botanical garden.

Some 3,000 citizens and numerous private and public organizations made direct contributions to À Fleur d'Eau (a flower of water), as the park was named, in the first five years. I visited the park with Réal in 2012, when Rouyn-Noranda was celebrating the 25th anniversary of its Healthy City project, and I can testify to the power of such a shared vision—it's a beautiful place.

But there is much more to their Healthy City initiative, including a remarkably successful initiative to reduce children's exposure to lead from the local smelter and actions addressing poverty and other social issues. Best of all, and a key indicator of success, Rouyn-Noranda Healthy City has survived five different mayors!

Woolwich Healthy Communities, Ontario[7]

The Township of Woolwich is a rural community of 23,000 people in the region of Waterloo, about 120 kilometres west of Toronto, in rich farmland. Woolwich Healthy Communities (WHC) is a volunteer group that "strives to promote and improve the health and well-being of our community, economy and environment." Formed in 1991, WHC began with a vision workshop; one of the most striking findings to emerge, which has been a central theme ever since, was that while the Grand River, which runs through St. Jacobs, was depicted in the images that people drew as being central to the life of the community—a place where people walked, swam, fished, played, and boated—that was not the reality. This led to the creation of a Clean Waterways workgroup, which is still active.

The Clean Waterways group improves water quality throughout Woolwich Township. Working with volunteers and landowners, they improve the health of Woolwich waterways by stabilizing and rehabilitating creek banks. Schools and community members have helped the core volunteers plant native trees and shrubs and install fencing along upper sections of the Canagagigue Creek. These activities reduce erosion and prevent pollutants from entering the waterway.[8]

In 2008 the Clean Waterways group was honoured by the Grand River Conservation Authority with a Watershed Award for helping farmers protect and improve the quality of the creeks flowing through their land. In addition to the Clean Waterways group, WHC in 2014 had four other working groups: trails, on-road cycling, environmental enhancement, and a coordinating committee. Other groups, such as a well-water–quality group and a sustainable community group, have sprung up from time to time to address particular needs and interests. In 2007, the Ontario Healthy Communities Coalition awarded WHC a Community Recognition Award for its work.

Intersectoral Collaboration

Municipal governments alone cannot make cities healthier; as the UN Habitat definition above notes, there are many other actors who must be engaged, both at a leadership level and at the community level. At a leadership level, an obvious step would be to create a Civic Leadership Council on Sustainable Human Development. Such a Council could bring together the civic leadership from across all sectors to find common purpose and drive common strategies to improve the city.

One important point here is to avoid making the Council the creation of one mayor or one municipal council, since the tendency is for new brooms to sweep clean. Accordingly, creating the Civic Leadership Council at arms-length from the municipal government may be a useful strategy to ensure longevity. How that is done will vary from place to place.

An interesting example is Horsens, in Denmark, one of the first—and in many ways the best—of the original WHO/Europe Healthy Cities; perhaps not coincidentally, it was also the smallest, with a population of about 70,000. The city government worked with a private foundation to establish and jointly fund a Healthy City Shop as a form of social entrepreneurship that became "a powerhouse of community action" but also acted as "a think tank for municipal bureaucrats" (de Leeuw, 1999). This "half-in, half-out" position may be a useful model for communities to adopt.

Re-establish Links with Urban Planning

Of particular importance in the process of creating a healthy community is the re-establishment of the close ties that once existed between public health and urban planning. The roots of urban planning in Canada lie in the work of the Public Health Committee of the Commission on Conservation in the early twentieth century (Hancock, 1997a), but over time the two disciplines drifted far apart. The re-creation of those links has been an important part of the Healthy Cities and Communities approach in Canada and elsewhere.[9]

When we did have a Canadian Healthy Communities project (1989–1992) it was based at the Canadian Institute of Planners (CIP), and the Steering Committee was chaired by the president of the CIP. The interest in healthy communities has continued at the CIP, on and off, ever since, and has been quite strong in recent years, with an active Healthy Communities Committee. The Committee notes that "promoting healthy communities is bound up with nearly all aspects of the built environments that planners help create" and offers several resources for planners.[10]

Of particular note is a *Healthy Communities Practice Guide* that took a broad approach to healthy community planning. The Guide begins by discussing the importance of establishing a vision. Topics covered included active transportation, open space planning, food systems, and green and healthy buildings. But most important is the section of the Guide entitled "Beyond land use planning," in which the issues of social development, mental health, and spiritual wellbeing are discussed. The Guide recommends

> a consideration of topics often in the realm of social planning, such as social development and mental health. It can also involve broadening the definition of well-being to include a truly holistic perspective on what makes us happy, successful, connected and healthy as human beings. This could involve exposure to a sense of wonder and awe, openness, authenticity, or spiritual contemplation. It is the stuff that makes us grow as a community and as individuals, and connects us to our neighbours and to the world around us. (Canadian Institute of Planners, n.d.)

Several other successful initiatives that bring together urban planning and public health in Canada are profiled in the Resources section at the end of this chapter.

Engage with the Social Entrepreneurship Sector

As I note in chapter 22, it makes no sense to make economic growth and development the central pillar of public policy. The focus must be on ensuring human and social development in a manner that is compatible with sustaining in perpetuity the natural systems that are the fundamental underpinnings of human wellbeing. But in addition to opposing the current harmful economic model, we also need to be supporting the emergence of a new economic model, one rooted in sustainable human development, in making a reasonable profit while improving the environment, strengthening community, and enhancing well-being and human development.

Thus, a new set of potential partnerships is emerging as we contemplate the challenge of living justly and in good health within the confines of the Earth's limited capacity, and that is partnering with the social entrepreneurs that are building a new economy compatible with those requirements; we must help to bring to life the new economy that we need for the twenty-first century.

The relationship between social entrepreneurship and health has recently attracted the attention of the CIHR's Institute of Population and Public Health, which held a workshop on this topic in 2015. The workshop report (CIHR, 2015) identified several common elements in various definitions of *social entrepreneur*:

- The primary purpose is for the common good, specifically to address social vulnerability;
- Trading is the main source of income (actual or aspirational);
- Profits are used for social or community benefit;
- Assets are locked for common benefit; and/or
- The approach includes being a good employer, being democratic, and empowering communities, cooperation, and social justice.

It is noteworthy—and of concern—that the concept of environmental sustainability is not explicitly included in these definitional elements, although it may be included under "community benefit."

At the local level, health promotion will mean identifying and working with the new and emerging social entrepreneurs who will do this. Hernandez, Carrion, Perotte, and Fullilove (2014) call for "public health entrepreneurship," which they define as "enterprises rooted in health promotion, disease prevention, health-care services, and the social determinants of health"; they are social entrepreneurs "with a specific emphasis on achieving health impacts." They also identify a number of industries "that are ripe for public health entrepreneurs," including the following:

- Real estate: Design/development of healthy homes and responsible urban revitalization
- Environmental services: Renewable products related to health and hygiene, such as water, waste, energy, and food production
- Nutrition: Healthy supermarket creation and retrofits, food co-ops, and cooking and food preparation classes
- Tourism and transportation: Alternative/active transportation options

Other industries they mention are education and social services, fitness and recreation, holistic health, information and communications, organizational support services and consulting, and product development. Clearly, there is much scope for health promoters both to work with and, indeed, work within these and other business and non-profit sectors that, collectively, are working to create the future we need.

From Community Engagement to Participatory Democracy

Another key Healthy Community strategy is community engagement, which is seen as health promoting, since it leads to personal and community empowerment (see chapter 2), which are—or should be—mutually reinforcing; empowerment (as long as it is not harmful to disadvantaged people or communities) has long been seen as good for health (Wallerstein, 1992). Healthy City projects always include a strong focus on this, although what is meant by citizen or community engagement or participation varies widely, depending on local political, cultural, and historical traditions; it can range from mere tokenism to true political empowerment.

It is time our notions of community engagement and empowerment progress from the usual focus on empowerment (often nebulously understood and described in broad "feel good" terms) to something more profound: broader democratic revitalization.

Of particular interest are models of participatory governance that have emerged in Brazil, notably the concept of participatory budgeting. Despite its current troubles at the national level, Brazil has been a hot-house for experiments in participatory engagement ever since the days of Paulo Freire (see chapter 2). In a report on participatory governance in the city of Belo Horizonte, Wampler (2012) noted that

Today, hundreds of thousands of Brazilian citizens are elected to public policy management councils. There is also the ongoing mobilization of citizens into participatory budgeting and policy conferences, thus greatly expanding how policies are debated in the public sphere.

In the case of Belo Horizonte, with its population of about 2.7 million, he reports there were 571 participatory venues (municipal and regional councils, and hundreds of local-level councils, such as schools and public health clinics), providing "more than 3,400 seats," to which citizens could be elected or appointed. On top of that, he adds, their 2009/2010 participatory budgeting process involved citizens in public meetings (more than 50,000 participants), multi-day policy workshops (at least 9,000 citizens) and digital voting (more than 110,000 votes in 2008); from these processes "nearly 1800 citizens were elected ... to monitor the program."

I cannot think of anything even remotely comparable in a major Canadian city. But equally interesting and impressive, in my opinion, was something I observed when I was in Belo Horizonte at about the same time: the city has a Deputy Secretary for Democratic Participation. Given the low rates of voting in municipal elections, and the generally low rates of municipal engagement, I have been suggesting ever since that every municipality in Canada needs a similar position. What could be more important for democracy, and for empowerment and wellbeing, than making democratic participation a major urban priority?

But we also need to consider what democracy should look like in the twenty-first century, in the age of social media and the Internet. One interesting example of the new power of the Internet is reflected in the concept of "crowdsourcing" of policy. I have become interested in the role of the Internet in the development of Iceland's new constitution and Finland's approach to the development of new legislation. This may be one way of engaging people more in the democratic process and in community engagement and participation, but what would that look like in a Canadian municipality?

If we are to "enable people to increase control over and improve their health" (WHO, 1986), health promotion must be part of the process of re-inventing democracy for the twenty-first century, especially at the local level. Government is only legitimate if it is democratically elected and—even more important—if people are engaged in the process not simply as occasional voters, but as ongoing participants.

Towards a "One Planet" Region

The relationship between "healthy" and "sustainable" cities has been clear for many years (Hancock, 1994, 1996, 1997b, 2000b), but as the recent international statements noted earlier have made clear, this is an issue of growing importance. One way our impact on the Earth can be understood is in terms of the ecological footprint (EF), which measures the amount of bio-productive land and sea needed to maintain our current way of life. As the Worldwide Fund for Nature noted in its 2014 *Living Planet Report*, "the high human development in developed countries has been achieved at the expense of a high ecological footprint. Decoupling and reversing this relationship is a key global challenge" (Worldwide Fund for Nature, 2014).

The EF of high-income countries such as Canada is the equivalent of four to five planets' worth of annual biocapacity, which is clearly unsustainable. It is also unjust; we are taking more than our fair share, which disadvantages low- and middle-income countries whose resources we use, thus limiting their own ability to use those resources for their own development. In addition, we are borrowing—some would say stealing—from our descendants; as the Planetary Health Commission put it, "we have been mortgaging the health of future generations to realise economic and development gains in the present" (Whitmee et al., 2015). This too is both unjust and unsustainable.

This is also true of Canada's cities; the EFs of the 20 largest cities (using 2001 data) ranges from 6.87 (Greater Sudbury) to 9.86 (Calgary CMA) hectares per capita (Anielski Management Inc., 2005). However, "the planet only has 1.9 hectares of nature (productive land and sea) available to meet the needs of each person" (Anielski Management Inc., 2005), which means in 2001 we consumed between 3.6 and 5.2 times the biocapacity that is available to us. If we only take the fair share of the Earth's ecosystem goods and services to which we are entitled—what the Worldwide Fund for Nature (2014) calls "One Planet" living—we need to reduce our EF in those municipalities by 75 to 80 percent, to between 27 and 19 percent of its current level; high-income groups in high-income countries, who have even larger footprints, would need to reduce their footprints considerably more.

One idea I have been pursuing recently is a way of integrating many of these ideas at a regional or metropolitan level in the form of a "One Planet" initiative. To this end, I have initiated a series of "Conversations for a One Planet Region" in Victoria, BC, where I live. So I was delighted to recently discover that Bioregional (2017)—a UK-based charity and social enterprise working around the world with developers and municipal governments, among others—created its One Planet Living initiative in 2003. Its ten One Planet Principles begin with "Health and Happiness" and also address other social concerns (e.g., "Culture and Community," "Equity and Local Economy") in addition to environmental and urban planning focus areas.

As people whose focus is health and wellbeing, the important question for health promoters is how do we maintain a high quality of life, with high life expectancy and good health, while doing this? Thus, my attention has been drawn to one of the alternative measures of national progress that is based on exactly these issues, and to its potential adaptation at the local level.

The Happy Planet Index (HPI) has been developed by the New Economics Foundation in the UK, a leading ecological economics think tank. It is a comparatively simple measure in principle, although challenging in some respects at a local level. Its four components capture the key themes of concern for population health promotion in the twenty-first century: life expectancy and life satisfaction (as a percentage), the product of which is considered to be life quality, and is equity-adjusted, all divided by the ecological footprint (EF). (Life satisfaction is measured in a standard international Gallup poll.) The sweet spot is a high and equitable life quality and a low EF. In the latest report (New Economics Foundation, 2016), the top five nations were Costa Rica, Mexico, Colombia, Vanuatu, and Vietnam; Canada was 85th and the US 105th out of 140 nations.

While designed for the national level, there is in principle no reason why the HPI cannot be applied to the local level, although to date this has only been done in one place: Caerphilly, in Wales (Caerphilly County Borough Council, 2008). However, it does require calculating the ecological footprint (EF), which can be challenging at a local level because the appropriate data are not always readily available. Fortunately, the EF has been calculated for 20 of the largest Canadian municipalities (Anielski Management Inc., 2005); and more recently, and in a more detailed, bottom-up, consumption-based approach, for Vancouver (Moore, Kissinger, & Rees, 2013; Moore, 2015).

What I anticipate is a process of local engagement amongst municipal governments, community organizations, NGOs, local academics, and others to measure the EF and the HPI. That would the first stage. The second stage would be to work with the community to envision a future where the region or municipality had a "One Planet" footprint, but a high quality of life. What would that look like? What social, technological, and economic changes would be necessary, what environmental results would be obtained, what would our future way of life look like, and how would we maintain—and even improve—our quality of life?

I see this as an essential step in getting to "One Planet" communities, because if we can't convincingly describe and show such a hopeful future, we are not going to find it easy to persuade people to move in that direction. It is, therefore, an eminently useful role for health promoters in the twenty-first century, as we embark on the creation of more just, sustainable, and healthy communities and a more just, sustainable, and healthy world.

CONCLUSION

In an urban world, the Healthy Cities and Communities approach should be a major strategy for health promotion, but it has remained somewhat marginal in many places. In the face of the challenges to health posed by our current economic system—damaging global ecological changes and global, national, and local inequality—as well as by low levels of real democratic participation, urban health promoters must partner with social, democratic, and economic reformers in many other sectors—public, private, community and citizen-based, and non-profit—who together create the conditions for health in cities and other urban settings. Together, we can and must create a vision of a more just, sustainable, and healthy future and then co-create the cities, towns, and villages that are compatible with that vision. It is perhaps the greatest health promotion challenge of the twenty-first century.

CRITICAL THINKING QUESTIONS

1. How can we make governance for health an important strategy for all levels of government in the twenty-first century?
2. How can health promoters work with local governments and multiple community partners to put health on, if not at the centre of, the agenda?
3. How should we measure progress, and what role can health promoters play in bringing about change in the way we measure progress at all levels?

4.   Who are the key community partners for health promoters in creating more just, sustainable, and healthy communities?
5.   How can health promoters play a role in renewing democracy at all levels, but especially at the local level, so that people can be enabled to increase control over and improve their health?

RESOURCES

Further Readings

Cities and Health: www.tandfonline.com/loi/rcah20
This newly established journal provides an innovative new international platform for consolidating research and know-how for city development to support human health.

Corburn, J. (2009). *Toward the healthy city: People, places, and the politics of urban planning.* Boston: MIT Press.
This book provides a detailed account of how city planning and public health practices can reconnect to address health disparities, and offers a new decision-making framework that reframes traditional planning and development issues and provides a new scientific evidence base for participatory action, coalition-building, and ongoing monitoring.

De Leeuw, E., & Simos, J. (2017). *Healthy cities—The theory, policy, and practice of value-based urban health planning.* New York: Springer.
This book models, critiques, and provides global examples that illustrate institutional change, community input, targeted assessment, and other means to address sources of urban health challenges. It contains several chapters by Canadian authors.

Frumkin, H., Frank, L., & Jackson, R. (2004). *The public health impacts of sprawl.* Washington, DC: Island Press.
The authors examine the direct and indirect impacts of sprawl on human health and wellbeing, and discuss the prospects for improving public health through alternative approaches to design, land use, and transportation.

Journal of Urban Health: www.springer.com/public+health/journal/11524
This journal provides a platform for interdisciplinary exploration of the evidence base for the broader determinants of health and health inequities needed to strengthen policies, programs, and governance for urban health.

Let's Start a Conversation About Health: Video User Guide: www.sdhu.com/health-topics-programs/health-equity/health-equity-resources#video
Video user guide on how to start a conversation about health with the public developed

by the Sudbury and District Public Health Unit. The site also includes other resources to help inform health equity action developed by the Unit as well as other organizations.

Relevant Websites

For those interested in establishing a healthy city or community initiative in Canada, the following are useful resources.

Healthy Community Networks in Canada
For more detail on each of these, see Hancock, Norris, Lacombe, and Perkins (2017).

BC Healthy Communities
bchealthycommunities.ca
   This website provides comprehensive information about BC Healthy Communities.

Mouvement Acadien des Communautés en Santé—A New Brunswick Francophone Network
www.macsnb.ca
   This website provides comprehensive information (in French) about the New Brunswick Francophone network.

Ontario Healthy Communities Coalition
www.ohcc-ccso.ca
   This website provides comprehensive information (in English and French) about the Ontario Healthy Communities Coalition.

Villes et villages en santé—The Québec network of Healthy Cities and Villages
www.rqvvs.qc.ca
   This website provides comprehensive information (in French) about the Québec network of Healthy Cities and Villages.

Urban Planning and Public Health Initiatives
For more detail on each of these see Hancock, Norris, Lacombe, and Perkins (2017).

BC Healthy Built Environment Alliance
www.phsa.ca/our-services/programs-services/population-public-health/healthy-built-environment
   This website, managed by the Provincial Health Services Authority, provides information for the BC Healthy Built Environment Alliance as well as the built environment in general, and tools such as the Healthy Built Environment Linkages Toolkit.

BC Healthy Communities' PlanH program

planh.ca/about-us

PlanH, implemented by BC Healthy Communities Society, facilitates local government learning, partnership development, and planning for healthier communities.

Healthy Canada by Design

While no longer funded, many of its key learnings were published in a special supplement of the *Canadian Journal of Public Health* in 2015: journal.cpha.ca/index.php/cjph/article/view/5009/2998

WHO and International Resources

International Society for Urban Health

www.isuh.org/home.html

ISUH is an interdisciplinary organization that advances the generation, exchange, and application of high-quality urban health knowledge across academics, policy makers, implementers, and communities to attain health equity in urban settings worldwide. The website provides information about their work as well as resources on urban health. ISUH also publishes the *Journal of Urban Health*.

WHO Collaborating Centre for Healthy Cities and Urban Policy Research, Tokyo, Japan

www.tmd.ac.jp/med/hlth/whocc/

The WHO Collaborating Centre for Healthy Cities and Urban Policy Research conducts research on Healthy Cities and urban policy, and performs various functions in support of the WHO. As is the case with the European Collaborating Centre, the website provides information about the activities of this Centre.

WHO Collaborating Centre for Healthy Urban Environments, Bristol, UK

www1.uwe.ac.uk/et/research/who.aspx

This WHO Collaborating Centre is one of two WHO Collaborating Centres in the world situated in a built environment faculty. It works with municipalities, planning consultancies, and health authorities in the UK and through the wider WHO Healthy Cities Network. The website provides information about the work of the Centre including research, publications, seminars, training, and conferences.

WHO/Europe—Urban Health

www.euro.who.int/en/health-topics/environment-and-health/urban-health

This website, managed by the European Office of the World Health Organization, provides information in news, events, policies, activities, publications, and partners in relation to urban health.

NOTES

1. This is not to deny the important health promotion issues in rural and remote settlements, where the issues and needs are often more serious and the resources to address them are fewer. But this chapter is focused primarily on the urban setting.
2. UNDP Human Development Index, hdr.undp.org/en/content/human-development-index-hdi
3. Both of these indicator sets also share many characteristics with the Canadian Index of Wellbeing, which tracks changes in eight quality of life categories. It was developed by an NGO and is now housed at the University of Waterloo, but sadly is not used by the Government of Canada. uwaterloo.ca/canadian-index-wellbeing
4. Edited, abridged, and used with permission from a case study authored by Fran Perkins, former Director, Toronto Healthy City Office (1993–1999), in Hancock, Norris, Lacombe, & Perkins (2017).
5. For a discussion of the Anthropocene and its relevance to health, see chapter 22.
6. Abridged from a case study authored by the late Réal Lacombe in Hancock, Norris, Lacombe, & Perkins (2017).
7. Adapted from www.healthywoolwich.org/ and from Hancock, Norris, Lacombe, & Perkins (2017).
8. Source: www.healthywoolwich.org/Clean%20Waterways.html
9. See for example the work of the WHO Collaborating Centre for Healthy Urban Environments in Bristol: www1.uwe.ac.uk/et/research/who.aspx
10. www.cip-icu.ca/Issues/Healthy-Communities

REFERENCES

Anielski Management Inc. (2005). *Ecological footprints of Canadian municipalities and regions.* Ottawa: Federation of Canadian Municipalities.

Armstrong, A. (1959). Thomas Adams and the commission of conservation. *Plan Canada, 1*(1), 14–32.

Bioregional. (2017). *One planet living.* www.bioregional.com/oneplanetliving/

Burris, S., Drahos, P., & Shearing, C. (2005). Nodal governance. *Australian Journal of Legal Philosophy, 30*, 30–58.

Caerphilly County Borough Council. (2008). *Living better, using less: Sustainable development strategy 2008.* Blackwood, Caerphilly, Wales: Author.

Canadian Institute of Planners. (n.d.). *Healthy communities practice guide.* Ottawa: Author. Available at www.cip-icu.ca/Files/Healthy-CommunitiesCIP-Healthy-Communities-Practice-Guide_FINAL_lowre.aspx

Canadian Institutes of Health Research (CIHR), Institute of Population and Public Health. (2015). *New pathways to health and well-being through social enterprise workshop—Executive summary.* Ottawa: Author. Available at www.cihr-irsc.gc.ca/e/49242.html

Canadian Public Health Association (CPHA). (1992). *Human and ecosystem health.* Ottawa: Author.

City of Vancouver. (2014). *A healthy city for all: Vancouver's healthy city strategy 2014–2025—Phase 1.* Vancouver: Author. Available at council.vancouver.ca/20141029/documents/ptec1_appendix_a_final.pdf

Commonwealth Human Ecology Council. (n.d.). *Human ecology brochure.* London: Author. (This brochure was produced at around the time the CHEC was established in 1969, but is no longer available.)

Commonwealth Human Ecology Council. (2017). *Mission statement.* www.checinternational.org/about-chec/who-we-are/

De Leeuw, E. (1999). Healthy cities: Urban social entrepreneurship for health. *Health Promotion International, 14*(3), 261–270.

Hancock, T. (1994). A healthy and sustainable community: The view from 2020. In C. Chu & R. Simpson (Eds.), *The ecological public health: From vision to practice.* Brisbane: Griffith University and Toronto: Centre for Health Promotion.

Hancock, T. (1996). Planning and creating healthy and sustainable cities: The challenge for the 21st century. In C. Price & A. Tsouros (Eds.), *Our cities, our future: Policies and action for health and sustainable development.* Copenhagen: WHO Healthy Cities Project Office.

Hancock, T. (1997a). Healthy cities and communities: Past, present and future. *National Civic Review, 86*(1), 11–21.

Hancock, T. (1997b). Healthy, sustainable communities: Concept, fledgling practice and implications for governance. In M. Roseland (Ed.), *Eco-city dimensions: Healthy communities, healthy planet.* Gabriola Island, BC: New Society Press.

Hancock, T. (2000a). *Urban ecosystems and human health.* Unpublished manuscript prepared for the "Seminar on CIID-IDRC and urban development in Latin America," Montevideo, Uruguay, April 6–7, 2000.

Hancock, T. (2000b). Healthy communities must be sustainable communities too. *Public Health Reports, 115*(2/3), 1516.

Hancock, T. (2014). The little idea that could! A global perspective on healthy cities and communities. *National Civic Review, 103*(3), 29–33.

Hancock, T. (2017). Healthy cities emerge: Toronto—Ottawa—Copenhagen. In E. De Leeuw & J.Simos, *Healthy Cities—The theory, policy, and practice of value-based urban health planning* (pp. 63–73). New York: Springer.

Hancock, T., Norris, T., Lacombe, R., & Perkins, F. (2017). Healthy cities and communities: The North American experience. In E. De Leeuw & J. Simos, *Healthy Cities—The Theory, Policy, and Practice of Value-Based Urban Health Planning* (pp. 215–240). New York: Springer.

Healthy Canada by Design. (2015). Special supplement. *Canadian Journal of Public Health, 106*(1) (Suppl. 1).

Hernandez, D., Carrion, D., Perotte, A., & Fullilove, R. (2014). Public health entrepreneurs: Training the next generation of public health innovators. *Public Health Reports, 129*, 477–481.

Howard, E. (1902). *Garden cities of tomorrow.* (Reprinted, edited with a Preface by F. J. Osborn and an Introductory Essay by L. Mumford). London: Faber and Faber [1946].

International Institute for Global Health (IIGH). (2016). People, planet and participation: The Kuching statement on healthy, just and sustainable urban development. *Health Promotion International.* doi: 10.1093/heapro/daw046

Kartmann, L. (1967). Human ecology and public health. *American Journal of Public Health, 57,* 737–749.

Kickbusch, I., & Gleicher, D. (2012). *Governance for health in the 21st century: A study conducted for the WHO Regional Office for Europe.* Copenhagen: WHO Regional Office for Europe.

Kuznets, S. (1934). *National Income, 1929–1932.* 73rd US Congress, 2nd session, Senate document no. 124, p. 7. library.bea.gov/u?/SOD,888

MacDougall, H. (1990). *Activists and advocates: Toronto's health department, 1883–1983.* Toronto: Dundurn Press.

Moore, J. (2015). Ecological footprints and lifestyle archetypes: Exploring dimensions of consumption and the transformation needed to achieve urban sustainability. *Sustainability, 7,* 4747–4763. doi:10.3390/su7044747

Moore, J., Kissinger, M., & Rees, W. E. (2013). An urban metabolism and ecological footprint assessment of Metro Vancouver. *Journal of Environmental Management, 124,* 51–61.

New Economics Foundation. (2016). *The Happy Planet Index 2016.* London: Author. Available at happyplanetindex.org

Place. (n.d.). In *Oxford Dictionaries.* Retrieved from en.oxforddictionaries.com/definition/place

Richardson, Sir B. (1875). *Hygeia: A city of health.* London: MacMillan.

Social space. (n.d.). In *Oxford Dictionaries.* Retrieved from en.oxforddictionaries.com/definition/social_space

United Nations, Department of Economic and Social Affairs, Population Division. (2014). *World urbanization prospects: The 2014 revision, highlights.* New York: United Nations.

UN Habitat. (2002). *Global campaign on urban governance—principles.* Available at mirror.unhabitat.org/categories.asp?catid=25

UN Habitat. (2016). *The new urban agenda.* Nairobi: Author.

Wallerstein, N. (1992). Powerlessness, empowerment, and health: Implications for health promotion programs. *American Journal of Health Promotion, 6*(3), 197–205.

Wampler, B. (2012). Participation, representation, and social justice: Using participatory governance to transform representative democracy. *Polity, 44,* 666–682. doi: 10.1057/pol.2012.21

Whitmee, S., Haines, A., Beyrer, C., Boltz, F., Capon, A. G., de Souza Dias, B. F., ... Yach, D. (2015). Safeguarding human health in the Anthropocene epoch: Report of The Rockefeller Foundation–Lancet Commission on Planetary Health. *The Lancet, 386*(1007), 1973–2028 dx. doi.org/10.1016/S0140-6736(15)60901-1

WHO/Europe. (1992). *Reflections on progress: A framework for the Healthy Cities Project Review.* Copenhagen: Author.

World Health Organization (WHO). (1986). *The Ottawa Charter for health promotion.* Copenhagen: Author.

World Health Organization (WHO). (2016a). *Health as the pulse of the new urban agenda: United Nations conference on housing and sustainable urban development, Quito, October, 2016.* Geneva: Author.

World Health Organization (WHO). (2016b). *The Shanghai Declaration on promoting health in the 2030 agenda for sustainable development.* Geneva: Author. www.who.int/healthpromotion/conferences/9gchp/shanghai-declaration.pdf?ua=1

World Health Organization (WHO) Commission on Social Determinants of Health. (2008). *Closing the gap in a generation: Health equity through action on the social determinants of health. Final report of the Commission on Social Determinants of Health.* Geneva, Switzerland: Author.

Worldwide Fund for Nature. (2014). *Living planet report.* Gland, Switzerland: WWF.

Yorke, K. M. (1915, July). Saving lives on the wholesale plan. *Maclean's Magazine, 28*(12).

CHAPTER 13

Promoting Educational Success, Health, and Human Development within Education: Making the Shift to a Systems Approach

Douglas McCall and Daniel Laitsch

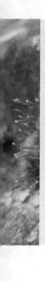

LEARNING OBJECTIVES

1. Understand Canadian approaches to school health and their origins
2. Understand that the evolution of school-based health promotion and social development, from programs to systems, is still in progress, with policy, practice, and research often still focused on the problems/programs of the day rather than long-term, sustainable strategies
3. Understand what a systems-based approach is and how it can better advance school health in Canada, particularly the integration of programs within education system mandates, constraints, and concerns

INTRODUCTION

Canadian schools have always been places where health, safety, social, and other concerns about children and youth have been addressed. In the 1800s, churches and charities created schools to guide children's moral, physical, and spiritual development as their parents left farms to join the industrial revolution. Community schools emerged in the 1950s as a hub to unite communities after World War II. Health education, home economics, physical education, and vocational/career education were all compulsory subjects as governments took over control and funding of schooling in the 1960s. They continued to be mandatory core curricula in most provinces and territories into the 1990s.

The first Canadian consensus statement proposing a "Comprehensive School Health" approach was published in 1990. This statement differed from the American model of several stipulated "coordinated" core programs as well as the values-driven statements from Europe (St. Leger, Kolbe, Lee, McCall, & Young, 2007). Ironically, this Canadian statement was not inspired by the 1986 *Ottawa Charter for Health Promotion*, as was the case in other parts of the world. Instead, it drew upon typically Canadian ideas and values such as shared responsibility across several ministries/agencies, equity, and child development. Rather than a mandatory set of components or programs as defined in the US, the Canadian consensus on school health and development (SH&D) was more of a planning framework, providing flexibility for jurisdictions or advocates on different health issues to develop their own models and terminology as they combined interventions such as policy, instruction, support services, physical environment, and different forms of social support.

Although valuable, these Canadian ideas about shared responsibility and flexibility only added to the early and ongoing confusion about goals, values, principles, components, systems, levels, agencies, professionals, programs, outputs, and capacities that should be included in school-based and school-linked health promotion and social development (WHO, 1997). (Please see the discussion and definition provided in the Appendix.) It is this absence of a consistent, comprehensive, and systems-based understanding and concomitant planned approach that is the greatest challenge for school health promotion in Canada and most other parts of the world.

THE WHOLE CHILD INSTEAD OF BODY PARTS

Albeit that schools in Canada have always played a role in socialization and that "comprehensive school health" has been recognized as an important concept in Canada since 1990 (McCall et al., 1999), most of the funding and initiatives in school health and development have been driven by various health or social issues. The first wave of progress in Canada (and the US) came from the HIV/AIDS crisis in the 1980s. Tobacco funding and alcohol/drugs support continued that momentum until the turn of the century when physical activity and nutrition dominated as the health sector responded to the obesity crisis. Mental health is now trending as a dominant concern, even shifting the language away from "health" towards "wellbeing." Often the attention on the crisis issues of the day has pushed aside the existing programs and sought new, separate funding, staffing, and structures for their issue. Consequently, duplication, restructuring, and competition often occur at multiple levels. Moreover, the sustainability of these targeted programs is at risk as soon as funding declines after the emergency aspects are addressed.

Advocates for a comprehensive approach have always tried to ensure that attention to overall health was maintained while still addressing the urgent problem of the day, but competing voices have always ensured that general "health" was subordinate to their more urgent and hence "more important" focus. Consequently, the research funding, program budgets, pilot projects, government and agency structures, professional and research expertise, and attention from senior health managers, politicians, and the public have also reflected the issue of the day and neglected the necessary infrastructure of stable policies, ongoing interorganizational partnerships, planned scope and sequence in a health, personal, and social development (HPSD) curriculum, and more.

More recently, educators in many jurisdictions have been able to secure support for an approach to schooling that educates the "whole child" (Brown, 2008) and countries such as England and the United States are redefining their educational goals in a more balanced way, seeking success for every child. This creates a wider opportunity for health and social programs as attention is moved away from a narrow academic focus on literacy and numeracy. However, this trend is not yet accompanied by a commitment to mandatory curricula/learning outcomes and a focus on teaching students specifically about their health and wellness.

Further, many jurisdictions, including several Canadian provinces, are reverting to very broad, generic, interdisciplinary curricula that expect students to develop "competencies" that could, but may not, include their health and social development. Given that many of these generic curricula models also include "personalized" pathways, many students could end up without a planned scope and sequence of HPSD learning.

Ironically, this trend in the education system comes at a time when health promotion (and school health promotion) has been restructured and diminished in many health ministries and agencies. Health promotion programs and staff are now often reporting to disease-focused managers responsible for chronic diseases or health services. The status of school health programs, as well as programs aimed at supporting other settings such as the workplace, cities, families, and others, has been reduced as part of this retreat from health promotion.

The absence of a holistic or salutogenic understanding of health—one that recognizes that health is not only intertwined with education and learning but also with welfare, personal and social development, equity, safety, and the environment—has also caused many health promotion efforts in Canada and elsewhere to ignore or end up competing with other sectors that also work with schools. These include social services that provide family supports, child protection and school-based social workers; justice, law enforcement, and private security sectors that prevent crime/drug use and assign police school resource officers or security guards; the municipal sector, which promotes recreation and sports activities that often overlap with schools; and the environmental sector, which includes human health as part of its mandate, thereby including schools in promoting sustainable development education.

These other sectors have their own multi-component approaches (MCAs), such as "community schools," "safe schools," and "eco-schools." These MCAs include policies, instruction, various services delivered through schools, changes to the physical environment, and engaging parents and students related to their respective goals and mandates. They all promote specific interventions that address the specific problems related to their mandates. Consequently, educators are often overwhelmed by the number of competing initiatives being pushed at their schools. Organizational development theory and real world experience clearly warn that "mission creep" and the constant pressure to find new funding will cause all sectors to compete for attention, infrastructure, and funding for their respective school programs. We can continue to use this competitive short-term strategy that is not sustainable without extensive, ongoing funding, or we can try something different.

MANY MODELS, INSUFFICIENT UNDERSTANDING AND INFRASTRUCTURE

Researchers, practitioners, and officials are now recognizing that the various multi-component frameworks and approaches are not being implemented, nor maintained (Deschenes, Martin, & Hill, 2003; Adamowitsch, Gugglberger, & Dür, 2014; Fathi, Hamid, Shaghaghi, Kousha, & Jannati, 2014). While there are many excellent projects, individual interventions, and several multi-intervention programs addressing broad issues such as physical activity, mental health, bullying, and others, there is little attention being paid to the status and effectiveness of the common core components or infrastructure elements that are needed to deliver such projects and programs.

The absence of attention to these core components is also prevalent in Canada. The core instructional component, a health, personal, and social development (HPSD) education curriculum, has been significantly reduced in several provinces. Further, there are few studies or surveys documenting the instruction that is delivered, and the education sector does not report on student learning in these areas. Minimum service levels, staffing, qualifications, and wait times for school-based or school-linked health and other services have not been defined or monitored. Key personnel to deliver these services, such as school nurses, school social workers, police resource officers, and others, operate without clear guidelines and their presence varies within and across school districts. Student perceptions about school and teachers are tracked in surveys but there are few reports and analyses connecting these survey results to school discipline and school climate programs. Participation rates in after-school and extra-curricular programs are not systematically monitored. Perceptions and levels of parent participation in school health and social development programs as well as in parent education and training are also not widely tracked.

There is a similar lack of research, policy, and program attention regarding the organizational or system capacities needed to implement and maintain the school-based or school-linked approaches. A systems-based approach requires both basic capacity in terms of funding and staffing as well as ongoing capacity-building at an organizational and systems level. Currently, most capacity-building is focused just on building the knowledge of front-line professionals. The revised 2007 version of *Canadian Consensus Statement on Comprehensive School Health* (Canadian Association for School Health, 2007) incorporated capacity-building as its primary new focus. But this change has not had an impact on practice or research. The statement adapted a capacity-based model that was originally published by the World Health Organization (2003). It contains eight key capacities:

- Over-arching policy and leadership from senior managers
- Assigning intersectoral coordinators at all levels
- Using formal and informal mechanisms to promote intersectoral cooperation/coordination

- Ongoing workforce development
- Ongoing knowledge development and exchange
- Regular monitoring, reporting, and continuous improvement focus on child/youth behaviours, system/organization policies and programs, and student learning
- Joint strategic planning to set priorities and manage emerging issues
- Explicit plans for the sustainability of programs and succession planning of key personnel

Most provinces/territories and local agencies have published supportive declarations on school health promotion and similar multi-component approaches (McCall et al., 1999) but, without any systematic monitoring, we do not know if the agencies and ministries have assigned coordinators at various levels, if there are effective inter-ministry and inter-agency agreements in place, whether there are long-term workforce development programs for teachers, nurses, and other personnel, or if there are agreements on joint priorities among ministries and agencies. There are small-scale school recognition/incentive programs for some schools in some provinces as well as an abundance of self-assessment tools, but no jurisdiction regularly monitors and reports on the status and reach of its policies and programs.

Despite the gaps in capacity in these areas, Canada has been a leader in one, namely knowledge development and exchange. In the early years of this century, prior to the introduction of significant cutbacks in federal programs and funding in 2010, Canadian programs, practitioners, and advocates benefited from a rapid growth in capacity at the national level. In 2004, as part of a federal-provincial/territorial accord on health care, a commitment was made by first ministers to promote health and development "working across sectors through initiatives such as Healthy Schools" (Health Canada, 2004) and an intergovernmental consortium was established. Funding from the Canadian Institutes for Health Research (CIHR) permitted researchers to define a research agenda that used an ecological and systems-based approach (Doherty & McCall, 2004). The Canadian Consensus Statement on Comprehensive School Health (Canadian Association for School Health, 2007), supported by more than 35 organizations, was updated. Canada hosted a global meeting with the World Health Organization in Vancouver in 2007 (Tang et al., 2009), which marked the shift towards contextualization, capacity-building, and ecological, systems-based approaches. A knowledge centre funded by the Canadian Centre for Learning supported the creation of an active knowledge exchange program using Web-based tools and several communities of practice (see www.canadianschoolhealth.ca and its international successor www.schools-for-all.org).

Canada has also been at the forefront in developing multi-component approaches to safe schools, community schools, and several multi-intervention programs that target bullying, physical activity, mental health, social and emotional learning, and other issues addressed within these multi-component approaches.

CANADIAN LEADERSHIP IN INTERNATIONAL, ONLINE EXCHANGES

Canadian researchers, practitioners, and advocates also hosted the formation of several international networks, including one on international school health in 2004, early childhood learning/development in 2005, and violence prevention in 1994.[1] It is interesting to note that Canada also hosted the revival of global interest in health-promoting universities when it published the *Okanagan Charter* in 2015 (see chapter 14). Much of the work of these international centres has been online, with innovative and effective uses of webinars and other Web-based tools. Incidentally, the networks on early childhood and on school health/development have used Wikipedia-style websites to develop, collaborate, and publish knowledge in the form of encyclopedias on early childhood and school health and development.[2]

As the second decade of the twenty-first century began, much of the discretionary and project-based funding disappeared with the federal cutbacks, leaving large parts of the collaborative infrastructure dormant. The result has been a return to issue-specific activity on topics such as mental health, bullying, and physical activity, but the coalition of non-governmental organizations, the research network, and other mechanisms promoting healthy schools, safe schools, and community schools are all quiet.

This is not to say that all activities have stopped. A cursory review of the ongoing compilation of Canadian school-related research and knowledge exchange done by the Canadian Association for School Health[3] since 2007 (McCall, 2016a) has identified more than 1,300 published journal articles, reports, and other analyses of the Canadian experience. The governments in Canada have expanded the sample size of the Health Behaviour in School-aged Children (HBSC) survey to permit provincial/territorial reporting. The researchers involved in the HBSC surveys (which have occurred regularly over several years) are publishing many more analyses of the trends. Provincial/territorial governments have continued to name school health coordinators and have published various policy papers and initiatives using the comprehensive approach. Indeed, there is a significant policy opportunity as the governments in Canada re-negotiate the 2004 Health Care Accord. Perhaps this is the time to expand the mandate and resources to the Pan-Canadian Intergovernmental Joint Consortium for School Health.[4]

FROM AN ECOLOGICAL ANALYSIS TO A SYSTEMS-BASED APPROACH

A systems-based approach can help to address the overlap, confusion, and competition within the health sector and with other sectors (see figure 13.1). By starting with a better understanding of how school systems truly work, by responding to the renewed education system interest in the whole child, and by working within the common ground and

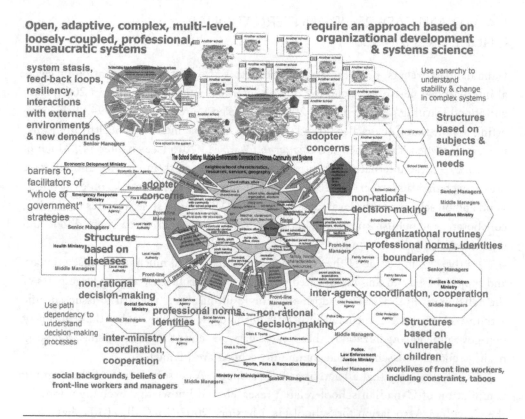

Figure 13.1: Complex, Confusing, Competing Systems: Systems Science Concepts Applicable to School Health Promotion and Social Development

Source: McCall, D. S. (2016b). *Ecological, systems-based understanding and approaches to school health, safety, equity, social & sustainable development.* Surrey, BC: International School Health Network (In Progress).

boundaries established by educators, it is more likely that the competition within the health sector and with other sectors can be managed more effectively. The competition for scarce resources will never stop because it is a function of public and private enterprise. However, by starting with the whole child, rather than body parts or narrow conceptions of health, we can redefine system goals, establish new organizational processes and routines, train professionals differently, and modify service and funding mandates and procedures while still responding to the issues of the day and assigning tasks across the public service agencies and ministries.

An earlier edition of this book (McCall, Deschesnes, & Laitsch, 2012) noted that Canada needs to make

a shift from only promoting evidence-based programs and building multi-intervention programs on selected health issues to sustaining those efforts through ecological, systems-based approaches (Canadian Association for School Health, 2007; Deschesnes, Trudeau, & Kebe, 2010; Deschesnes, Couturier, Laberge, & Campeau, 2010; Doherty & McCall, 2004; Laitsch, Taylor, & Rootman, 2006; McCall, 2006; Palluy, Arcand, Choinière, Martin, & Roberge, 2010). These new ideas suggest that school health promotion is more than simply implementing a program or set of programs in the school setting. Instead, it is more about combining interventions at multiple levels across several systems to improve the health of the entire setting (Dooris et al., 2007).

This Canadian team of researchers (Doherty & McCall, 2004) also noted that sorting out this complexity requires new thinking and new types of research. The CIHR project even developed a somewhat disturbing diagram that illustrates the many people, places, and processes that are present in the ecology of schools. This 2012 diagram is part of an expanded and updated diagram above, which places the school more effectively within several systems. Poland, Krupa, and McCall (2009) provide a framework for understanding and using this kind of complexity.

Despite these efforts to make a paradigm shift towards a systems-based approach, in Canada, an "over focus on promoting packaged programs in the form of evidence-based programs (EBPs) does not successfully integrate the knowledge of settings and persons toward maximal impact" (Atkins, Rusch, Mehta, & Lakind, 2016). The authors suggest a shift "from an emphasis on how to bring *this program to that setting* [emphasis in the original] toward an ecologically driven science that prioritizes the needs and resources of settings that matter most to youth and families."

A preliminary review (McCall, 2016a) of the school-related research published about Canadian programs is depicted in the following table. As we move downwards through the categories in table 13.1, we move closer to the ecological, systems-based approach that is now recommended by the emerging research, by reports on the sustainability of programs, and by practitioner advice. This review indicates that most of the research remains focused on reports on the health status and behaviours of individuals, the characteristics of those individuals that affect their behaviours, and various social influences on their behaviours. The attention in Canadian research is also on the effectiveness and implementation of individual interventions rather than on comprehensive approaches that coordinate such interventions. Studies examining the complexities of working across sectors or in building the capacities of systems/organizations are also minimal. Most of the articles that examine how such programs can be integrated within education systems are published in educational journals and may not be considered by the health or other sectors.

The proportions within the categories of the 1,909 research articles, shown in table 13.1, have remained roughly the same between October 2011 and October 2016.

Table 13.1: Preliminary Review of Canadian Research, 2011–2016

Categories	Number of items	Percent
Overall status of child & adolescent health, development, welfare, & well-being	7	0.3
Reports & analysis of health/social problems, behaviours, child/adolescent status prevalence, burden of the problems	272	14.2
Individual characteristics, correlates related to behaviours	268	14.0
Social influences, including parents, peers, friends, media, community, etc.	246	12.9
Social determinants, including economic, race, culture, geography, discrimination, education level, and others	109	5.7
Indigenous populations and interventions focused on their needs, context	177	9.3
Influence of the physical and social environment/routines of the school	96	5.0
Influence, impact of macro-policies on health, wellness, children (including schools) on behaviours, policies, or program status or program reach	91	4.8
The effectiveness and impact of individual programs/interventions	168	8.9
The effectiveness or impact of a multi-intervention program addressing a broad health or social issue	34	1.8
The quality of the implementation of programs or approaches	98	5.1
Reports, analysis, or commentaries on the capacities of systems or organizations to deliver programs	44	2.4
Reports, analysis, or commentaries on specific types of organizational/system capacity such as policy/leadership, coordination mechanisms, workforce development, knowledge exchange, monitoring/reporting/surveillance	46	2.4
Reports, analysis, commentary on intersectoral cooperation (all sectors)	12	0.6
Reports, analysis, commentary on the effective integration of health & social programs within the core mandates, constraints, or concerns of education systems	113	5.9
Applications, analysis of ecological approaches, complexity, systems thinking or science	55	2.9
Discussion of research methods, tools for knowledge exchange or policy development	73	3.8

INTEGRATION OF HEALTH AND SOCIAL PROGRAMS WITHIN EDUCATION SYSTEMS

Given that Canada has often been at the forefront of global developments related to school health promotion and social development, it is not surprising that Canadian health and social development organizations are participating in a global dialogue that is being led and facilitated by education-sector organizations representing teachers, school leaders, and education ministry officials seeking to integrate health and social programs more effectively within the core mandates, constraints, and concerns of education systems. Canadian and American leaders have endorsed a global consensus statement (ASCD, Education International, & International School Health Network, 2013), met in forums and workshops, and identified strategies and examples of policies, programs, and practices that are based on a true understanding of education systems rather than continuing efforts to persuade educators, school by school, to teach more, care more, or do more. Educators understand that healthy, safe, and supported children learn more effectively but they are not persuaded that it is their primary job to take on the responsibilities of other ministries, agencies, parents, nurses, social workers, police officers, and other personnel in delivering services in schools. This call for a new type of partnership requires health, social, and other systems to invest in school-based or school-linked programs and staffing for the long-term, to focus on educational as well as health or social goals, to cooperate with other sectors seeking to access schools, and to address specific problems within a whole child, life-course approach. This call for better integration within, not simply with, education needs to be rooted in a systems-based approach and not just appeals to individual schools or teachers or other volunteer "champions."

A Systems Approach Helps to Address Disadvantage

A systems-based approach reflects the deeper ecological understandings about health, development, and learning by recognizing the contextual factors and systemic barriers that aggravate disadvantage and deprivations caused by poverty, geographical isolation, and discrimination based on race, religion, or language. This emerging research in this area reflects the real-world experiences that practitioners and officials have lived with for too many years.

Two examples of such adaptations of systemic planning have been identified and articulated in Canada. The first of these systems-based models is focused on how schools can address the needs of disadvantaged communities through a coordinated combination of specific policies, programs, and practices. The Canadian Association for Community Education and the Canadian Association for School Health organized a consultation, organized a community of practice, and published an agenda of topics for future knowledge development. The resulting Consensus Statement[5] was subsequently adopted at an international symposium convened by the International School Health Network (2010) in Geneva.

This statement notes that an adapted, harmonized version of the strategies used to alleviate disadvantage and reduce disparities used by proponents of safe schools, healthy schools, and community schools would be the best starting point. The statement then goes on to identify the strengths (14), urgent challenges/issues (10), and programs and policies (43) that are specifically relevant to disadvantaged communities.

The school health community in Canada also initiated a consultation among Indigenous nations around the world to develop a culturally relevant model for school health and development. Funded by the National Collaborating Centre on Aboriginal Health and the Canadian Council on Learning Knowledge Centre on Aboriginal Learning, this project included a Community of Practice, a series of webinars, an inventory of better practices, a discussion paper, and the publication of *A Framework for Indigenous School Health* (Tagalik, Corless, & McCall, 2010).

The final report[6] noted that "Essential cultural differences can be found in the basic ideas that drive school health programs. For example, the western cultural view of 'health' is as a personal possession—a resource for daily living, while most Indigenous cultures define health as a set of relationships and responsibilities held across a continuum, and which include the environment, families, the tribe and ancestors. The challenge facing health educators and practitioners today is one of decolonizing existing curricula and programs so there is a cultural fit for the Indigenous client."

These two school-related projects on disadvantaged and Indigenous communities are both conceptual and practical. They defined a need, set a course, and offered practical advice on programs and steps or pathways to take. These two publications preceded much of the current Canadian and global discussion consisting mostly of general ideas and over-arching models that address social determinants and the needs of Indigenous populations. Unfortunately, in Canada, the ongoing generalized discussions about lofty principles and concepts continue while these two early starts on how schools could actually take action remain on the shelf.

SYSTEMATIC MONITORING, REPORTING, AND IMPROVEMENT

A systems-based approach can also facilitate and support systematic monitoring, reporting, and improvement across and at all levels within the different ministries, agencies, and front-line entities that support educational success by delivering health and development programs. A paradigm shift to a systems-based approach would significantly affect the purposes and nature of current and previous monitoring and reporting efforts.

Most of these efforts in Canada and in other countries have been narrowly focused on specific health or social problems. They have often consisted of sporadic, one-time surveys of child and adolescent behaviours or perceptions. They have been oriented to a health sector approach to surveillance and reporting rather than the education sector preference for using data for continual improvement. Since the data are collected in schools, the ensuing discussion is more often on what the education sector is doing about the health and social issues of the day rather than the actions of the other sectors involved.

As well, in Canada, there is a plethora of surveys and one-time studies, much without any tracking of subsequent policy/program improvements or relevance and with few secondary analyses. It is only recently that some of these surveys have opened up access to their data for other researchers and others.

There is very little, if any, tracking of the status of policies and programs in the various levels of the systems involved. Where there is any assessment of policy/program capacity and status, it is done by publishing various self-assessment tools or small-scale school recognition programs with the hope that more than a small minority of already interested schools will use them. Like almost every other country in the world, no Canadian province or territory tracks student learning outputs in health and social development, even though such curricula and learning are mandatory in most jurisdictions.

The first consequence of a shift to a systems approach would be a fundamental change of purposes; moving away from monitoring/surveillance towards a continual improvement model that enables and supports the practitioners, local agencies, ministry units, and other parts of the systems to identify and be accountable for specific improvements in their operations each year. This moves away from uniform testing or criteria that are usually focused and narrow in scope, towards using data for more local or school-based decision-making.

This model is much more compatible with current practices in many education systems, where high-stakes testing of a few academic subjects has been largely discredited. It is also closer to the quality-management systems used in large corporations and increasingly in the private sector.

The second consequence of a systems approach to monitoring, reporting, and improvement is a requirement that a proper monitoring system be established. A group of experts was supported by the Division of Adolescent and School Health, Centers for Disease Control and Prevention, to develop a description of such a system. Their summary (McCall et al., 2009) noted the following:

> A Monitoring and Reporting (M&R) System uses carefully selected indicators based on reliable data sources to produce regular reports on system/organizational performance over time as a tool to focus system reform and improvement. The goals of monitoring/reporting systems are to assess the effectiveness and efficiency of a system, agency or coordinated set of programs in order to improve performance as well as provide a mechanism for accountability. M&R systems provide enhanced information for improved planning, policy, practice and decision-making. Effective M&R systems record changes over time in the local context, inputs, processes (programs, policies, practices) and outputs (short term health/social status, behaviours, knowledge, skills, attitudes). These outputs can lead to positive lifelong outcomes in health, social development and education provided that similar supportive conditions or interventions are available over the life course.

M&R systems related to health and development should include three essential areas: (1) student health/development including health status, behaviours and conditions affecting health, (2) the quality, reach and capacity of the health, social, law enforcement and education systems (ministries, school boards/agencies, schools and staff/professionals) to deliver support and (3) the learning outcomes (knowledge, attitudes, beliefs, skills and intentions) achieved by students through their core studies in health, personal/social development, family studies/home economics and physical education.

Canada has a good base upon which to make progress in systematic monitoring and improvement. There are two types of surveys of child and adolescent behaviours that are now administered regularly, so comparisons can be made over time. The Health Behaviour in School-aged Children (HBSC) survey has been done several times over two decades. The many provincial surveys on youth risk behaviours and alcohol and drug use include very similar questions and can therefore form a national picture on a regular basis. The intergovernmental consortium on school health has developed a set of indicators and measures (Hussain, Christou, Reid, & Freeman, 2013) to understand how a comprehensive school health approach can enhance student achievement. The Joint Consortium for School Health has also developed a school-level self-assessment tool that could be expanded to cover the other levels, including regional agencies/authorities and ministries in other systems such as health, social services, and others.

The Council of Ministers of Education, Canada (n.d.) has an established process for monitoring student learning and educational outputs through its data and research program. This is a natural home for assessments of student learning in health and social development.

At the global level, the Organisation for Economic Co-operation and Development (OECD, 2016) is currently exploring indicators related to student wellness as part of its PISA monitoring of academic achievement. The UN, through its 2030 Sustainable Development Goals, has created a space and is developing indicators and targets within Goal #4 (Quality Education) for student learning in student health, personal, and social development as part of a broader concern for the quality of education.

There are also three relatively new international multi-level, multi-system self-assessment tools that can be used to monitor progress regarding policies and programs. Several UN agencies and global organizations have developed a basic assessment of the core components of a school health and development approach (FRESH, 2012). The World Health Organization (n.d.) is adapting the American School Health Policies and Practices Study (SHPPS) for use in other countries. The World Bank (n.d.) includes a set of questions on school health as part of its systems-based school effectiveness monitoring system (SABER).

These Canadian and international tools could be used to establish a systems-based monitoring, reporting, and improvement process and program in Canada.

CONCLUSION

The articulation of a comprehensive approach to school health promotion is now 25 years old in Canada. Like many other developments in Canada's culture and history, the evolution of that approach has been moderate, mushy, and motivating. Like many other countries, the movement forward has been possible through the efforts of several volunteers who pioneered the initial shift from a focus on one type of intervention, health education, to an aspiration of a comprehensive, multi-component approach. The knowledge about individual behaviours has grown to now consider social influences and, eventually, social determinants as part of the interacting, complex ecologies that affect children's lives.

Our deeper understanding of the open, adaptive, and complex environment of the school has led us to the inevitable conclusion that we must work with many organizations, operating at many levels, within many systems. As we mature, we often realize what we don't know, so many of the emerging scholars, practitioners, and officials are now looking to organizational development strategies and systems science. We have also realized that if the work is to occur within schools, then we must be prepared to integrate our efforts within the mandates, constraints, and concerns that drive education systems.

As in real life, we must now accept that we have and continue to make mistakes. Despite our models and principles, our work in school-based and school-linked health promotion and social development is still occurring in silos separated by topic expertise, structures, and boundaries. We continue to work in short-term, disconnected projects, often developing narrowly focused programs with little attention to scaling up or sustaining the effort.

This is the challenge of the next generation of leaders, researchers, practitioners, and officials: To not only make the paradigm shift to systems-based approaches, but to implement and maintain that shift in policy and practice.

APPENDIX: GUIDE TO TERMS

The following terms and operational definitions are used in this chapter. They are included here as a means to reduce some of the ongoing confusion that confounds research and practice.

Settings-Based Health Promotion and Social Development

According to the WHO Health Promotion Glossary,[7] a setting for health is a place or social context in which people engage in daily activities in which environmental, organizational, and personal factors interact to affect their health and wellbeing. These settings are often called places where people live, learn, work, or play. Settings can normally be identified as having physical boundaries, a range of people with defined roles, and an organizational structure. Examples of settings include schools, work sites, hospitals, villages, and cities as well as hybrid settings (community gardens) or virtual settings (socially oriented websites or services). In this chapter on educational settings, we extend the concept of "health" to include several aspects of human development because there are several sectors beyond the health care/public health sector that also work with schools and because the health sector itself often includes issues that are more accurately the purview of those other sectors. These different aspects of human development include access to schooling; lifelong learning, education, and training; health; welfare; safety; security; crime prevention; environmental citizenship and sustainability; reducing disparities; promoting equity and economic development for those in poverty; inclusion of people with disabilities; personal, social, moral, and spiritual/religious development; human rights; diversity; and global awareness. Action to promote health through different settings can take many forms but should include a focus on multiple coordinated interventions that modify the physical, social, economic, instructional, recreational, or other aspects of that setting. Actions in settings-based health promotion also often involve some level of organizational development, including changes to the physical or social environment or to the organizational structure, administration, and management. Settings can also be used to promote health as they are vehicles to reach individuals, to gain access to services, and to synergistically bring together the interactions throughout the wider community. Dooris (2006) has pointed out that this basic difference in goals (individual or setting) has caused confusion between the concepts of doing health-promoting programs aimed at modifying individual behaviours within a setting as opposed to multiple interventions aimed at modifying the conditions of the setting, or even the factors or conditions underlying the setting. Poland et al. (2009) have addressed this by providing a framework for planning and delivering multiple interventions in settings that are aimed at the whole setting or underlying conditions.

Interventions, Multi-Intervention Programs, Multi-Component Approaches in School-Based and School-Linked Health Promotion and Social Development

Intervention: a policy, instructional program, service, or organizational or professional practice to prevent a problem behaviour/condition or promote health or development on a specific issue, behaviour, or risk/protective factor or condition.

Multi-Intervention Program (MIP): a set of different types (policy, instruction, services, social support, physical conditions) of coordinated interventions (programs, services, policies, practices) to address a broad education, health, social, or economic issue such as sanitation/hygiene, child protection/exploitation, school dropout, physical activity, bullying, sexual health, healthy diet, mental health, and others, or to address the needs of a specific sub-population such as Indigenous or disadvantaged communities, sexual minorities, and others.

Multi-Component Approach (MCA): a set of core components, pillars, or infrastructure that includes a macro-policy requiring a multi-intervention approach; a mandatory health, personal, and social development curriculum and instruction; a minimum set of health, social, and other services; minimum physical conditions and safety/ sanitary standards; a minimum social environment delivered in and with schools through education systems in cooperation with other sectors/ministries; and sets of corresponding agencies/authorities. To be considered a distinct multi-component approach in this text, these multi-faceted strategies need to have a distinct primary partner sector. These include the Healthy Schools model with the health sector, Community Schools with the economic and social planning sectors, Safe Schools with law enforcement/youth justice, Eco-schools with the environment sector, Education in Emergencies working with relief aid agencies and donors, School Health and Nutrition working with development aid agencies and donors, Child Friendly Schools working with the human rights sector, and others. Often the descriptions of the multiple components are accompanied by a list of system, organizational, and professional capacities/standards such as leadership, workforce development and training, staff assigned to coordination, regular monitoring, and reporting, and similar concepts. As well, some MCAs include cross-cutting themes such as community participation or youth engagement as a part of their core. Sometimes a multi-intervention program (MIP) on a vital issue such as nutrition is also considered to be a key component.

An MCA should be comprehensive (delivered at multiple levels, in multiple systems, on multiple issues) and include several coordinated agency–school district programs at the regional level. However, many models are focused only at the school level in whole-school strategies that involve only educators as the delivery agents and, consequently, do not truly use a comprehensive approach. MCAs are often confused with similar descriptions of various planning frameworks that often combine various interventions or components to respond to one or more clusters of problems and issues. These planning frameworks and models sometimes obscure the need for establishing and maintaining a core set of components or infrastructure.

CRITICAL THINKING QUESTIONS

1. To your knowledge or based on your experience, is it important that agencies and sectors work together to align their efforts and programs that they wish to be adopted by schools? If so, what are the barriers and facilitators of that type of alignment?
2. Do you think that Canadian schools and other agencies have truly implemented and maintained comprehensive approaches to promoting health, safety, or other forms of human development through schools? Or does that goal still remain elusive in most schools and communities?
3. Do you agree that the systems-based approach suggested in this chapter should be developed further by practitioners, researchers, and officials in the future? If so, what are some of the immediate steps that could be considered?

RESOURCES

Further Readings

ASCD, Education International, International School Health Network. (2013). *Consensus statement on the integration of health & social programs within education systems.* Alexandria, VA: ASCD. www.wholechildeducation.org/about/globalschoolhealthstatement
This consensus statement has initiated a global dialogue, led by educator organizations, that has included workshops in several parts of the world, discussion among UN agencies and integrational organizations, a Twitter feed, several webinars, and, currently, the preparation of a White Paper/e-book listing examples of more than 50 policies, program modifications, and revised processes/procedures to support better integration of programs within the core mandates, constraints, and concerns of education systems.

Atkins, M. S., Rusch, D., Mehta, T. G., & Lakind, D. (2016). Future directions for dissemination and implementation science: Aligning ecological theory and public health to close the research to practice gap. *Journal of Clinical Child & Adolescent Psychology, 45*(2), 215–226. dx.doi.org/10.1080/15374416.2015.1050724
This article calls for a paradigm shift of health promotion practice and policy that would move "away from an overemphasis on promoting program adoption towards an approach that fits interventions within settings that matter most to children's healthy development and for utilizing and strengthening available community resources." The limits of traditional paradigms such as diffusion of innovation theory and social network theory applied to the adoption of innovations within organizations are noted, as well as the application of organizational theory (explaining how various organizational characteristics will affect the implementation and maintenance of programs). The article illuminates a pathway towards getting beyond the current discussions of "ecological approaches," which are often more aptly seen as more "ecological analysis" of the complex, multi-level factors that influence behaviour rather than "ecological action," which explain how to modify those factors.

Deschesnes, M., Martin, C., & Hill, A. J. (2003). Comprehensive approaches to school health promotion: How to achieve broader implementation? *Health Promotion International, 18*(4), 387–396. doi: 10.1093/heapro/dag410
This groundbreaking analysis was part of an investigation into the implementation and sustainability of multi-component approaches to school health promotion undertaken in Québec that led to a significant shift away from an issue/program focus towards a systems-based approach. The analysis shows that the Health Promoting School/ Comprehensive School Health Approach has remained more of an aspiration than a reality, noting that implementation is often focused only on instruction or on a couple of key health issues rather than a comprehensive approach. Four conditions for sustainability are identified: (1) negotiated planning and coordination to manage the required coordination;

(2) true intersectoral partnerships based on reciprocal benefits; (3) political and financial support for the coordinated approach (rather than single issues or elements); and (4) on-going evaluation of the implementation and maintenance strategies being used to support the approach.

Carey, G., Malbon, E., Carey, N., Joyce, A., Crammond, B., & Carey, A. (2015). Systems science and systems thinking for public health: A systematic review of the field. *BMJ Open, 5*(12). doi:10.1136/bmjopen-2015-009002

This review examines if and how concepts and strategies derived from systems science are used to guide health promotion strategies. The article helps us to move along the pathway that began a decade ago regarding "systems thinking" about implementing interventions in large complex organizations and systems towards a more practical and disciplined use of established scientific concepts such as systems modelling. This is the new frontier in research and practice for school health promotion.

Relevant Websites

The Canadian School Health Community

www.canadianschoolhealth.ca

A website tracking Canadian research and events, along with resources from several Canadian projects.

Schools for All

www.schools-for-all.org

A Wikipedia-style website with hundreds of summaries, webinars, and other resources prepared by experts from around the world.

Videos and Modules

Complexity Science: 3 Systems Thinking

www.youtube.com/watch?v=AP7hMdnNrH4

A module, part of an online course on systems thinking.

Systems Thinking and Evaluation

www.youtube.com/watch?v=2vojPksdbtI

An animated video depicting systems thinking.

Systems Thinking White Boarding Animation Project

www.youtube.com/watch?v=lhbLNBqhQkc

A great animated video explaining systems concepts.

Wicked Problems, Dynamic Solutions: The Ecosystem Approach and Systems Thinking

www.unep.org/ecosystems/resources/tools/wicked-problems-dynamic-solutions-ecosystem-approach-and-systems-thinking

A MOOC developed for the UN on systems-based planning and science.

NOTES

1. For international school health, see www.internationalschoolhealth.org; for early childhood development, see earlylearning.ubc.ca/about/help-internationally/; for violence prevention, see www.cdc.gov/violenceprevention/youthviolence/index.html

2. For childhood development, see www.child-encyclopedia.com; for school health and development, see www.schools-for-all.org

3. The Canadian Association for School Health regularly extracts Canadian articles from more than 400 journals, more than 150 media outlets, and more than 100 social media sources and publishes them in monthly reports at www.canadianschoolhealth.ca as well as in a Canada-focused Twitter news/resources news feed.

4. For the Joint Consortium on School Health, see jcsh-cces.ca

5. For Consensus Statement, see www.schools-for-all.org/page/Addressing+Health+%26+Equity+through+Schools

6. For a copy of the Indigenous School Health Framework, see www.nccah-ccnsa.ca/en/publications.aspx?sortcode=2.8.10&publication=42

7. For the WHO Health Promotion Glossary, see www.who.int/healthpromotion/about/HPG/en/

REFERENCES

Adamowitsch, M., Gugglberger, L., & Dür, W. (2014). Implementation practices in school health promotion: Findings from an Austrian multiple-case study. *Health Promotion International*. doi: 10.1093/heapro/dau018

ASCD, Education International, & International School Health Network. (2013). *Consensus statement on the integration of health & social programs within education systems*. Alexandria, VA: ASCD. www.wholechildeducation.org/about/globalschoolhealthstatement

Atkins, M. S., Rusch, D., Mehta, T. G., & Lakind, D. (2016). Future directions for dissemination and implementation science: Aligning ecological theory and public health to close the research to practice gap. *Journal of Clinical Child & Adolescent Psychology, 45*(2). dx.doi.org/10.1080/15374416.2015.1050724

Brown, J. L. (2008). *Educating the whole child*. Alexandria, VA: Association for Supervision and Curriculum Development (ASCD). www.ascd.org/Publications/Books/Overview/Educating-the-Whole-Child.aspx

Canadian Association for School Health. (2007). *Comprehensive school health: A Canadian consensus statement* (2nd ed.). Surrey, BC: Author.

Council of Ministers of Education, Canada. (n.d.). Education Data & Research Program, Operated in cooperation with the Canadian Education Statistics Council, Toronto, CMEC. cmec.ca/143/Programs-and-Initiatives/Education-Data--Research/Overview/index.html

Deschesnes, M., Couturier, Y., Laberge, S., & Campeau, L. (2010). How divergent conceptions among health and education stakeholders influence the dissemination of healthy schools in Quebec. *Health Promotion International, 25*(4), 435–443.

Deschesnes, M., Martin, C., & Hill, A. J. (2003). Comprehensive approaches to school health promotion: How to achieve broader implementation? *Health Promotion International, 18*(4), 387–396. doi: 10.1093/heapro/dag410

Deschesnes, M., Trudeau, F., & Kebe, M. (2010). Factors influencing the adoption of a Health Promoting School approach in the province of Quebec, Canada. *Health Education Research, 25*(3), 438–450.

Doherty, M., & McCall, D. S. (2004). *Developing a research agenda in school health promotion.* Surrey, BC: School Health Research Network. drive.google.com/file/d/0B76Y7Zl6A-eBS2lUQldmLVU4M1E/view?usp=sharing

Dooris, M. (2006). Health promoting settings: Future directions. *Promotion & Education, 13*(1), 2–4.

Dooris, M., Poland, B., Kolbe, L., de Leeuw, E., McCall, D., & Wharf-Higgins, J. (2007). Healthy settings: Building the evidence for whole system health promotion—Challenges and future directions. In D. McQueen & C. M. Jones (Eds.), *Global perspectives on health promotion effectiveness* (pp. 327–352). New York: Springer.

Fathi, B., Hamid A., Shaghaghi, A., Kousha, A., & Jannati, A. (2014). Challenges in developing health promoting schools' project: Application of global traits in local realm. *Health Promotion Perspectives, 4*(1), 9–17. doi: 10.5681/hpp.2014.002

FRESH. (2012). *Monitoring & evaluating school health programmes.* Paris: UNESCO. www.unesco.org/new/en/education/themes/leading-the-international-agenda/health-education/fresh/me-indicators/

Health Canada. (2004). *First ministers meeting on the future of health care 2004: A 10-year plan to strengthen health care.* Retrieved from www.scics.gc.ca/CMFiles/800042005_e1JXB-342011-6611.pdf

Hussain, A., Christou, G., Reid, M., & Freeman, J. (2013). *Development of the Core Indicators and Measures (CIM) Framework for school health and student achievement in Canada.* Summerside, PE: Pan-Canadian Joint Consortium for School Health (JCSH).

International School Health Network. (2010). *Creating and maintaining schools for all: Addressing determinants, reducing disparities and alleviating disadvantages: An initial identification of priority issues, related strengths and relevant programs for disadvantaged students in high resource countries.* A Consensus Statement adopted by participants in the global school health symposium held in Geneva on July 9–10, 2010. www.schools-for-all.org/page/Linking+Health%2C+Equity+%26+Sustainability+in+Schools+%28July%2C+2010%29

Laitsch, D., Taylor, M., & Rootman, I. (2006). *Systems thinking, capacities and change.* Keynote panel presentation at the 2006 National Invitational Conference and Seminars of the Joint Consortium for School Health, May 25, Vancouver, BC, Canada.

McCall, D. (2006). *An ecological and systems approach to school health promotion.* Surrey, BC: School Health Research Network, Canadian Council on Learning. drive.google.com/file/d/0B76Y7Zl6A-eBVGRBZ0NYLVJ1U2M/view?usp=sharing

McCall, D. S. (2016a). *An analysis of the published research and reports on school-based and school-linked health promotion and social development in or about Canadian students, parents, programs and comprehensive, systems-based approaches.* Surrey, BC: International School Health Network (In Progress).

McCall, D. S. (2016b). *Ecological, systems-based understanding and approaches to school health, safety, equity, social & sustainable development.* Surrey, BC: International School Health Network (In Progress). www.schools-for-all.org/page/Ecological%2C+Systems-based+Understanding+%26+Approaches+to+Schools+%28EE%29

McCall, D. S., Beazley, R., Doherty-Poirier, M., Lavato, C., MacKinnon, D., Otis, J., & Shannon, M. (1999). *Schools, public health, sexuality and HIV: A status report.* Toronto: Council of Ministers of Education, Canada. cmec.ca/9/Publications/index.html?searchCat=37&searchYr=1999

McCall, D. S., Deschesnes, M., & Laitsch, D. (2012). Addressing complexity, capacity and context to support educators: School health promotion in Canada. In I. Rootman, S. Dupéré, A. Pederson, & M. O'Neill (Eds.), *Health promotion in Canada: Critical perspectives on practice* (3rd ed.) (p. 176). Toronto: Canadian Scholars' Press.

McCall, D. S., Lee, A., Beyer, C., Hudson, N., Currie, C., & Berkenow, V. (2009). *Monitoring & reporting systems in promoting health, learning & social development through schools.* Surrey, BC: International School Health Network. www.schools-for-all.org/page/Monitoring+%26+Reporting+Systems+%28HS%29

Organisation for Economic Co-operation and Development (OECD). (2016). *PISA 2015 results (Volume I): Excellence and equity in education.* Paris: OECD Publishing. doi: dx.doi.org/10.1787/9789264266490-en

Palluy, J., Arcand, L., Choinière, C., Martin, C., & Roberge, M. C. (2010). *Réussite éducative, santé et bien-être: Agir efficacement en contexte scolaire. Synthèse de recommandations.* Montréal: Institut national de santé publique du Québec. Retrieved from www.inspq.qc.ca/pdf/publications/1065_ReussiteEducativeSanteBienEtre.pdf

Poland, B., Krupa, G., & McCall, D. S. (2009). Settings for health promotion: An analytic framework to guide intervention design and implementation. *Health Promotion Practice, 10*(4), 505–516.

Roberge, M.-C., & Choinière, C. (2009). *Analyse des interventions de promotion de la santé et de prévention en contexte scolaire québécois: Cohérence avec les meilleures pratiques selon l'approche École en santé.* Montréal: Direction développement des individus et des communautés de l'Institut national de santé publique du Québec. www.inspq.qc.ca/pdf/publications/958_RapAnaPPIntEES.pdf

Saito, J., Keosada, N., Tomokawa, S., Akiyama, T., Kaewviset, S., Nonaka, D., … Jimba, M. (2015). Factors influencing the National School Health Policy implementation in Lao PDR: A multi-level case study. *Health Promotion International, 30*(4), 843–854. dx.doi.org/10.1093/heapro/dau016

St. Leger, L., Kolbe, L., Lee, A., McCall, D. S., & Young, I. M. (2007). School health promotion: Achievements, challenges and priorities. In D. V. McQueen & K. Jones (Eds.), *Perspectives on health promotion effectiveness* (pp. 107–124). Saint Denis: Springer. link.springer.com/chapter/10.1007%2F978-0-387-70974-1_8

Tagalik, S., Corless, G., & McCall, D. S. (2010). *A framework for Indigenous school health: Foundations in cultural principles.* Prince George, BC: National Collaborating Centre for Aboriginal Health. www.nccah-ccnsa.ca/docs/nccah%20reports/NCCAH_CASH_report.pdf.

Tang, K. C., Nutbeam, D., Aldinger, C., St. Leger, L., Bundy, D., Hoffman, A. M., … Heckert, K. (2009). Schools for health, education and development: A call for action. *Health Promotion International, 24*(1), 68–77. doi: 10.1093/heapro/dan037

World Bank. (n.d.). *SABER: Systems approach for better education results.* New York: Author. saber.worldbank.org/index.cfm

World Health Organization (WHO). (1997). *Promoting health through schools.* Report of a WHO Expert Committee on Comprehensive School Health Education and Promotion. Geneva, Switzerland: Author. apps.who.int/iris/bitstream/10665/41987/1/WHO_TRS_870.pdf

World Health Organization (WHO). (2003). *Rapid assessment and action planning process (RAAPP): A method and tools to enable ministries of education and health to assess and strengthen their capacity to promote health through schools.* Geneva: World Health Organization, Department of Non-Communicable Disease Prevention, & Health Promotion Division of Global School Health Initiative.

World Health Organization. (n.d.). *Global school health policies and practices survey.* Presentation to a meeting convened by the SEARO regional office. www.searo.who.int/entity/noncommunicable_diseases/events/global-shpps-overview-slides.pdf

CHAPTER 14

Health Promoting Universities: Shifting from Health Education to Social Innovation[1]

Paola Ardiles, Crystal Hutchinson, Alisa Stanton, Rosie Dhaliwal,
Michelle Aslan, and Tara Black

LEARNING OBJECTIVES

1. Understand the Health Promoting Universities concept
2. Identify promising practices, key barriers and enablers, and methods of measurement in whole-system approaches to health promotion within a Canadian higher education setting
3. Explore how to apply a system approach to health promotion within a Canadian higher education setting

Universities and colleges are in best positions to foster health literate citizens as transformed learners and future leaders, committed and capable of sustaining and growing the health promotion movement

—Fayed, 2016, p. 4

INTRODUCTION

As knowledge and citizen creators, post-secondary institutions hold ample socio-political powers, which can be leveraged to advance the health promotion agenda (Fayed, 2016). The Health Promoting University concept, based on the setting approach, has been well established in many parts of the world, including the development of Health Promoting Universities networks across the United Kingdom, Germany, and Iberoamerica (Tsouros, Dowding, Thompson, & Dooris, 1998; Suarez-Reyes & Van den Broucke, 2015). Much has been theorized in the literature about Health Promoting Universities, emphasizing the importance of systems thinking and of adopting a whole-system perspective (focusing on how the system works as an entire entity) (Newton, Dooris, & Wills, 2016). Although most universities and colleges are working towards similar goals, there is a lack of documentation in terms of how these initiatives have been implemented in the various contexts (Suarez-Reyes & Van den Broucke, 2015).

Canada has played a significant role as a global convener for important international conferences and milestones achieved in this Health Promoting Universities movement. In 2005, the *Edmonton Charter for Health Promoting Universities and Institutions of Higher Education* was developed with international input, articulating principles and goals for higher education to strive towards creating a health promotion culture and a sustainable working, living, and learning environment (Edmonton Charter, 2005). A decade later, an international delegation provided input into the creation of the *Okanagan Charter: An International Charter for Health Promoting Universities and Colleges* in 2015. The *Okanagan Charter* calls on universities and colleges to embed health in all aspects of campus culture, administration, operations, and academic mandates as well as to lead health promotion action more broadly. It provides a framework to guide a whole-systems approach and implementation. Some institutions were already paving the way for system-level change in Canada, including University of British Columbia (UBC) and Simon Fraser University (SFU) in British Columbia, Canada. This chapter will focus on some of these initiatives, as well as the barriers and enablers in terms of implementation of a Health Promoting University settings approach.

FROM HEALTH EDUCATION TO WHOLE-SYSTEMS APPROACHES

There is growing support for addressing the challenges to health and wellbeing in post-secondary settings through a systemic approach (Dooris & Doherty, 2010; Washburn, Teo, Knodel, & Morris, 2013; Keeling, 2014; Okanagan Charter, 2015; Georgetown University, 2011; Simon Fraser University, 2012). Currently, a number of Canadian higher education institutions are working to initiate and advance whole-campus, comprehensive health promotion initiatives. Despite the increasing national momentum, universities and colleges still grapple with how to translate theory into action. The following section will feature promising practices exemplifying how higher education institutions and related organizations are implementing a settings approach. These examples also demonstrate leadership and innovation in health promotion action within a Canadian higher education context.

Making the Case

Higher education institutions grapple with the tension of focusing on specific health topics, disease prevention and management efforts, and promoting health at a systems level. A settings approach requires a paradigm shift in how to design social, organizational, and physical environments that promote health and wellbeing using a whole-campus and whole-person approach. This requires institutions to shift from health education initiatives aimed primarily at individual outcomes, to addressing higher education contexts

themselves (Poland, Krupa, & McCall, 2009). The higher education institutions themselves become the object of inquiry and intervention by embedding health and wellbeing
into their core mandates. As is the case with other health-promoting setting approaches,
alignment between bottom-up action and top-down commitment is critical in effective
implementation of a Health Promoting University approach (Suarez-Reyes & Van den
Broucke, 2015). A recent systematic review of healthy universities around the world identified that a key challenge is convincing academic leadership of the responsibility institutions
have to promote health, particularly when their core mandates are education and research
(Suarez-Reyes & Van den Broucke, 2015). This is no different in the Canadian context,
especially since there is limited data to make the case on the connection between student
health and learning outcomes in higher education.

Canadian institutions started to take notice of the results from the National College
Health Assessment (NCHA) 2008 survey, revealing that isolation, stress, depression,
and anxiety were significantly impacting post-secondary students in the US and Canada
(American College Health Association [ACHA], 2008). In 2013, a Canadian cohort of
colleges and universities participated in the NCHA survey and results indicated that stress
was the most common barrier to academic achievement; more than 57 percent of students
reported above-average levels of stress related to academics, finances, and sleep problems (ACHA, 2013). The results from this survey resulted in mental health becoming a
priority issue for post-secondary institutions in Canada. The data enabled a broad group
of stakeholders across campuses to seriously consider taking collective action on mental
health. In 2016, a Canadian cohort again participated in the NCHA survey, obtaining
data from 43,000 students at 41 Canadian institutions (ACHA, 2016). Results indicated
that mental health continues to be a concern, and in fact, results are generally worse than
in 2013, with 13 percent of respondents having seriously considered suicide, 67 percent
feeling very lonely, 44 percent feeling so depressed that it was difficult to function, and 65
percent feeling overwhelming anxiety within the last 12 months (ACHA, 2016). Stress
(42%), anxiety (33%) and depression (20%) continue to have considerable negative impacts
on academic achievement (ACHA, 2016). Interestingly, growing concern related to mental
health problems served as a catalyst for many Canadian institutions to look for innovative
ways to address concerns related to student health and wellbeing.

In 2012, the University of British Columbia in Vancouver demonstrated leadership in
this area and released a *Mental Health and Wellbeing Strategy*, a new service delivery model
that connected mental health and wellbeing to learning and academic success for students.
The model identified various objectives across the continuum of care, from promotion,
prevention, and early identification to case management and treatment (UBC, 2012). Some
of the goals outlined included the expansion of educational opportunities outside the classroom (e.g., community service learning, co-op placements, and international practicums)
and personal development goals to support students' wellbeing. This strategy provided a
holistic perspective of health and was critical in moving UBC towards thinking about the
system, beyond clinical health services.

At a provincial level, Healthy Minds Healthy Campuses has been an important initiative of the Canadian Mental Health Association (CMHA), BC Division and the Centre for Addictions Research of British Columbia (CARBC) to implement a community of practice approach in mental health and substance use at the campus level. They have provided a platform where diverse stakeholders across various colleges and universities can share knowledge, exchange new ideas, and obtain technical skill development in order to facilitate self-management, early detection and prevention of mental health and substance use issues, as well as the promotion of mental health using a determinants of health approach. In 2013, the Canadian Association for College and University Student Services and the Canadian Mental Health Association collaborated on the *Post-Secondary Student Mental Health: A Guide to a Systemic Approach* (Washburn, Teo, Knodel, & Morris, 2013). This drew attention to the importance of a broad approach to address the issue of campus mental health.

One of the most significant areas of social determinants of mental health and substance use identified by this community of practice is the very nature of higher educational settings, built upon traditions, expectations, and assumptions that create a toxic culture (Personal Communication, 2016).[2] Hierarchical and bureaucratic systems affect staff/faculty relations and ultimately have an impact on the whole campus. The "publish or perish" competitive environments extend well beyond faculty, into the classroom. Academic institutions are faced with competing priorities, financial cutbacks, and an increasingly corporate culture aimed at attracting "the best" and producing "the best" students. They are accountable for "producing" the innovators and future leaders able to solve society's toughest challenges such as climate change, growing disparities between rich and poor, technological shifts, and political and economic instability worldwide. Yet, until the *Okanagan Charter* there was little support at the top executive levels for a whole-systems approach to promote health and wellbeing as a key enabler of academic success (Personal Communication, 2016).

In 2010, Simon Fraser University's (SFU) Health Promotion unit was prompted to adopt a systemic approach to health promotion and developed the Healthy Campus Community Framework based on literature and best practices from workplace and school settings (Simon Fraser University, 2015a). The framework shown in figure 14.1 highlights six Action Areas.

The main focus of the SFU Healthy Campus Community initiative is to create an environment that enhances staff, faculty, and student wellbeing through policies, practices, spaces, teaching, and programs, and specific projects have been developed to facilitate action. SFU's Health Promotion unit was able to engage faculty members and the Teaching and Learning Centre to support the implementation of the Well-being in Learning Environments project, to support a positive classroom culture and teaching practices that create conditions for wellbeing (Stanton, Zandvliet, Black, & Dhaliwal, 2016). This project has resulted in new research studies providing insight into the students' lived experiences of wellbeing in learning environments (Stanton et al., 2016). Findings from some of this work reveal that experiences of social connection, flexibility, and learning for a purpose (outside of obtaining a grade) may contribute to greater engagement, deeper learning, happiness, and satisfaction (Stanton et al., 2016).

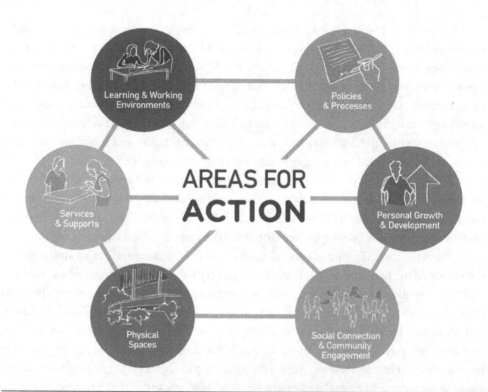

Figure 14.1: SFU Healthy Campus Community Areas for Action, 2013

Source: Simon Fraser University Health Promotion Unit . (2015). Areas of action. In *Simon Fraser University's vision for a healthy campus community.* Burnaby: Simon Fraser University Health Promotion Unit.

Creating Conditions for Wellbeing in Higher Education Learning Environments

Health and wellbeing are widely considered important elements for effective learning (Caulfield, 2007; El Ansari & Stock, 2010; Stanton et al., 2016); however, there is increasing evidence that Canadian post-secondary students are not experiencing optimal mental health (American College Health Association, 2016). Learning experiences can have either a positive or a negative impact on health and wellbeing (Hammond, 2004; Stanton et al., 2016), and there is an opportunity to contribute to student wellbeing through the design and delivery of learning experiences. Evidence from elementary, secondary schools, and higher education settings note that classroom culture, course design, curriculum, assessment, assignments, and instructors themselves may all have the ability to impact student wellbeing (Adriansen & Madsen, 2013; Byrd & McKinney, 2012; Cohen, 2006; Fink, 2014; Seligman, Ernst, Gillham, Reivich, & Linkins, 2009). Traditionally, challenges to personal wellbeing "have been addressed in residential halls, campus clinics, and counselling centers—everywhere but the classroom" (Georgetown University, 2011, p. 3). Learning environments are an essential setting for creating supportive environments in post-secondary institutions as they have a profound impact on students' personal experiences. A letter to the editor of the *New York Times* states, "As a student who has suffered from depression and anxiety as a result of the crippling race towards academic "achievement," I find it disheartening that academic success continuously trumps learning—which is about experience, not perfection" (as cited in Gitlin, 2016, p. 87).

Across Canada, efforts are underway to enhance post-secondary learning environments in order to better support student wellbeing. At Simon Fraser University (SFU), Well-being in Learning Environments is a partnership project that started in 2012 between Health Promotion and the Teaching and Learning Centre (TLC). This innovative project involves working with instructional staff to create conditions for wellbeing within learning environments. These conditions, based on a literature review and feedback from students, faculty, staff, and partners at SFU include the following:

- Social connection
- Inclusivity
- Real-life learning
- Optimal challenge
- Flexibility
- Instructor support
- Services and supports
- Positive classroom culture
- Civic engagement
- Personal development

An interactive website, available for others to use and adapt, offers examples of teaching practices and resources that faculty members can use to create these conditions, whether it be through course design, delivery, or assessment (SFU, 2014). To date more than 100 campus members have been engaged in the award-winning project. A complementary research project has explored students' experiences of wellbeing in the learning environment and highlighted learning experiences that promote connection, flexibility, and learning for purpose as significant (Stanton et al., 2016). Similar projects are being developed at other Canadian institutions (Camosun College, 2016; George Brown College, 2016; University of British Columbia, 2016a) and together these projects provide a timely and important opportunity to design and deliver learning experiences in ways that enhance student wellbeing.

Application of the Optimal Learning Environment Tool to Enhance Students' Wellbeing in a University Setting

SFU's Well-being in Learning Environments project has inspired several initiatives, including the development of the Optimal Learning Environment tool (Aslan, 2016) aimed to foster a culture of wellbeing in the classroom. This tool takes into consideration the student experience within the learning environment and each student's unique learning style. It is designed to support empowerment in the classroom and capture assessments by both the instructor and the learners. Students assess their own knowledge, and grade themselves on class participation while providing the instructor important feedback on their class experience. The tool consists of specific learning activities that build student skills one step at a time, building on existing strengths, reinforcing competency layer by layer with a sophisticated understanding of the relevance of the subject, and finally leading to a full utilization of the knowledge in their own lives. The learning activities are specifically designed to support the process of the unfolding lesson plan and curriculum in a conscious and focused manner to enhance learning and students' wellbeing. The self-evaluation component in the tool allows students to monitor their own progress and be proactive in evaluating their learning activities. The Optimal Learning Environment tool allows educators to create personalized learning experiences for their students, and the different learning activities address the students' unique learning styles. This tool is an instructional resource for educators in helping them enhance their students' strengths rather than focusing on their weaknesses.

The Optimal Learning Environment tool was implemented in a 2016 graduate course at the Faculty of Health Sciences, at Simon Fraser University. Ninety-eight percent of the students rated the Optimal Learning Environment tool as a 6 (with 6 being the highest score and 1 being the lowest score). The feedback that was captured by students clearly indicated that the learning activities, physical energizers, weekly feedback, critical reflection, self-grading, and self-evaluation reduced their anxiety, created a safe learning environment, enhanced their learning, and played a vital role in their physical wellbeing.

If the goal as educators is for students to flourish and succeed, then wellbeing must be incorporated in their everyday learning. Addressing mental health proactively by emphasizing wellbeing within the curriculum enables educators to introduce available resources and supports early on for individuals facing mental health challenges. It also gives students the opportunity to seek support through individual counselling, mentorship programs, and peer support groups. The Optimal Learning Environment tool enables educators to revise and reform the curriculum to reflect wellbeing in the classroom and adapt to reflect the current needs of the students.

Wellbeing through Physical Spaces

There is an increasing body of research that demonstrates linkages between built environments and health status. In recent years, building design in health care, the corporate sector, and education have intentionally included enhancements in order to create a built environment that promotes health. Physical space features directly impact psychosocial, mental, and physical health. A poorly designed space can result in distracted behaviour, irritability, physical discomfort, increased stress levels, and increased blood pressure. In contrast, well-designed spaces have the ability to positively impact mood, creativity, social connectedness, and learning. In a post-secondary setting, a supportive physical space is important for fostering student wellbeing and success overall. As a result, physical environments within higher education settings present a strategic opportunity to impact student learning and wellbeing.

SFU's focus on wellbeing through physical spaces is innovative within the Canadian higher education context. Developed prior to the release of the WELL Building Standard (Delos Living LLC, 2014), the Wellbeing through Physical Spaces project aims to enhance psychosocial wellbeing through the design of built environments. The project aligns with the *WELL Building Standard* (Delos Living LLC, 2014) and with the *Okanagan Charter for Health Promoting Universities and Colleges* (2015), which identifies creating supportive campus environments and working cross-departmentally to enhance student wellbeing.

The Wellbeing through Physical Spaces project was developed in 2013. A literature review process indicated the quality of physical learning environments has a significant and measurable impact on student achievement, productivity, satisfaction, and wellbeing (Earthman, 2002; Hill & Epps, 2010; Lippman, 2010; Brooks, 2010; Young, Green, Roehrich-Patrick, Joseph, & Gibson, 2003; Schweitzer, Gilpin, & Frampton, 2004; Strange & Banning, 2001). Data were collected and analyzed from focus groups and existing undergraduate student surveys in order to examine students' perceptions of physical spaces on campus in relation to their wellbeing. The SFU Health Promotion Unit identified seven features—air quality, lighting, furniture, temperature, nature, art and colour, and opportunities for social connection and inclusivity—as key considerations when designing health-promoting spaces. Momentum for this work was built through the development of strategic partnerships with relevant campus stakeholders including Campus Development and Planning and the Simon Fraser Student Society. Subsequently, support was provided to campus partners in considering and incorporating the above-mentioned features through SFU Health Promotion's input and recommendations related to design plans.

Another noteworthy aspect of this project is that it uses a human-centred design approach. SFU Health Promotion actively facilitates the ongoing engagement of space users by collecting feedback to inform space design projects at SFU to ensure community needs are being met. Approximately 500 students' feedback has shaped design decisions and has informed more than 15 campus spaces including classrooms, lounges, and lecture theatres. Wellbeing was also an important consideration in the design of SFU's first student union building. The success of new spaces within higher education settings is not just dependent on resources, stakeholder support, and design expertise, but also the involvement of space users, namely students. In order to ensure that newly created or renovated campus spaces meet the needs of the community, the participation of community members in the design process is necessary (Strange & Banning, 2001). A clear understanding of the input and interplay between campus design and campus community members is necessary for the implementation of effective and supportive learning spaces that physically and socially contribute to the wellbeing of all.

Beyond the Classroom: Students as Agents for Health Promotion Change

The *Okanagan Charter for Health Promoting Universities and Colleges* calls on institutions to partner on and off campus in order to lead action for health promotion locally and globally (*Okanagan Charter*, 2015). In building community partnerships that extend beyond the immediate campus context, institutions must create opportunities for civic engagement and the development of future citizens "with the capacity to act as agents for health promoting change beyond campuses" (*Okanagan Charter*, 2015).

In the fall of 2016, 30 undergraduate students from Simon Fraser University took part in the Health Change Lab, an experimental course based in Surrey and developed by the Faculty of Health Sciences and RADIUS Social Innovation Laboratory of the Beedie School of Business. The Health Change Lab is designed so that students can develop innovative and entrepreneurial solutions to complex health problems in the community. The City of Surrey, one of the most diverse and fastest-growing cities in Canada, faces growing and complex social and health challenges, such as increasing prevalence of chronic diseases, food insecurity, social exclusion, and an aging population.

This social innovation course in health was based on interdisciplinary team projects and provided students an opportunity for experiential learning, design thinking, community engagement, and application of systems thinking to address particular health issues in a community setting. As part of their engagement with the Surrey community, students were tasked with finding potential solutions for some key community health issues, while learning from and being mentored by staff from the City of Surrey, Fraser Health Authority, SFU Surrey Campus, and various community partners. Students spent one day a week in Surrey, conceiving ideas and creating projects designed to impact health and wellbeing in the community. This 30-student cohort actively engaged in learning about applying health promotion values and principles in conjunction with social entrepreneurship skills. Seven interdisciplinary teams tackled issues in Surrey such as food security, refugee resettlement, mental health and substance use, cultural safety, and active transportation by taking a wide view that focused on root causes rather than symptoms. Students embarked on a "deep dive" into prototyping and tested their early stage ideas, giving demos and making presentations along the way. SFU's Health Change Lab highlights how innovative educational programs in health promotion can impact community health through the design of interdisciplinary team approaches that are solution-focused and promote civic action and social innovation outside the classroom and in the surrounding community.

ENABLERS AND BARRIERS OF WHOLE-SYSTEM APPROACHES

While specific examples of health promotion action within higher education may vary, the promising practices featured above illustrate growing national momentum in enacting whole-system approaches. The *Okanagan Charter* was developed in order to guide and inspire action by providing a framework that higher education institutions can draw upon, founded in current concepts, processes, and principles relating to health-promoting universities. Using a settings and whole-systems approach is a fundamental principle outlined in the Charter, and can be operationalized through a set of key action areas outlined.

Although the *Okanagan Charter* has the potential to be a key enabler, building action for health-promoting universities in the Canadian context has not been a coordinated, national effort as it has in other parts of the world where there are strong networks, as previously mentioned. However, a new Canadian Health Promoting Universities Network Committee was established in 2016 and has generated interest and momentum for the *Okanagan Charter*, with six university and college presidents having formally adopted the Charter and committed to specific actions within their campuses. The hope is that with a national committee and intentional focus on activating the *Okanagan Charter*, sharing knowledge, and building a network, efforts for enhancing higher education settings will advance within Canada. A new International Health Promoting Universities Working Group has also been established with the purpose of inspiring and catalyzing further action towards the creation of health-promoting universities and colleges at an international level.

Not surprisingly, key enablers of this whole-campus approach in BC include both grassroots support from students and staff, leadership from the top, and faculty champions using research approaches that have added legitimacy to this work within academic institutions. Moreover, both SFU and UBC have had dedicated staff and resources (both internal and external funding) to sustain health-promoting efforts over the years, and continue building momentum. Because of the complex nature of systems and culture change, positioning of health promotion efforts within higher education is important. Traditionally, Health Promotion units and health educators have been situated within Student Services, for which students are the mandate. UBC has implemented a new model whereby efforts within Student Services continue, with a focus on student wellbeing, but a new position reporting to a number of vice-presidents has been added in order to focus on systemic action.

Participatory Approaches and Engagement

One of the key principles and enablers of the Health Promoting Universities approach is the use of participatory approaches (see chapter 21). For decades, the University of British Columbia (UBC) Okanagan has used a community-based participatory action model to generate interest, research, and action across campus and stakeholders. Every year they conduct surveys and community dialogues to better understand the needs and priorities of the diverse stakeholders, which include students, faculty, staff, student services, facilities, health and safety, landscapers, chefs, and business administrators. Using an asset-based approach they create opportunities for everyone to have a voice and get involved in various campus-wide working groups tackling issues like sexual assault, mental health, smoking, and cafeteria food. More than 150 students participate every year in this work and obtain course credit and/or research opportunities (Personal Communication, 2016).

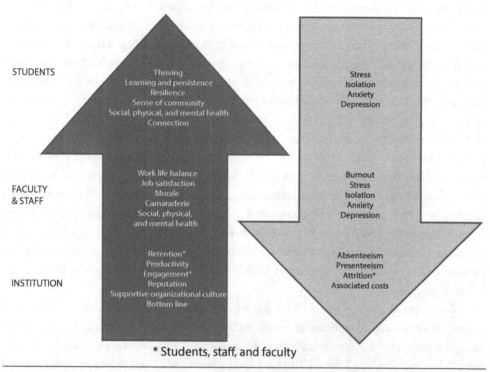

STUDENTS

Thriving
Learning and persistence
Resilience
Sense of community
Social, physical, and mental health
Connection

Stress
Isolation
Anxiety
Depression

FACULTY
& STAFF

Work life balance
Job satisfaction
Morale
Camaraderie
Social, physical,
and mental health

Burnout
Stress
Isolation
Anxiety
Depression

INSTITUTION

Retention*
Productivity
Engagement*
Reputation
Supportive organizational culture
Bottom line

Absenteeism
Presenteeism
Attrition*
Associated costs

* Students, staff, and faculty

Figure 14.2: Individual and Institutional Benefits of Enhancing Wellbeing, 2015

Source: Adapted from Simon Fraser University Health Promotion Unit. (2015). Appendix A: Individual and institutional benefits of enhancing well-being. In *Simon Fraser University's vision for a healthy campus community.* Burnaby: Simon Fraser University Health Promotion Unit.

In an academic institution it is vital to engage staff, faculty, and students in creating a supportive and healthy campus community. One of the core values of the Health Promotion unit at Simon Fraser University is to engage and empower students and other stakeholders to participate in the healthy campus initiative. The students play a crucial role in shaping and implementing the initiative through collecting student feedback and engaging the student community in ongoing dialogue around wellbeing. SFU students are encouraged to be a part of the health advisory committee or become peer health educators. The health and wellbeing champions at SFU work tirelessly to create community engagement and social connections through dialogue. Campus stakeholders who exemplify systemic action are recognized annually through SFU's Champions for a Healthy Campus Community award.

One of the main challenges of applying a systems or whole-campus approach has been to incorporate staff and faculty health and wellbeing initiatives, in part because student learning outcomes are the primary focus of higher educational institutions. Yet, a whole-campus approach necessarily involves all stakeholders, as there are benefits and consequences for staff, faculty, and students as shown in figure 14.2.

MEASUREMENT AND MONITORING

Universities and colleges understand that investing in the health and wellbeing of students enhances academic performance, yet the evidence base is only beginning to emerge in Canada. Monitoring and evaluation is key in order to make the social and economic case to effectively implement this work across campus. Yet there are significant challenges in building the evidence base in these settings, as students are on a four-year cycle (or less) and students start to graduate and leave while new ones enter the system. As in most health promoting settings, monitoring and evaluating system-level change is very challenging as it involves various stakeholders (administration, facilities, academic departments, health providers, student services, etc.) operating at various levels of the system, who do not necessarily interact on a regular basis. Moreover, they have very distinct, siloed organizational cultures (e.g., academic departments function as their own mini-organizations) that often are removed from the classroom itself (e.g., administrative and operational staff). In these scenarios with such diverse interests and complex cultures and expectations, it is very difficult to track changes and develop population-level outcomes that can be tied back to impact measurement systems.

These challenges outlined above may be mitigated with the release of the *Okanagan Charter* in 2015, as there is growing interest from key academic and administrative leaders to participate and collaborate in whole-campus approaches to promote health and wellbeing across Canadian institutions. Such is the case at the University of British Columbia, which recently established the Wellbeing at UBC initiative in 2015 across both campuses (Vancouver and Okanagan) to better connect health promotion with the sustainability agenda in order to gain more support across the university. This whole-campus initiative views the university as a living lab, a setting where one can test new solutions on designing the social, natural, and built environments (UBC, 2016b). Students are able to work on sustainability projects with researchers across a wide range of disciplines. One of the most important enablers of this initiative is senior leadership at the executive academic level and an investment in core staff to ensure this is embedded in all areas of governance, teaching, and administration (Personal Communication, 2016).

CONCLUSION

The vision outlined in the *Okanagan Charter* is for health-promoting universities and colleges to be an integral part of the transformation of the "health and sustainability of our current and future societies, strengthen communities and contribute to the well-being of people, places and the planet" (*Okanagan Charter*, 2015). The examples provided in this chapter point to a growing body of theoretical and practical evidence of the use of the *Okanagan Charter* principles for implementation, such as using settings and participatory approaches to engage students and others.

In the next decade, Canadian institutions have an opportunity to build an evidence base and focus on some key principles of implementation not yet fully realized, such as (1) valuing local and Indigenous communities' contexts and priorities; (2) developing trans-disciplinary collaborations and cross-sector partnerships; and (3) ensuring health promotion action embodies principles of social justice, equity, dignity, and respect for diversity while recognizing the interconnectedness between people's health and health determinants, including social and economic systems and global ecological change (*Okanagan Charter*, 2015). There is also opportunity to enhance the role of higher education institutions to lead health promotion action and collaboration locally and globally as emphasized in the *Okanagan Charter*. Recently, a student leader noted that "by promoting intra and inter-campus collaborations, the Okanagan Charter builds a shared vision for health within campus communities as well as the larger society and globe. This not only creates an internal equilibrium, but also cultivates a strong collective political impact to propel the health promotion movement further" (Fayed, 2016, p. 4).

The *Okanagan Charter for Health Promoting Universities and Colleges* has the potential to galvanize support for a health promotion agenda that capitalizes on the mutual benefits between health and education, to create a sustainable infrastructure for strengthening, creating, and mobilizing socio-political capital (Fayed, 2016). Yet it is important to recognize that social innovation requires leadership and creativity in order to break down power structures and shift the knowledge base towards sustained change over time. As such, it will be critical for staff and faculty at post-secondary institutions to lead by example, support, and make way for the leadership development of students to act as change agents for health promotion action within and beyond the walls of universities and colleges.

CRITICAL THINKING QUESTIONS

1. What are some of the key elements of a systems approach to wellbeing in the university campus setting?
2. What are some of the key enablers and barriers in implementing a systems approach in this setting?
3. Give some examples of what your campus has done to promote health and wellbeing for (a) students, (b) staff, and (c) faculty. Identify areas for improvement.
4. In what ways do you see the *Okanagan Charter* being an important contribution to implementing this vision in your own post-secondary environment?
5. How can you support the implementation of the *Okanagan Charter* in your current role (as student, staff, faculty, or community member)?

RESOURCES

Further Readings

Cawood, J., Dooris, M., & Powell, S. (2010). Healthy Universities: Shaping the future. *Perspectives in Public Health, 130*(6), 259–260.
This article outlines the potential for universities and colleges to further advance the Healthy Universities movement through ecological and whole systems action.

Harward, D. (2016). *Well-being and higher education. A Strategy for change and the revitalization of education's greater purpose.* Washington, DC: Bringing Theory to Practice.
This book provides a series of essays exploring the interconnections between wellbeing, deep learning, and the core purposes of higher education.

Keeling, R. (2014). An ethic of care in higher education: Well-being and learning. *Journal of College & Character, 15*(3), 141–148.
This article outlines the importance of working collaboratively to create an ethic of care within higher education institutions. The benefits to students and institutional outcomes are discussed.

Stanton, A., Zandvliet, D., Black, T., & Dhaliwal, R. (2016). Understanding students' experiences of wellbeing in learning environments. *Higher Education Studies, 6*(3), 90–99.
This article provides a qualitative exploration of students' lived experiences of wellbeing in learning environments and identifies three pathways through which learning experiences can influence student wellbeing. Specific examples of how teaching practices can support wellbeing are shared.

Relevant Websites

Canadian Health Promoting Universities and Colleges Network
www.healthpromotingcampuses.ca
   Through this website, higher education professionals, students, and external partners can become part of a Canadian Network on Health Promoting Universities and Colleges.

Canadian Mental Health Association (CMHA) BC Division and the Centre for Addiction Research of BC
healthycampuses.ca
   This initiative serves to bring a wide range of stakeholders from across British Columbia together to advance collective action on campus mental health and substance

use. The website serves as a platform to engage the Healthy Minds Healthy Campus community around various projects, learning events, online resources, and reports.

The WELL Building Standard
www.wellcertified.com/well

The WELL Building Standard provides evidence-based approaches and best practice guidelines for designing buildings that support holistic health and wellbeing.

Healthy Universities—A National Toolkit
www.healthyuniversities.ac.uk/

Developed by the Healthy Universities National Network in the United Kingdom, this website provides a self-review tool for higher education institutions interested in adopting Healthy University work. Guidance packages that support project development are shared, along with links to relevant publications.

Okanagan Charter: An International Charter for Health Promoting Universities and Colleges
internationalhealthycampuses2015.sites.olt.ubc.ca/files/2016/01/Okanagan-Charter-January13v2.pdf

The *Okanagan Charter* was a product of the 2015 International Conference on Health Promoting Universities and Colleges/VII International Congress. It outlines a transformative vision for health promoting universities and colleges and provides an action framework that includes both specific calls to action and key principles.

NOTES

1. A special recognition and thank you for all the thoughtful contributions from Monica Suarez-Reyes, Doug McCall, Johnny Morris from the Canadian Mental Health Association, and our colleagues at the University of British Columbia, including Melissa Feddersen, Patty Hambler, Matt Dolf, and Cheryl Washburn. This book chapter is dedicated to the memory of Claire Budgen PhD RN, a colleague and friend we lost in January 2017 when we were finalizing this chapter. Claire was an inspirational leader to many including the authors, for her foundational work at the University of British Columbia–Okanagan in promoting the healthy universities movement. Her work had impact at a local and global level and she leaves the legacy of the *Okanagan Charter for Health Promoting Universities and Colleges* for us to continue.

2. Personal Communication (2016) cited in text relates to information gathered from key informant interviews in 2016 as part of the research for this book chapter. The key informants were selected experts from the academic and NGO sector who were active in the healthy universities movement in British Columbia but their names are not disclosed for confidentiality purposes.

REFERENCES

Adriansen, H. K., & Madsen, L. M. (2013). Facilitation: A novel way to improve student well-being. *Innovative Higher Education, 38*(4), 295–308.

American College Health Association (ACHA). (2008). *American College Health Association National College Health Assessment Spring 2007 Reference Group Data Report* (Abridged). Linthicum: Author.

American College Health Association (ACHA). (2013). *National College Health Assessment II: Canadian Reference Group Report Spring 2013.* Linthicum: Author.

American College Health Association (ACHA). (2016). *National College Health Assessment IIb: Canadian Reference Group Report Fall 2016.* Linthicum: Author.

Aslan, M. (2016). *Optimal learning environment tool.* Unpublished Manuscript. Simon Fraser University.

Brooks, D. C. (2010). Space matters: The impact of formal learning environments on student learning. *British Journal of Educational Technology, 42*(5), 719–726.

Byrd, D., & McKinney, K. (2012). Individual, interpersonal and institutional level factors associated with the mental health of college students. *Journal of American College Health, 60*(3), 185–192.

Camosun College. (2016). *Student mental health and well-being strategy.* Retrieved from camosun.ca/about/mental-health/documents/MentalHealthStrategyBooklet.pdf

Caulfield, S. (2007). Student health: Supporting the academic mission. Student Health Spectrum, 3–24. The Chickering Group.

Cohen, J. (2006). Social, emotional, ethical and academic education: Creating a climate for learning, participation in democracy and well-being. *Harvard Educational Review, 76*(2), 201–237.

Delos Living LLC. (2014). *The WELL Building Standard* (1.0). New York: Delos Living LLC.

Dooris, M., & Doherty, S. (2010). Healthy universities: Current activities and future directions: Findings and reflections from a national level qualitative research study. *Global Health Promotion, 17*(3), 6–16.

Earthman, G. I. (2002). *School facility conditions and student academic achievement.* Los Angeles: UCLA's Institute for Democracy, Education and Access (IDEA).

Edmonton Charter for Health Promoting Universities and Institutions of Higher Education. (2005).

El Ansari, W., & Stock, C. (2010). Is the health and wellbeing of university students associated with their academic performance? Cross sectional findings from the United Kingdom. *International Journal of Environmental Research and Public Health, 7,* 509–527.

Fayed, S. (2016). *Reflections on health promotion.* Unpublished. Simon Fraser University.

Fink, J. (2014). Flourishing: Exploring predictors of mental health within the college environment. *Journal of American College Health, 62*(6), 380–388.

George Brown College. (2016). *Staff & faculty shaping a healthy campus.* Retrieved from www.georgebrown.ca/healthycampus/staff/

Georgetown University. (2011). *Englehard project overview.* Retrieved from cndls.georgetown.edu/engelhard/join/

Gitlin, T. (2016). Education for well-being. In D. Harward (Ed.), *Well-being and higher education: A Strategy for change and the revitalization of education's greater purpose* (pp. 87–90). Washington, DC: Bringing Theory to Practice.

Hammond, C. (2004). Impacts of lifelong learning upon emotional resilience, psychological and mental health: Fieldwork evidence. *Oxford Review of Education, 30*(4), 551–568.

Hill, M. C., & Epps, K.K. (2010). The impact of physical classroom environment on student satisfaction and student evaluation of teaching in the university environment. *Academy of Educational Leadership Journal, 14*(4), 65–79.

Keeling, R. (2014). An ethic of care in higher education: Well-being and learning. *Journal of College & Character, 15*(3), 141–148.

Lippman, P. C. (2010). Can the physical environment have an impact on the learning environment? *Centre for Effective Learning Environments Exchange, 13*, 1–6.

Newton, J., Dooris, M. T., & Wills, J. (2016). Healthy universities: An example of a whole-system health-promoting setting. *Global Health Promotion, 23*(1), 57–65.

Okanagan Charter: An International Charter for Health Promoting Universities and Colleges. (2015). Retrieved from internationalhealthycampuses2015.sites.olt.ubc.ca/files/2015/10/Okanagan_Charter_Oct_6_2015.pdf

Poland, B., Krupa, G., & McCall, D. (2009). Settings for health promotion: An analytic framework to guide intervention design and implementation. *Health Promotion Practice, 10*(4), 505–516.

Schweitzer, M., Gilpin, L., & Frampton, S. (2004). Healing spaces: Elements of environmental design that make an impact on health. *The Journal of Alternative and Complementary Medicine, 10*(1), 71–83.

Seligman, M. E. P., Ernst, R. M., Gillham, J., Reivich, K., & Linkins, M. (2009). Positive education: Positive psychology and classroom interventions. *Oxford Review of Education, 35*(3), 293–311.

Simon Fraser University. (2012). *Rationale and background on SFU's Healthy Campus Community Initiative.* Retrieved from www.sfu.ca/healthycampuscommunity/abouthcc.html

Simon Fraser University (SFU). (2014). *Well-being in learning environments.* Retrieved from www.sfu.ca/healthycampuscommunity/learningenvironments/WLE.html

Simon Fraser University (SFU). (2015a). *Rationale for embedding conditions for well-being in academic settings.* Retrieved from www.sfu.ca/healthycampuscommunity/academic-settings

Simon Fraser University (SFU). (2015b). *Simon Fraser University's vision for a healthy campus community.* Retrieved from www.sfu.ca/healthycampuscommunity/vision.html

Stanton, A., Zandvliet, D., Black, T., & Dhaliwal, R. (2016). Understanding students' experiences of well-being in learning environments. *Higher Education Studies, 6*(3), 90–99.

Strange, C. C., & Banning, J. H. (2001). *Educating by design: Creating campus learning environments that work.* San Francisco: Jossey-Bass.

Suarez-Reyes, M., & Van den Broucke, S. (2015). Implementing the Health Promoting University approach in culturally different contexts: A systematic review. *Global Health Promotion, 23*(1), 46–56.

Tsouros, A. D., Dowding, G., Thompson, J., & Dooris, M. (1998). *Health promoting universities: Concept, experience and framework for action.* Retrieved from www.euro.who.int/__data/assets/pdf_file/0012/101640/E60163.pdf

University of British Columbia (UBC). (2012). *Mental health and wellbeing strategy.* Working document Student Development and Services, University of British Columbia, Vancouver.

University of British Columbia (UBC). (2016a). *First year wellness in the classroom project.* Retrieved from blogs.ubc.ca/firstyearwellness/

University of British Columbia (UBC). (2016b). *Well-being at UBC.* Retrieved from www.wellbeing.ubc.ca

Washburn, C., Teo, S., Knodel, R., and Morris, J. (2013). *Post-secondary student mental health: A guide to a systemic approach.* Vancouver: Canadian Association of Colleges and University Student Services (CACUSS) & The Canadian Mental Health Association (CMHA).

Young, E., Green, H. A., Roehrich-Patrick, L., Joseph, L., & Gibson, T. (2003). *Do K-12 school facilities affect education outcomes?* Nashville, TN: Tennessee Advisory Commission on Intergovernmental Relations.

CHAPTER 15

Health Promotion in Clinical Care

Katherine Bertoni and Geneviève Dubé

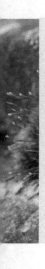

LEARNING OBJECTIVES

1. Understand the role of social determinants of health within health promotion practice
2. Identify how the social determinants of health can be addressed at the patient, practice, and community levels
3. Identify the relationship between health literacy and health promotion practice
4. Understand the role of family theory and family-centred care when implementing health promotion into practice
5. Reflect upon integrating health promotion into practice when transitioning from student to practitioner

INTRODUCTION

When writing this chapter, the question of whether or not the practice of health promotion in the clinical setting needed improvement was posed. The answer to this question is that there is always room for improvement. As the landscape of health care changes, so must our practice, to meet the needs of our patients, families, and communities. Students in practice are often telling me to provide examples that can help them visualize and understand the concepts of health promotion more concretely. This chapter was written to address health promotion in the clinical setting for health professionals who promote optimal health in their practice in Canada.

Rootman, Dupéré, Pederson, and O'Neill (2012) define *health promotion* as the "planned change of health-related lifestyles and life conditions through a variety of individual and environmental strategies" (p. 23). Individual strategies may include taking daily walks for 20 minutes, eating more vegetables and less red meat, or quitting smoking. Environmental strategies may include building healthy public policy, developing community partnerships, and creating a supportive environment for change. These are all fundamental to good health. Those involved in many different aspects of health care provision, including medicine, nursing, and allied health, can also define the term *health promotion* and apply it to their clinical practice. Asking individual questions, offering care specific to the patient's individual or family needs, or referring to/consulting with the appropriate resources, are all examples of how to do this. This alludes to identifying and addressing the economic and social conditions that shape the health of individuals and their communities, otherwise known as the social determinants of health (Raphael, 2016). Primary prevention measures such as immunizations can be implemented to help reduce the incidence of disease, and bicycle or helmet safety help to prevent injury. Disease progression can be controlled through preventive health screening measures, modifying risk factors, and altering lifestyle behaviours or environmental factors. Politi, Wolin, & Legare (2013) suggest that clinicians use shared decision-making when engaging patients in promoting health through these examples. This entails collaborating with patients when making health care treatment decisions and engaging them in conversation. Promoting health behaviours and empowering patients to actively participate in their health care choices can lead to improved psychological, developmental, and behavioural outcomes, and thus a healthier social environment (Ryan & Deci, 2000; Deci & Ryan, 2008). In an attempt to take control of and manage one's own health, an individual must be health literate (Rootman & Gordon-El-Bihbety, 2008). In this chapter, we will explore and discuss the relationship between the social determinants of health and health literacy, and health promotion in a clinical setting. We will also provide suggestions on how to implement health promotion in practice using family theory and family-centred care. Finally, we will contextualize health promotion as an essential component of clinical practice, including the perspective of a student, explore related trends and issues, and offer advice for the future.

One of the ways to provide health promotion is to educate individuals about what is considered "healthy" behaviour. Whitehead (2004) defines *health education* as actions that inform the individual on the nature and cause of health and illness and their own level of risk associated with their lifestyle behaviour; it also attempts to motivate individuals to accept a process of behavioural changes by influencing their values, beliefs, and attitude systems (p. 313). It is necessary, however, to move beyond the primary level of health education toward the broader concept of health promotion. Through the practice of health promotion, clinicians are not only providing health education, but also enabling patients to "increase control over their own health" (WHO, 2016a, para. 1). This requires more involvement in legislative reform at both the municipal and federal levels; advocating for disadvantaged individuals, particularly for those with low levels of health literacy or who cannot petition for themselves; and ultimately empowering communities to institute healthy public policy changes. One of the initial steps to achieving this goal is to fully comprehend and appreciate the power of the social determinants of health (SDOH); see chapter 8.

SOCIAL DETERMINANTS OF HEALTH

Food, shelter, education, income, a stable environment, sustainable resources, social justice, and equity can be considered essential health resources, as noted in the *Ottawa Charter for Health Promotion*. It is postulated that any improvement in one's health status requires "a secure foundation in these basic prerequisites" (WHO, 1986). Thus, it is imperative that we, as health professionals, address these prerequisites through the SDOH. Simply acknowledging the importance of a patient's community and the implicating social conditions is not enough. As clinicians, our level of knowledge and understanding of what the SDOH are and how they apply to each patient, and then knowing how to address their social needs, must be on a deeper and more active level (S. Dupéré, personal communication, November 25, 2016).

The SDOH are defined by the World Health Organization (WHO, 2016b) as "the conditions in which people are born, grow, work, live and age and the wider set of forces and systems shaping the conditions of daily life" (para. 1). These include income and social status, social support networks, education and literacy, employment and working conditions, social environments, physical environments, personal health practices and coping skills, healthy child development, biology and genetic endowment, health services, gender, and culture (Public Health Agency of Canada, 2011). Health promotion strategies then need to be directed according to one's life experience. The aim is to improve upon and maintain good quality of life.

Andermann (2016a) proposes that while clinicians are already engaging in preventive practices and intervention, there is an increasing need for us to also address the SDOH "early and broaden the scope of interventions to make entire families and communities healthier" (p. 2). She suggests that the SDOH should be examined at three levels: the patient level, the practice level, and the community level. We will briefly present how these determinants of health can be addressed in clinical care at each of those levels.

Patient Level

Health professionals need to take a broader look at the populations that they are working with. Andermann (2016b) suggests that questions be worked into the patient encounter by asking patients about their social challenges. Use simple screening questions such as "Do you work?" "Where is your money coming from?" (e.g., regular employment with or without benefits, social services) "Where do you get your food from?" (e.g., shelter, food bank, grocery store, restaurant, or dumpster diving) and "Where is home for you?" (e.g., house, apartment, shared residence, street). Offer advice; map out and facilitate access to community services such as local food sources, legal aid, educational resources, housing support, and social work; and act as a reliable resource throughout their care. Asking patients in a socially and culturally respectful way helps them work through these issues; by not asking, we are going "down the wrong route" rather than providing good clinical care (Andermann, 2016b). When a patient presents to a clinic with bruises or other signs of abuse or even broken bones, we ask questions to rule out violence or abuse in the home. As clinical instructors, we teach our students to have a heightened awareness of clinical red flags in practice such as acute chest and abdominal pain, the "worst headache of my life," suicidal ideation, and so on. The same must apply to the patients' social and physical challenges. There must be a heightened awareness of what's going on in their life. Clinical practice guidelines can be used as a reference when dealing with specific populations and specific determinants of health. These are included in the further readings for this chapter.

Practice Level

Health promotion strategies can be introduced and maintained at the practice level within the health care clinic. Andermann (2016b) advises going "beyond the provider-patient interaction" and introducing practice- or organizational-level interventions such as facilitating access to clinic services, reducing barriers, and navigating the health care system for their patients who require this assistance. She cites examples such as offering bus fare and/or child care to make it easier for marginalized patients to attend regular clinic appointments or to see a specialist, and implementing system navigators or life coaches to help guide the health care of the patient, particularly those with low literacy or cultural differences. Interpreters can be provided, language preferences can be documented, clinic hours can be extended, and/or satellite clinic hours offered closer to where patients live, according to Andermann (2016b). Patient experience surveys or a community-led board of directors can also be useful when responding to patients' needs and re-designing clinical practices (Royal College of General Practitioners Health Inequities Standing Group, 2008, as cited in Andermann, 2016b). This type of system has been adopted in community health centres in Ontario. Community health centres and family health teams offer a variety of health services, including nursing, allied health, access clinics, and afterhours clinics, under one roof. This organizational structure change facilitates access to health and social services and enables the patient to navigate the system more effectively. Other suggestions from Andermann (2016b) include offering a welcoming and culturally safe environment, providing targets and benchmarks for improving outcomes for vulnerable patients, and creating community and outreach programs to local schools and to the homeless population and shelters. It is our opinion that, more often than not, patients are aware of what their needs are but require support with navigating the system to learn what programs are offered and how to gain access to the services they want and need. Appropriately navigating a complex health care system as an active member of society requires proficiency in reading, writing, listening, communicating, and understanding the information that is being offered (Sorensen et al., 2012, as cited by Kickbusch, Pelikan, Apfel, & Tsouros, 2013). Without these skills, patients will obviously struggle to meet their needs.

An example is a nurse practitioner who worked in a tertiary diabetes clinic in southwestern Ontario. One of her patients was a 56-year-old female who was on long-term disability, related to chronic health problems, including diabetes and mental health. Her education was at the grade 5 level; she could not differentiate between her two insulins. She did not have Internet access or knowledge, nor did she have a cellphone. She lived with her husband, who was also chronically ill, in a tiny apartment in a remote community 90 minutes away from the clinic. They did not own a car and could not afford transportation. With little combined income, they relied on the local food bank. Their diet mainly consisted of canned foods (high in salt), fruit drinks and pop (high in sugar), and very little fresh produce. Combined with her life stressors (mental health concerns, little money, feeling unwell), her lifestyle did not benefit her diabetes, which itself was out of control. The more her insulin was increased to target her sugars, the more weight she gained, and her health further declined. Strategies that were implemented to motivate this woman to make changes towards better health included arranging transportation with another patient who lived in the same rural community who also attended the clinic. Appointments were combined when she came to the clinic; this included seeing the nurse practitioner, dietician, and psychologist in one trip, alternating with the endocrinologist, dietician, and kinesiologist the next trip. At one of these appointments, the nurse practitioner and patient together made a few telephone calls to connect her with a free swimming program three times per week at a community pool that the patient could walk to. The insulin company was contacted for compassionate supply on a yearly basis to help with the cost of her insulin, and a government application was completed for funds to help with the cost of needles and BG test strips. She was given different coloured insulin pens that helped her distinguish between mealtime insulin and bedtime insulin. Pictures of low-carbohydrate foods were put onto her refrigerator. When the patient's health started to improve, telephone visits were incorporated into the care plan every other visit.

Community Level

Andermann (2016b) believes that health professionals have a powerful voice and can use their collective influence to create a supportive environment in the community. Strategies to accomplish this include developing partnerships with public health resources and community groups at the local, provincial, and federal levels, using clinical experiences and research to advocate for social change, and becoming actively involved in community health assessment and planning. Examples of this include introducing programs to prevent violence, to facilitate healthy eating in schools, and to initiate community gardens (Andermann, 2016b). Health clinicians cannot do this alone; they require the expertise, resources, and endorsement from community leaders (S. Dupéré, personal communication, November 25, 2016). By partnering with community leaders, broader social change can be achieved.

HEALTH LITERACY

Health literacy has been defined in Canada as "the ability to access, comprehend, evaluate and communicate information as a way to promote, maintain and improve health in a variety of settings across the life-course" (PHAC, 2014, para. 1). This means using health information that is provided in health care clinics, pharmacies, schools, in the media, and in communities. It is often part of our normal practice to offer written literature to our patients or direct them to reputable Internet sources for education; however, if they cannot read or comprehend this information, then our efforts are futile.

Education and literacy are social determinants of health and are directly related to health status. A high level of education and literacy keeps Canadians healthy by improving their ability to access, understand, and evaluate information (PHAC, 2013). It is estimated that 60 percent of adults and 88 percent of seniors in Canada have low levels of health literacy (PHAC, 2014, para. 1). Poor literacy has been shown to directly affect health literacy and thus overall health outcomes (WHO, 1998). By improving an individual's capacity to access and use health information effectively, their health literacy becomes a component of their empowerment (WHO, 1998). One of the first steps is for the health professional to identify those who are at risk of low health literacy. These may include people over age 65; recent immigrants; those with low income and low education; Indigenous populations; people of diverse cultures; those whose primary language is other than English or French; people who are unable to read and write; and people with learning disabilities (Mitic & Rootman, 2012; Rootman & Ronson, 2005; Rootman & Gordon-El-Bihbety, 2008). Clinical assessment tools such as the REALM (Rapid Estimate of Adult Literacy in Medicine) test or Newest Vital Sign can be used to assess the level of the patient's ability to read and understand health terms.[1] Another option is to use an introductory sentence such as, "Many people have difficulty reading and understanding medical information, so please feel comfortable asking questions if there is something you don't understand" (Hoffman-Goetz, Donelle, & Ahmed, 2014, p. 191). Other strategies include the following:

- Using other technologies to provide information, rather than just printed sources
- Using teaching materials that are appropriate to the patient's education level, culture, and language
- Taking time when providing education to ensure that the patient understands what is being taught, as patients may not ask questions or clarify if the health professional is rushing
- Avoiding the use of medical jargon
- Providing an environment that is calm and quiet, as a crowded and noisy environment is not conducive to effective learning and information retention
- Ensuring the patient has time to sit and focus on new learning and doesn't have to be somewhere else in a hurry
- Assessing if the patient is ready to focus on learning and isn't affected by pain, anxiety, or medication side-effects
- Using a "teach-back" method, in which the patient reiterates and/or demonstrates what they have just learned
- Not providing too much information at once; keeping the message simple (Rootman & Ronson, 2005; Gilboy & Howard, 2009; Nielsen-Bohlman, Panzer & Kindig, 2004; Hoffman-Goetz et al., 2014)

It is our responsibility to find out what patients already know and what they want to know, and then facilitate that transfer of knowledge efficiently. This implies reaching a level of knowledge, personal skills, and confidence that propels individuals to strive to improve personal and community health by changing their lifestyles and living conditions accordingly (WHO, 1998). This also means communicating and networking efficiently and respecting cultural preferences with every patient encounter. By addressing health literacy, health is promoted and inequities are reduced (Health Disparities Task Group, 2005; Murthy, 2009, as cited in Hoffman-Goetz et al., 2014). This is especially true for those at risk that were discussed earlier in the chapter. Clear and effective communication is essential.

CARE MODELS AND HEALTH PROMOTION IN CLINICAL CARE

With this awareness, addressing the social determinants of health and health literacy represents a key strategy in clinical practice. When assessing social determinants of health for patients and families, the meaning of family must be considered. Successful implementation of health promotion in clinical practice also involves having a clear understanding of family theory and family-centred care.

Family Theory

Bowen's Family Systems Theory proposes a higher level of understanding of the interactions and influence of the family system within the context of health, rather than focusing on just the individual. Wright and Leahey (2013) propose that applying the concepts of Family Systems Theory can not only guide health care assessment and intervention, but also promote the understanding that behaviour is best understood from a circular view rather than linear causality.

Application of these concepts can further guide health promotion strategies in the clinical setting. Doane and Varcoe (2014) suggest that "relational inquiry directs us to carefully consider the distinctions and judgments we make about people and families" (p. 204). Family can be defined according to one's own frame of reference, value, judgment, or discipline. In other words, the family is what the individual considers it to be. It can be assumed then that each individual experiences a unique meaning of family and health. While a low-income, single, divorced mother with three kids is considered high risk, the family itself may not share the same outlook. The Calgary Family Assessment Model (CFAM)[2] can also be used to understand this scenario. The CFAM is a multi-dimensional framework based on structural, developmental, and functional categories that supports a more in-depth understanding of the individual and the family and provides guidance towards developing an effective plan of care. For instance, in the structural category, this family may be part of a large extended family and thus have a large support network. For the developmental category, the single mother may have recently left an abusive relationship.

For the functional category, she may have a history of depression. With this contextual information, strategies for health promotion and disease prevention may vary. A referral to a counsellor or social worker could be initiated with the patient's consent or free bus passes could be offered so the family can access the local community recreation centre's free resources more easily. As a result, the clinician not only understands the SDOH, but also engages on a deeper level. Understanding this, we are better equipped to educate and provide resources specific to the patient's and family's needs.

Applying family theories in clinical practice generates advantages for health promotion with patients and families. A greater understanding of the individual and the family promotes better health care and likely will result in empowering the patient and family towards the goal of improved quality of life. Family theories guide the development of a systematic and organized approach when working with patients and their families and allow for a more organized assessment of families through systems. Although many resources are available, as mentioned earlier, current practice must direct more focus towards the SDOH.

Family-Centred Care

Family-centred care is an approach to the provision of health care. It is a partnership between the health care provider and the family in their health care planning. Family-centred care is considered the standard of health care in many clinical practices (Kuo et al., 2012). Understanding family-centred care can be facilitated through the core concepts described by the Institute for Patient and Family-Centered Care (2016):

- Respect and dignity: listen to and honor patient and family perspectives and choices, with incorporation of core values, beliefs and cultural backgrounds into the planning and delivery of care.
- Information-sharing: ensure communication is timely and share complete, accurate and unbiased information with patients and families in ways that are affirming and useful so that patients and families can effectively participate in their care and decision-making.
- Participation: encourage and support patients and their families to participate in their care and decision-making at the level they choose.
- Collaboration: collaborate with patients and families in policy and program development, implementation, and evaluation; in health care facility design; and in professional education, as well as in the delivery of care.

The collaborative relationship developed between health professionals and the family becomes the basis of health care interactions. Family-centred care aims to address the concerns of the family and also provide information and support. Through this partnership, health professionals are better equipped to assess the social determinants of health and understand the meaning of health and illness for families, but also to develop goals and strategies that are realistic and attainable for the family at the centre of care (Burns, Dunn, Brady, Barber Starr, & Blosser, 2013; Kozier et al., 2010). Family-centred care is a vector facilitating health promotion.

NURSING STUDENT PERSPECTIVE ON HEALTH PROMOTION IN CLINICAL CARE

By Geneviève Dubé

It is my interpretation that the concept of health promotion evolves as students progress through their education. As students learn about health promotion, they often face moments of understanding and confidence mixed with moments of disillusion and challenge. Based on our experience, nursing students gradually develop awareness of health promotion as they work through the undergraduate curriculum. Their understanding will change as they start clinical practice, and it will evolve further in those choosing to pursue graduate education. This section of the chapter explores the student perspective around health promotion in clinical care. I am a recent nurse practitioner graduate, after having practised as a registered nurse for a decade. Throughout this journey, I have observed how my knowledge and understanding shifted. I also noticed how much the role for health promotion in nursing is broad and diversified.

Health promotion is fundamental to nursing practice (Chambers & Thompson, 2009). The concept is addressed early on and consistently in the nursing education journey. Health promotion is either covered as part of basic curriculum courses in the undergraduate programs, or as a dedicated course (Université Laval, 2016). Nurses are taught the essential elements of health promotion and how to implement it in practice. For instance, they are taught a definition of health promotion and the difference between health promotion and health education (see chapter 2). Students then use these concepts and learn ways to put them into practice (e.g., assisting patients in improving their blood glucose levels with education on what a healthy diet is and how to access dietary resources rather than rely solely on medications, or empowering patients to be more physically active and offering specific but achievable weekly targets). These practices are also what made me feel, as a nursing student, that I could make a significant difference in someone's health. It is empowering to learn about concepts and tools conducive to improving the health of individuals, groups, and populations.

Depending on a new graduate's area of clinical practice, fully integrating health promotion concepts might prove more or less challenging. Health promotion and disease prevention practices are mostly based in the community setting, compared to acute care, where disease management is the focus. It is estimated that 13.3 percent of nurses in Canada practise in the community while 71.6 percent of them practise in acute and long-term care (CIHI, 2011; CIHI, n.d. a; CIHI, n.d. b). Since the majority of nurses work in acute care, there are limited opportunities for nurses to fully explore and apply health promotion as taught in school. This imbalance is a challenge for nurses to engage in meaningful health promotion activities. Nonetheless, there are opportunities for health promotion in acute care using both individual and environmental strategies (Rothstein, 2014). Such activities are optimized using a multi-disciplinary approach including nurses, nurse practitioners, occupational therapists, nutritionists, physiotherapists, and other allied health professionals.

While health promotion is a cornerstone of health care, students usually notice the gap between what is taught in school and what the clinical reality holds when they graduate and transition into practice. Nursing students believe they have a professional responsibility in health promotion and they are aware that this concept extends beyond the individual they are working with. However, Halcomb (2010) reported that students do not see themselves performing this role in the future. As explored here, there are barriers preventing not only students from fully engaging in health promotion clinical care activities, but practising clinicians as well.

Chambers and Thompson (2009) suggest that even though health promotion is a core theme in nursing education, the theory taught to students is not consolidated when the transition to practice occurs. They studied how nurses use the concept of empowerment in health promotion. From their study, they explain that there are two types of nurse health promotion practitioners: Type I divergent nurses and Type II convergent nurses. They differ in the type of empowerment practices they use with individuals, and because the majority are convergent thinkers, so are the students' role models and mentors. Consequently, they influence students to adopt this narrow mode of thinking about health promotion. According to Chambers and Thompson (2009), convergent practitioners, as opposed to divergent practitioners, steer health promotion activities away from ideal practice by disempowering patients, which results in sub-optimal health outcomes.

They suggest that convergent nurse health promotion practitioners assume a more biomedical approach based on the ideology that patients are incapable of their own decision-making. As a result, the nurse controls the behaviour change and defines the terms of the interaction. They disempower patients who then become "recipients" of health promotion. Convergent health promotion nurses focus on simplistic answers to problems rather than explore the complexity of contributing factors. They focus on changing an individual's behaviour through fear and blame so that patients fit the medically defined behaviours. The right to self-determination of patients is generally not respected when the concept of empowerment is replaced by that of "informed choice" (Chambers & Thompson, 2009).

In contrast, divergent nurse health promotion practitioners employ a reflexive and holistic approach (Chambers & Thompson, 2009). They conceptualize health as part of the social context and understand that their social environment influences patients' actions. Their reflexive thinking includes a range of possible solutions while trying to understand the social and interpersonal factors influencing people's health. Divergent practitioners analyze the intersectionality between health, illness, culture, and the social determinants of health. As a result, they avoid linear thinking and the use of stereotypes (Chambers & Thompson, 2009). The outcome is to empower individuals in identifying health promotion strategies that meet their needs and capacities.

Thus, our learning processes are influenced by concomitant experiences. One of the most influential factors on our ability to incorporate health promotion into practice is the quality of our preceptorship. Walthew and Scott (2012) suggest that ideal role models for students in practice are those preceptors who have a strong knowledge base and understanding of the community they work in, and a supportive attitude. However, with medical concepts and approaches being ubiquitous in nursing education and the clinical environment, it is inevitable that nursing will be affected by some elements of the medical

Box 15.1: Advanced Nursing Practice and Nurse Practitioner Practice

Advanced nursing practice represents an advanced level of clinical nursing practice. Advanced practice nurses (APN) complete graduate education to acquire advanced skills, knowledge, and expertise. They maximize the use of their in-depth knowledge and expertise to meet the health care needs of individuals, families, groups, communities, and populations. APNs are either clinical nurse specialists or nurse practitioners (CNA, 2008). In Canada, nurse practitioners have integrated into the health care systems at different levels, but the majority are Family Nurse Practitioners working in primary care settings. Family nurse practitioners provide community-based primary health care to patients of all ages while keeping a focus on health promotion and disease prevention. They provide "timely, accessible, cost-effective and quality health care for all Canadians" (CNA, 2006, p. 3). This includes autonomously diagnosing, ordering, and interpreting diagnostic tests, prescribing pharmaceuticals, and performing certain procedures. Family nurse practitioners have the competencies to function as primary care providers. With advanced nursing education and training and non–fee for service remuneration, they have flexibility in integrating health promotion activities, making them an asset to the Canadian health care system. Through their holistic practice, nurse practitioners are able to contextually understand how to apply health promotion principles and practices. They are also well positioned in the system to influence policy and system improvements that improve health promotion activities overall (CNA, 2008). With their advanced education in theory, policy, and leadership, they take an active role in our health care system. Nurse practitioners are dynamic agents of change who seek effective ways to practise and improve delivery of health care. For example, their role in relation to health promotion includes advocating for patients, mentoring nursing colleagues and students, promoting accessibility to health care, and understanding and engaging in legislative and socio-political initiatives (CNA, 2008). Nurse practitioners are well positioned within the system in terms of understanding the system view to promote health for Canadians.

model. In relation to health promotion, the "traditional medical model of health education ... assumes that knowledge informs attitudes, which in turn lead to certain behaviour" (Chambers & Thompson, 2009, p. 135). Therefore, we tend to focus on health and illness more often. We sometimes fail to embrace the concept of patient empowerment and how it is central to health promotion practices. The medical model, while used in nursing education, limits the use of a more holistic approach, subsequently shifting health promotion practices further away from optimal patient empowerment (Chambers & Thompson, 2009). In order for health promotion to be holistic, divergence must prevail.

TRENDS AND ISSUES IN TRANSLATING HEALTH PROMOTION INTO PRACTICE

Health promotion, as with other areas of health care, evolves over time and the concept adapts to the reality of the current health care era. As we dynamically adapt the concept of health promotion to the current health care model, we also, at times, face issues with its translation into clinical care.

Health practitioners generally consider that health promotion practices are part of their scope of practice. Nevertheless, when it is time to put the concept into routine practice, clinicians face barriers. For instance, integrating health promotion practices in acute care settings is a challenge. Care providers mention barriers such as time constraints, the focus on patient discharge, and the skepticism towards effectiveness of health promotion activities (Walkeden and Walker, 2015). In primary care, the barriers to health promotion are different. For instance, practitioners mention a lack of health promoting programs in communities (their waitlist or their lack of continuity), an insufficient collaboration between acute care settings and primary care, a lack of patient motivation to initiate and maintain lifestyle changes, and insufficient proven effectiveness of interventions (Visscher, Geense, Glind, & Achterberg, 2013).

The health promotion movement emphasizes the concept of empowerment as foundational. Empowerment is a process where individuals are encouraged to assert their autonomy and self-management to identify their own health agendas (MacDonald, 1998, as cited in Chambers & Thompson, 2009). Patients need to believe they have a significant influence on themselves, their lives, and their own futures. In addition, they need to trust that health professionals are committed to sharing power with them (Labonté, 1994, as cited in Chambers & Thompson, 2009). The expected outcome is an improved quality of life, increased engagement in health decisions, and a reduced use of acute care services. Empowerment in health promotion optimizes equality and quality in health promotion practices (Chambers & Thompson, 2009; MacDonald, 1998). Patient empowerment is a fundamental part of nursing practice and fits well with the concept of health promotion (Ashton & Rodgers, 2005). For empowerment to occur, clinicians must be able to analyze the relationships between health, illness, socio-economic, and cultural influences (Walthew & Scott, 2012).

STRATEGIES FOR THE FUTURE

Health practitioners have a responsibility to understand the concept of health promotion and remain current on practices promoting health. They also need to contribute in carrying health promotion forward while making it applicable to clinical practice. Clinicians are accountable to develop and engage in strategies for the future of health promotion in order to achieve optimal outcomes for individuals, families, and communities. Although barriers to the promotion of health have been mentioned in this chapter, there are also solutions that exist and that we need to work on implementing.

The WHO (2008) has advocated for practitioners to move away from focusing exclusively on illness and disease, and consider both health promotion and disease prevention in the health care of their patients. Strategies targeting an optimal approach to health promotion start with the education of new health practitioners. Students entering into practice not only need to learn the definition of health promotion, but must be provided with support to "engage in and navigate a range of broad health promotion arenas" (Whitehead, 2007, p. 235). As instructors and preceptors, we can help facilitate this through teaching and ensuring an understanding of theories—for example, the family theories presented in this chapter—and by demonstrating how to apply them to their practice. On this note, it is important not to limit the knowledge of health promotion to individuals, but to expand it to groups, communities, and populations to obtain a comprehensive and holistic understanding. Students need to be taught that there is not a single universal definition of health promotion in the current literature, but many (Halcomb, 2010; see chapter 2).

There are also recommendations on didactic strategies. To help bridge the gap felt by students when transitioning into practice, authors suggest avoiding premature exposure to in-depth health promotion concepts and instead gradually integrating health promotion constructs throughout the nursing curriculum. This would help students acquire a foundational basis first, then gradually build upon this with increasingly in-depth concepts (Mooney, Timmins, Byrne, & Corroon, 2011).

Because the transition into practice is challenging, increased accessibility to practicum experiences for students is suggested (Walthew & Scott, 2012). These authors propose that, ideally, these practicums should include activities that aim at influencing physical environment and economic conditions, but also at making and changing policies and social conditions. If students experience working in the expanded role of health promotion during their education, they might be able to see themselves performing these activities in the future (Halcomb, 2010; Walthew & Scott, 2012).

Being part of political processes is fundamental to many spheres of our lives, including health promotion. Whether we are students or practising clinicians, we need to learn about, understand, and be part of the advocacy involved in health promotion practices (Halcomb, 2010). For instance, health practitioners can advocate at the municipal and provincial levels to implement safe injection sites, or increase access to public toilets and showers for the homeless population. Another example is to politically support measures facilitating physical activity, such as developing park space, improving urban design, increasing access to bicycle paths and sidewalks, ensuring adequate lighting at night, and controlling wildlife. Being politically engaged in health promotion also means working to decrease the gap in health inequities (refer to chapter 8 for more discussion on this topic).

Strategies related to education not only target undergraduate students in health care programs, but also graduated practitioners. It is recommended that education programs continue health promotion education at the graduate level. Nurses and other allied health professionals should also include health promotion in their continuing education plan. The outcome of graduate and continuing education would improve students' and practitioners' knowledge about health promotion, thereby making them positive role models for future students, but also improving their clinical skills (Chambers & Thompson, 2009; Walthew & Scott, 2012). This would allow nurses and other health professionals to develop as practitioners with the ability to understand the nuances and apply them effectively.

As always in a scientific field of practice, research remains a cornerstone to develop knowledge and improve practices. Scientific research is an essential strategy to ensure that the development of health promotion practices evolves along with the needs of the Canadian population. We encourage clinicians to identify gaps in knowledge related to the promotion of health, and to lead or participate in scientific research initiatives.

While it is important to maximize the promotion of health in clinical care, it is unavoidable for practitioners to face frustration at times. However, let us be reminded that organizational change is most likely to happen when front-line clinicians persevere and focus on strategies leading to optimal health outcomes for individuals and communities by influencing system-level policies.

CONCLUSION

The practice of health promotion in the clinical setting improves the health of individuals, families, and the community. It is our belief that we, as health professionals, need to become acutely engaged in the health and wellbeing of the populations and communities that we serve. Such engagement implies that health professionals believe what they are doing and, in turn, demonstrates positive reinforcement. We are in an ideal position to facilitate this movement with health education and empowerment. It will become necessary to find a way to overcome barriers to health promotion with innovation and a multi-disciplinary approach. More work can be done to educate students from various health care fields to transition their knowledge of health promotion into clinical practice, in both acute and community care settings, and to strengthen their understanding of the social determinants of health. Opportunities ought to be taken where health promotion becomes a routine part of the patient encounter. The focus must remain on the lived experience and patients need to be empowered to make changes that suit their needs. This can be facilitated through a shared approach where the trust is mutual. The fundamental objective will be to facilitate a healthier and less vulnerable population that the community can invest in.

CRITICAL THINKING QUESTIONS

1. Is there a difference between health promotion and disease prevention? If there is, what is the difference?
2. The terms *family-centred care* and *patient-centred care* are sometimes used interchangeably. Do you agree that they are one and the same?
3. How do you envision addressing the social determinants of health at the patient level, the practice level, and the community level in the area that you practise?
4. Are you a convergent or divergent health promotion practitioner? What evidence supports your answer?
5. How do you see yourself, as a health promotion practitioner, become a positive role model for students and new graduates in your clinical practice? What do you need to learn? How would you change your practice?

RESOURCES

Further Readings

Andermann, A. (2016). Taking action on the social determinants of health in clinical practice: A framework for health professionals. *Canadian Medical Association Journal*. doi:10.1503/cmaj.160177.
This article provides a framework on how to adopt the social determinants of health approach into practice.

Doane, G. H., & Varcoe, C. (2014). *How to nurse: Relational inquiry with individuals and families in changing health and health care contexts*. Baltimore: Wolters Kluwer Health/ Lippincott Williams & Wilkins.
This volume examines using relational inquiry and theoretically informed nursing practice in a contemporary health care landscape.

Kickbusch, I., Pelikan, J. M., Apfel, F., & Tsouros, A. D. (Eds.). (2013). *Health literacy: The solid facts*. Copenhagen: World Health Organization, Regional Office for Europe.
This publication identifies health literacy as a key determinant of health and discusses using an intersectoral approach to improving health literacy in various settings.

Politi, M. C., Wolin, K. Y., & Legare, F. (2013). Implementing clinical practice guidelines about health promotion and disease prevention through shared decision making. *Journal of General Internal Medicine, 28*(6), 838–844.
This article outlines how to use shared decision-making as one solution to linking practice guidelines to health promotion in clinical practice.

Raphael, D. (2016). *Social determinants of health: Canadian perspectives* (3rd ed.). Toronto: Canadian Scholars' Press.

This book summarizes how socio-economic factors affect the health of Canadians, surveys the current state of the social determinants of health across Canada, and provides an analysis of how these determinants affect Canadians' health.

Relevant Websites

CLEAR Toolkit

www.mcgill.ca/clear/download

The CLEAR toolkit is a clinical decision aid to help health care practitioners attend to the social determinants of health in clinical practice. The toolkit includes a trainer's manual, is available in more than ten languages, and can be downloaded free of charge.

CMAJ Podcast

soundcloud.com/cmajpodcasts/160177-rev

This CMAJ Podcast features an author interview with Dr. Anne Andermann. She discusses how social determinants can be addressed in the day-to-day practice of physicians and allied health care workers.

Poverty Tool

effectivepractice.org

The Poverty Tool is a clinical screening tool for primary care providers to use with particularly vulnerable populations including new immigrants, women, and Indigenous and LGBTQ populations. It is accessed through the Centre for Effective Practice.

NOTES

1. Toolkit for Newest Vital Sign available at www.pfizer.com/health/literacy/public_policy_researchers/nvs_toolkit

2. Calgary Family Assessment Model available at internationalfamilynursing.org/2015/01/30/calgary-family-assessment-model-cfam-and-calgary-family-intervention-model-cfim/

REFERENCES

Andermann, A. (2016a). Taking action on the social determinants of health in clinical practice: A framework for health professionals. *Canadian Medical Association Journal*. doi: 10.1503/cmaj.160177

Andermann, A. (2016b). Taking action on social determinants of health (CMAJ Audio podcast). Retrieved from www.cmaj.ca/content/early/2016/08/08/cmaj.160177/suppl/DC2

Ashton, H., & Rodgers, J. (2005). A health promoting empowerment approach to diabetes nursing. In A Scriven (Ed.), *Health promotion practice: The contribution of nurses and allied health professionals* (pp. 45–56). Basingstoke: Palgrave Macmillan.

Burns, C. E., Dunn, A. M., Brady, M. A., Barber Starr, N., & Blosser, C. G. (2013). *Pediatric primary care* (5th ed.). St. Louis: Saunders.

Canadian Institute for Health Information (CIHI). (2011). *Regulated nurses—Canadian trends, 2007 to 2011.* Retrieved from secure.cihi.ca/free_products/Regulated_Nurses_EN.pdf

Canadian Institute for Health Information (CIHI). (n.d. a). *Acute care.* Retrieved from www.cihi.ca/en/types-of-care/hospital-care/acute-care

Canadian Institute for Health Information (CIHI). (n.d. b). *Primary health care.* Retrieved from www.cihi.ca/en/types-of-care/primary-health-care

Canadian Nurses Association (CNA). (2006). *Report of 2005 dialogue on advanced nursing practice.* Ottawa: Author.

Canadian Nurses Association (CNA). (2008). *Advanced nursing practice—A national framework.* Retrieved from www.cna-aiic.ca/~/media/cna/page-content/pdf-en/anp_national_framework_e.pdf

Chambers, D., & Thompson, S. (2009). Empowerment and its application in health promotion in acute care settings: Nurses' perceptions. *Journal of Advanced Nursing, 65*(1), 130-138. doi:10.1111/j.1365-2648.2008.04851.x

Deci, E. L., & Ryan, R. M. (2008). Facilitating optimal motivation and psychological well-being across life's domains. *Canadian Psychology, 49*(1), 14–23. doi: 10.1037/0708-5591.49.1.14

Doane, G. H., & Varcoe, C. (2014). *How to nurse: Relational inquiry with individuals and families in changing health and health care contexts.* Baltimore: Wolters Kluwer Health/Lippincott Williams & Wilkins.

Gilboy, N., & Howard, P. K. (2009). Comprehension of discharge instructions. *Advanced Emergency Nursing Journal, 31*(1), 4–11.

Halcomb, K. A. (2010). *Health promotion and health education: Nursing students' perspectives.* University of Kentucky Doctoral Dissertations, Paper 13. Retrieved from uknowledge.uky.edu/gradschool_diss/13

Health Disparities Task Group. (2005). *Reducing health disparities—Roles of the health sector.* Discussion paper. Retrieved from www.phac-aspc.gc.ca/ph-sp/disparities/ddp-eng.php

Hoffman-Goetz, L. Donelle, L., & Ahmed, R. (2014). *Health literacy in Canada.* Toronto: Canadian Scholars' Press.

Institute for Patient and Family-Centered Care. (2016). *Advancing the practice of patient- and family-centered care in primary care and other ambulatory settings: How to get started.* Retrieved from www.ipfcc.org/resources/GettingStarted-AmbulatoryCare.pdf

Kickbusch, I., Pelikan, J. M., Apfel, F., & Tsouros, A. D. (Eds.). (2013). *Health literacy: The solid facts.* Copenhagen: World Health Organization, Regional Office for Europe.

Kozier, B., Erb, G., Berman, A., Snyder, S. J., Bouchal, D. S. R., Hirst, S., ... Buck, M. (2010). *Fundamentals of Canadian nursing: Concepts, process, and practice.* Toronto, ON: Pearson.

Kuo, D. Z., Houtrow, A. J., Arango, P., Kuhlthau, K. A., Simmons, J. M., & Neff, J. M. (2012). Family-centered care: Current applications and future directions in pediatric health care. *Maternal Child Health Journal, 16*(2), 297–305.

MacDonald, T. H. (1998). *Rethinking health promotion: A global approach.* New York, London: Routledge.

Mitic, W., & Rootman, I. (Eds). (2012). *An inter-sectoral approach for improving health literacy for Canadians.* A discussion paper. Retrieved from www.cpha.ca/uploads/portals/h-l/intersectoral_e.pdf

Mooney, B., Timmins, F., Byrne, G., & Corroon, A. M. (2011). Nursing students' attitudes to health promotion: Implications for teaching practice. *Nurse Education Today, 31*, 841–848.

Murthy, P. (2009). Health literacy and sustainable development. *UN Chronicle Online, XLVI*(1/2).

Nielsen-Bohlman, L., Panzer, A. M., & Kindig, D. A. (Eds.). (2004). *Health literacy: A prescription to end confusion.* Washington DC: National Academies Press.

Politi, M. C., Wolin, K. Y., & Legare, F. (2013). Implementing clinical practice guidelines about health promotion and disease prevention through shared decision making. *Journal of General Internal Medicine, 28*(6), 838–844.

Public Health Agency of Canada (PHAC). (2011). *What determines health?* Retrieved from www.phac-aspc.gc.ca/ph-sp/determinants/index-eng.php

Public Health Agency of Canada (PHAC). (2013). *What makes Canadians healthy or unhealthy?* Retrieved from www.phac-aspc.gc.ca/ph-sp/determinants/determinants-eng.php

Public Health Agency of Canada (PHAC). (2014). *Health literacy.* Retrieved from www.phac-aspc.gc.ca/cd-mc/hl-ls/index-eng.php#tabs-2

Raphael, D. (2016). *Social determinants of health: Canadian perspectives* (3rd ed.). Toronto: Canadian Scholars' Press.

Rootman, I., Dupéré, S., Pederson, A., & O'Neill, M. (2012). *Health promotion in Canada: Critical perspectives on practice* (3rd ed.). Toronto, ON: Canadian Scholars' Press.

Rootman, I., & Gordon-El-Bihbety, D. (2008). *A vision for a health literate Canada: Report of the expert panel on health literacy.* Toronto: Canadian Public Health Association.

Rootman, I., & Ronson, B. (2005). Literacy and health research in Canada: Where have we been and where should we go? *Canadian Journal of Public Health, 96*, S62–77.

Rothstein, M. A. (2014). Promoting public health in health care facilities. *American Journal of Public Health, 104*(6), 965–967. doi:10.2105/AJPH.2014.301885

Ryan, R. M., & Deci, E. L. (2000). Self-determination theory and the facilitation of intrinsic motivation, social development, and well-being. *American Psychologist, 55*(1), 68–78. doi: 10.1037/0003-066X.55.1.68

Université Laval. (2016). *Baccalauréat en sciences infirmières (formation initiale)—Activités de formation continue.* Retrieved from www2.ulaval.ca/les-etudes/programmes/repertoire/details/baccalaureat-en-sciences-infirmieres-formation-initiale-b-sc.html#description-officielle&structure-programme

Visscher, T. L., Geense, W. W., Glind, I. M. v. d., & Achterberg, T. V. (2013). Barriers, facilitators and attitudes influencing health promotion activities in general practice: An explorative pilot study. *BMC Family Practice, 14*(1), 20. doi:10.1186/1471-2296-14-20

Walkeden, S., & Walker, K. M. (2015). Perceptions of physiotherapists about their role in health promotion at an acute hospital: A qualitative study. *Physiotherapy, 101*(2), 226–231. doi:10.1016/j.physio.2014.06.005

Walthew, P., & Scott, H. (2012). Conceptions of health promotion held by pre-registration student nurses in four schools of nursing in New Zealand. *Nurse Education Today, 32*(3), 229–234. doi:10.1016/j.nedt.2011.04.013

Whitehead, D. (2004). Health promotion and health education: Advancing the concepts. *Journal of Advanced Nursing, 47*, 311–320.

Whitehead, D. (2007). Reviewing health promotion in nursing education. *Nurse Education Today, 27*(3), 225–237. doi:10.1016/j.nedt.2006.05.003

World Health Organization (WHO). (1986). *The Ottawa Charter for health promotion*. Retrieved from www.who.int/healthpromotion/conferences/previous/ottawa/en/

World Health Organization (WHO). (1998). *Health promotion glossary*. Geneva: Author.

World Health Organization (WHO). (2008). *Primary health care now more than ever*. Geneva: Author.

World Health Organization (WHO). (2016a). *What is health promotion?* Retrieved from www.who.int/features/qa/health-promotion/en/

World Health Organization (WHO). (2016b). *What are the social determinants of health?* Retrieved from www.who.int/social_determinants/en/

Wright, L. M., & Leahey, M. (2013). *Nurses and families: A guide to family assessment and intervention* (6th ed.). Philadelphia: F. A. Davis.

CHAPTER 16

Digital Media and Health Promotion Practice

Laura L. Struik, Rebecca J. Haines-Saah, and Joan L. Bottorff

LEARNING OBJECTIVES

1. Understand the role of digital media in Canadian health promotion practice
2. Identify benefits of using digital media for health promotion practice
3. Identify challenges associated with integrating digital media in health promotion practice
4. Critically evaluate the role of digital media in health promotion practice

INTRODUCTION

Searching for health information online is one of the most frequent ways that people use the Internet. Indeed, digital health technologies are now ubiquitous, and as the saying goes, for any health-related practice you can imagine—from physical activity trackers to mindfulness mediation podcasts—"there's an app for that." While health promotion delivered through digital media holds promise for reaching and engaging a variety of populations using innovative approaches, the myriad of information and platforms delivering such content has also created its own set of unique challenges for the field. For example, although people are responding positively to receiving health information via new technologies, the avalanche of health information provided online can be difficult for the average user to navigate. As digital networks are profoundly shifting the ways that we work, connect to each other, and share information in almost all aspects of our daily lives, so too has the context of health promotion practice shifted: in terms of how we disseminate health information, how we target communities or populations, and also in terms of how we carry out research and evaluation of our programs and initiatives in the context of "virtual" as opposed to "real life" settings or communities. By delivering content through graphic and interactive formats that may appeal to users from different backgrounds and with disparate levels of health literacy, digital technologies have been lauded for their potential to expand the reach and uptake of health promotion interventions. However, as we explore in this chapter, gaps in access to digital technologies and the focus of interventions targeted almost exclusively to effecting health behaviour change at the individual level are some limitations of existing digital approaches.

In highlighting key aspects of the digital context for health promotion, this chapter will present some of the most important implications of online initiatives for the field, and also raise some critical questions about how the shift to digital practice has added complexity, and in some instances has prompted concerns in relation to reach, representation, and user/community engagement. Drawing from specific examples from our work in digital contexts related to tobacco use, we present examples of promising practices that highlight the advantages—but also the potential drawbacks—of working through online platforms, most notably the potential to engage so-called hard-to-reach populations through using "youth-friendly" and gender-specific online approaches. To conclude this chapter, we highlight the benefits of approaching eHealth promotion from a critical perspective, bringing attention to challenges in the convergence of the online and offline world in health promotion, as well as user-driven initiatives that both positively and negatively impact health promotion. It must be noted that, rather than a complete review of the digital health promotion arena, this chapter is intended to provide readers with a broad introduction to eHealth promotion, share some examples of how digital technology has been taken up by the field, and highlight some of the implications of this shift for research and practice.

AN OVERVIEW OF DIGITAL HEALTH PROMOTION IN CANADA

The use of digital media in health care is also frequently known as eHealth, and has inarguably pervaded every area of the health sector, including health promotion. Gunther Eysenbach (2001), the editor of the *Journal of Medical Internet Research*, has provided the following comprehensive definition of eHealth:

> eHealth is an emerging field in the intersection of medical informatics, public health and business, referring to health services and information delivered or enhanced through the Internet and related technologies. In a broader sense, the term characterizes not only a technical development, but also a state-of-mind, a way of thinking, an attitude, and a commitment for networked, global thinking, to improve health care locally, regionally, and worldwide by using information and communication technology. (p. 1)

The introduction of personal computing and the proliferation of Internet use during the 1990s began the eHealth movement, whereby telehealth, telemedicine, and online health discussion forums were developed, and since then, new mobile devices, digital apps, and social media platforms have flooded the market, providing a proliferation of opportunities for people to find health information, share experiences, and collect and analyze their own biometric data (Lupton, 2016). From an institutional perspective, the benefits of innovations in health technologies and digital media are seen as almost exclusively positive for health promotion, as they provide a new set of tools for practitioners and organizations focused on developing and implementing interventions for positively influencing health behaviours (Public Health Agency of Canada, 2014a). However, the drivers of digital innovation in health promotion are complex and have been driven by multiple social, institutional, and commercial forces within and outside the field, making it difficult to disentangle how the spread and uptake of technology has led to changes that promote health and health behaviour change at the individual and community levels. For example, we might call into question whether or not the ability to access and engage with health information and supports through digital and online delivery modes actually contributes to better health, or just to greater use of technology? Similarly, there are also legitimate concerns about the capacity of digital practice to exacerbate social and health inequities; even as the goal is empowering through technology, having access to and the skills and ability to use digital technologies is far from universal and is shaped by factors including socio-economic status, geography, and "e-literacy." Even as many people actively choose and prefer to engage with digital health apps and information, there is also unease amongst consumers and privacy "watchdogs" about how the personal data collected online and through mobile apps is used and shared by the corporate, government, and health promotion entities involved.

Yet, in that they are user-driven and offer flexibility and portability, and many people interact with technologies on a habitual basis, digital health promotion interventions provide tools that may be attractive to individuals with a preference for self-monitoring shifts in their health practices such as dietary intake, physical activity, and substance use. Capitalizing on the scalability of eHealth approaches to the population level and the capacity to tailor and customize interventions to diverse groups, eHealth has the potential to improve access to and efficiency of health promotion efforts aimed at encouraging the prevention and self-management of chronic diseases. This has emerged as a priority for health promotion authorities in Canada who have been challenged to find equitable, actionable solutions to trends showing that more Canadians than ever are living with chronic diseases, with four out of five people at risk of developing diseases such as cancer, type 2 diabetes, and heart disease (Public Health Agency of Canada, 2016). In this context, there are novel ways that digital media has been used to develop outreach and prevention efforts for promoting health behaviour change, when "traditional" or offline strategies for engaging people and communities have not seen major successes in shifting the so-called modifiable lifestyle factors that lead to poor health outcomes.

One of the most significant contributions of digital media to health promotion practice is that it has provided new means to deliver health promotion information and interventions, with the aim of increasing capacity for health literacy. Review evidence has suggested the feasibility of eHealth interventions for improving health literacy on a range of different health conditions and with populations from diverse socio-economic backgrounds (Jacobs, Lou, Ownby, & Caballero, 2016). As a result, nearly all new health information and education campaigns make use of digital media as a primary mode of communication and delivery, and many older initiatives have been re-packaged from traditional (e.g., paper, radio, television) to digitized formats (e.g., websites, social media, text messaging, apps). In Canada, health promotion researchers have been at the forefront of eHealth innovation, with pioneering work in domains of practice such as smoking cessation and tobacco control. A well-known initiative that began in Canada is Web-Assisted Tobacco Interventions (WATI), developed in 2004 to support the research on implementation and evaluation of online tobacco control interventions (Norman & Huerta, 2006). This initiative helped to establish the new transdisciplinary field of eHealth research in Canada, through using Web-based technologies to support smoking prevention and cessation, and to influence policy development and knowledge translation for health promotion (Norman, McIntosh, Selby, & Eysenbach, 2008). Used as a solo intervention, to complement other interventions, or as an integrated component within a larger intervention, WATI resources focused on four key areas: cessation, prevention, social support, and providing professional development and training online (Norman et al., 2008). Some early examples of successful WATI resources that were pioneering online interventions for their time include the youth-focused prevention and cessation website The Smoking Zine, and the adult-oriented QuitNet program (Best et al., 2003; Norman et al., 2008). This shift to modes of online practice was significant for tobacco control, where standard interventions in the field had typically been developed from medical (i.e., nicotine replacement therapies) or behavioural (i.e., one-to-one or group counselling) models, and were frequently challenged with finding ways to decrease smoking rates amongst groups seen as "hard to reach" (e.g., adolescents and "hard core" smokers resistant to quitting).

While concerns about the privacy of personal information are persistent in online contexts, in some specific instances, digital media have facilitated less invasive, more private ways to deliver health promotion interventions, providing channels ideally suited for engaging with communities around potentially sensitive health topics. The Get Tested. Why Not? campaign launched in 2011 by Ottawa Public Health is an example of how digital media were used to increase sexually transmitted infection (STI) testing for chlamydia and gonorrhea, as well as increase access to health information among youth and young adults (aged 15–29 years) (Mann, Uddin, Hendriks, Bouchard, & Etches, 2013). The campaign used a bilingual, youth-friendly website that provided information and enabled visitors to assess their risk for STIs and their appropriateness for testing. Users were able to download a testing requisition from the website and use it to submit a urine sample to a local laboratory, thereby eliminating the need to visit a primary care provider prior to being tested, which youth might resist due to the persistent shame and social stigma of STIs. After the first year of the campaign, survey participants indicated increased knowledge about STI risks, testing, and services, and said that they would change their behaviours (e.g., ask partners to use condoms) (Mann et al., 2013). Ottawa Public Health also launched a website called Sex It Smart, which aimed to support safer sex practices by encouraging testing, as well as by increasing access to condoms by enabling site visitors to order free condoms mailed directly to their home or preferred public health agency (Ottawa Public Health, 2014: Healthy Sexuality and Risk Reduction Program, Ottawa Public Health; Personal Communications on Sex It Smart online program, August 27, 2014).

Moving beyond the didactic model of one-way information delivery, digital and online media also offer interactive tools (e.g., calculators to monitor health improvements and savings) and platforms (e.g., social media, photo-sharing and video messaging apps) to enhance user engagement and interactions. Given that user engagement has been consistently documented as a predictor of health behaviour change (e.g., Bricker et al., 2014), capitalizing on interactive technologies has become a major focus in eHealth promotion, especially in light of evidence that traditional health communication interventions have often failed to show an effect (Neuhauser & Kreps, 2010).

At the level of the individual, advances in mobile technologies (e.g., smartphones, tablets, personal wearable devices) have sparked the rapid development of mobile health-related applications (mHealth apps), expanding eHealth interventions through mobile devices. mHealth technologies extend user engagement beyond websites, social media, and text-messaging by supporting a multitude of complex functionalities, including hosting both static and interactive multimedia, enabling interactive self-monitoring (e.g., tracking cigarettes smoked over time), connecting to virtual support networks and online communities, and inferring context through internal sensors (e.g., geographical location, movement, etc.) (BinDhim, McGeechan, & Trevena, 2014; Dennison, Morrison, Conway, & Yardley, 2013). With these developments, the mHealth app market has rapidly expanded, bringing with it concerns about the evidence-base for health-oriented apps and the need for quality control. For example, according to the IMS Institute for Healthcare Informatics (2015), there are more than 165,000 mHealth apps available in the Apple iTunes and Android app stores, 90,000 of which are in the Apple iTunes store, reportedly double the number from 2013. The introduction of mHealth apps in health promotion practice, whether they are solo interventions or accompany a campaign or website, have also been seen as shifting the user experience of interventions from passive to active, whereby interventions are not limited to information delivery, but also prompt users to reflect and learn about obstacles to changing their behaviour (Kennedy et al., 2012).

In Canada, federal health authorities have developed mHealth technology in a novel attempt to increase immunization rates and to address parental and caregiver confusion around what has become a socially contentious public health issue—that of the schedule and timing of childhood immunizations. A partnership between Immunize Canada, the Canadian Public Health Association, and the Royal Ottawa Hospital, the bilingual (French and English) ImmunizeCA app was released in March 2014 to help Canadians track and manage their immunization records more easily (Immunize Canada, 2014). In addition to providing "expert-approved" vaccination information and personalized sched-ules for an entire family or household, the app offers tools such as vaccination appointment reminders and alerts to local outbreaks (Public Health Agency of Canada, 2014b). In April 2016, the Minister of Health announced a $3.5-million investment of three years for enhancing and expanding ImmunizeCA in an effort to improve immunization reporting to public health authorities (Public Health Agency of Canada, 2016). While such an app might be useful in providing a portable digital record of vaccinations and be helpful for parents who are unclear about when to immunize their children, this type of initiative relies on the idea that information alone will lead to positive behaviour change. Moreover, in that it circumvents the contentious social issue of vaccine hesitancy and refusal amongst some parents, the app represents investment in a digital health promotion initiative that may be "preaching to the converted," while, ironically, perhaps reinforcing the fears about state intervention and monitoring that is prevalent among those termed "anti-vaxxers" (Bowes, 2016).

Another example of the collusion of eHealth, corporate interests, and public health surveillance is seen through Canada's first "wellness rewards program" released in March 2016: the Carrot Rewards app. First launched in British Columbia, the app rewards residents for making an effort to lead a healthier lifestyle with consumer loyalty points, such as those available for travel and at gas or retail outlets. The development of the app was supported by a partnership that included the Public Health Agency of Canada, BC Ministry of Health, Social Change Rewards, the Heart and Stroke Foundation, the Canadian Diabetes Association, and YMCA Canada. After downloading a free app, users are able to earn their choice of loyalty points for completing activities centred on making "healthier lifestyle choices," which include completing a health profile, partici-pating in learning activities (e.g., surveys and quizzes), and doing activities such as going to the gym or eating a healthy meal. Beyond user inputs, the app was also designed to link up with "wearable tech" physical activity tracking devices to monitor and reward behaviour and achieve "daily step goals" (Public Health Agency of Canada, 2016). On the website for the app's founding company, Carrot Insights, their mission is defined as "to completely reinvent sustainable behaviour on a mass scale" (Carrot Insights, 2016) although a cynic might argue that such an approach is merely part of a neo-liberal trend towards incentivizing and individualizing the responsibility for healthy behaviours. Moreover, an emphasis on "step counting" is necessarily ableist, and does not account for barriers to physical activity within people's social and built environments, such as the lack of "walkability" in cities and safe and accessible ways for people to accumulate their daily step counts.

So while eHealth technologies are encouraging developments, a critical perspective on health promotion considers that virtual engagement alone is likely insufficient for sus-taining change and fostering empowerment, whereby people and communities still face multiple and complex social and political obstacles in the "real world" that influence health status and limit their ability to create "healthy" changes.

IMPACT OF EHEALTH PROMOTION

It is clear that digital media innovations have been taken up in many different ways by health promotion. However, as we have already alluded to, questions persist about how to measure the effectiveness of these interventions for promoting—and sustaining—health behaviour change and whether or not the impact is the same across the population. While evaluative evidence has yet to keep up with the constant outpouring of new eHealth promotion initiatives (Baker, Gustafson, & Shah, 2014), there is some research on effectiveness emerging. The Public Health Agency of Canada conducted a literature review to assess the different types of eHealth interventions being used to promote health (Valaitis et al., 2014). The review included international studies that aimed to address a range of public health issues, such as increasing physical activity, smoking cessation, healthy eating, sexual health promotion, immunization uptake, and substance abuse via Web-, mobile-, and desktop computer–based approaches. The Canadian studies included covered a wide range of health issues and focused mostly on Web-based or online programs, and one text-messaging intervention. Over half of the Canadian studies targeted adolescents and young adults.

Overall, study results indicated that eHealth interventions provide a promising avenue for engaging individuals in monitoring and improving health behaviours. While not yet tested in "real world" settings, within the contexts of the research studies reviewed, individuals demonstrated interest in using the technologies. Also notable was that the efficacy of the interventions varied by health topic (alcohol use and sexual health studies demonstrated mostly positive outcomes, whereas smoking cessation and multiple-risk-factor studies demonstrated both positive and negative outcomes), and the biggest predictors of efficacy regardless of health topic were the use of mixed components (e.g., website plus face-to-face support), tailoring in relation to individual characteristics or behaviours (e.g., personalized feedback), and the integration of behaviour change theory in intervention design. It is also important to keep in mind that effects of the interventions were demonstrated in the short-term (less than six months), but not in the long-term, or outside of the study context. While emerging evidence is encouraging, the lack of conclusive, long-term evidence of the uptake and impact of eHealth initiatives is sobering. With the constant outpouring of eHealth interventions and a continued lack of evidence in relation to uptake and impact (Baker et al., 2014), the risks of taking health promotion practice in unproductive directions, or worse, harmful directions, looms.

Perhaps the biggest challenge for eHealth promotion efforts is sustainability, especially in light of the constantly evolving nature of existing technologies and platforms, as well as the introduction of new ones. There is growing frustration expressed in the eHealth literature that more often than not, eHealth interventions are one-off events (Bergmo, 2015). In this regard, eHealth promotion requires media-savvy skill sets, long-term investment, and adaptability in an ever-changing context. An example of one such initiative from the tobacco cessation field is British Columbia's QuitNow website and suite of online resources. An initiative of the BC Lung Association that has had an online presence since 2004, QuitNow BC offers a range of supports for users including a personalized Web-based dashboard, an interactive quit plan, live chats and Facebook interactions with a Quit Coach (cessation expert from the Quit Line), and email tips tailored to a user's quit date. QuitNow has continually innovated to develop new technologies to engage smokers in cessation, including QuitNow's text support, Canada's first mobile text service providing interactive cessation support accessible via "short code" (Context Research, 2016). The expansion of QuitNow services has also been based on active partnerships with researchers to ensure evidence-informed cessation approaches as seen through the development of the online resource QuitNow Men in 2014, a website that provides gender-specific online resources to support men in cessation through the lens of a "men-centred" approach that was identified as a key gap within tobacco control and health promotion practice (Bottorff et al., 2016).

In addition to issues of evaluation and sustainability, digital media bring forward new equity concerns (see box 16.1). eHealth and mHealth interventions carry the potential to increase health inequities, especially for people without ready access to computers or mobile devices and Internet service, contributing to what has been described as a "digital divide" or "digital inequalities" (Robinson et al., 2015). Although Canadians have the highest rates of Internet use globally, there are marked differences in Internet access by income. A 2014 report from the Canadian Internet Registration Authority found that only 62 percent of Canadians in the lowest income quartile have Internet access, compared to 95 percent in the highest income quartile (Freeman, 2014). Reliable high-speed Internet connectivity (broadband) is increasingly viewed as a "necessity" for working and accessing services but remains out of reach to low-income Canadians, especially those living in rural and remote communities (Goodyear, 2016). For example, in all but one of the mHealth interventions included in the review by Valaitis and colleagues (2014), participants had to have a cellular phone, and often a data plan. Conceptualizing the notion of the digital divide as a form of digital inequity and "digital exclusion" (Baum

Box 16.1: Digital Health Theorist: Lupton and the Digital Self

Australian sociologist Deborah Lupton is one of the most well-known scholars in the critical sociology of public health and health promotion, highly cited for her writings on how "the new public health" in late modernity has constructed the prevention and management of health risks as the individual's responsibility (Lupton, 1995). In recent years, Lupton's (2016) work has turned to theorizing the implications of the "digital self" and how new "self-tracking" health technologies in the form of user-driven monitoring apps and "wearable tech" are blurring the lines between the personal and public, in terms of the potential for individuals' health information to be exploited by commercial or governmental bodies that collect and use the data generated by health apps.

et al., 2014), other critical perspectives from health promotion draw attention to factors beyond access and socio-economic status that may constrain or exclude populations from eHealth uptake, such as comfort and skill with technology amongst older adults and the capacity for technology to adapt to the needs of persons with disabilities. As such, eHealth interventions also hold the potential to increase disparities in health literacy, an equity issue it was hoped that eHealth could address.

A final consideration associated with the current state of eHealth promotion is the demand for adapting and developing research practices to suit the digital media context. While many new online research designs have been developed and implemented, they come with challenges associated with recruiting, enrolling, and retaining participants, thereby jeopardizing the power and significance of eHealth research (Lane, Armin, & Gordon, 2015). In addition, new ethical challenges arise for conducting online research, such as ensuring privacy, obtaining informed consent, and ensuring professionalism within the interventions (Dyer, 2001).

That eHealth promotion worldwide, and in Canada specifically, is beginning to demonstrate a positive effect is encouraging. However, it is important to keep in mind that, amidst the excitement over digital media as a much-needed solution to help address many areas of health behaviour change (e.g., diet, physical activity, sexual health), the fact remains that most digital media strategies employ a consumerist model that targets practices at the individual level. A key gap therefore remains in that these innovations do little to address the determinants of health inequities such as poverty, racism, and other structural influences that are shown to be key contributors to chronic illness, as well as people's ability to engage in "positive" and health-promoting practices. In this context, apps or e-interventions that adopt a more "upstream" approach to health promotion are virtually nil, with the exception of social media "movements" and virtual communities created by consumers and the lay public that raise awareness and advocate for health equity issues

Box 16.2: Position of the Consumer in Active Interventions

There is much excitement about the transition from passive to active interventions as mobile technologies continue to advance and become increasingly more intelligent (i.e., learning and automating user preferences), with demands for user input becoming less and less. It is important, however, that the push-pull nature required of these interventions (Kennedy et al., 2012) is carefully considered such that the user does not inadvertently become positioned as passive. It has been stressed in the literature that users should feel in control of the intervention (e.g., Gibbons et al., 2009), which raises some critical questions in relation to the continued development of eHealth interventions (e.g., When is an intervention too "heavy-handed" or intrusive? How can a balance between user and intervention control be established?) These are questions that only end-users can answer, a key evaluative component that is often overlooked.

(i.e., campaigns against racism or poverty, or for LGBTQ rights). However, a common limitation to both market- and user-driven online initiatives is that evaluation data and evidence of impact may be absent or not systematically collected.

PROMISING DIGITAL PRACTICES: EXAMPLES FROM YOUTH AND YOUNG ADULT TOBACCO CONTROL

Tobacco use remains one of the biggest public health concerns in Canada, particularly among youth and young adults, with smoking rates over 18 percent for young adults aged 20 to 34 years and just under 11 percent for youth aged 15 to 19 years (Reid, Hammond, Rynard, & Burkhalter, 2015). Efforts to address tobacco use for these groups have populated every media channel available, including the most recent avenues made available via digital media. Youth and young adults, traditionally hard-to-reach populations, may be particularly responsive to eHealth and mHealth initiatives since they are the largest adoptors of innovative technologies (Lenhart, 2015; Anderson, 2015). Delivering tobacco control initiatives via Web- and mobile-based technologies enables tobacco control programming to essentially meet young people where they are at, something that "traditional" tobacco control efforts had not been able to do, as reflected in the underutilization of such services by these populations (Lane, Leatherdale, & Ahmed, 2011; Suls et al., 2012). While evaluative evidence is still emerging, there are some promising developments in this area in Canada.

Web-Driven Initiatives

The Supporting Tailored Approaches to Reducing Tobacco (START) program is an example of how an online intervention was successfully employed to deliver tobacco control messages describing the link between second-hand smoke and breast cancer to youth aged 13 or older in Canada (Schwartz et al., 2014). Guided by health behaviour theory and the notion that puberty presents as a teachable moment for health behaviour change, brief Web-based infographic-style messages, tailored according to gender and Aboriginal status, were delivered to youth through the British Columbia Adolescent Substance Abuse Survey (BASUS) in 2011–2012. The development of these messages was informed by focus groups with the target youth populations (Bottorff et al., 2014). A prospective randomized controlled trial was used to evaluate the START messages, compared to a standard control message by Health Canada, among 618 non-smoking girls aged 13 to 15 years in 74 Canadian secondary schools six months after the delivery of the messages. The results revealed that girls who received the START messages were significantly more likely to report exposure to cigarette smoke as a possible cause of breast cancer and that being exposed to second-hand smoke increases their risk for breast cancer (Schwartz et al., 2014). The use of brief, tailored Web-based messages in this study demonstrates how the Internet can be harnessed to deliver health promotion messages as well as the importance of developing sensitive messages based on an understanding of youth perspectives (e.g., related to age, gender, and health issues) and the involvement of youth. Given that tailoring tobacco control materials to youth populations and delivering them through youth-friendly media (e.g., Internet) has been identified as the most promising strategy for approaching tobacco control among youth (Borland & Schwartz, 2010), the START messages provide a useful model.

Following the initial START study, a range of online resources were developed for youth, parents, and educators, including quizzes, YouTube videos, teaching guides, and factsheets, and were hosted on a website designed to appeal to youth. Youth-centred efforts like this are increasingly important to counter unregulated messages promoting the use of tobacco products online by the tobacco industry and pro-tobacco content shared by youth themselves (Struik, Bottorff, Jung, & Budgen, 2012; Richardson, Ganz, & Vallone, 2015; Richardson & Vallone, 2014).

In 2011–2012 a feasibility study was conducted to assess Picture Me Smokefree, an online tobacco reduction and cessation intervention for Canadian young adults that combined Facebook and digital photography (Haines-Saah, Kelly, Oliffe, & Bottorff, 2015). The design was underpinned by photovoice, whereby participants documented their tobacco use and cessation experiences via photography. Sixty young adult smokers aged 19 to 24 participated in the private online Facebook group for 12 consecutive weeks. Young adults reported an appreciation for the anonymous and easily accessible nature of the intervention, the peer-to-peer interaction, and the user-driven nature of the intervention. Many participants reported that this self-reflective and community-like experience helped in their reduction and cessation efforts. While recruitment and retention of young adult smokers proved challenging, Picture Me Smokefree is an example of how the interactive

Box 16.3: Digital Photo Methods in Health Promotion

In the mid-90s, Wang and colleagues (1998) from the University of Michigan School of Public Health pioneered the method of photovoice. The aim was to provide people with an opportunity to document and share their perspectives on local health and social issues through taking photographs and writing explanatory captions. The approach can be seen as a precursor to the now ubiquitous photo-posting, captioning, and sharing that takes place on social networks and on apps that stream live real-time video clips, digital technologies that are frequently used by health promoters and the lay public alike to share health-related content and campaigns online. Health promotion practitioners and researchers have also been early adopters of "digital storytelling" as a research and community mobilization practice. This method consists broadly of training and guiding users to create and share their own mini-documentaries (short video clips) using digital video editing. While images and digital stories shared online can be powerful for the creator and viewer alike, there is a need for care in their dissemination so that the content (and the story creator) is represented accurately and ethically.

features of social media (e.g., connecting with others, live newsfeeds, documenting, and posting) can be harnessed to positively engage young adults who smoke, a feat for tobacco control efforts directed towards this population. Not only was Picture Me Smokefree successful in reaching this population, but it was also successful in engaging them, which is key to behaviour change.

Mobile-Driven Initiatives

Not surprisingly, mHealth interventions have emerged as the fastest-growing area for smoking reduction and cessation, especially apps. Very few of the many cessation apps available, however, use evidence-based clinical practice guidelines (Abroms, Westmaas, Bontemps-Jones, Ramani, & Mellerson, 2013). It has been suggested, therefore, that apps that reflect clinical practice guidelines as well as behaviour change theories in their design may be able to produce higher quit rates (Bricker et al., 2014; Choi, Noh, & Park, 2014), and there is emerging evidence to support this (see, for example, Bricker et al., 2014).

Crush the Crave, a smartphone app directed towards young adult smokers (ages 19 to 29 years), is an example of a Canadian smoking cessation app targeting young adults that takes up both evidence and theory in its design (Baskerville et al., 2015), a first of its kind. Crush the Crave was developed in 2012 by a team of experts at the University of Waterloo and a media development team, and incorporated best practice guidelines for treating tobacco use and dependence, and principles of persuasive technology for behaviour change. Development of the app was also informed by the target end-users through the use of eight focus groups to establish functionality, look and feel, and usability. Crush the Crave, therefore, is one of the most comprehensive, evidence-informed apps to date and enables a variety of activities to mobilize young adults' quit smoking efforts, including a tailored quit plan, the ability to track and receive feedback on their tobacco use patterns, awards, access to information and distractions, and connection to others to share experiences and receive support (e.g., via social media). A prototype was pilot-tested by more than 300 smokers, and revealed substantial engagement. While results from the randomized controlled trial have yet to be published, the strong evidence base and use of theory presents Crush the Crave as a promising addition to tobacco control efforts targeting the largest population of smokers in Canada.

CONCLUSION

As this chapter has shown, there is the potential for both benefits and pitfalls with digital health promotion. While the research literature strikes a mostly positive tone about the capacity for eHealth and mHealth interventions to attract users and to increase health literacy by delivering content using interactive and innovative approaches, more evidence is still needed about whether or not digital interventions are effective for sustaining "real world" behavioural change outside of the contexts of intervention studies. Through our examples, we have provided illustrations of how "going digital" can provide health promotion with new technologies with which to engage so-called hard-to-reach populations, such as youth smokers, and may also have advantages for addressing health promotion topics that are potentially sensitive, such as encouraging people to get tested for sexually transmitted infections. Yet, as digital health promotion has largely focused on engagement and health behavioural change at the individual level, we should also be cautious that a focus on eHealth and mHealth does not shift too much attention from addressing core principles in health promotion, such as strengthening communities and building neighbourhood capacities for health, as well as focusing upstream on intervening on the social determinants of health and health inequities. Indeed, as access to health information and services increasingly shifts to delivery through online and mobile platforms, access to digital technology hardware, the affordability and reliability of Internet service provision, and capacity for e-literacy might also be considered determinants of health in their own right. Questions around "digital inequity" are complicated further by the issue of app development in mHealth, as this rapidly expanding domain of technology development has been driven by commercial industries that for the most part have been outside of health promotion research and practice. Therefore, to the extent that innovations in the field may be motivated by profit motives of private corporations rather than informed by research evidence of best practice, there are also possibilities for consumers to be misled, as the market becomes saturated with apps and online portals claiming they can improve health, but that are not necessarily supported by rigorous evaluation or informed by health promotion principles. As Lupton's (2015) critical theorizing on digitized health has cautioned, the advent of such technologies has resulted in a blurring of the boundaries between government strategies, commercial interests, and the work of professional health promotion, and brought with them concerns about the ways users' personal data is collected, monitored, and shared, which make it difficult to argue that eHealth and mHealth are not top-down practices that provide little space to empower consumers.

Although an in-depth examination was not possible within the scope of this chapter, a third arena at play in the digital health context are the organic, user-driven online campaigns and communities (some with charity or even profit-generating aspects themselves) that spring up around issues within the domain of health promotion. For example, beyond the use of mHealth apps, there are a range of different online settings where people interact around health and health behaviour change, such as message boards, group chats, and social media groups where users share information and experiences, and support other members. For example, in relation to mental health promotion engagement and activism online, "stigma-busting," peer supports, and suicide prevention has coalesced around well-known campaigns such as Live Through This and To Write Love on Her Arms (TWLOHA), both initiated by an individual with lived experience. In addition to their reach with users online, what is significant about these campaigns is that they can shift relatively quickly from ad-hoc online movements driven by a social media hashtag or blog post to include a more formal offline presence as non-profit organizations, especially when the people behind these campaigns emerge as advocates for public perception and policy change.

In that they often "talk back" to dominant approaches within the field, or aim to represent issues or people that may feel marginalized or misrepresented by mainstream health promotion, these user-driven movements can be empowering through promoting visibility (raising the profile of a health issue to the general public) and inclusion (connecting users who want to remain anonymous, or users from across disparate communities or geographic locations). While some such campaigns "go viral" and achieve a great deal of online and media attention, it may be difficult to measure the impact on changes in the public's perception of health issues and their potential to shift health behaviours, beyond their "raising awareness." Yet the experience is not always positive for everyone, as online campaigns also have potentially negative effects for their originators and users, in that they generate online harassment in the form of abusive and defamatory comments and backlash (known as cyberbullying and trolling) on users' sites and more broadly online. This is a particular concern with regards to sharing personal stories and imagery as posts to online communities, where there is the potential for users' accounts or posts to be hijacked, and material can be misrepresented and re-distributed without their consent.

Finally, there is also a more problematic aspect of how health promotion issues are taken up in online contexts by a lay public, in that online contexts provide virtual and viral contexts for the proliferation of health "myths" and misinformation such as unsupported claims about practices that promote health or fight illness (e.g., the "miracle cure" of the week). Perhaps even more worrisome is that the Internet is increasingly playing a major role in the growth and dissemination of controversial stances from activist groups (e.g., those opposed to vaccination or community water fluoridation) who use online platforms to rally support for activism that works *against* public health and health promotion. This may be the biggest challenge professional health promotion organizations will face from the digital realm going forward, in terms of leveraging their authority and capacity as trusted online sources, in order to compete against the rapid expansion of digital innovations from corporate sources, and to be heard amongst the din of voices—some perhaps health-promoting and some perhaps health-harming—that have been empowered through digital technologies and social media channels. While the shift to digital engagement requires that those working as researchers and practitioners in health promotion possess digital technology and social media skills—as well as an awareness of the online contexts where health promotion issues are taken up—the need to ground our work in the "offline" community and social contexts where health practices are shaped remains.

APPENDIX: GUIDE TO TERMS

Social Networking Sites: These are sites that are based on user-driven membership (profiles) for generating content and posting. Features of these sites allow users to form communities around shared interests and also to promote causes or products. Social networks have also emerged as a parallel news stream (hence the term *social media*), as channels or feeds for sharing images and video of social unrest or conflict zones, and making digital connections globally when an event occurs. While some social networking sites are used around the world, there is regional variation in terms of site popularity as well. For example, in North America Facebook dominates, and in China QZone and Sina Weibo are the most widely used. Instant messaging applications (such as WhatsApp or WeChat) are also sometimes referred to as social networks.

eHealth and mHealth: Broadly speaking, eHealth refers to all aspects of online, digital, and "electronic" health interventions and programs. Some of these programs refer to arenas where information is managed by health professionals, such as a system of electronic medical records (EMR) that is implemented across a health organization or system. By contrast, mHealth typically refers to user-driven mobile (smartphone or tablet) applications (apps).

The Digital Divide: This refers to the idea that online access has not always been equally distributed within contexts such as Canada, due to an uneven technology infrastructure and income constraints that keep digital devices out of reach. While the expansion of mobile Internet access through smartphones and tablets has made access less expensive and available to a broader swath of the population, access to high-quality broadband is still limited in rural and remote areas. More recently, the field has moved towards "digital equity" to represent the fact that, although many people have access to online technologies, digital literacy is lower for populations such as older adults and people with disabilities.

Trolls/Trolling: This label refers to the negative side of online behaviours. This can consist of deliberately inflammatory and often offensive and harassing comments and postings that can proliferate on online platforms, such as social networking, and in the context of comments posted to a blog or online news article. "Don't feed the trolls" is a frequently used call to ignore or to not spend a great deal of time in rebuttal with postings that are seen as "trolling" for a response.

CRITICAL THINKING QUESTIONS

1. How do we strike the right balance in health promotion between working digitally/ online and "real life" or face-to-face in order to effect health behaviour change and to create healthier communities?
2. Do you think there could be health equity implications related to a focus on consumer- or individually driven apps (mHealth) geared towards changing health behaviours?
3. How do user-driven health campaigns have the potential for both positive and negative consequences for participants, and for the representation of a group or issue (e.g., sharing potentially sensitive health information on social media)?

RESOURCES

Further Readings

Kreps, G. L., & Neuhauser, L. (2010). New directions in eHealth communication: Opportunities and challenges. *Patient Education and Counseling, 78*(3), 329–336.
A comprehensive description of the promise of digital media for health communication. The authors describe responsibilities to the consumer that must be met in order to actualize the promise.

Lupton, D. (2015). Health promotion in the digital era: A critical commentary. *Health Promotion International, 30*(1), 174–183.
This article provides a critical commentary on digitized health promotion and argues that digitized health promotion strategies focus on individual responsibility for health and fail to recognize the social, cultural, and political dimensions of digital technology use.

Norman, C. D., & Skinner, H. A. (2006). eHealth literacy: Essential skills for consumer health in a networked world. *Journal of Medical Internet Research, 8*(2), e9.
The authors assert the importance of paying attention to the eHealth literacy skills of potential consumers targeted by eHealth innovations.

RELEVANT WEBSITES

Crush the Crave
www.crushthecrave.ca
A Canadian mobile app for helping young adults quit smoking.

Immunization Canada
www.canimmunize.ca/en/home
A Canadian mobile app that provides information, scheduling, and recording of vaccinations.

Live Through This
livethroughthis.org
A website that brings forward a collection of portraits and stories of suicide attempt survivors, as told by those survivors.

QuitNow
quitnow.ca/
A Web-based program designed to help Canadians quit smoking.

QuitNow Men
men.quitnow.ca/
   A gender-specific version of QuitNow dedicated to helping men quit smoking.

Sex It Smart/Get Tested Why Not?
www.sexitsmart.com/
   An online condom campaign for Canadian youth.

START
start.ok.ubc.ca
   A Canadian website dedicated to raising awareness about the link between tobacco smoke and breast cancer risk.

To Write Love on Her Arms
twloha.com
   An American website dedicated to helping people who struggle with depression, addiction, self-injury, and suicide.

REFERENCES

Abroms, L. C., Westmaas, J. L., Bontemps-Jones, J., Ramani, R., & Mellerson, J. (2013). A content analysis of popular smartphone apps for smoking cessation. *American Journal of Preventive Medicine, 45*(6), 732–736.

Anderson, M. (2015, October). *Technology device ownership: 2015*. Washington, DC: Pew Research Center. Retrieved from www.pewinternet.org/2015/10/29/technology-device-ownership-2015

Baker, T. B., Gustafson, D. H., & Shah, D. (2014). How can research keep up with eHealth? Ten strategies for increasing the timeliness and usefulness of eHealth research. *Journal of Medical Internet Research, 16*(2), e36.

Baskerville, N. B., Struik, L. L., Hammond, D., Guindon, G. E., Norman, C. D., Whittaker, R., … Brown, K. S. (2015). Effect of a mobile phone intervention on quitting smoking in a young adult population of smokers: Randomized controlled trial study protocol. *JMIR Research Protocols, 4*(1), e10.

Baum, F., Newman, L., & Biedrzycki, K. (2014). Vicious cycles: Digital technologies and determinants of health in Australia. *Health Promotion International, 29*(2), 349–360.

Bergmo, T. S. (2015). How to measure costs and benefits of eHealth interventions: An overview of methods and frameworks. *Journal of Medical Internet Research, 17*(11), e254.

Best, A., Moor, G., Holmes, B., Clark, P. I., Bruce, T., Leischow, S., … Krajnak, J. (2003). Health promotion dissemination and systems thinking: Towards an integrative model. *American Journal of Health Behavior, 27*(Suppl. 3), S206–S216.

BinDhim, N. F., McGeechan, K., & Trevena, L. (2014). Assessing the effect of an interactive decision-aid smartphone smoking cessation application (app) on quit rates: A double-blind automated randomised control trial protocol. *BMJ Open, 4*(7), e005371.

Borland, T., & Schwartz, R. (2010). *The next stage: Delivering tobacco prevention and cessation knowledge through public health networks*. A literature review prepared by the Ontario Tobacco Research Unit for the Canadian Public Health Association. Ottawa: Canadian Public Health Association. Retrieved from www.cpha.ca/uploads/progs/substance/tobacco/cpha_litreview.pdf

Borrelli, B., Bartlett, Y. K., Tooley, E., Armitage, C. J., & Wearden, A. (2015). Prevalence and frequency of mHealth and eHealth use among US and UK smokers and differences by motivation to quit. *Journal of Medical Internet Research, 17*(7), e164.

Bottorff, J. L., Haines-Saah, R., Oliffe, J. L., Struik, L. L., Bissell, L. J., Richardson, C. P., ... Hutchinson, P. (2014). Designing tailored messages about smoking and breast cancer: A focus group study with youth. *CJNR (Canadian Journal of Nursing Research), 46*(1), 66–86.

Bottorff, J. L., Oliffe, J. L., Sarbit, G., Sharp, P., Caperchione, C. M., Currie, L. M., ... Stolp, S. (2016). Evaluation of QuitNow Men: An online, men-centered smoking cessation intervention. *Journal of Medical Internet Research, 18*(4), e83.

Bowes, J. (2016). Measles, misinformation, and risk: Personal belief exemptions and the MMR vaccine. *Journal of Law and the Biosciences, 3*(3), 718–725.

Bricker, J. B., Mull, K. E., Kientz, J. A., Vilardaga, R., Mercer, L. D., Akioka, K. J., & Heffner, J. L. (2014). Randomized, controlled pilot trial of a smartphone app for smoking cessation using acceptance and commitment therapy. *Drug and Alcohol Dependence, 143*, 87–94.

Carrot Insights. (2016). *Story*. Retried from www.carrotinsights.com/en/story/

Choi, J., Noh, G. Y., & Park, D. J. (2014). Smoking cessation apps for smartphones: Content analysis with the self-determination theory. *Journal of Medical Internet Research, 16*(2), e44.

Context Research. (2016). *Work*. BC Lung Association: QuitNow Management Program. Retrieved from www.contextresearch.ca/work/work/1.php

Dennison, L., Morrison, L., Conway, G., & Yardley, L. (2013). Opportunities and challenges for smartphone applications in supporting health behavior change: Qualitative study. *Journal of Medical Internet Research, 15*(4), e86.

Dyer, K. A. (2001). Ethical challenges of medicine and health on the Internet: A review. *Journal of Medical Internet Research, 3*(2), e23.

Eysenbach, G. (2001). What is e-health? *Journal of Medical Internet Research, 3*(2), e20.

Freeman, S. (2014, March 20). Canada's digital divide persists, CIRA report shows. *Huffington Post Canada*. Retrieved from www.huffingtonpost.ca/2014/03/20/digital-divide-canada-broadband-access_n_4995560.html

Gibbons, M. C., Wilson, R., Samal, L., Lehman, C. U., Dickersin, K., Lehmann, H. P., ... Bass, E. B. (2009). Impact of consumer health informatics applications. *Evidence Report/Technology Assessments, 188*, 1–546. Retrieved from www.ncbi.nlm.nih.gov/books/NBK32638/

Goodyear, L. (2016, February 8). Digital divide: Is high-speed internet access a luxury or a right? *CBC News*. Retrieved from www.cbc.ca/news/technology/internet-access-digital-divide-1.3433848

Haines-Saah, R. J., Kelly, M. T., Oliffe, J. L., & Bottorff, J. L. (2015). Picture Me Smokefree: A qualitative study using social media and digital photography to engage young adults in tobacco reduction and cessation. *Journal of Medical Internet Research, 17*(1), e27.

Immunize Canada. (2014, March 21). *A Canadian first: One-of-a-kind mobile app puts vaccination information in the hands of Canadians.* Ottawa: Immunize Canada. Retrieved from immunize.ca/sites/default/files/Resource%20and%20Product%20Uploads%20(PDFs)/Media%20and%20News%20Releases/2014/app-media-release_e.pdf

IMS Institute for Healthcare Informatics. (2015). *Patient adoption of mHealth—Availability and profile of consumer health care apps.* Danbury, CT: IMS Health Global Headquarters. Retrieved from www.imshealth.com/files/web/IMSH%20Institute/Reports/Patient%20Adoption%20of%20mHealth/mHealth-Apps-by-Category-2015.pdf

Jacobs, R. J., Lou, J. Q., Ownby, R. L., & Caballero, J. (2016). A systematic review of eHealth interventions to improve health literacy. *Health Informatics Journal, 22*(2), 81–98.

Kennedy, C. M., Powell, J., Payne, T. H., Ainsworth, J., Boyd, A., & Buchan, I. (2012). Active assistance technology for health-related behavior change: An interdisciplinary review. *Journal of Medical Internet Research, 14*(3), e80.

Lane, N. E., Leatherdale, S. T., & Ahmed, R. (2011). Use of nicotine replacement therapy among Canadian youth: Data from the 2006–2007 national youth smoking survey. *Nicotine & Tobacco Research, 13*(10), 1009–1014.

Lane, T. S., Armin, J., & Gordon, J. S. (2015). Online recruitment methods for web-based and mobile health studies: A review of the literature. *Journal of Medical Internet Research, 17*(7), e183.

Lenhart, A. (2015, April 9). *Teens, social media & technology overview 2015.* Washington, DC: Pew Research Center. Retrieved from www.pewinternet.org/2015/04/09/teens-social-media-technology-2015/

Lupton, D. (1995). *The imperative of health: Public health and the regulated body* (Vol. 90). London: Sage Publications.

Lupton, D. (2015). Health promotion in the digital era: A critical commentary. *Health Promotion International, 30*(1), 174–183.

Lupton, D. (2016). *The quantified self.* New Jersey: John Wiley & Sons.

Mann, T. A., Uddin, Z., Hendriks, A. M., Bouchard, C. J., & Etches, V. G. (2013). Get tested why not? A novel approach to internet-based chlamydia and gonorrhea testing in Canada. *Canadian Journal of Public Health, 104*(3), e205–e209.

Neuhauser, L., & Kreps, G. L. (2010). eHealth communication and behavior change: Promise and performance. *Social Semiotics, 20*(1), 9–27.

Norman, C. D., & Huerta, T. (2006). Knowledge transfer and exchange through social networks: Building foundations for a community of practice within tobacco control. *Implementation Science, 1*(1), 20.

Norman, C., McIntosh, S., Selby, P., & Eysenbach, G. (2008). Web-assisted tobacco interventions: Empowering change in the global fight for the public's (e) Health. *Journal of Medical Internet Research, 10*(5), e48.

Norman, C. D., & Skinner, H. A. (2006). eHealth literacy: Essential skills for consumer health in a networked world. *Journal of Medical Internet Research, 8*(2), e9.

Public Health Agency of Canada. (2014a, September). *The Chief Public Health Officer's report on the state of public health in Canada, 2014: Public health in the future.* Ottawa: Her Majesty the Queen in Right of Canada, as represented by the Minister of Health. Retrieved from www.phac-aspc.gc.ca/cphorsphc-respcacsp/2014/tech-eng.php

Public Health Agency of Canada. (2014b, March 21). *Fact sheet—Free mobile app helps Canadians keep track of their vaccinations.* Retrieved from www.phac-aspc.gc.ca/media/nr-rp/2014/2014_0320f-eng.php

Public Health Agency of Canada. (2016, March 3). Canada's first wellness rewards program launches in BC—New online app to reward users' healthy behaviour with popular loyalty points (News Release). Retrieved from news.gc.ca/web/article-en.do?nid=1037789&tp=1

Reid, J. L., Hammond, D., Rynard, V. L., & Burkhalter, R. (2015). *Tobacco use in Canada: Patterns and trends* (2015 ed.). Waterloo, ON: Propel Centre for Population Health Impact, University of Waterloo. Retrieved from tobaccoreport.ca/2015/TobaccoUseinCanada_2015_Accessible.pdf

Richardson, A., Ganz, O., & Vallone, D. (2015). Tobacco on the web: Surveillance and characterisation of online tobacco and e-cigarette advertising. *Tobacco Control, 24*(4), 341–347.

Richardson, A., & Vallone, D. M. (2014). YouTube: A promotional vehicle for little cigars and cigarillos? *Tobacco Control, 23*(1), 21–26.

Robinson, L., Cotten, S. R., Ono, H., Quan-Haase, A., Mesch, G., Chen, W., … Stern, M. J. (2015). Digital inequalities and why they matter. *Information, Communication & Society, 18*(5), 569–582.

Schwartz, J., Bottorff, J. L., Ratner, P. A., Gotay, C., Johnson, K. C., Memetovic, J., & Richardson, C. G. (2014). Effect of web-based messages on girls' knowledge and risk perceptions related to cigarette smoke and breast cancer: 6-month follow-up of a randomized controlled trial. *Journal of Medical Information Research Protocols, 3*(3), e53.

Struik, L., Bottorff, J. L., Jung. M., & Budgen, C. (2012). Reaching adolescent girls through social networking: A new avenue for smoking prevention messaging. *Canadian Journal of Nursing Research, 44*(3), 84–103.

Suls, J. M., Luger, T. M., Curry, S. J., Mermelstein, R. J., Sporer, A. K., & An, L. C. (2012). Efficacy of smoking-cessation interventions for young adults: A meta-analysis. *American Journal of Preventive Medicine, 42*(6), 655–662.

Valaitis, R., Hunter, D., Lam, A., Murray, N., Spark, R., & Valaitis, R. F. (2014, February 24). *Technology to encourage the adoption of health promoting/protecting behaviours: A comprehensive literature review* (Prepared for the Public Health Agency of Canada). Unpublished.

Wang, C. C., Yi, W. K., Tao, Z. W., & Carovano, K. (1998). Photovoice as a participatory health promotion strategy. *Health Promotion International, 13*(1), 75–86.

World Health Organization (WHO). (2016, June). *Tobacco (Fact sheet).* Retrieved from www.who.int/mediacentre/factsheets/fs339/en/

PART III

CRITICAL REFLECTIVE PRACTICE IN HEALTH PROMOTION

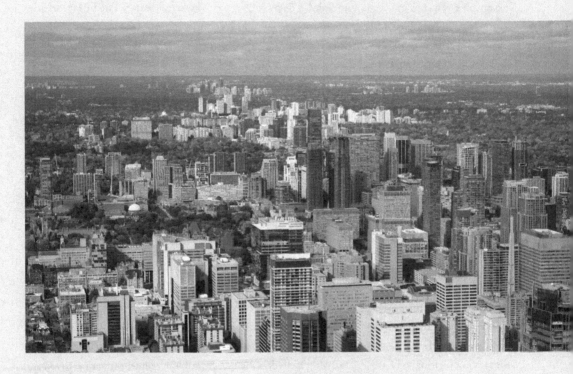

In Part III, we turn to a critical element in twenty-first century health promotion, that of reflective practice. Reflective practice has been introduced into health promotion as a means of generating knowledge from experience for the improvement of practice and research. In fact, reflective practice can be conceived of as an intended and conscious intellectual investigation in which individuals (or groups) question their experiences to develop new understandings and knowledge that are ultimately reinvested to transform their actions. In this part of the book we use reflective practice as a jumping-off point for discussions about a wide set of topics, including health promotion ethics, participatory practice, the Anthropocene, and promoting health in a globalized world.

In chapter 17, Boutilier and Mason kick off the section by giving the contours of what is known as reflexivity and reflective practice. They signal several themes inherent to this form of practice; power relations and the messiness of collaborative work are a few. These themes are then picked up by many of the authors in this section. Boutilier and Mason offer advice on why and how health promotion practitioners (whether their job is in intervention, research, policy-making, or even teaching contexts) would benefit from being reflexive about it, providing some practical hands-on examples.

Chapter 18 by Shankardass, Hemsing, and Greaves is about what has been called "health in all policies" (HiAP). This approach to addressing the matter of "healthy public policy" advocated in the *Ottawa Charter for Health Promotion* though intersectoral action has recently been advocated and adopted by progressive governments. The chapter elaborates on the intersectoral nature of HiAP, provides a historical account of the concept, and describes examples of its use in Canada and globally, as well as some key challenges. The latter includes improving the understanding and measurement of an economic argument for HiAP and generating a critical workforce in policy-making.

In chapter 19 by Potvin, a long-time leader in health promotion in Canada and the editor of the *Canadian Journal of Public Health*, she argues that because health promotion is an action-oriented field it lacks direction in research and has borrowed from many other disciplines. She suggests that the new and emerging field of population health intervention research (PHIR) "may serve as a starting point to develop and promote a research agenda that would support health-promoting practice." Based on her analysis in the chapter, she concludes that a large part of PHIR is directly relevant to health promotion, but that there are "some problem/related research topics that need to be addressed by health promotion" (e.g., positive health, empowerment, and participation) that do not necessarily have to be linked to intervention research.

In chapter 20, Knight and Shoveller address a relatively new and growing topic that is all too often forgotten in health promotion practice—its ethical dimension. They introduce the burgeoning area of health promotion ethics and underscore myriad reasons why health promotion practitioners and researchers should be concerned with the ethical ramifications of their everyday practice. They demonstrate that health promotion, being an area of intervention (largely by the state) on people, is compelled to address tensions by identifying the best (i.e., the most ethical) relationship between the individual, the community, and the state. Issues such as the means by which health promotion *can* (empirically) and *should* (ethically) address the tensions that occur between a variety of values, including freedom and paternalism, education and persuasion, coercion and liberty, autonomy and social justice, are discussed. In so doing, Knight and Shoveller delineate what makes health promotion ethics a field distinct from bioethics, or other forms of medical ethics, and makes a plea for the further development of this area in health promotion scholarship and practice.

In chapter 21, Springett and Masuda use reflexivity to explore what they call transformative participation, which, in contrast to "practical" participation, begins where people are, rather than where we desire them to be. They describe a process of participation that endeavours to confront the power relations normally present in health promotion practice and evaluation by encouraging respectful dialogue between health promotion practitioners/researchers and those they aim to serve, along with joint critical reflection. Participatory health promotion puts the "relational" at the centre of the work for social change, valuing trust, reciprocity, diversity, mutual respect, dignity, and equality as well as focusing on the processes of co-learning and consciousness-raising to shift power relations. They conclude with three case studies of participatory practice that illustrate their position.

In chapter 22, Hancock makes a timely plea for health promotion to "take off the blinders" and engage with issues confronting the planet's environment based on the notion of the Anthropocene, the epoch in which we live, defined as one in which human activities have made a significant global impact on the Earth's geology and ecosystems. He makes an impassioned argument that we need to go back to the *Ottawa Charter* and adopt a socio-ecological approach to health, or what is now more often called an eco-social approach. Hancock gives a full explanation of what the Anthropocene entails and the importance of shifting our thinking in health promotion, bringing an end to the separation of the ecological from the social and encouraging more interdisciplinary work with disciplines such as ecology, urban planning, and others.

In chapter 23, Labonté muses on changes having taken place in the context of health promotion since the first edition of this book, namely the globalization of health. He enumerates the massive changes that have taken place in the last 20-plus years including global pandemics and the worldwide spread of health problems such as obesity through the corporate infusion of unhealthy Western commodities. Labonté details both globalization's successes and failures from a health perspective, giving greater weight to the latter and arguing that neo-liberalism's effects on health will continue to be deeply problematic if certain steps are not taken at a global level. As with all of the authors of this section, Labonté ends with the suggestion that health promotion lead the way in being reflexive about how our political economy affects the health of our population (including the widening of inequities) and work towards a more equitable and salubrious society.

The final chapter, written by the editors, reflects on the content of the book and offers the editors' thoughts on what the future of health promotion may look like, bearing in mind factors that will impact on the development of health promotion in Canada and elsewhere. Finally, the book closes with an afterword by Ronald Labonté that challenges health promoters to strengthen their efforts and voices to address the important issues that affect the health and wellbeing of people in Canada and around the world.

At the end of this third part, the reader will have reflected on several key dimensions important for the practice of health promotion and, hopefully, will have seen, in a reflexive way, how this can have an impact on his or her own current or future practice.

CHAPTER 17

The Reflexive Practitioner in Health Promotion: From Reflection to Reflexivity

Marie Boutilier and Robin Mason[1]

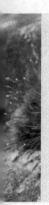

LEARNING OBJECTIVES

1. Understand and distinguish between reflection, reflection in action, and reflective practice
2. Be familiar with some tools/strategies to support reflective practice
3. Recognize the ways in which reflection in action can be used to improve health promotion activities and programs
4. Understand how reflection may illuminate professional relationships, group dynamics, power hierarchies, and one's own practice

INTRODUCTION

When we were invited to write this chapter on reflective practice in health promotion, we expected to draw heavily upon our previous experience and writings to distill lessons and guidelines for others. Now, as we finish, we are reminded of how risky it is to act on assumptions at a project's beginnings. Upon reflection, we have found that we brought different disciplines, questions, and writing styles to this project, and this has led us to examine reflexivity in health promotion as both a solitary and collaborative process, practised within different modes and mediums. In this chapter we review some understandings of and foci for reflection, and focus on the "how to" of reflective practice in health promotion in different modes—verbal and visual—and the ways in which our own reflections might shed light on the reflective process for others.

CYCLES AND SPIRALS: REFLECTION AND REFLECTIVE PRACTICE

Historically, reflection was initially defined as the "active persistent and careful consideration of any belief or supposed form of knowledge in the light of the grounds which support it" (Dewey, 1933, p. 118), emerging from a state of doubt and involving "the kind of thinking that consists in turning a subject over in the mind and giving it serious thought" (Moon, 1999, p. 12). In this model, reflection is a cycle that concludes with the testing or evaluation of a determined action and then begins again—the inspiration for Lewin's (1946) spiral of action research. Later, Schön (1983) recognized that in the action of real-life problem solving, professionals must "reflect *in* action" when faced with complex problems. Thoughtful experimentation becomes part of the process of problem solving—a form of "research"—occurring in an iterative and cyclical process.

The act of questioning and experimenting with strategies occurs in an ongoing cyclical process until the question is reframed (often in collaboration with others) and change occurs. Not only does reflection expand the professional's tacit knowledge tool kit for problem-solving, it can contribute to theory development, self-development, decision-making, empowerment, and other outcomes that are unexpected as new ideas or images are applied in practice (Moon, 1999). In addition, it serves as a preventive process in being drawn into repetitive and routine thinking and solutions, missed opportunities, and boredom or burnout (Schön, 1983).

There is the risk that reflexivity may become too inward-looking, self-absorbed, and over-individualized in "hermeneutic narcissism" (Maton, 2003), losing its intent of transformative knowledge development. It can "become a disembodied process because it involves turning ourselves into objects of study" (Cunliffe & Easterby-Smith, 2003, p. 34). Or, "the often lofty theoretical justifications for greater reflexivity can manifest themselves as a license to write about our most beloved topic—ourselves ... shad[ing] into personal therapy" (Haggerty, 2003, p. 159). In plain language, the risk is that our reflexive undertakings will focus on our personal emotions and psyches rather than being accompanied by critical analysis of our practice and its context. Haggerty points out that the assumption of self-awareness requisite to reflexivity sidesteps the truism (following Freud) that we cannot be fully aware of our assumptions and, in reflexivity, we may unwittingly "rationaliz[e] unconscious motivations and prejudices" (Haggerty, 2003, p. 159). For this reason, we offer the caveat that reflexivity is meant to focus largely on professional practice, with some boundaries drawn by the individual between personal and professional issues. This is integral to "professionalism" for most people and becomes more or less intuitive, but is a point that bears articulation.

For health promoters, the challenges for reflection are found in the combination of collaboration, multidisciplinary strategies, and values (including a professional ethic of service to communities), all practised within the context of the employing organization. When health promotion entails evaluation research, it draws on professional training, but can also be grist for reflection and creativity.

FOCI FOR REFLECTION IN HEALTH PROMOTION: POWER AND COLLABORATION

Health promotion practice often requires the "messiness" of collaboration. Collaboration is seldom defined, but involves working across differences of discipline, culture, community, and practice. Challenges to collaboration include power, expertise, and control (Gondolf,

Box 17.1: "What If?" Questions for Individual and Collaborative Reflection

The most important question that professionals ask might be "What if?" (Schön, 1983, p. 145). The question opens the door to creativity, artistic strategies, tacit knowledge, and "the swampy lowlands." Consider what questions could be asked in your reflections that highlight issues of values, discipline-based knowledge, tacit knowledge, resources, power, and collaborations in health promotion. These questions can be asked individually or collaboratively.

Examples of "what if" questions about collaborations include the following:

- What if different partners had collaborated? Who else should be here?
- What if you, for example, lived in this neighbourhood, had a child at this school, or worked in this hospital? How would the issue change for you?
- What if all the collaborators were employed by the same organization? Shared visible characteristics (e.g., race, gender, ability)? Had the same medical health issue? Lived in your neighbourhood? How do these differences shape our perspectives?
- What if all of your collaborators were at the same professional level, or paid the same amount as you are? Would it change the power dynamics?
- What if the collaborators don't share the same language? What if they are uncomfortable with writing? What images would capture the project vision? The process? How do partners' visions differ and what is shared? Why?
- What if you had been guided by a different theory or a different discipline-based training? What would you have done differently? Would the process and outcome be different? What have you read or heard about that is similar?
- What if you were to be engaged in this project for years to come? How would you feel? How would that change your strategies?
- What if you met in a different place? On different "turf"? How does place and space affect your collaboration?
- What if you had a different form of reporting about your project? For example, what would you emphasize in a documentary film on your project? In a play or short story? What is the narrative?
- What if you were working on a very short-term contract? What if you worked from home? What if you had a permanent job? How does career ambition and/or tenure colour some of your and your collaborators' perspectives?
- What and who are your most helpful resources? What are the biggest challenges?
- What if you were asked to do this again? Would you do it differently?

Yllo, & Campbell, 1997; Rovegno & Bandhauer, 1998; Boutilier, Cleverly, & Labonté, 2000); different work cultures, language of practice, time constraints, and outcome expectations (Buckeridge et al., 2002); and discipline and institutional expectations (Mason & Boutilier, 1996). The current acceptance of "professional-community collaboration" has led to "new roles" in community health (e.g., community trainers), with complex relationships negotiated around differences in power, skills, and understanding, and requiring increasingly critical reflection on the "messiness" of collaborative work (Dugdill, Coffey, Coufopoulos, Byrne, & Porcellato, 2009). Regular individual and collective engagement in the process of reflection can help bring problematic or contentious issues to light, while honest commitment to the process also supports the development of trust in the individuals and organizations participating in the collaboration.

While reflective practice is usually an individual activity, the collaborative and interprofessional practices common in health promotion also lend themselves to reflection as a collaborative activity (O'Neill & Dupéré, 2006). Collaborative reflection involves collective consideration of issues, actions, and questions, including those that affect group interactions (Barr, 2005). Collaborative reflection offers the possibility of creating effective, successful working relationships, but requires investments of time, energy, and trust. As some caution, "rigourous [*sic*] reflection, especially when done in a process of social interaction with others, can be both exhilarating and painful. The question is, 'can collaborations succeed without it?'" (Bray, Lee, Smith, & Yorks, 2000, p. 11).

When individuals engage in reflective practice, they deliberately examine their situations, behaviour, practices, and effectiveness within specific situations *after the fact*, so they become wiser at working within the complex and dynamic world of practice. Experienced professionals also engage in reflection *during action*, forming judgments, acting and reacting in the moment on the basis of past experience and learning—Schön's "reflection-in-action" (1983). When decisions are made on the basis of experience and the aims, means, and context are considered against the actual situation and probable outcomes, however, reflection may be considered to have begun *before the action* (Clarke, James, & Kelly, 1996). This kind of reflection also builds on learnings from previous projects, merging with reflection-in-action. Not to be taken lightly are the resources needed for both kinds of reflective practice: the time and space to ask questions and speculate upon the answers.

MOVING BEYOND PROJECTS: BECOMING A REFLECTIVE HEALTH PROMOTION PRACTITIONER

In this section we will explore some of the tools that can assist in becoming a reflexive practitioner. The literature offers some examples of how to begin, including: role-playing, video or audiotaping practice sessions, utilizing client feedback, and working with peer or mentor supervision (Evans, 1997; Kottkamp, 1990). There are also resources in participatory research evaluations that will also often apply to health promotion, such as group reflections and storytelling (Labonté & Feather, 1996; Ellis, Reid, & Barnsley, 1990).

The most frequently used and easily accessible tool for health promoters is writing (Health Promotion Resource System, 2010). Writing is a powerful tool for learning from and reflecting upon experience. First, the act of writing itself engages both hand and brain integrating the right and left hemispheres in the action. Second, the physical act of converting thoughts into words upon a page demands the slowing down of thought; it allows for moving back into the past and invites musing about the future. While writing, we can pause the action, go back and revisit a thought, consider options and reformulate a sentence; in this way writing is itself often a reflective process (Kottkamp, 1990).

There is also an increasing interest in the relationship between art and health, reflecting understandings both of different modes of learning and knowing, and of the mind-body relationship as seen, for example, in the online *International Journal of the Creative Arts in Interdisciplinary Practice* (www.ijcaip.com). Recent commentaries on Schön's work on reflective practice highlight the new strategies and professional roles in health, which endeavour to reflect and collaborate with communities (Dugdill et al., 2009), and construct new narratives drawing on arts-based knowledge (Bold & Chambers, 2009). Thus, apart from written journals, "new conversations" are emerging in different modes of professional reflection (Overby, 2009). These include photography (Bhosekar, 2009; Lemon, 2007), drawing-based journals (Tokolahi, 2010; Deaver & McAuliffe, 2009), other visual documentations (Jaruszewica, 2006), spatial poetics and imagery (McIntosh, 2008), weblogs (Hagerman, 2010; Sharma, 2010), and can be individual or collaborative (O'Neill & Dupéré, 2006). Visual modes of reflection are also appropriate where community members need to reflect but are reluctant to write (Ghaye et al., 2008), or in cultural contexts where visual images better articulate reflections, or where access to and use of pens and papers are problematic (Williams, 2009).

Writing, Writing, Writing ...

There are different forms that writing can take, including diaries, case records, or journals. While a diary is a list of daily activities with little space set aside for review of those activities, a case record contains detailed description of specific situations or projects. Kottkamp (1990) describes a case record as based on a problematic situation that includes responses to basic questions about the nature of the situation, the action taken, the alternatives considered, and the hoped-for outcomes. Another useful layout involves a factual description of an event in one column and later reflections in a second column (Moon, 1999), akin to reflection on action. Journal writing shares features with case records, but expands the scope of reflection beyond problematic situations.

A journal contains the ongoing consideration of the individual in relation to others, the emotions evoked, the values in harmony or collision, and the skills possessed or wanting, in addition to questions about specific situations, the actions taken, the alternatives considered, and the hoped-for outcomes. A journal may contain conversations, poetry, drawings, or songs that assist in making thoughts or feelings clear.

Box 17.2: Aids to Written Reflection

- Questioning what, why, and how one does things
- Asking what, why, and how others do things
- Seeking alternatives
- Keeping an open mind
- Comparing and contrasting
- Seeking the framework theoretical basis or underlying rationale
- Viewing from varying perspectives
- Asking for others' ideas and viewpoints
- Using prescriptive models only when adapted to the situation
- Considering consequences
- Hypothesizing
- Synthesizing and testing
- Seeking, identifying, and resolving problems

Source: Roth, R. (1989). Preparing the reflective practitioner: Transforming the apprentice through the dialectic. *Journal of Teacher Education, 40*(2), 31–35.

In addition to the descriptive documentation of situations and events, alternatives considered, and possible outcomes had these been followed, the journal includes a critical analysis of the political context in which actions unfold, one's knowledge, skills, expertise, values, and assumptions. It becomes the means by which observing, questioning, critiquing, synthesizing, and acting are integrated into daily practice, or reflection-in-action. From reflecting on the specifics of a project or problematic situation and in the midst of making choices in daily practice, one shifts into reflection as a way of encountering the world.

To begin journaling, one should set aside a block of time. Many find it works best to begin the entry with the date, place, and a summary of a specific situation, activity, or focus of reflection. Consider issues and questions such as the "What if" ones noted above. Emotional reactions are important considerations in that reality. If reflecting on a specific event or situation, consider the emotions related to the entry, during the situation and now, upon reflection.

Reflections Past and Present: Journals and Diagrams

In writing this chapter we have inevitably reflected on our own reflective processes. One of us (RM) is a fairly consistent journal writer while the other (MB) uses journals more selectively and more often engages in diagrams that map out relationships and ideas, leading to decisions and strategies. We offer below examples drawn from our own reflections.

Journal Reflections (RM)

My career path has taken me to work in community social service settings, research centres, and a hospital. I have worked collaboratively on projects to address local hunger, youth unemployment, newcomer settlement issues, an organizational policy on intimate partner violence (IPV), and curriculum development. I have frequently found journaling a useful way of organizing my thoughts and experiences. In the excerpts below, written during a collaborative initiative focused on integrating education on IPV into a hospital setting, I consider the "place" and "ownership" of education in the larger hospital environment. At the time, I was the facilitator of an ad-hoc group of front-line practitioners who decided to design and disseminate across the hospital a curriculum on IPV to improve care for patients who had experienced abuse. However, within the larger institutional structure,

Box 17.3: Case Study: Reflections on a Practical Situation

May 30, 2001

Our group won an award for medical education. What a boost this was to group morale. And [it was] a lot of fun to get to go out to the award dinner. A number of people [named] stopped to congratulate the group. This should make it somewhat harder for them (the senior hospital administrators) to ignore us or take the program from us to Organizational Development as has been suggested via the rumour mill. Dr. A.A. said we should know there was tremendous support behind us. I don't know if this means behind the award or for the program itself.

June 12, 2001

The politics could kill you or, kill the project. Last week (June 7) at a formal meeting of [managers], Dr. B.B. quickly presented a series of overheads on women's health indicators for the hospital—one of which was based on the policy our group had developed—the indicator was a projected 75 percent of staff as attending one of our trainings. She turned to me and asked if I had anything to say. There had been no consultation or invitation to comment on the plan before the meeting and I was taken by surprise. Certainly in the wake of the earlier meeting it helped explain why they want to roll it out through the Organizational Development office. Our group doesn't have the support or resources to achieve 75 percent attendance. After the meeting I wrote her a note explaining how process, content, and values drive our project and the difficulties inherent in making it a mandatory program. Have to wait and see if there's a response. Then yesterday, C.C. came to see me from [a community organization] and told me that our formalizing education and trying to expand the training to organizations outside the hospital would create animosity and divisiveness among other hospitals and organizations.... Frustrating ... we wanted to share it with others, but it's just too competitive around funding and resources. I need to stay focused on the issue—helping and providing services to women. I think I better pull back from the community a bit and stay focused on the internal dissemination.

our group—and thus the project—were vulnerable; there was no funding for the group or the education program we had developed, no clear lines for reporting or accountability, and our group did not appear on any organizational chart. While I was a salaried employee and represented the group at meetings, neither my job title nor role profile included this group or the educational initiative; nor did any of the other members have "educator" listed in their role profiles or job responsibilities. However, there was an organizational policy that stated that responding to disclosures of IPV was everyone's responsibility, and that the institution was required to provide the education to support staff. So our group operated in a grey area both within and outside the traditional professional hierarchies and institutional structures. The policy said that staff members were to be educated about the issue, but no one had said that it was our group that should be fulfilling that mandate.

In order to preserve the anonymity of those to whom I refer in the journal, names and other identifiers have been removed. The original entries are marked by the border.

In rereading these two excerpts I am aware now of the responsibility I felt for ensuring our group's collaborative way of working was upheld in the face of a sometimes overwhelming bureaucracy and hierarchy. I believed an enormous trust had been placed in me to represent and speak out for the group; it was as their representative that I found my power and courage to speak out in meetings with senior administrators. Representing the group also meant becoming highly attuned to (and even preoccupied by) the organizational politics and power dynamics. As an insider/outsider (a status achieved by default because the lines of reporting were unclear) I was afforded more power than other group members—for example, I did attend the same meetings as those who made key decisions for the organization—yet I had no access to the resources or infrastructure to help our group achieve its goals.

I also remember how conflicts with community partners added to my general frustration. As the first line of the second excerpt shows, I was exasperated by the politicking, which seemed to govern every aspect of my daily work life. In rereading this excerpt now, I recognize how reconciled I have become to the politics surrounding practice. The issue itself (IPV) is a politically sensitive one and those who work on it, particularly in hospital environments, are not usually accorded the support or recognition afforded those who specialize in other health issues. On the community side, the tension between comparatively well-resourced hospitals and poorly resourced community partners continues, although in my community we have developed ways of collaborating and supporting each other's work. I believe too that these collaborations have resulted in better understanding on each side of the demands and constraints of working in these very different sectors.

Visual Reflection (MB)
There are many modes of visual reflection, but diagramming with simple pen and paper, similar to journal writing, is accessible to most health promoters. Reflections need not follow a prescribed format, but it may be helpful to observe how diagrams change and evolve over time within a project. My own diagrams often take on a "layering" effect

over time, with expanded relationships and understandings eventually consistent with the spiral metaphor.

Rather than the traditional path of doctorate to academic post, my career has focused solely on research in different capacities and in a range of organizations and working arrangements. My written professional reflections have been somewhat sporadic and I have moved in and out of practice reflections, depending on the projects I worked on, stages of the projects, whether I am employed or working in a volunteer capacity, and the urgency of other dimensions of my life. My reflections have thus incorporated the logistics and "political economy of research," that is, how the structures of the university mesh with research funding models and the division of labour in research (McQueen, 1994). This contingent nature of formal written reflections may hold for many people—the need for written reflection subsides when work is more or less routine, but a crisis or a decision point will stimulate the reflective process. The irony of this is that it is at these moments of possible crises that the time needed for reflection is in short supply.

As seen in Figure 17.1, my reflections often take the form of charting ideas and building models that first lay out and then link different dimensions of projects and issues. This reflective process goes through stages, with early diagrams having arrows flying in all directions as issues, collaborators, and readings are all brought together. Stepping back to look at the initial collage of ideas, organizations, interests, and so on leads to second or third diagrams that are cleaner and more legible. At this point it is often helpful to share the diagram with a colleague and work on it iteratively until we reach some conclusion or decision. Bringing in "fresh eyes" then helps us to understand where interests and perspectives intersect and diverge, and where possible future action lies, possibly building models or narratives to assess and guide the project.

The diagram included here was intended to capture relationships in a participatory research project and requires contextualization. It was an early diagram, drawn late in the project, trying to distill "lessons learned" for a conference presentation (Boutilier et al., 1995). I was a research associate with a health promotion research unit, North York Community Health Promotion Research Unit (NYCHPRU), itself a partnership of the local public health unit and the University of Toronto. The project included a group of unemployed young people from Toronto's Jane-Finch neighbourhood who worked on federally funded literacy projects with Frontier College. NYCHPRU's Community Action Research Group (CARG) included two academics, named on the diagram: Irv (Rootman) and Ann (Robertson), nursing managers, two public health nurses, and Robin (Mason). The arrows indicate relationships and directions of influence and power.

Looking back, first, I remember how complex and exhilarating the project was, partly due to the non-academic emotional elements the young people brought—noted on the diagram as "anger, hope, and play." While Robin and I initially came to meetings ready to "work," we soon learned they needed time to joke around and "play" before talking about the research, which included expressions of anger and hope for change. Second, I notice the arrows from Frontier College are labelled "support" rather than

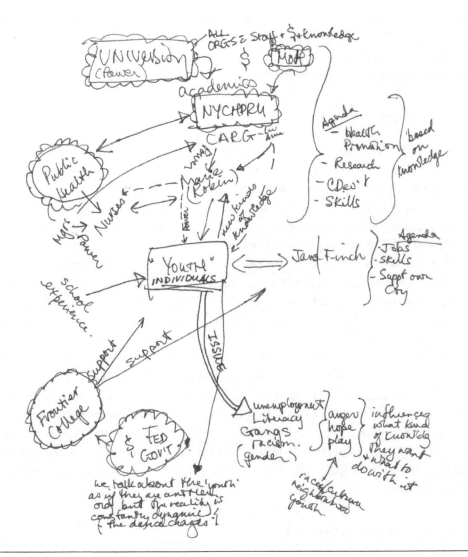

Figure 17.1: Reflective Diagram

"power" and now wish I had explored the dynamic of that distinction more at the time. Finally, Robin's name was in brackets because her involvement lasted several months on a student contract basis. In my mind it partially exempted her from some of the power dynamics and gave her a more neutral perspective. I now reflect that since then, I have been on contracts so I may be "bracketed" on research teams and power relationships, leading me to ask how that generates unique contributions to other projects. Thinking further about how this influenced my health promotion "practice," this project directly led to my observation that there are four "arenas" of health promotion practice: health and social services; community activism; policy (Boutilier, Cleverly, & Labonté, 2000); the fourth being research itself, especially when it is participatory (Boutilier, 1996). The question remains for research as health promotion practice: How is "insider/outsider" status conferred in different spheres, e.g., am I an intellectual "insider" but an "outsider" to organizational politics, and how are specific interests (health-related, political, intellectual, social) integrated in each project?

CONCLUSIONS

We have examined health promotion reflection, how to reflect, and considered how the process of reflection can illuminate relationships, power, hierarchies, and improve practice. Reflection is integral to the repertoire of knowledge and understanding of what it means to promote health in a context of multiple interests. It becomes a key resource for health promoters as they develop expertise over time, becoming a part of one's professional identity and way of being a reflexive practitioner.

On reflection, the writing of this chapter itself has shaped our representation of reflexivity. While emphasizing the principles and values outlined in the *Ottawa Charter*, we are mindful of the practice of health promotion as lived experience for professionals committed to the health of the communities they serve. Reflection requires resources and facilitators, not the least of which is time.

We have focused on health promoters, but the processes of reflective practice described here apply to professional work in general. In health promotion, the importance of collaboration begs the question of whether processes and foci of reflection and reflexivity may differ across disciplines and professions, as influenced by their respective assumptions and values. While we see collaborative reflection as part of the health promotion reflective process, each individual and health promotion initiative will be unique according to the diversity of individual, interests, organizations, values, personalities, and goals involved.

Afterword: Further Reflections

Prior to beginning work on this chapter, it had been several years since our last professional collaboration. In the interim we had each worked on other projects and in new collaborative relationships. In starting to work together again we found we could not immediately take up where we last left off. We found that we were challenged to re-examine our assumptions about our professional identities and ways of working together. We learned that we had benefited in different ways from our diverse experiences and now came together with new tacit knowledge that needed articulation for this new endeavour. Predictably, we required time and had to create a space in which to reflect, individually and together, in order to collaborate on this chapter. We recognize that the time and space to creatively explore and articulate ideas are critical in facilitating reflexivity.

CRITICAL THINKING QUESTIONS

1. What are the underlying disciplines that form the bases of the knowledge and theoretical frameworks with which you frame questions and issues in health promotion?
2. What is the difference between reflecting on an issue and becoming a reflexive professional?
3. If you were to organize a collaborative reflection process, who would you involve? How would it happen? What questions would you start with?
4. What values are important to you in your work/professional life? Can you imagine a situation in which these are challenged in your work? What would be your first steps in working through it?
5. If you were designing a type 2 diabetes educational initiative for an urban hospital setting, which stakeholders representing which interests would you consider as you developed your program? Who would be the target audience for the program? If you were designing a similar program for a low-income housing complex, which stakeholders representing which interests would you need to consider? In what ways would the program change depending upon where it was being delivered?

RESOURCES

Further Readings

Gould, J., & Nelson, J. (2005). Researchers reflect from the cancer precipice. *Reflective Practice, 6*(2), 277–284.
Two researchers at a cancer research unit reflect together about the difficult emotional issues involved in working with cancer patients, power relations, and privilege, as well as facets of identity—race, class, gender, cultural capital, and personal biography.

McIntosh, P. (2010). *Action research and reflective practice: Creative and visual methods to facilitate reflection and learning*. London: Routledge.
Part one provides a historical overview of evidence-based medicine, and argues that evidence-based practice and research in health and social services must evolve to incorporate reflection; part two offers philosophical and practical guidance.

Reynolds, M., & Vince, R. (Eds.). (2004). *Organizing reflection*. Aldershot: Ashgate Publishing Ltd.
This collection examines reflection as important in organizational development. It applies reflection to communities of practice, collective reflection, critical reflection, and reflexivity; it also includes discussions of power relations, experience, and emotions.

Schön, D. (1983). *The reflective practitioner: How professionals think in action*. Boston: Basic Books.

This seminal work in the literature on reflective practice provides a "sociology of knowledge" approach to expertise and expert power. It rests on meticulous case studies of how professionals learn; its historical perspective maintains it as a paradigm-shaping work and a continuing resource for professionals, their teachers, and managers.

Relevant Website

ItsLife
www.itslifejimbutnotasweknowit.org.uk/RefPractice.htm
   UK teacher education site; extensive bibliography on reflective practice.

NOTE

1.   Authorship is alphabetical.

REFERENCES

Barr, C. (2005). *Effective interprofessional education: Arguments, assumptions, and evidence*. Oxford: Blackwell.

Bhosekar, K. (2009). Using photographs as a medium to create spaces for reflective learning. *Reflective Practice, 10*(1), 91–100.

Bold, C., & Chambers, P. (2009). Reflecting meaningfully, reflecting differently. *Reflective Practice, 10*(1), 13–26.

Boutilier, M. (1996). *The effectiveness of community action in health promotion: A research perspective*. International Symposium on the Effectiveness of Health Promotion, European Office of the World Health Organization, Toronto.

Boutilier, M., Cleverly, S., & Labonté, R. (2000). Community as a setting for health promotion. In B. Poland, I. Rootman, & L. Green (Eds.), *Settings for health promotion* (pp. 250–279). Thousand Oaks: Sage Publications.

Boutilier, M., & Mason, R. (1994). Paper presented at Health and Behaviour 1994, Queen's University, Kingston, March 1994.

Boutilier, M., Mason, R., Rootman, I., Robertson, A., Bresolin, L., Panhuysen, N., … Marz, C. (1995). Can the 2-step become a square dance? Participatory action research with community residents, agencies, public health, and the university. Annual Meeting of the Ontario Public Health Association.

Bray, J., Lee, J., Smith, L., & Yorks, L. (2000). *Collaborative inquiry in practice: Action, reflection, and meaning making*. Thousand Oaks: Sage Publications.

Buckeridge, D., Mason, R., Robertson, A., Frank, J., Glazier, R., Purdon, L., … Wright, R. (2002). Making health data maps: A case study of a community/university research collaboration.

Social Science & Medicine, 55(7), 1189–1206.

Clarke, B., James, C., & Kelly, J. (1996). Reflective practice: Reviewing the issues and refocusing the debate. *International Journal of Nursing Studies, 33*(2), 171–180.

Cunliffe, A., & Easterby-Smith, M. (2003). From reflection to practical reflexivity: Experiential learning as lived experience. In M. Reynolds & R. Vince (Eds.), *Organizing reflection* (pp. 30–46). Burlington: Ashgate Publishing Co.

Deaver, S., & McAuliffe, G. (2009). Reflective visual journaling during art therapy and counselling internships: A qualitative study. *Reflective Practice, 10*(5), 615–632.

Dewey, J. (1933). *How we think.* Boston: Heath & Co.

Dugdill, L., Coffey, M., Coufopoulos, A., Byrne, K., & Porcellato, L. (2009). Developing new community health roles: Can reflective learning drive professional practice? *Reflective Practice, 10*(1), 121–130.

Ellis, D., Reid, G., & Barnsley, J. (1990). *Keeping on track: An evaluation guide for community groups.* Vancouver: The Women's Research Centre.

Evans, D. (1997). *Reflective learning through practice-based assignments.* Paper presented at the British Educational Research Association Annual Conference, September 11–14. Retrieved from www.leeds.ac.uk/educol/documents/000000468.htm

Ghaye, T., Melander-Wikman, A., Kisare, M., Chambers, P., Bergmark, U., Kostenius, C., & Lillyman, S. (2008). Participatory and appreciative action and reflection (PAAR)—democratizing reflective practices. *Reflective Practice, 9*(4), 361–397.

Gondolf, E. W., Yllo, K., & Campbell, J. (1997). Collaboration between researchers and advocates. In G. K. Kantor & J. L. Jasinski (Eds.), *Out of the darkness: Contemporary perspectives on family violence* (pp. 255–267). Thousand Oaks: Sage.

Hagerman, K. (2010). *At the very root of it.* Retrieved from attheveryrootofit.wordpress.com/

Haggerty, K. (2003). Ruminations on reflexivity. *Current Sociology, 51*(2), 153–162.

Health Promotion Resource System. (2010). *HP-101, Health promotion online course.* Retrieved from www.ohprs.ca/hp101/about_course_faq.htm

International Journal of the Creative Arts in Interdisciplinary Practice. Retrieved from www.ijcaip.com

Jaruszewica, C. (2006). Opening windows on teaching and learning: Transformative and emancipatory learning precipitated by experimenting with visual documentation of student learning. *Educational Action Research, 14*(3), 357–375. Retrieved from www.informaworld.com/smpp/title~db=all~content=t716100708~tab=issueslist~branches=14 - v14

Kottkamp, R. B. (1990). Means for facilitating reflection. *Education and Urban Society, 22*(2), 182–203.

Labonté, R., & Feather, J. (1996). *Handbook on using stories in health promotion practice.* Cat. no. H39-378/1996E. Ottawa: Minister of Supply and Services.

Lemon, N. (2007). Take a photograph: Teacher reflection through narrative. *Reflective Practice, 8*(2), 177–191.

Lewin, K. (1946). Action research and minority problems. *Journal of Social Issues, 2*, 34–46.

Mason, R., & Boutilier, M. (1996). The challenge of genuine power sharing in participatory research: The gap between theory and practice. *The Canadian Journal of Community Mental Health, 15*(2), 145–152.

Maton, K. (2003). Reflexivity, relationism & research: Pierre Bourdieu and the epistemic conditions of social scientific knowledge. *Space & Culture, 6*(1), 52–65.

McIntosh, P. (2008). Poetics and space: Developing a reflective landscape through imagery and human geography. *Reflective Practice, 9*(1), 69–78.

McQueen, D. (1994, June 16). *Visions of health promotion research.* Keynote address, Third Conference on Health Promotion Research, Calgary.

Moon, J. (1999). *Reflection in learning and professional development.* London: Kogan Page.

O'Neill, M., & Dupéré, S. (2006). Du carré à la spirale: Réflexions sur quelques années de participation du comité avec du collectif pour un Québec sans pauvreté. *The Canadian Journal of Program Evaluation, 21*(3), 227–234.

Overby, A. (2009). The new conversation: Using weblogs for reflective practice in the studio art Classroom. *Art Education, 62*(4), 18–24.

Reynolds, M., & Vince, R. (2004). *Organizing reflection.* Burlington: Ashgate Publishing Co.

Roth, R. (1989). Preparing the reflective practitioner: Transforming the apprentice through the dialectic. *Journal of Teacher Education, 40*(2), 31–35.

Rovegno, I., & Bandhauer, D. (1998). A study of the collaborative research process: Shared privilege and shared empowerment. *Journal of Teaching in Physical Education, 17,* 357–375.

Schön, D. (1983). *The reflective practitioner: How professionals think in action.* Boston: Basic Books.

Sharma, P. (2010). Enhancing student reflection using weblogs: Lessons learned from two implementation studies. *Reflective Practice, 11*(2), 127–141.

Tokolahi, E. (2010). Case study: Development of a drawing-based journal to facilitate reflective inquiry. *Reflective Practice, 11*(2), 157–170.

Williams, C. (2009). *A critical and participatory approach to gender equity among youth in Kibera, Kenya.* Thesis submitted to College of Nursing, University of Saskatchewan, Saskatoon.

CHAPTER 18

Health in All Policies

Ketan Shankardass, Natalie Hemsing, and Lorraine Greaves

LEARNING OBJECTIVES

1. Understand the concept of health in all policies (HiAP) and how it came to prominence
2. Understand the relationships between the social determinants of health, intersectoral action, and HiAP
3. Appreciate some of the challenges of using HiAP to address health equity

INTRODUCTION

As we grow to learn about the ways that social determinants of health (SDOH) influence population genetics and behaviours, we should ask, How can governments sustainably incorporate knowledge to make health promoting public policy outside of the health sector? Governments that adopt this objective use what is increasingly referred to as *health in all policies* (HiAP) (Shankardass, Solar, Murphy, Greaves, & O'Campo, 2012). In this chapter, we elaborate on the intersectoral nature of HiAP, provide a historical account of the concept, and describe some examples. We identify some of the key challenges for implementing HiAP, while emphasizing a critical view of the limitations of using this approach to improve health equity. Finally, we conclude with ideas about the future of this relatively new health promotion practice in Canada.

Marmot (2005) notes that because "the major determinants of health are social, so must be the remedies" (p. 1103). So how are the SDOH themselves shaped? In 2008, the World Health Organization's (WHO) Commission on Social Determinants of Health (CSDH) published a framework of *structural* determinants of health that includes social, economic, and political mechanisms that "generate, configure and maintain social hierarchies" (p. 36) of income, gender, occupation, education, social class, and race/ethnicity (among other factors) (Solar & Irwin, 2007). In other words, the structural determinants of health shape our experience of the SDOH by creating socio-economic positions within society.

Some of the key structural determinants of health outlined in the CSDH framework are policies that address macro-economics, labour markets, housing, land use, education, health care, and social protection, along with governance processes that produce those policies. Governments that adopt HiAP develop and implement long-term strategies to engage diverse sectors in the development of healthy and equitable policies (i.e., laws, budgets, programs, etc.) (Freiler et al., 2013; Baum et al., 2014). This could mean, for example, that a new transportation policy would be assessed and potentially modified in relation to its impacts on the distribution of commuting options, safety, physical activity, exposure to air pollution, and property values, along with implications for gentrification and social inclusion. In this way, applying the HiAP approach to transportation could produce better population health, support health-promoting initiatives, and possibly reduce health inequities.

A SHORT HISTORY OF HEALTH IN ALL POLICIES

The term *health in all policies* was introduced by Finland during their presidency of the Council of the European Union in 2006. The Council defined some of the key concepts related to HiAP and encouraged action by the Union and Member States to utilize HiAP as a means to improve health equity (Ståhl, Wismar, Ollila, Lahtinen, & Leppo, 2006; Bauman, King, & Nutbeam, 2014). The HiAP approach builds on a range of health promotion concepts that grew in popularity in the 1980s, such as "intersectoral action for health," "healthy public policy" (De Leeuw & Peters, 2015), and "joined up government" (Delany et al., 2014). It also embodies some key health promotion reports and events, including the 1974 Lalonde Report (Lalonde, 1974), which identified health determinants; the 1978 WHO *Declaration of Alma-Ata* (UNICEF), and the subsequent "Health for All" movement, which identified health equity concerns and the need for intersectoral action.

In 1986, participants in the First International Conference on Health Promotion produced the *Ottawa Charter for Health Promotion*. The *Ottawa Charter* drew attention to the notion of intersectoral action, where no single sector can be expected to have the capacity and knowledge to solve complex health issues, so that action is required by multiple sectors of government and civil society, including through the development of health-promoting policies and practices (De Leeuw & Peters, 2015). Although HiAP and intersectoral action are sometimes regarded as synonymous, HiAP is best understood as a specific form of intersectoral action for health equity. As distinguished by Freiler et al. (2013), "if intersectoral action is the coordination of various sectors towards the improvement of health equity, HiAP should be considered the most administratively integrated, formal and systemically-focused form of intersectoral action" (p. 1069). HiAP is particularly concerned with policy-making, including consideration of the actors and levels of government involved in decision-making and health system provision (Leppo, Ollila, Pena, Wismar, & Cook, 2013). Unlike HiAP, intersectoral action for health equity can include more ad hoc activities that do not depend on formal governance structures (Shankardass et al., 2012).

Although there are examples of intersectoral action for health equity from before the 1980s, there seems to have been a growth in this approach through the 1990s, and especially in the 2000s (Shankardass et al., 2012; Leppo et al., 2013). There is a long history of intersectoral action to address environmental issues, and that effort has often relied on use of tools (e.g., environmental impact assessment) to assess the impact of current or potential projects or policies on the outcome (e.g., environment). Similarly, health impact assessment (HIA) tools feature prominently in the governance approach to HiAP and have been more recently expanded to focus on health equity outcomes (i.e., health equity impact assessment, or HEIA) by considering and incorporating the SDOH (Saint-Pierre, Lamarre, & Simos, 2014). Environmental, health, and health equity impact assessment tools have been used to support intersectoral action in the WHO Healthy Cities projects, with the health sector engaging with municipalities and urban planning to promote health within cities (Leppo et al., 2013).

Despite these developments, the adoption of HiAP remains the exception rather than the rule. A recent scoping review by Shankardass et al. (2011) described the use of HiAP in country and province/state levels in a small but diverse group of jurisdictions, including South Australia, Finland, Québec, Thailand, and Iran. This lack of widespread uptake may reflect a failure by many governments to seriously embrace health promotion and health equity as a part of the political agenda, as noted in the final report of the Commission on Social Determinants of Health (CSDH, 2008). In 2010, at the International Meeting on HiAP in South Australia, the *Adelaide Statement on HiAP* was produced, which drew attention to the need for leadership at the highest levels of government with support from the civil service, and recognizes the challenge of implementing HiAP alongside the political agendas of other sectors (Government of South Australia and World Health Organization, 2010). In 2013, at the International Conference on Health Promotion in Finland, the *Helsinki Statement on HiAP* reiterated this call while articulating specific actions that governments should adopt to move the HiAP agenda forward (WHO, 2014).

HEALTH CONCEPTS IN HEALTH IN ALL POLICIES

In a WHO (2014) definition, HiAP is "an approach to public policies across sectors that systematically takes into account the health implications of decisions, seeks synergies and avoids harmful health impacts in order to improve population health and health equity" (p. 2). Thus, HiAP initiatives frame population health and equity as influenced by a variety of factors operating at multiple levels, from individual to ecological (Baum et al., 2014). What distinguishes HiAP governments from governments using intersectoral action in an ad hoc manner is that they recognize the value of embedding health and health equity considerations in a wide range of policy decisions (Baum et al., 2014; Delany et al., 2014).

While many scholars have emphasized the technical and political processes of inter-sectoral action (Shankardass et al., 2012), others have noted that the concept of HiAP aligns well with the *Universal Declaration of Human Rights*, the *United Nations Millennium Declaration*, and principles of good governance. These principles include legitimacy, ac-countability, transparency and access to information, participation, sustainability, and collaboration across sectors and levels of government (De Leeuw & Peters, 2015).

The aspirational basis of HiAP often means that there is no single, specific way to conceptualize and implement HiAP. In fact, most initiatives do not even refer explicit-ly to HiAP in the mandate (see table 18.1). Yet, when a government decides to enact a HiAP-like approach, they generally formulate some specific mandate (e.g., adopting a new law or long-term strategy) that outlines how and why politicians, civil servants, and other non-governmental partners ought to integrate governance of health equity. Hence, it is possible to discern some general models for health governance when using a HiAP approach. Table 18.1 describes four general approaches to health governance across seven recently enacted cases of HiAP.

The implementation of HiAP does not stop at the technical processes of policy-making. As a social justice intervention, there are also political processes that will be crit-ical in determining whether or not it is pursued in a sustainable manner. A clear example occurred in 2003 in Sweden when the Swedish Public Health Objectives Bill, with a "vision" of addressing upstream and midstream determinants of health, shifted following

Table 18.1: Description Of Health Governance Approaches Across Seven Health in All Policies (HiAP) Jurisdictions (Including Initial Mandate)

Jurisdiction	Initial Mandate for HiAP (Year of Initiation)	Health Governance Approach of HiAP
Québec	Public Health Act (2003)	Use of health impact assessment tools to embed intersectoral action on new, poten-tially harmful policies/projects
Thailand	National Health Act (2007)	
Sweden	Swedish Public Health Objectives Bill (2003)	Coordinating intersectoral action on strate-gic health objectives over a fixed period
Finland	Health 2015 Strategy (2001)	
California	HiAP Task Force Executive Order (2010)	Coordinating intersectoral action on health objectives to achieve other strategic objectives, e.g., growth, sustainability, quality of life
South Australia	HiAP Unit (2007)	
Iran	Supreme Council for Health and Food Security (2006)	Community-driven needs-based strategy for coordinating intersectoral action

a change in government in 2006. The new right-wing government had a different "political and theoretical orientation" and the bill was amended to shift the focus away from a universal vision that broadly addressed structural determinants to one that emphasized the "individualization of health" and tackled the lifestyles of vulnerable groups (Shankardass, Oneka, Molnar, & Muntaner, 2014). In effect, there was a shift to use HiAP to intervene on more downstream (and often individual-level) determinants of health, which are less likely to address the root causes of health inequities; this problem has been referred to elsewhere as "lifestyle drift" (Hunter, Popay, Tannahill, & Whitehead, 2010).

CANADIAN AND INTERNATIONAL CASE STUDIES OF HEALTH IN ALL POLICIES

In Canada, examples of HiAP have been implemented at various jurisdictional levels in several provinces. These cases illustrate the widely different approaches that can be taken to HiAP. For example, in 2002, Québec revised its Public Health Act by mandating health impact assessment (HIA) as a routine part of developing any policy that may potentially impact population health (section 54), and giving public health directors the power to compel changes to policies where they deemed ameliorable solutions to exist (section 55) (Pinto, Molnar, Shankardass, O'Campo, & Bayoumi, 2015). This approach to HiAP is based on informed decision-making by using HIA to prospectively assess and address any potentially negative health impacts of policies and programs (Pinto et al., 2015). The Ministère de la Santé et des Services Sociaux (MSSS) and the Institut National de Santé Publique du Québec support the use of HIA by providing training and expertise to assist with the decision-making process (Poirier, 2014).

The municipality of Chatham-Kent sits next to the county of Elgin and the city of St. Thomas along the northwest bank of Lake Erie in Ontario, Canada. Governments in these settings have adopted long-term strategies to use intersectoral action to improve equity in the quality of life of all residents. These initiatives are being driven by "community leaders' cabinets" that include political and bureaucratic leaders (e.g., mayors and chief administrative officers) as well as public health leadership (e.g., medical officers of health) and other community stakeholders (e.g., Local Health Integration Network chief executive officers, First Nations chiefs, presidents of industries) (Municipality of Chatham-Kent, 2016; St. Thomas Elgin Community Leaders' Cabinet, 2016). There are some important differences in what HiAP looks like in these in two jurisdictions; for example, in Chatham-Kent, the Board of Health is a part of the municipal government, while they are autonomous in St. Thomas/Elgin.

The Peterborough County-City Health Unit has a history of using intersectoral action for health equity (e.g., King, 2011). Its 2013–2017 strategic plan includes the use of a rapid health equity assessment tool to develop policy recommendations, and analysis to inform and support public policy initiatives (Peterborough County-City Health Unit, 2013). Importantly, although the Board of Health is autonomous from the City and County governments, it is one of the only boards of health in the province with First Nations, municipal, and provincial representatives. Compared with the community leaders' cabinets used in Chatham-Kent and Elgin, the type of HiAP emerging in Peterborough involves stronger leadership from public health, who work in a more opportunistic manner to foster intersectoral action for health equity.

Health in All Policies has also been used by many diverse governments internationally (Shankardass et al., 2011). The government of South Australia formally adopted a HiAP approach in 2008 under the leadership of the Department of the Premier and Cabinet and the Health Department (Delany et al., 2016). A HiAP Unit was created that engages with partners in different sectors to seek "win-win" opportunities for intersectoral action (Delany et al., 2016). A recent publication describes how the unit has worked with 13 departments and agencies (Delany et al., 2014). A health lens analysis (HLA) process is used to collaboratively and systematically plan for health equity in ways that are relevant to South Australia's Strategic Plan (e.g., Aboriginal education—early years) (Delany et al., 2014).

For example, Delany et al. (2014) describe how the HiAP Unit and Education Department engaged in interviews with parents of students at four schools with a student base that was primarily Aboriginal and living on a low income, to identify effective processes and parental engagement strategies to develop a theory of change that informed policy changes.

CHALLENGES IN IMPLEMENTING HEALTH IN ALL POLICIES

One of the key challenges of implementing HiAP is creating transformative change in governance. Fafard (2013) refers to this transformation as "integrated governance," which does not come naturally to governments that are large, complex systems with short, politicized mandates. Typically, policy-making occurs within policy "silos" where departments and ministries are given specific mandates to achieve along with an earmarked implementation budget. It can be very challenging to convince policy makers to integrate health equity considerations because it is likely not an objective that exists in their silo.

The implementation of HiAP involves *sustained work* by the civil service to engage a range of partners, both inside and outside government, and to get buy-in to design health equity interventions and embed them in a range of policies. At the same time, politicians need to be engaged *across electoral cycles* to lead potentially difficult intersectoral initiatives over the middle- to long-term. This ongoing work involves multiple levels of government, which multiplies the challenges of implementing HiAP.

There are at least three challenging tasks required of governments as they pursue sustainable integrated governance: (1) getting buy-in for HiAP and setting the agenda for health equity considerations from partners across diverse sectors inside and outside of government; (2) providing financial resources, expertise, and human resources needed to implement HiAP; and (3) evaluating the population health and economic implications of implementing HiAP.

Agenda-Setting for HiAP

Agenda-setting processes are critical to the implementation of HiAP including acquiring buy-in. For example, how can urban planning and infrastructure development departments be convinced to collaborate on developing better walkability in neighbourhoods or less polluting transport systems? This process may be particularly difficult where there are conflicting political objectives among policy sectors. As noted by Rudolph, Caplan, Mitchell, Ben-Moshe, & Dillon (2013), addressing the SDOH requires reflection on and challenging of the "underlying assumptions about the way society is organized" (p. 17).

The promotion and success of HiAP clearly depends on political and economic factors (Kokkinen, 2015). Ideological concerns also directly affect the uptake of HiAP, the influence of business interests, and the level of interest in addressing the SDOH in a structural fashion (rather than one focused on individual-level factors). Indeed, the success or failure of HiAP is often dependent upon the power relations that exist within and between the government and external sectors. The values of and tensions between these actors will influence the implementation and realization of the goals of HiAP. In particular, budget issues and economic growth questions that relate to particular HiAP issues will be different for each sector, actor, or level of government. And, has been seen in Canadian HiAP efforts, local and regional pressures and issues, as well as differences in leadership, will have an impact on the launching and focus of HiAP.

Ollila (2011) has described four key approaches for setting the agenda with diverse policy sectors: (1) *health at the core*, in which health objectives are the primary focus of the policy activity; (2) *win-win*, in which the focus is on developing policies and actions that benefit all sectors; (3) *cooperation*, in which the health sector supports other sectors to achieve their goals, while promoting health through ongoing and cooperative relationships; and (4) *damage limitation*, in which the goal is to limit or reverse the negative health consequences of policies in areas other than health.

A recent study by Molnar et al. (2016) found that the win-win approach is often the most useful, while other approaches can be productive when used in combination with the win-win approach, but not alone. This may be explained by the perception of "health imperialism" which can make a HiAP initiative seem like an expansion of the power of health actors over other departments in government, especially given the large budgets health sectors control (Nutbeam, 1994).

Capacity-Building for HiAP

Another challenge for governments is structuring and supporting the civil service through the transformation towards integrated governance. What should be done to make it feasible for sectors to consider health equity objectives, especially if they don't have an understanding of the relevant evidence base or expertise with the tools being used to implement HiAP? Carey, Crammond, and Keast (2014) describe the "supportive architecture" required to facilitate intersectoral action within government. Mandates from central government, dedicated staff-ing and resources, and legislative frameworks that support intersectoral collaboration towards shared goals have all been identified as key contributors to HiAP (Baum et al., 2014). Such features ideally require active decision-making, resources, and committed leadership that reflects a societal vision, transcending government mandates or leaders.

The success of HiAP also relies on the ability of non-health sectors to recognize how their work affects population health and for all to work to dismantle silos and build part-nerships for the promotion of health equity (Rudolph et al., 2013). Many HiAP initiatives use decision-support tools like HIA to facilitate such policy coordination. There are often new technologies that actors across sectors need to learn in order to conduct assessments, and governments need to provide staff with the necessary time to conduct assessments (Harris-Roxas et al., 2012). Tools like HIA also require evidence to inform decision-making, which may not be readily accessible to civil servants in different sectors. Further, there may only be limited (if any) baseline data on population health variation and risk factors of interest.

More recently, health *equity* impact assessment (HEIA) tools have emerged which bring clearer focus to considerations of how proposed changes will impact on priority vulnerable populations and various equity outcomes. For example, the Ministry of Health and Long-Term Care in Ontario has developed an HEIA tool that is currently employed on an ad-hoc basis by health authorities and health units (Ministry of Health and Long-Term Care, 2016). The tool is supported by a workbook and supplements for public health organizations and French-language users. The Ministry also helps to facilitate a commu-nity of interest for users in the province to support each other in using the tool (www.porticonetwork.ca/web/heia/heiacoi).

But such tools are blunt instruments, as they do not teach or measure critical thinking skills in their users. Despite their popularity, a key fault of tools such as HIA and HEIA is that they are often gender blind, in that they do not typically include sex- and gender-related factors in their tool structure *in a mainstreamed* or thorough manner. For example, HIA tools that ignore the impact of gender- and sex-related factors when considering how a neighbourhood could be more walkable may not recognize how certain built environment forms can heighten fear of sexual assault or lessen safety for women. Some tools, including the Ontario one, include gender and/or sex in a checklist alongside other demographic factors like age or culture. But in reality, all social determinants of health (SDOH) and features and categories of populations are gendered and need to be assessed accordingly, not merely nodding to gender as an add-on consideration. In addition, those governments that have mandated sex- and gender-based analysis policies need to overtly link them to all other policy improvement mechanisms, such as HiAP, and then fashion tools such as HIA and HEIA accordingly.

There are many examples where regional population characteristics and issues demand a more complex assessment process than provided by checklists and tools. Harris-Roxas et al. (2012) suggest that there are opportunities to improve HIA tools by considering knowledge alternatives (how we understand the issue/problem), institutional alternatives (different options for partnering/working at the organizational level), and goal alternatives (how success is framed and achieved). When health equity is also an explicit goal, as in HEIA, consciously improving and re-developing tools to measure health equity is required. On the contrary, at present these tools are rarely "living" documents but rather rely on straightforward training and implementation processes.

Evaluation of HiAP

One of the key barriers to more rapid deployment of HiAP initiatives is the lack of supportive and convincing evaluation and economic evidence. To date, there have been few evaluations of either health equity outcomes or economic impacts of HiAP (Baum et al., 2014; Bauman et al., 2014; Pinto et al., 2015). This may be a function of such health impacts occurring over a long time period, coupled with a lack of methodology for tracing economic costs over such a timeline, as well as the overarching difficulty in measuring and disentangling the impact of shifting underlying SDOH. Hence, there is relatively limited understanding of how and why HiAP efforts are successful or not in improving health equity and economic sustainability.

By its nature, HiAP and the related SDOH improvements reflect long-term goals and require consistent follow-up and longitudinal research. Further, HiAP is inherently a complex process and requires measures assessing all elements of HiAP, such as content and process from issue to leadership to timing to engagement. Sufficiently comprehensive evaluation frameworks are often missing when HiAP initiatives are launched. Thus, although adopting HiAP may make sense to governments that recognize the importance of SDOH, sustaining the approach may require the demonstration of favourable impacts, which in turn requires more attention paid to evaluation, especially economic evaluations.

The ultimate effects of HiAP and SDOH improvements take years or even generations to accrue, and may be more difficult to measure as they are not represented as direct health care costs, but more likely in costs averted across sectors. While governments are often motivated by reducing health care costs, there is often less attention to long-term health promotion or prevention policies and initiatives. Further, bureaucratic processes within governments are often not infused with demanding critical-thinking processes, and may be more likely to reinforce the status quo, departmental, or divisional mandates; reflect political realities and tensions; and maintain budgets and territory. Finally, and perhaps as a result, there are few long-term models that illustrate the economic impact of HiAP that could support arguments for involving partners and sectors, and for convincing governments of any ideological stripe to support HiAP (Greaves & Bialystok, 2011).

Pinto and colleagues (2015) also suggest that further research is required on "the political economy of implementing HiAP policies" (p. 7). This includes considering the political agendas of government sectors, the power of individual departments, and the economic context and its impact on funding and resource provision to support HiAP.

CONCLUSION

There is pan-Canadian concern about the sustainability of health care systems in the coming decades and the need to either flatline or reduce the cost curve. This critical point in health reform in Canada could put greater emphasis on the need for governments and researchers to support the transition to integrated governance for health equity, using approaches such as HiAP. The uptake of HiAP has historically been spurred on by strong political leadership, but this commitment needs to transcend, and be appropriated by, all political parties in Canada.

As described, current intersectoral governance structures and tools, such as impact assessment tools or lenses, are considered to be key to underpinning HiAP approaches. However, a more farsighted and effective approach may be "transectoral" approaches, designed explicitly to overarch existing siloes and departments and create a brand new approach to complex health problems (Greaves & Bialystok, 2011). Thus, as the challenges of achieving integrated governance emerge and persist, transectoral governance structures may become more common as an embedded approach to health equity. For example, in Ecuador, the Buen Vivir strategy coordinates diverse sectors through the leadership of a so-called *coordinating ministry*, the Secretaría Nacional de Planificación y Desarrollo (SENPLADES), which oversees more traditional sectors such as environment and national defence (Monni & Pallottino, 2015).

Such a transectoral shift will require strong leadership and vision, long-term thinking, and shared data collection across platforms and siloes, in order to create original and effective approaches to difficult and intransigent health equity issues. In Canada, that would mean premiers and cabinets would need to lead and measure progress on HiAP. As many health equity issues are reflective of SDOH, such as income, education, environments, or gender, long-term policy positioning is required well past the average life cycle of a government. These factors require that Canadian political leaders reach past typical ideological positioning and look for common evidence-based levers to create social and economic change.

Some suggest that reaching the "long game" for HiAP will require leaders to do a better job of recognizing linkages with economic sustainability and other common societal goals to address multiple problems at once.

While there is clear potential to link HiAP with long-term economic gains, as well as sustainability and other common societal goals such as equity, a collective vision is required. Rudolph et al. (2013) argue the need for an intersectoral approach that combines health, equity, and sustainability, such as in California, where a Strategic Growth Council has the primary function of ensuring inter-agency coordination on sustainability issues including oversight of a HiAP task force. Harris-Roxas et al. (2012) also identify the potential to integrate health impact assessments with sustainability assessments to enable a more holistic assessment approach; however, this must be balanced against the risk of health concerns being buried beneath other priorities. On a practical level, Delany et al. (2016) suggest that the long-term contributions of HiAP to the economy may be enhanced by building in evaluation milestones to recognize achievements over the course of the project.

In addition to a lack of long-term evaluation and economic research on HiAP, there has been little meaningful engagement and involvement of non-governmental, community-based organizations in its implementation; yet community engagement is necessary for strong health equity interventions to be identified, designed, and implemented. In 2016, on the 30th anniversary of the *Ottawa Charter for Health Promotion*, the *PEI Declaration* was signed at the 6th Global Forum for Health Promotion, which called for stronger inclusion of civil society partners in health promotion efforts. If implemented, we may well see a demand for HiAP initiatives to be more community-engaged, demanding a renewed approach to agenda-setting.

In Canada, and elsewhere, few disagree with the underlying notion of HiAP, but it can suffer from poor implementation, operationalization, and measurement. As Greaves and Bialystok suggest, HiAP in Canada has suffered from "All talk, but little action" (2011). But as health care costs continue to escalate, in some cases approaching 50 percent of provincial budgets, there may come a breaking point when governments are forced to address health very differently. If researchers provide data to form an economic argument for HiAP, and courageous and visionary political leaders campaign on innovations in addressing health, the stage will be set. At that time, perhaps, a pan-Canadian commitment will emerge to generate effective comparative analyses of HiAP, and grow more critical policy-making workforces in the process. Only then will we see an effective Canadian vision that could transform idealistic support for HiAP into real change for all citizens.

CRITICAL THINKING QUESTIONS

1. The ideas underlying health in all policies related to the social determinants of health and the need for intersectoral action are not new, so what is it about health in all policies that is innovative?

2. What distinguishes health in all policies from other forms of intersectoral action for health?

3. The use of health in all policies implies a number of technical and political challenges for government. Under what conditions might technical or political challenges be harder or easier to overcome?

RESOURCES

Further Readings

Freiler, A., Muntaner, C., Shankardass, K., Mah, C. L., Molnar, A., Renahy, E., & O'Campo, P. (2013). Glossary for the implementation of health in all policies (HiAP). *Journal of Epidemiology and Community Health, 67*, 1068–1072.

A collection of terms for understanding agenda-setting and capacity-building aspects of the implementation of health in all policies initiatives.

Solar, O., & Irwin, A. (2007). *A conceptual framework for action on the social determinants of health: Discussion paper for the Commission on Social Determinants of Health.* Geneva: World Health Organization.

A theoretical framework for understanding why governance approaches such as health in all policies are critical for health equity.

Wismar, M., McQueen, D., Lin, V., Jones C. M., & Davies, M. (2013). Rethinking the politics and implementation of health in all policies. *Israel Journal of Health Policy Research, 2*, 17. doi: 10.1186/2045-4015-2-17

A case study of Israel's National Programme to Promote Active, Healthy Lifestyles that indicates the role of politics in the implementation of health in all policies initiatives.

Relevant Website

World Health Organization, Health in All Policies: Framework for Country Action
www.who.int/healthpromotion/frameworkforcountryaction/en/

Current recommendations from the World Health Organization on using a health in all policies approach.

REFERENCES

Baum, F., Lawless, A., Delany, T., Macdougall, C., Williams, C., Broderick, D., Wildgoose, D., Harris, E., Mcdermott, D., Kickbusch, I., Popay, J., & Marmot, M. (2014). Evaluation of health in all policies: Concept, theory and application. *Health Promotion International, 29*(Suppl. 1), i130–i142.

Bauman, A. E., King, L., & Nutbeam, D. (2014). Rethinking the evaluation and measurement of health in all policies. *Health Promotion International, 29*(Suppl. 1), i143–i151.

Carey, G., Crammond, B., & Keast, R. (2014). Creating change in government to address the social determinants of health: How can efforts be improved? *BMC Public Health, 14*, 1087.

CSDH. (2008). Closing the gap in a generation: Health equity through action on the social determinants of health, Final Report of the Commission on Social Determinants of Health. Geneva: World Health Organization.

Delany, T., Harris, P., Williams, C., Harris, E., Baum, F., Lawless, A., Wildgoose, D. Haigh, F., MacDougall, C., & Broderick, D. (2014). Health impact assessment in New South Wales & Health in all policies in South Australia: Differences, similarities and connections. *BMC public health, 14*(1), 1.

Delany, T., Lawless, A., Baum, F., Popay, J., Jones, L., McDermott, D., Harris, E., Broderick, D., & Marmot, M. (2016). Health in all policies in South Australia: What has supported early implementation? *Health Promotion International, 31*(4), 888–898.

De Leeuw, E., & Peters, D. (2015). Nine questions to guide development and implementation of health in all policies. *Health Promotion International, 30*(4), 987–997.

Fafard, P. (2013). Health in all meets horizontal government. First International Conference on Public Policy. Grenoble.

Freiler, A., Muntaner, C., Shankardass, K., Mah, C. L., Molnar, A., Renahy, E., & O'Campo, P. (2013). Glossary for the implementation of health in all policies (HiAP). *Jounral of Epidemiology and Community Health, 67*, 1068–1072.

Government of South Australia and World Health Organization. (2010). *Adelaide statement on health in all policies: Moving towards a shared governance for health and well-being.* Geneva: WHO. www.who.int/social_determinants/hiap_statement_who_sa_final.pdf

Greaves, L. J., & Bialystok, L. R. (2011). Health in all policies—all talk and little action? *Canadian Journal of Public Health, 102*(6), 407–409.

Harris-Roxas, B., Viliani, F., Bond, A., Cave, B., Divall, M., Furu, P., Harris, P., Soeberg, M., Wernham, A., & Winkler, M. (2012). Health impact assessment: The state of the art. *Impact Assessment and Project Appraisal, 30*(1), 43–52.

Hunter, D. J., Popay, J., Tannahill, C., & Whitehead, M. (2010). Getting to grips with health inequalities at last? *British Medical Journal, 340*, c684.

King, A. (2011). Health, not health care—changing the conversation: 2010 annual report of the Chief Medical Officer of Health of Ontario to the Legislative Assembly of Ontario (Catalogue No. 016748). MoHaLTC. Toronto, ON: Queen's Printer for Ontario.

Kokkinen, L. (2015). Taking health into account in all policies. *The Lancet Global Health, 3*(10), e594.

Lalonde, M. (1974). *A new perspective on the health of Canadians.* Ottawa: Government of Canada.

Leppo, K., Ollila, E., Pena, S., Wismar, M., & Cook, S. (2013). *Health in all policies. Seizing opportunities, implementing policies.* Helsinki, Finland: Ministry of Social Affairs and Health.

Marmot, M. (2005). Social determinants of health inequalities. *The Lancet, 365*(9464), 1099–1104.

Ministry of Health and Long-Term Care. (2016). *Health equity impact assessment.* Retrieved from www.health.gov.on.ca/en/pro/programs/heia/

Molnar, A., Renahy, E., O'Campo, P., Muntaner, C., Freiler, A., & Shankardass, K. (2016). Using win-win strategies to implement health in all policies: A cross-case analysis. *PLoS One, 11*(2), e0147003.

Monni, S., & Pallottino, M. (2015). Beyond growth and development: Buen vivir as an alternative to current paradigms. *International Journal of Environmental Policy and Decision Making, 1*(3).

Municipality of Chatham-Kent. (2016, September 12). *Chatham-Kent Community Leaders' Cabinet.* Retrieved from www.chatham-kent.ca/Mayor/CommunityLeadersCabinet/Pages/CKCommunityLeadersCabinet.aspx

Nutbeam, D. (1994). Inter-sectoral action for health: Making it work. *Health Promotion International, 9*(3), 143–144.

Ollila, E. (2011). Health in all policies: From rhetoric to action. *Scandinavian Journal of Public Health, 39*(Suppl. 6), 11–18.

Peterborough County-City Health Unit. (2013). *Strategic plan 2013–2017.* Peterborough: Author.

Pinto, A. D., Molnar, A., Shankardass, K., O'Campo, P. J., & Bayoumi, A. M. (2015). Economic considerations and health in all policies initiatives: Evidence from interviews with key informants in Sweden, Quebec and South Australia. *BMC Public Health, 15*, 171.

Poirier, A. (2014). Implementing HiAP: The Quebec experience. Ontario Public Health Association & Nutrition Resource Centre 2014 Annual Conference. Toronto, Ontario.

Rudolph, L., Caplan, J., Mitchell, C., Ben-Moshe, K., & Dillon, L. (2013). *Health in all policies: Improving health through intersectoral collaboration*. Washington: National Academy of Sciences.

Saint-Pierre, L., Lamarre, M., & Simos, J. (2014). Health impact assessments (HIA): An intersectoral process for action on the social, economic and environmental determinants of health. *Global health promotion, 21*(Suppl. 1), 7–14.

Shankardass, K., Oneka, G., Molnar, A., & Muntaner, C. (2014). Ideological conflict in the implementation of health in all policies: A multiple case study of Quebec, Sweden and South Australia. 23rd World Congress of Political Science. Montréal, Québec, Canada.

Shankardass, K., Solar, O., Murphy, K., Freiler, A., Bobbili, S., Bayoumi, A., & O'Campo, P. (2011). *Health in all policies: Results of a realist-informed scoping review of the literature. Getting started with health in all policies: A report to the Ontario Ministry of Health and Long Term Care*. Toronto: Centre for Research on Inner City Health. Retrieved from www.stmichaelshospital.com/crich/reports/hiap/

Shankardass, K., Solar, O., Murphy, K., Greaves, L., & O'Campo, P. (2012). A scoping review of intersectoral action for health equity involving governments. *International Journal of Public Health, 57*(1), 25–33.

Solar, O., & Irwin. A. (2007). A conceptual framework for action on the social determinants of health: Discussion paper for the Commission on Social Determinants of Health. Geneva, World Health Organization.

Ståhl, T., Wismar, M., Ollila, E., Lahtinen, E., & Leppo, K. (Eds.). (2006). *Health in all policies: Prospects and potentials*. Finland: Ministry of Social Affairs and Health.

St. Thomas Elgin Community Leaders' Cabinet. (2016, June 22). *St. Thomas Elgin Community Leaders' Cabinet*. Retrieved from www.stthomaselginclc.ca/

UNICEF. (1978). *The declaration of Alma-Ata*. International Conference on Primary Health Care. Alma-Ata: United Nations Children's Fund and World Health Organization.

World Health Organization (WHO). (2014). Health in all policies: Helsinki statement. Framework for country action. Geneva: Author. Retrieved from www.who.int/healthpromotion/frameworkforcountryaction/en/

CHAPTER 19

Developing a Health Promotion Research Agenda: Learning from Population Health Intervention Research

Louise Potvin

LEARNING OBJECTIVES

1. Understand population health intervention research (PHIR) and its origins
2. Understand the differences between PHIR and evaluation research
3. Understand the potential contributions of PHIR to health promotion research

INTRODUCTION

Health promotion (WHO, 1986) is essentially an action-oriented field. Its foundational document, the *Ottawa Charter for Health Promotion* (WHO, 1986), does not propose much in terms of research. It chiefly elaborates on strategies, areas of action, and supporting values for the collective project of improving health and equity (Potvin & Jones, 2011). Despite, or because of, this lack of direction, research in health promotion has developed through a wide variety of topics. A perusal of any health promotion journal would highlight this point. Health promotion has borrowed from many disciplinary perspectives, and aside from clear reference to the *Ottawa Charter* it may be difficult to clearly delineate what constitutes health promotion research and how it informs health promotion interventions.[1]

One could argue that in an action-oriented field this absence of problematization about the role of research is inconsequential, but this is false. Failing to clearly identify the kind of scientific knowledge that should inform intervention and practice, in addition to the values and principles of the *Ottawa Charter*, makes health promotion more akin to an ideology than to a legitimate area of public action (and spending). In addition, there are examples of calls to action that clearly identify the role of research. For example, the call to "close the gap in a generation" (CSDH, 2008) made by the WHO Commission on Social Determinants of Health identified three priorities of action, one of which was clearly concerned with research: "Measure and understand the problem and assess the impact of action" (CSDH, 2008, p. 2).

In this chapter, I will show that there are many areas of overlap between the new and emerging fields of population health intervention research and health promotion. I will propose that the former may serve as a starting point to develop and promote a research agenda that would support health-promoting practice.

WHAT IS POPULATION HEALTH INTERVENTION RESEARCH?

For a little more than ten years, researchers, knowledge users, and research funders—mainly from Canada but also from the UK, Australia, US, and a few European countries—have attempted to define, profile, and advocate for a new field of scientific inquiry, population health intervention research (PHIR) (Institute of Population and Public Health, 2012). PHIR is defined as the use of scientific methods to produce knowledge about all relevant aspects of interventions in the form of programs and policy that aim at shifting the distribution of health or its determinants in a population (Hawe & Potvin, 2009). Such interventions may be initiated and operated from within or outside of the health sector. Because it uses health and health-related indicators as the main characteristics of the interventions it studies, PHIR is part of the broader domain of health research.

PHIR: A Science of Solution

There are many ways in which one can represent the widespread domain of health research. The graph in figure 19.1 emphasises two dimensions. The horizontal axis identifies a continuum of analytical scales on which health can be appraised. It ranges from the infinitely small biochemical components of the human body to the encompassing ecosystems in which human populations are embedded. The vertical axis represents a continuum of research development that ranges from the more fundamental research that defines/documents a "new" problem to the very applied research that studies the scaling up of solutions and their generalized applications. Implicit in this representation is that at any analytical scale along the continuum, research can either focus on the problems and their causes or on solutions, their development, and large-scale implementation. Instead of contrasting fundamental to applied or developmental research, as is often the case, or a science of discovery to that of delivery as Catford (2009) did, I propose, as illustrated in figure 19.2, to contrast a science of problems to a science of solutions recognizing also that the two may have some areas of overlap. More specifically, a science of solutions investigates a whole range of solution-related questions: how interventions (whatever the scale at which their target is located) produce their intended and unintended effects; how they are effectively planned, implemented, sustained, and scaled up; how delivery systems and contexts facilitate or impede these processes; and probably many others that will emerge as this kind of research develops.

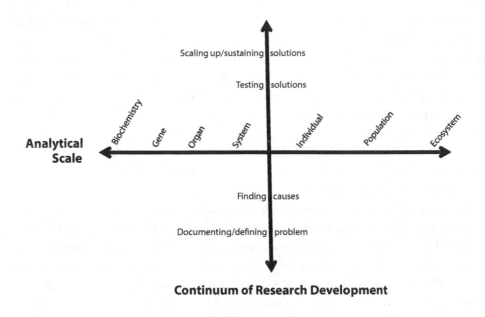

Figure 19.1: Representation of Health Research Domains

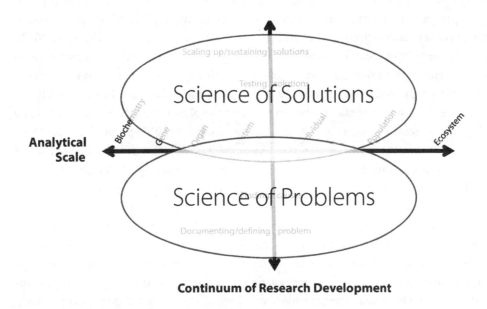

Figure 19.2: A Science of Problems and a Science of Solutions

Increasingly, public health decision makers recognize that although knowledge and evidence[2] about the prevalence, causes, and consequences of health problems are necessary for designing and implementing effective health programs and policy, they remain largely insufficient (Butler-Jones, 2009). Knowing what causes a problem does not automatically provide insight into appropriate solutions and how to implement them. In many developed countries, following the rapid expansion of evidence-based medicine, there has been an increasing demand for the production, dissemination, and integration into professional practice of scientific evidence about public and population health interventions (Kohatsu, Robinson, & Torner, 2004), including in health promotion (Juneau, Jones, McQueen, & Potvin, 2011).

The nascent field of population health intervention research would occupy a large part of the top right quadrant as illustrated in figure 19.3. On the vertical axis, PHIR is concerned by issues related to interventions development, implementation, sustainability, and scaling up both in terms of processes (how they work) and outcomes (changes they produce). PHIR is explicitly concerned with developing knowledge about interventions designed and operated by delivery systems in real-life situations (in vivo) as opposed to interventions designed and operated by a research team to test hypotheses in controlled situations (in vitro) (CIHR-IPPH, 2007).

Situating PHIR on the horizontal axis appears to be more problematic. At the core is the concept of human population, defined as a group of human beings linked together through governance, economic, social, and cultural institutions. Populations have emerging properties that cannot be reduced to the sum of constituting individuals' properties. A population is thus constituted of individuals and their interrelationships (Krieger, 2012). Towards the right of the horizontal axis, most would agree that PHIR includes interventions that encompass whole ecosystems containing other species. Indeed, public health has been increasingly concerned with the pervasive relationships between human health and environmental issues that affect other species and the planet as a whole, such as climate change. In a recent report, Hancock, Spady, and Soskolne (2015) propose an eco-social framework for public health action (see chapter 22). Given that human-created social systems and natural systems are in constant interaction and strongly influence each other as well as population health, the eco-social framework proposes that public health interventions should promote ecological as well as socio-economic changes.

On the left-hand side, whether the field of PHIR would stop short of including individual-level interventions remains a contentious issue. To change the distribution of ill health or risk in a population, interventions must address system-level conditions that shape their distribution (Hawe, 2015). Therefore, for some, interventions aiming at changing individual risk and behaviour, one individual at a time, will never constitute population intervention even if they reach lots of individuals (Hawe, Di Ruggiero, & Cohen, 2012). Others argue that individual-level interventions that provide adapted services for underserved segments of the population have the potential to change the distribution of health in the overall population. This is partly so because such interventions require some organizational changes

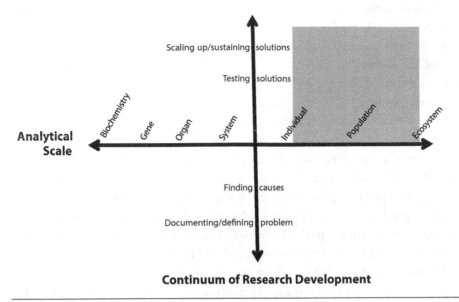

Continuum of Research Development

Figure 19.3: The Conceptual Space of PHIR

in the service-delivery system. In this perspective, a post-natal home-visiting nursing program that targets hard-to-reach households would constitute a population health intervention because of its potential impact on health inequality (Jack et al., 2012). Obviously there are still grey zones in defining what constitutes population health interventions, but what seems to be clear is the exclusion of clinical interventions addressing individuals from the general population and the focus on system-level interventions.

This conceptualization of PHIR as a science of solution that takes interventions as objects of inquiry raises two issues relevant for better integrating research in health promotion, a field already invested in by practitioners. The first relates to the role of those practitioners in the constitution of PHIR and the second concerns the distinction between PHIR and an already existing applied field of science: evaluation research.[3]

A Favourable Context for an Innovation in Science

One critical distinction between a science of solutions (such as PHIR) and a science of problems is the necessary collaborative relationship between research and practice implied in the former. Producing scientific knowledge about how interventions are developed, implemented, sustained, and scaled up means coupling research with an intervention delivery system (Potvin & McQueen, 2008), both operating in a shared social space that implies they interact with each other. For example, researchers who are not the primary targets of the intervention may participate in activities implemented by intervention staff in order to collect data about this activity. In the same vein, researchers may also be interacting with interventions' beneficiaries to collect information to document potential impact.

Conversely, intervention staff will have to devote some of their precious intervention time to support data collection and research activities. There are two critical conditions for such collaborations to be possible: researchers must have the opportunity for conducting this kind of applied research, and practitioners and decision makers must have incentives for integrating scientific knowledge into their practice.

The development of PHIR in Canada at the turn of the twenty-first century corresponds to the creation of two institutions that facilitated the simultaneous emergence of these two conditions: the Canadian Institutes for Health Research (CIHR) and the Public Health Agency of Canada (PHAC). The almost simultaneous creation of these two institutions reflects the fact that Canada was increasing its investments in both the capacity to conduct public health research and in the demand for high-quality research results to inform public health practice and programs. Models in knowledge transfer would frame this as an increase in both the push (the research side) and the pull (the knowledge-user side) for scientific evidence (Lavis, Ross, McLeod, & Gildiner, 2002).

CIHR was created in 2000 to replace and expand the Medical Research Council (MRC) as the funding agency for medical/health research. Much broader than that of the MRC, CIHR's mandate encompasses the whole range of health research, which is organized in a continuum anchored into four pillars: biomedical/fundamental; clinical; health systems and services; and social/cultural/environmental population health. One of the 13 founding institutes, the Institute of Population and Public Health (IPPH) was closely aligned to the fourth pillar, which further heightened the profile of public health research and allowed for the development and implementation of critical strategic funding initiatives. One such initiative, repeated several times and in collaboration with several other institutes, was the "intervention research operating grant" opportunity that funded research involving collaborations between researchers and intervention implementers in order to study various relevant aspects of these interventions (CIHR-IPPH, 2007). Fully aligned with the idea of natural experiments in which researchers develop a study about an intervention they do not control (Petticrew et al., 2005), this initiative even excluded projects wherein researchers were the main drivers of the intervention.

The other critical institution created at the turn of the century is the Public Health Agency of Canada (PHAC), whose mission is to "Promote and protect the health of Canadians through leadership, partnership, innovation and action in public health" (PHAC, 2016). Importantly, one part of PHAC's mandate is to foster quality in public health practice through increasing the use of scientific evidence in public health interventions (PHAC, 2016). Concretely, in 2005, PHAC established a network of six National Collaborating Centres for Public Health (NCCPH) with the mandate to collect, synthesize, and disseminate evidence about public health interventions and facilitate the uptake of evidence to inform public health programs and decisions. The NCCPH constitutes a broker for increasing the quality and volume of exchange between researchers and knowledge users (NCCPH, 2016).

It is within this context of enhanced capacity for public health research and of an increasing demand for evidence that a group of health researchers, knowledge users, and research funders gathered in a broad coalition and developed the Population Health Intervention Research Initiative for Canada (PHIRIC) aiming at increasing the quantity, quality, and use of population health intervention research (Sullivan, 2009). PHIRIC's ambition was nothing less than building a new field of research and, to this end, it developed strategic objectives and implemented a work plan (Institute of Population and Public Health, 2012). PHIRIC's activities have certainly enhanced the profile of PHIR, a domain in which books are being published (see for example Harrington, McLafferty, & Elliot, 2016), international conferences organized, and mainstream research funding competitions created (see for example Institut National du Cancer, 2016).

Distinguishing Population Health Intervention Research from Evaluation Research

For the past 50 years or so, the field of program evaluation has gained much notoriety and prominence in Western countries, especially with the generalized implementation of auditing systems that require that publicly funded programs show evidence that they produce their expected outcomes. With the publication of specialized textbooks and scientific journals and the creation of graduate training programs, evaluation has become a thriving scientific activity. Given the existence of such a field and its penetration into the health domain, one may question the necessity of creating a new field of scientific research such as PHIR.

There are indeed large areas of overlap between evaluation and PHIR (Hawe & Potvin, 2009). Both involve the use of scientific methods to produce knowledge about interventions that aim at improving the human condition. There are, however, two main advantages in developing PHIR as a distinct field from that of evaluation (Potvin, Di Ruggiero, & Shoveller, 2013).

First, contrary to the field of evaluation, which is relevant to a broad range of applied fields such as public administration, education, and many others, PHIR is a deliberate effort to define and circumscribe a specific object for scientific inquiry: population health intervention. Over and above the idea of providing evidence for practice, the emergence of PHIR is the result of a collective attempt to clearly problematize what constitutes a population health intervention as a specific class of objects for research. PHIR emphasizes that population health interventions are complex systems embedded in context and, as such, they pose a series of research problems that cut across a number of disciplinary and applied fields that, taken as a whole, form a unique set of issues (Hawe, 2015). Beyond the traditional distinction between process and outcomes, which is pervasive in the literature on evaluation, PHIR broadens the spectrum of questions particularly relevant to population health interventions (Hawe &Potvin, 2009).

Coming from the Latin words *inter*, which means in-between, and *venir*, which means to come, intervening means literally coming in between events in a process in order to change its likely outcome (Hawe & Potvin, 2009). It is a deliberate attempt to alter the foreseeable future by changing the current state of affairs. Increasing health has always been a highly legitimate reason for public institutions to intervene in peoples' lives. Anthropologists such as Didier Fassin (1996) have described in ample detail how early human communities created specialized functions such as shamans and wizards with the authority to "intervene" in cases of sorcery or ill-health in order to prevent further disorders. Later on, health, and more specifically public health, played an important role in legitimating the nascent nation-state of the nineteenth century to intervene in and regulate the public sphere and limit individuals' freedom.

Attempts to create a science of population health intervention bring to the forefront a very specific type of intervention: population health interventions. Those seek to change the distribution of health in populations, as whole entities in their contexts. PHIR encompasses all aspects of these interventions, including effective mechanisms, implementation challenges, interaction with contexts, and others (Hawe, 2015).

Second, and more importantly, PHIR switches the emphasis away from the idea of making decisions about the future of a singular evaluated intervention, as it is the case in most definitions of evaluation (Potvin & McQueen, 2008). It indicates an intention to develop a whole body of cumulative knowledge about population health interventions as a class of objects: a science of population health interventions. The underlying assumption is that there are patterns and regularities in ways in which interventions are planned, implemented, sustained, scaled up, and evaluated and a cumulative knowledge base can be developed regardless of the specific objectives of each intervention studied (McQueen & Anderson, 2001). This, in turn, opens up critical areas of investigation that cut across numerous interventions, irrespective of their specific substantive aim.

Examples of recent crosscutting inquiries deal with questions such as what makes, and how to account for, intervention complexity (Craig et al., 2008; Hawe, Shiell, & Riley, 2004); how to appraise context and context-intervention interactions (Shoveller et al., 2015; Poland, Frohlich, & Cargo, 2008); what constitutes an intervention's core or active components that can be transferred to other contexts (Villeval et al., 2016); and how interactions between intervention implementers and researchers influence its implementation and research results (Israel, Schulz, Parker, & Becker, 1998; Bilodeau et al., 2012).

The interest in creating a new field of applied scientific inquiry defined by its specific object is not unique to PHIR. Recently, and stemming mainly from research on health care systems, *implementation research* has been defined as "the scientific study of methods to promote the systematic uptake of proven clinical treatments, practices, organisational, and management interventions into routine practice, and hence to improve health" (Implementation Science, 2016). Clearly, implementation research intersects with PHIR, as it includes population health interventions among various types of health interventions as possible subjects of research. It is distinct from PHIR, however, as it seems to exclude research on interventions designed and controlled by researchers to test hypotheses.

RELEVANCE OF PHIR FOR HEALTH PROMOTION

Over the past 20 years there has been a strong movement within the field of health promotion to evaluate its effectiveness. In most countries, as is the case in Canada, health promotion is located within a Department of Health and, in most instances, it is framed as one of the mandates of public health. PHAC, for example, identifies seven roles in its mandate; one of them is to promote health (PHAC, 2016). Thus, having to compete with other mandates such as health care for the scarce resources of the public health sector, health promotion decision makers felt the need to promote and advocate for a widespread use of evaluation in order to (1) justify spending money on it, because it is an effective way to invest in achieving better health at the population level (McQueen & Jones, 2007); and (2) provide evidence to practitioners on which to base interventions (PHAC, 2014). Given the importance of evaluation in the health promotion research agenda, and also because PHIR claims to encompass health promotion, it is interesting to examine more closely four dimensions of overlap between health promotion and PHIR.

PHIR and Health Promotion Pursue the Same Overarching Goal

PHIR's goal is ultimately to contribute to better health for populations (Institute of Population and Public Health, 2012). To this end, PHIR's working hypothesis is that a cumulative knowledge base about how to change population health determinants through interventions can be elaborated using scientific methods from a variety of relevant disciplines. Such a knowledge base would support the elaboration of theoretical propositions about the planning, implementation, and future development of population health interventions. Obviously, in order to maintain their heuristic function, such theoretical propositions would need to be adapted to local conditions and context, like all theoretical propositions. Nevertheless, empirically derived theoretical propositions that can be tested scientifically are thought to be better guides for public health interventions than ideology and beliefs.

An example of such a theoretical proposition is Hawe and colleagues' distinction between an intervention's essential function and its contextualized form (2004). According to them, an intervention's effective mechanism does not equate to the formal activities implemented. Such activities represent ways of locally adapting and contextualizing more fundamental mechanisms, which they call essential functions. In a school-based intervention, for example, an essential function could be to involve students in the planning of activities. The forms this function takes would vary and be locally adapted to each school's studentship, history, culture, and so on.

Health promotion's overarching goal is to increase health and equity, which is very similar to that of PHIR. To this end the *Ottawa Charter* proposes strategies and values to guide the action of those engaged in this goal. In all of its declarations, charters, or statements produced through the various WHO health promotion conferences over the past 30 years, research has never been identified as a valued strategy to increase health and equity. At best, the *Bangkok Charter for Health Promotion in a Globalized World* invites health promoters to use health promotion intervention with proven effectiveness, without defining criteria for what constitutes proof (WHO, 2005).

Fortunately, health promotion is much more than WHO-led initiatives and documents. The number of scientific peer-reviewed journals that have health promotion in their titles, the number of graduate research training programs that propose degrees in health promotion or related fields, and the number of research infrastructures from chairs to research centres that implement health promotion research programs all testify that health promotion research is alive and well. However, health promotion has yet to take stock of the range of topics and methods that characterize it as a distinct field. Potvin and McQueen (2008) argued that given the action and solution-oriented nature of the field of health promotion, an important part of health promotion research should be about interventions and evaluation. In addition to the most-needed evaluation of health promotion "which uses methods and paradigms which belong to the outside perspective from which the field is evaluated" (Potvin & McQueen, 2008, p. 32), they advocate for the development of evaluation in health promotion, defined as "the borrowing and adaptation by health promotion of conceptual and methodological tools developed in other scientific domains to enhance its own capacity to better understand its own object" (p. 32). PHIR may be an opportunity to further develop this idea of evaluation in health promotion and develop a cumulative knowledge base that would provide empirically derived knowledge about the planning, implementation, sustainability, scaling up, and evaluation of health promotion interventions.

PHIR and Health Promotion Embrace a Collective Perspective about Health

As previously mentioned, PHIR is about population health interventions. The class of objects that it seeks to better understand (and eventually improve) is coordinated actions and resources that involve a variety of social actors and that aim at changing health and its determinants at the population and ecosystem level (Hawe, 2015). Whether it includes interventions to support individual change may still be debatable but even excluding them would still leave huge areas of overlap with health promotion.

Since the *Ottawa Charter*, there has been a lively debate in health promotion about whether the level of action is individual or collective. The *Ottawa Charter* embraces a collective perspective on health and its determinants. The Charter's perspective on health is populational because its emphasis on inequalities suggests a distributional dimension of health: one's health is influenced by that of the population to which one belongs and by one's status in this population (Rose, 1985). To understand what makes an individual healthy, one needs to understand and take into account the conditions that shape the health of the group to which this individual belongs. The Charter's perspective on health is also societal. It proposes that health is mostly produced in everyday life using resources whose local availability and accessibility are highly dependent on the ways in which societies are organized (Bambra, 2016). Thus, promoting health means mobilizing a variety of actors from various sectors to develop and implement programs and policies to modify the largely social conditions that influence health. As a matter of fact, among the five health promotion strategies identified in the *Ottawa Charter*, four involve social processes (creating supportive environments, re-orienting health services, building healthy public policy, and strengthening community action). So health promotion is mostly an agenda for transforming the social conditions that affect health, which does not, however, exclude actions at the individual level, as shown by the fifth strategy of action identified by the *Charter* (i.e., developing personal skills).

PHIR and Health Promotion Favour Collaboration

As previously mentioned, PHIR has emerged out of a preoccupation with increasing the relevance of research results for practitioners and decision makers, which means that studied interventions have to be aligned as closely as possible with real-life program or policy implementation conditions. This involves collaborative partnerships between research teams and implementation systems. The favoured approach is that of integrated knowledge translation and exchange,[4] which integrates the principles of knowledge translation throughout the entire research process (CIHR, 2012). The main intention is to increase research relevance for knowledge users, but collaborative research[5] with integrated knowledge translation and exchange is also key for producing valid conclusions when studying interventions implemented by organizations whose mandate is primarily to intervene in populations. Although PHIR does not automatically reject the possibility that research teams are the main drivers of the intervention, it emphasizes the need to conduct rigorous research in real-life situations. Thus, PHIR involves a collaborative partnership between delivery systems that operate an intervention and a research team that produces knowledge about this intervention. This is acknowledged within the set of required competencies for PHIR that clearly identifies working in partnership with implementation systems as a core competency for PHIR (Riley, Harvey, Di Ruggiero, & Potvin, 2015).

Together with empowerment, collaboration and participation are also key values and principles of action for health promotion (Rootman, Goodstadt, Potvin, & Springett, 2001). There is an explicit assumption that the role of health promotion experts is one of enabler for change and not necessarily the main driver. Typically, health promotion interventions are not planned and implemented in isolation from the input of those who benefit from them. Participation ensures interventions' relevance with regard to local needs and conditions.

PHIR and Health Promotion Require Methodological Pluralism and Adaptation to Context

Conducting research about interventions developed and implemented in real-life situations is key in PHIR to ensure maximum relevance for practice (Green, 2006) and ultimately to facilitate evidence-based practice. This is so because of the critical role of local, contextual conditions, not only on the emergence and causes of the problem to be solved, but also as they interact with the intervention to produce expected (as well as unexpected) outcomes (Shoveller et al., 2015). As a consequence, any research methodology that aims to control for, or take away, the role of context and implementation conditions runs the risk of obliterating key effective intervention dimensions (Potvin & McQueen, 2008). Understanding how an intervention works and for whom largely means capturing and taking into account the role of context vis-à-vis the intervention. This cannot be achieved by a randomized control trial wherein individuals are the units of assignment and taken out of their context to be given an intervention. In population health intervention research, whole settings have to be assigned to interventions, randomly as in cluster randomized trials (Oakes, 2004), or taking advantage of "natural" variations as in natural experiments (Petticrew et al., 2005). In all cases, intervention effects have to be conceived as resulting from the interaction between the intervention and the various contexts of implementation, and need to be estimated at the setting level. In this perspective, it is usually recommended that studies estimating an intervention's effects be complemented with observational implementation studies that document the intervention/context interactions and the resulting variation in intervention forms (Hawe et al., 2004). Briefly, the use of multiple methods adapted to the research questions and the intervention contextual conditions is characteristic of PHIR.

Health promotion is also characterized by attention and local adaptation of methods to contextual conditions (Poland et al., 2008). Health promotion interventions are conceived as being constantly created and recreated through their adaptation to local conditions. Even in the case of interventions proven effective, research has shown that their successful implementation is often associated with adapting them to their new implementation context (Juneau et al., 2011). Therefore, health promotion does not advocate for one-size-fits-all intervention methods. On the contrary, it identifies a whole range of strategies of action and invites practitioners to use those that are most relevant to the intervention context.

CONCLUSION

Although one is primarily concerned with producing knowledge and the other with transforming people's living conditions, this chapter shows that there are large areas of overlap between population health intervention research and health promotion. However, a systematic analysis of these similarities highlights the lack of a unified and coherent perspective about the role and function of research in health promotion. Given the large overlaps between the two fields, figure 19.3 can be used as a starting point to a mapping exercise for health promotion research. Obviously, there is a large part of PHIR that is directly relevant to health promotion. On the vertical axis, creating a scientific knowledge base on the development, sustainability, and scaling up of health promotion interventions is critical for the field. But health promotion research would not only be a science of solutions. There are some problem-related research topics that need to be addressed by health promotion. For example, research that attempts to problematize and operationalize key health promotion concepts such as positive health, empowerment, and participation without necessarily linking them to intervention is critical for the advancement of the field.

CRITICAL THINKING QUESTIONS

1. Is there a need for health promotion to develop cumulative knowledge about interventions?
2. Should all research in health promotion be concerned with interventions? If not, what are the other research topics specific to health promotion?
3. To what extent do health promotion researchers need to exercise control over the various aspects of health promotion interventions in order to provide valid results?

RESOURCES

Further Readings

Ferron, C., Breton, E., & Guichard, A. (2013). Recherche interventionnelle en santé publique: Quand chercheurs et acteurs de terrain travaillent ensemble. *La santé en action, 425.*

This collection of articles presents various issues related to population health intervention from both researchers' and practitioners' perspectives. France is one European country where population health intervention research has gained much attention in the past five years.

Frankish, J., Bruce, T., Beanland, H., Di Rugiero, E., Muhajarine, N., Potvin, L., & Van Winsberghe, R. (2012). Population health intervention research: Advancing the field. *Canadian Journal of Public Health, 103*(Suppl. 1).

This is a collection of studies conducted by Canadian researchers about various population health interventions in Canada. This provides examples of a broad range of population health intervention research.

Harrington, D., McLafferty, S., & Elliott, S. (Eds.). (2016). *Population health intervention research. Geographical perspectives.* New York: Routledge.

This book presents a broad range of examples of population health intervention research conducted in various countries. It provides in-depth discussions of concepts borrowed from geography, such as context and place.

Institute of Population and Public Health, Canadian Population Health Initiative. (2011). *Population health intervention research casebook.* www.cihr-irsc.gc.ca/e/documents/ipph_casebook_e.pdf

This casebook presents short vignette examples of population health intervention research organized to illustrate crosscutting issues of population health intervention research.

Potvin, L., Di Ruggiero, E., & Hawe, P. (2009). The Population Health Intervention Research Initiative of Canada. *Can J Public Health, 100*(1), Special insert.

This series of four articles is the first collection of papers about PHIR that was published by PHIRIC to launch the initiative. The article by Hawe and Potvin provides a definition and a first discussion of PHIR.

RELEVANT WEBSITES

National Collaborating Centre for Public Health
ncchpp.ca/en/

This site is the introduction to the network and is a portal to the six centres that compose the network. Of particular importance for this chapter is the NCC for Methods and Tools (www.nccmt.ca), which contains a great number of resources on knowledge translation interventions and the promotion of public health evidence-based practice.

Population Health Intervention Research Initiative for Canada
www.cihr-irsc.gc.ca/e/38731.html

This is PHIRIC's website, hosted by CIHR Institute of Population and Public Health. It hosts all documents produced by the initiative and related to PHIR.

NOTES

1. An intervention is a set of coordinated actions supported by dedicated resources in the pursuit of an objective that aims at transforming existing conditions or changing the course of a process.

2. Evidence is knowledge that is mobilized and formatted to support an argument. Scientific evidence, specifically, is a collection of facts drawn from empirical research in support of a decision or intervention development.

3. Evaluation research is a type of research aimed at producing knowledge about a specific intervention (program or policy).

4. Knowledge translation and exchange (KTE) is a set of activities that aim at both formal and informal increasing of exchanges and sharing between researchers and knowledge users.

5. Collaborative research implies a collaborative relationship between a team of researchers and a group of knowledge users. In PHIR and health promotion research, knowledge user partners are usually those responsible for intervention delivery and implementation.

REFERENCES

Bambra, C. (2016). *Health divides. Where you live can kill you.* Bristol, UK: Policy Press.

Bilodeau, A., Gendron, S., Bédard, J., Couturier, Y., Bernier, J., & Lefebvre, C. (2012). Les opérations de la recherche participative et leurs finalités: Trois cas de recherche interventionnelle. In F. Aubry & L. Potvin. (Eds.), *Construire l'espace sociosanitaire: Expériences et pratiques de recherche dans la production locale de la santé* (pp. 45–74). Montréal: Presses de l'Université de Montréal.

Butler-Jones, D. (2009). Public health science and practice: From fragmentation to alignment. *Canadian Journal of Public Health, 100,* i3–i4.

Canadian Institute for Health Research (CIHR). (2012). *Guide to knowledge translation planning at CIHR: Integrated end-of-grant approaches.* Ottawa: COHR. Retrieved from cihr-irsc.gc.ca/e/45321.html

Catford, J. (2009). Advancing the "science of delivery" of health promotion: Not just the "science of discovery." *Health Promotion International, 24*(1), 1–5. DOI:10.1093/heapro/dap003

CIHR-IPPH. (2007). Operating grant—Intervention research. Retrieved from www.researchnet-recherchenet.ca/rnr16/vwOpprtntyDtls.do?prog=399&view=browseArchive&browseArc=true&progType=CIHR-12&type=EXACT&resultCount=25

Craig, P., Dieppe, P., Macintyre, S., Michie, S., Nazareth, I., & Petticrew M. (2008). Developing and evaluating complex interventions: The new Medical Research Council guidance. *BMJ, 337,* a1665.

CSDH. (2008). *Closing the gap in a generation: Health equity though action on the social determinants of health. Final Report of the Commission on Social Determinants Health.* Geneva: World Health Organization.

Fassin, D. (1996). *L'Espace politique de la santé. Essaie de généalogie.* Paris: Presses universitaires de France.

Green, L. W. (2006). Public health asks of systems science: To advance our evidence-based practice can you help us get more practice-based evidence? *American Journal of Public Health, 96,* 414–423.

Hancock, T., Spady, D. W., & Soskolne, C. L. (Eds.) (2015). *Global change and public health: Addressing the ecological determinants of health: The report in brief.* Retrieved from www.cpha.ca/uploads/policy/edh-brief.pdf

Harrington, D. W., McLafferty, S., & Elliot, S. J. (2016). *Population health intervention research: Geographical perspectives.* New York: Routledge.

Hawe, P. (2015). Lessons from complex interventions to improve health. *Annual Review of Public Health, 36,* 307–323.

Hawe, P., Di Ruggiero, E., & Cohen, E. (2012). Frequently asked questions about population health intervention research. *Canadian Journal of Public Health, 103,* e468–e471.

Hawe, P., & Potvin, L. (2009). What is population health intervention research? *Canadian Journal of Public Health, 100*(1), i8–i14.

Hawe, P., Shiell, A., & Riley, T. (2004). Complex interventions: How "out of control" can a randomised controlled trial be? *BMJ, 328,* a1561.

Implementation Science. (2016). *Description*. Retrieved from link.springer.com/journal/13012

Institute of Population and Public Health. (2012). *Population health intervention research initiative of Canada*. Retrieved from www.cihr-irsc.gc.ca/e/38731.html

Institut National du Cancer. (2016). *La recherche interventionnelle en santé des populations*. Retrieved from www.e-cancer.fr/Professionnels-de-la-recherche/Recherches-en-sante-des-populations/Recherche-interventionnelle

Israel, B. A., Schulz, A. J., Parker, E. A., & Becker, A. B. (1998). Review of community-based research: Assessing partnership approaches to improve public health. *Annual Review of Public Health, 19*, 173–202.

Jack, S. M., Busser, D., Sheehan, D., Zwygers, E., Gonzalez, A., & MacMillan, H. (2012). Adaptation and implementation of the nurse-family partnership in Canada. *Canadian Journal of Public Health, 103*(Suppl. 1), S42–S48.

Juneau, C-E., Jones, C. M., McQueen, D. V., & Potvin, L. (2011). Promotion de la santé basée sur des données probantes: Un domaine émergeant. *Global Health Promotion, 18*(1), 122–133.

Kohatsu, N. D., Robinson, J. G., & Torner, J. C. (2004). Evidence-based public health: An evolving concept. *American Journal of Preventive Medicine, 27*, 417–421.

Krieger, N. (2012). Who and what is a population? Historical debates, current controversies and implications for understanding population health and rectifying health inequities. *The Milbank Quarterly, 90*, 634–681.

Lavis, J., Ross, S., McLeod, C., & Gildiner, A. (2002) Measuring the impact of health research. *Journal of Health Services Research & Policy, 8*, 165–170.

McQueen, D. V., & Anderson, L. M. (2001). What counts as evidence: Issues and debates. In I. Rootman, M. Goodstadt, B. Hyndman, D. V. McQueen, L. Potvin, J. Springett, & E. Ziglio (Eds.), *Evaluation in health promotion. Principles and perspectives* (pp. 63–81). Copenhagen: WHO Regional Publications, European Series, No 92.

McQueen, D. V. & Jones, C. (Eds.). (2007). *Global perspectives on health promotion effectiveness*. New York: Springer.

National Collaborating Centres for Public Health (NCCPH). (2016). *About us*. Retrieved from www.nccph.ca/about-us/

Oakes, M. (2004). The (mis)estimation of neighbourhood effects: Causal inference for a practical social epidemiology. *Social Science & Medicine, 58*, 1929–1952.

Petticrew, M., Cummins, S., Ferrell, C., Findlay, A., Higgins, C., Hoy, C., Kearns, A., & Sparks, L. (2005). Natural experiments: An underused tool for public health? *Public Health, 119*, 751–757.

Poland, B., Frohlich, K., & Cargo, M. (2008). Context as a fundamental dimension of health promotion program evaluation. In L. Potvin, & D. V. McQueen (Eds.), *Health promotion evaluation practice in the Americas: Values and research* (pp. 299–318). New York: Springer.

Potvin, L., Di Ruggiero, E., & Shoveller, J. A. (2013). Pour une science des solutions: La recherche interventionnelle en santé des populations. *La santé en action, 425*, 13–16.

Potvin, L., & Jones, C. M. (2011). Twenty-five years after the Ottawa Charter: The critical role of health promotion for public health. *Canadian Journal of Public Health, 102*, 244–248.

Potvin, L., & McQueen, D. V. (2008). Practical dilemmas for health promotion evaluation. In L. Potvin & D. V. McQueen (Eds.), *Health promotion evaluation practices in the Americas: Values and practices* (pp. 25–45). New York: Springer.

Public Health Agency of Canada (PHAC). (2014). Canadian best practices portal. Retrieved from cbpp-pcpe.phac-aspc.gc.ca/

Public Health Agency of Canada (PHAC). (2016). *About the agency*. Retrieved from www.phac-aspc.gc.ca/about_apropos/index-eng.php

Riley, B., Harvey, J., Di Ruggiero, E., & Potvin L. (2015). Building the field of population health intervention research: The development and use of an initial set of competencies. *Preventive Medicine Report*s, *2*, 854–857. doi:10.1016/j.pmedr.2015.09.017

Rootman, I., Goodstadt, M., Potvin, L., & Springett, J. (2001). A framework for health promotion evaluation. In I. Rootman, M. Goodstadt, B. Hyndman, D. V. McQueen, L. Potvin, J. Springett, & E. Ziglio (Eds.), *Evaluation in health promotion. Principles and perspectives* (pp. 7–38). Copenhagen: WHO regional publications, European series, No 92.

Rose, G. (1985). Sick individuals and sick populations. *International Journal of Epidemiology, 14*, 32–38.

Shoveller, J., Viehbeck, S., Di Ruggiero, E., Greyson, D., Thomson, K., & Knight, R. (2015). A critical examination of context within research on population health interventions. *Critical Public Health, 26*, 487–500.

Sullivan, L. (2009). Introduction to the Population Health Intervention Research Initiative of Canada. *Canadian Journal of Public Health, 100*, i5–i6.

Villeval, M., Bidault, E., Shoveller, J., Alias, F., Basson J-C., Frasse, C., Génolini, J-P., Pons, E., Verbiguié, D., Grosclaude, P., & Lang, T. (2016). Enabling the transferability of complex interventions: Exploring the combination of an intervention's key functions and implementation. *International Journal of Public Health, 61*, 1031–1038.

World Health Organization (WHO). (1986). *Ottawa Charter for Health Promotion*. Ottawa: WHO. Retrieved from www.who.int/healthpromotion/conferences/previous/ottawa/en/

World Health Organization (WHO). (2005). *The Bangkok Charter for Health Promotion in a Globalized World*. Geneva: Author. Retrieved from www.who.int/healthpromotion/conferences/6gchp/bangkok_charter/en/

WHO Commission on Social Determinants of Health. (2008). *Closing the gap in a generation: Health equity through action on the social determinants of health*. Geneva: WHO. Retrieved from www.who.int/social_determinants/thecommission/finalreport/en/

CHAPTER 20

Health Promotion Ethics

Rodney Knight and Jean Shoveller

LEARNING OBJECTIVES

1. Identify and interrogate the ethical issues that arise within the practice of health promotion
2. Compare and contrast health promotion ethics with other areas of health ethics (e.g., medical ethics, population and public health ethics)
3. Propose and analyze solutions to dilemmas based on the values and principles that underpin health promotion

INTRODUCTION

If the epidemiological and social sciences have it "right," socially just societies will seek to minimize social inequities in health—not just because they *can* (i.e., empirically feasible), but because they *should* (i.e., an ethical obligation). Key philosophical questions remain, however, including, What is the "best"—that is, the most ethical—approach to health promotion (e.g., "upstream" versus "downstream" approaches)? Should individual freedoms be restricted in order to improve health? How should the distribution of health and social impacts of health promotion interventions be assessed? These are the kinds of issues that health promotion ethics is compelled to address.

Ethics

Before we can begin a discussion about "what is" and "how to do" health promotion ethics, it is helpful to understand how the various areas of scholarship and practice within the field of ethics more broadly inform and relate to health promotion ethics. Ethics is a branch of philosophy that aims to answer questions such as, What is right and what is wrong? What is the right or wrong action to take in response to a specific ethical dilemma? These are the sorts of questions that are not subject to empirical measurement alone (though the empirical realm can be used to inform our ethical deliberation; see Knight, 2016), but instead rely on philosophical inquiry. *Normative ethics* is the branch of ethics that seeks to answer these ethical questions (i.e., determine the ethically right course of action) through the use of theory and philosophical methods. Applied ethics is the practice of applying the various ethical theories, values, and principles that are developed within normative ethics in response to real-world ethical issues that need answering and action. Both normative and applied ethics are of importance to and within the practice of health promotion.

FROM BIOETHICS TO HEALTH PROMOTION ETHICS: MAPPING THE TERRAIN

Bioethics broadly refers to "all ethical issues relating to the creation and maintenance of the health of living things" (Dawson, 2010, p. 218). With a definition so broad, the field of bioethics has an enormous task—from determining whether a specific medical procedure (e.g., a Caesarean section) is the ethically appropriate course of action, to identifying what strategies should be put in place to address health inequity regarding a given chronic illness (e.g., diabetes). Since the 1960s, much "progress" has been made in bioethics, including the establishment of a variety of ethical values and principles that—in Canada today—are frequently taken up as the hallmarks of medical ethics. For example, Beauchamp and Childress's (2008) four principles (beneficence, non-maleficence, autonomy, and justice) are studied by students across Canada to inform decision-making in the practice of medicine. Similarly, in the realm of research ethics in Canada, the *Tri-Council Policy Statement 2: Ethical Conduct for Research Involving Humans* (Government of Canada, 2014) has continued to evolve over the years to provide what is largely held to be the "best" guidance for the Canadian research community based on the following three principles: respect for persons, concern for welfare, and justice.

Contemplating the ethical issues that arise within the practice of health promotion can be somewhat more complex than many of the issues that occur in other areas of medicine or public health. Measures to contain a pandemic (e.g., quarantine practices), or to ensure that people are not getting contaminated water pumped into their houses, tend to be more straightforwardly justified than policies that are designed to encourage people to change features of their day-to-day lifestyle (e.g., encouraging people to eat particular diets through tax policies; "discouraging" teenagers from becoming sexually active). To complicate matters further, liberal democracies like Canada tend to view government policy that "sways" human behaviour with a degree of suspicion, thereby making the kinds of policies that are used within health promotion at times difficult to justify. These questions can become ever more complex as we assess whether various measures should be advanced to ensure the appropriate life conditions are available for communities to live a healthy life, including what kinds of actions ought to be taken (or not be taken) to move "upstream" and address the social determinants of health (e.g., addressing gender inequity, poverty, or racism).

While a formal literature on health promotion ethics has existed since the advent of the field (e.g., Bayer & Moreno, 1986; Doxiadis & Blaney, 1987), since the early 2000s there has been an upsurge in the theorization of many of the key questions and ethical dilemmas that arise within health promotion, and much of this has transpired in the field of public health ethics. Public health ethics first arose, in part, due to a series of infectious disease outbreaks that exposed the insufficiency of some of the contemporary bioethical frameworks at the time (e.g., quarantine practices during the SARS outbreaks in the absence of diagnostic tests) (Bayer & Fairchild, 2004). As the field grew, much of this literature also began to "take up" the issues that often arise in the practice of health promotion, including the explicit interrogation of the ethical issues related to the planned pursuit of changing lifestyles and life conditions of individuals and communities to improve health.

Despite the recent popularity of this field, many questions remain unanswered and confusion often remains about the ethically appropriate course of action for those practising health promotion. Key philosophical questions continue to merit reflection by those practising health promotion, including the following:

- Who should try to change the health behaviour of individuals and communities, and how?
- What should the role of the state be in providing the best life conditions for producing good health?
- When an individual claims to have "autonomously" decided to engage in a "health-damaging" behaviour (e.g., consuming high rates of alcohol or tobacco), should the state intervene and behave paternalistically?
- How should health promotion implementation and evaluation strategies be selected, particularly when the evidence base regarding a specific intervention may be limited, complex, and implicitly value-laden?
- Is it ethical to design health promotion policy that accepts that health inequity is unjust and the result of "upstream" factors (e.g., poverty), while continuing to intervene on "downstream" risk factors (e.g., "health-damaging" behaviour)?

In real-world and applied contexts, these questions occur in contexts in which conflicts frequently arise between the values held by a society (e.g., a liberal democracy that features some of the tenets of liberalism, including a desire for limited state intervention and the value placed on freedom of choice) and the "public" values that inform health promotion (e.g., equity, justice). Here, it is important to distinguish the difference between *morals*—the values and beliefs that individuals and groups have about an ethical issue (e.g., people's views on abortion)—from *ethics*—the use of reasoning to determine what *ought* to be done about an ethical issue, regardless of what people happen to believe. Health promotion ethics is compelled to address these and other tensions by identifying the best (i.e., the most *ethical*) relationship between the

> **Box 20.1:** Health Promotion Ethics in Canada
>
> Canadian institutions, scholars, and practitioners have emerged as global leaders in terms of engaging in the ethical issues that arise in the practice of health promotion, and this is reflected in the lexicon that we use in the Canadian setting to refer to this area of practice and scholarship: *population health ethics* (Canadian Institutes of Health Research, 2012). According to the Canadian Institutes of Health Research, population health ethics differ from (and often build upon) traditional orientations of bioethics in that these approaches aim to (1) emphasize moral evaluations related to the population, alongside those of the individual; (2) acknowledge that many "upstream" interventions and influences on health occur both inside and outside of the health care system (e.g., from political and legal sectors); and (3) emphasize the *prevention* of illness and disease (in addition to the treatment of illness). Health promotion ethics is a branch of ethics—both applied and normative—that exists within and builds upon the theorization and applied practice of bioethics (including branches of population health ethics and medical ethics) and that focuses specifically on the questions that arise in the planned pursuit of changing lifestyles and conditions to improve community health.

individual, the community, and the state that can be applied to all Canadians. This process involves continually reflecting upon the means by which health promotion *can* (empirically) and *should* (ethically) address the tensions that occur between a variety of values, including freedom and paternalism, education and persuasion, coercion and liberty, autonomy and social justice.

ETHICAL ISSUES THAT ARISE IN HEALTH PROMOTION INTERVENTIONS

It is important for practitioners of health promotion to be aware of and reflect upon the ethical issues that frequently arise in the practice of health promotion in order to determine the appropriate course of action. Below, we discuss and offer insights into how three interdependent ethical themes can be normatively assessed and reflected upon in a variety of applied scenarios:

1. How should the tensions that can occur between values, value-laden evidence, and the practice of health promotion be negotiated?
2. How should the interests of individuals and the broader collective be "balanced" in the practice of health promotion?
3. How should the distribution of health and social impacts of health promotion interventions be assessed (e.g., unintended consequences, including stigmatization or "victim-blaming")?

1. Values and Evidence in the Practice of Health Promotion

In the practice of health promotion, ethical dilemmas can arise when the consequences of health promotion interventions infringe upon the values espoused by society. Embedded within many health promotion interventions are taken-for-granted assumptions about how to best intervene, and these value-laden (normative) dimensions need to be both interrogated and made transparent. For example, the values we hold (both as a society and in the field of health promotion) can create a tendency for different circles to favour specific "kinds" of evidence that, in turn, lead to the rollout of interventions that are "driven" (e.g., epistemologically or politically) in one direction or another.

Consider how many health promotion practices arise in the realm of teen pregnancy. In Canada and abroad, enormous amounts of public resources go into the *prevention* of teen pregnancy, and the vast majority of these interventions tend to be executed at the level of the individual, with many health promotion actions targeting the "potential" teen mother (e.g., social marketing campaigns). For example, some of these interventions aim to show adolescent girls the "dangers" of becoming pregnant, thereby presupposing that so-called scare tactics are efficacious and, ultimately, underpinned by a taken-for-granted assumption that teen parenthood is a morally inappropriate outcome.

As this sort of critical interrogation begins to reveal, underlying assumptions or values can influence how health promotion interventions are designed, implemented, and evaluated. For example, while "evidence-based" approaches to intervention may tend to be characterized as being "value neutral," the intervention responses may in fact reflect an approach to health promotion that, albeit implicitly, arises from a set of inherent political or ideological motivations (e.g., those that arise from neo-liberal ideals that de-responsibilize the state and foist responsibility onto the individual). While the ethical merits of focusing interventions at the level of the individual are debatable, values that inform health promotion, such as the need for transparency and justifiability, require those practising health promotion to address the extent to which various approaches to intervention may default to the valorization of individualism and personal responsibility *over* other values that could likewise be used in efforts. For example, in the realm of preventing unwanted pregnancies, there are many other intervention strategies that could rely less on foisting responsibility onto young women and instead focus on cultivating more gender-equitable relations (e.g., providing the conditions for young people, including adolescent boys, to negotiate and use contraceptives).

Regardless of the health issue, the ethical communication of "risk" to the public represents an ongoing challenge for those practising health promotion. While the public has a right to know about the factors that can influence their health and those practising health promotion have a duty to inform, questions remain about the extent to which various health promotion strategies ought to describe evidence surrounding a specific "risk" so that individuals can make informed decisions. However, given much of the evidence that we rely on in health promotion is complex, equivocal, or limited, health promotion ethics needs to determine at what point an intervention communicating "risk" or "nudging" a specific lifestyle is morally appropriate. To complicate matters, public understandings of risk (e.g., binary understandings in which risk is present or absent) are unlikely to align with epidemiological assessments of risk (e.g., statistical probabilities). This leaves those in health promotion with the task of developing the most ethical approach to risk communication.

So how does one assess and act upon the tensions that can arise between inherently value-laden evidence-based approaches and the duty to inform individuals so they can make autonomous decisions? Just as the evidence surrounding a particular risk needs to be dutifully translated, the values that inform health promotion also need to be made as transparent as reasonably possible. This includes addressing assumptions about the kinds of evidence that are used to assess a given health "problem" and/or "solution." But this also requires normative deliberation and transparency at each stage of the decision-making process, including those in health promotion:

- Identify the health problems that require intervention. There are, after all, many health issues that could benefit from health promotion interventions. How is the evidence base used to identify some health problems for intervention or action, while others are disregarded? How have the values and principles that inform the practice of health promotion influenced this process? How has the broader political and social discourse influenced this process?

- Determine the "best" approach to intervention. There are many ways to intervene on a health issue, and each approach to health promotion intervention implies different value assumptions. These assumptions need to be interrogated and made transparent. Integrating health promotion ethics into practice requires the skills to interrogate the extent to which interventions are put forth on values and how interventions relate to the evidence base, and this includes an interrogation of how choices are made among competing strategies to intervention (e.g., gains over the short- versus long-term; population-level gains versus individually oriented benefits; gains experienced only by more advantaged subgroups versus health equity–enhancing improvements for all).

- Evaluate the effectiveness of health promotion interventions. Outcomes are central for both the evaluation of an intervention's effectiveness, as well as the ethical assessment of the various consequences. The measures and indicators that are used to assess success or failure are inherently value-laden. Ethical evaluations of health promotion interventions need to account for more than the "positive" indicators (e.g., health benefits), including, for example, social outcomes that relate to the unintended consequences of the intervention (e.g., stigmatization).

2. How Should the Interests of Individuals and the Broader Collective Be Negotiated in the Practice of Health Promotion?

When considering the appropriateness of government policy that aims to change or influence personal behaviour, no issue has received more attention than that of individual autonomy and concerns about the incursion of individual freedom. Perhaps the most justifiable form of paternalism occurs in instances where interventions are designed to prevent people from harming others, rather than harming themselves. To that end, John Stuart Mill's (1859) *On Liberty* is frequently invoked to suggest that "the only purpose for which power can be rightfully exercised over any member of a civilized community, against his will, is to prevent harm to others" (p. 22). Yet, this kind of justification remains insufficient for many of the actions that take place in the planned pursuit of changing lifestyles and life conditions. How then, does health promotion negotiate the tensions that can arise between the values we place on both paternalism and autonomy?

Within the practice of medicine, these kinds of tensions are often resolved quite directly through the attainment of informed consent (Beauchamp & Childress, 2008). In the practice of health promotion, when the merits of individual autonomy are sufficiently attained—mainly, that it is both easy *and* economically feasible to "opt out"—it is often argued that paternalistic actions can also be ethically justified, even within societies that value limited state intervention (e.g., libertarian-oriented societies) (Nys, 2008). Consider, for example, a law in which healthier foods are placed in easier-to-access sections of a supermarket. While some may worry that this practice represents a form of manipulation, it nonetheless remains easy and economically free to "opt out" if one wishes to buy the less healthy alternatives.

Many policy actions that occur in the practice of health promotion, however, make both consent and easy opt out difficult or even impossible to attain (Carter, Cribb, & Allegrante, 2012). How could (or *should*) health promotion practitioners go about asking for consent at the level of the community, particularly when there is disagreement within the community? Consider, for example, the complexity of attaining community consent for taxation policies designed to discourage the consumption of high-fat and sugary foods or drinks. It seems highly doubtful that consent can be attained from every individual affected by such a policy. In health promotion ethics, we must ask, Does this policy represent an incursion on free choice and, if so, how might we justify this action, given our society's commitment to autonomy and liberty?

To answer this, health promotion practitioners need to interrogate the values held both by society and those that are used to inform the practice of health promotion. This process involves the assessment of a given policy or intervention, accounting for limitations and determining how health promotion interventions can (or cannot) align with societal values, while continuing to be critically conscious of both the intended and unintended effects of health promotion values and intervention outcomes. In doing these kinds of ethical interrogations, practitioners can identify how societal values can underpin health promotion actions that enhance equity and justice, including, at times, actions that require the limitation of free choice.

In other situations, paternalism can be somewhat more straightforwardly justified without the attainment of individual or community consent, including in situations in which it can be empirically demonstrated that so-called voluntary behaviour is the result of either (1) misinformation or (2) irresistible compulsion (Bayer & Moreno, 1986). One could argue, for instance, that individuals either do not understand the risks associated with consuming high-fat and sugary foods or drinks, or that they cannot resist the urge to buy and consume them—that is, consuming these items is inconsistent with what they wish to happen. In these cases, it is often suggested that a justified paternalism would seek to protect an individual from engaging in behaviour that they would not choose to do were they truly and autonomously expressing freedom of choice.

There is ongoing philosophical and social scientific work in this area that aims to better understand how individuals make theoretically autonomous decisions at the structure-agency interface. For instance, ethicists working in this area have recently argued that ethical deliberation in this area should not reduce towards a "dogma of autonomy" in which autonomy is upheld as the moral arbiter of how decisions are made with regards to public health and health promotion interventions (Dawson, 2010). For example, various feminist perspectives argue that the concept of *autonomy* is a far more complex theoretical construct that is currently bound within inherently "masculinist" (e.g., men-centred) assumptions or value traits (e.g., assumptions about "self-hood" that may counter the concerns of subordinate or marginalized members of society, including some groups of women and men). These perspectives argue that analyses regarding individual autonomy need to meaningfully take into account the *relationality* of an individual's social relationships, as well as the broader social and structural conditions in which individuals live and make theoretically autonomous decisions (Baylis, Kenny, & Sherwin, 2008). Consider, for example, how an individual with a high-paying job, a strong social network, and a home in a safe neighbourhood is more "meaningfully" autonomous than an individual who has none of these things.

Many of these arguments suggest support for an alternative approach that is frequently evoked within the justification of various health promotion actions and interventions that may involve the limiting of free choice: the *capability approach* (see Sen, 1989; Nussbaum, 2011). This approach argues that people ought to have real opportunities to achieve well-being and to do and be what they value. The approach diverges from those that suggest an individual needs to be left alone or act independently; instead, there is a careful analysis and reflection on the extent to which individual behaviour and decision-making is structurally embedded and that individuals therefore have a "stake" in how life conditions (e.g., social, relational, economical) "shape" individual behaviour. This approach to conceptualizing autonomy leaves us asking not only "Is this person able to be autonomous?" but also "Does this person have the opportunities that they value to live the best life possible?" In doing so, these approaches move beyond both liberal frameworks (e.g., those that prioritize autonomy above other values, such as solidarity) and utilitarian approaches that emphasize the maximization of health outcomes over other concerns (e.g., experiential

Box 20.2: Paternalism and Coercion

Health promotion interventions deploy a variety of actions that have implications for individual liberties, including the prohibition of specific health behaviours (e.g., smoking indoors), assertive health promotion campaigns (e.g., campaigns urging individuals to quit smoking), or mandatory practices (e.g., vaccinations, fluoridation of water supplies). In health promotion ethics, we need to distinguish between the implications that can arise through both *paternalistic* and *coercive* policies or practices. Paternalism involves interfering with a person's freedom *for their own good*— it is an inherently beneficent action, and it represents the conflict of two important values that we hold in liberal democracies such as Canada: the value we give to autonomy and the value we place on promoting health.

Coercion represents actions that overrule an individual's competent choice, including through the use of threats or force. It is widely accepted that many interventions should avoid coercive policies or practices, and this is largely related to the tainted legacy of previous interventions that undermined public confidence and trust in these practices (e.g., the mandatory testing of HIV before the advent of effective treatment in some settings). However, there are other interventions that might qualify as coercive, yet still can be determined to be ethically appropriate. Consider, for example, seat belt or bicycle helmet laws in which individuals are required to comply through the use of state-sanctioned enforcement (e.g., policing).

dimensions of living a "good" life). For example, rather than focusing just on concerns about individual liberties (e.g., autonomy, freedom of choice), a capabilities approach would view policies that aim to regulate human behaviour as providing the capacity for individuals to achieve the various goals that they value (e.g., remaining healthy throughout the life-course; getting a good education). As such, in certain cases paternalistic actions are required to support the life conditions or lifestyle changes that can best support individuals in accomplishing their goals.

3. How Should the Distribution of the Health and Social Impacts (Intended and Unintended) of Health Promotion Interventions be Assessed?

Given the emphasis on equity within the Canadian model of health care provision (e.g., all citizens are legally entitled to the same level of health care), and owing to the fact that health and illness are distributed along a social gradient (e.g., both communicable and non-communicable diseases tend to be concentrated among socially and economically disadvantaged populations), in health promotion it is largely held that there is an ethical obligation to reduce health and social inequities. Powers and Faden's (2006) theory of *social justice* has been an influential approach in terms of theorizing *how* the state ought to fairly distribute resources, opportunities, and wellbeing by moving "upstream" and attending to the social structures (e.g., neo-liberal economic systems) that systematically cluster disadvantage within various populations. For example, this approach suggests that the field of health promotion is ethically obliged to interrogate and address how individual-level health factors (e.g., biology; behaviour) are embedded within the broader social structures and environmental conditions. Therefore, it is often held that socially just health promotion interventions ought to mitigate—to the largest extent possible—the broader social and structural influences that shape health inequity.

These approaches to health promotion imply a particular way of understanding the distribution of health and illness and, in doing so, suggest the question, Is it ethical to design health promotion policy that accepts health inequity is unjust and the result of "upstream" factors (e.g., socio-economic deprivation), while continuing to intervene on "downstream" risk factors (e.g., smoking, drinking, exercise)? This trend is often referred to as a *lifestyle drift* effect.[1] For example, the "at-risk" and targeted approaches to health promotion intervention—whereby a specific population is targeted with an intervention due to the group's higher level of a given risk exposure—have been criticized for not fully addressing (or considering) the fundamental causes for health risks (e.g., social and economic influences) (Frohlich & Potvin, 2008; Raphael, chapter 8 in this book) and some have raised moral concern regarding their use (Goldberg, 2009).

In practice, many health promotion interventionists also continue to report only implementing interventions that have generally neglected the social determinants of health in favour of risk aversion and behaviourally oriented health promotion approaches (Brassolotto, Raphael, & Baldeo, 2014). This may be the result, in part, of the difficulty in terms of implementing structural interventions that can be politically unfavourable for those who have the power to make policies that can improve the life conditions of individuals and communities experiencing disadvantage. For example, structural interventions (e.g., the redistribution of wealth) can evoke images of status loss to those with power and can therefore be unpopular within some circles. In Canadian society, for example, the influence of neo-liberalism often reinforces a view that illness is "self-inflicted" and the direct result of lifestyle "choices," rather than a result of the life conditions available to an individual. The unfortunate result is that these viewpoints are highly moralizing and result in the stigmatization (e.g., labelling, status loss, discrimination) of individuals and/or population subgroups who engage in various behaviour (e.g., smoking) or who experience various disabilities or illnesses. Those practising health promotion are compelled to address the distribution of social and health impacts of these stigmatizing views, as well as how health promotion interventions can best remedy these kinds of social outcomes.

Regardless of one's philosophical approach or a society's given political and moral underpinnings, health promotion practitioners need to address a critical question in all pursuits of the promotion of health: Who does a given intervention benefit and who does it exclude (or potentially disadvantage)? A criticism of health promotion is that many of the interventions that become available are most likely to reach the proverbial "low-hanging fruit"—that is, the already most-advantaged members of society. Moreover, many health promotion interventions have also been critiqued for burdening specific population sub-groups with an intervention, while aiming to benefit those not explicitly targeted through a *dispersion of benefits* (e.g., reducing disease prevalence in a population will reduce the likelihood of disease acquisition among those not targeted) (O'Neill, 2011). As such, many individualist interventions can have the unintended effect of enhancing health inequity (intervention-generating inequalities) (Lorenc, Petticrew, Welch, & Tugwell, 2012). We suggest that, regardless of whether focusing on lifestyle factors or life conditions, socially just health promotion interventions are obliged to continually provide opportunities for a "levelling up" of the social gradient (or at the very least, avoid a "levelling down"). The benefits of interventions should therefore be distributed equally or preferentially with-in disadvantaged societies whenever possible. For example, Benach, Malmusi, Yasui, & Martinez (2013) argue that universal approaches to intervention may be most effective at reducing inequity if they include approaches that increase resource distribution as disad-vantage increases (e.g., by socio-economic status)—an intervention approach referred to as *universal proportionalism*.

APPLYING HEALTH PROMOTION ETHICS

We have learned that health promotion ethics must go beyond describing or applying approaches that Canadians happen to feel is the right thing to do (a descriptive endeav-our—what "is") to determining what "should be" (a normative endeavour). For health promotion practitioners, this process is analytic (identifying and assessing the morally relevant issues), reflective (reflecting on how one's own moral intuitions and one's own professional ethics influence decision-making), applied (results in the professional response that is deemed to be the ethical course of action), and requires ongoing evaluation (includ-ing evaluation of both the intended and unintended health *and* social outcomes). Health promotion ethics should not be left for the philosophers alone; health promotion practi-tioners must continually engage in questions about the various ethical implications that arise within and across each program of intervention. Developing skills in ethical reflection and understanding how to apply these skill sets are critical competencies that are required in the practice of health promotion.

To inform the practice of health promotion ethics, those working in this field have called for ethical codes to be developed (Bull, Riggs, & Nchogu, 2012). Recently, the International Union for Health Promotion and Education released the Ethical Principles of the IUHPE Health Promotion Accreditation System (see box 20.3), an accreditation process that aims to promote core competencies and standards in health promotion. The Accreditation System is underpinned by the ethical values and principles of equity and social justice, as well as respect for the autonomy and choice of individuals and commu-nities. Importantly, this process also stresses the value of working in collaborative and consultative ways, including ways that engage community-based participation.

Box 20.3: Ethical Principles of the IUHPE Health Promotion Accreditation System

The ethical values and principles underpinning the IUHPE Accreditation System include a belief in equity and social justice, respect for autonomy, and collaborative and consultative ways of working. Ethical health promotion practice is based on a commitment to the following:

- Health as a human right, which is central to human development.
- Respect for the rights, dignity, confidentiality and worth of individuals and groups.
- Respect for all aspects of diversity including gender, sexual orientation, age, religion, disability, ethnicity, race, and cultural beliefs.
- Addressing health inequities, social injustice, and prioritising the needs of those experiencing poverty and social marginalisation.
- Addressing the political, economic, social, cultural, environmental, behavioural and biological determinants of health and wellbeing.
- Ensuring that Health Promotion action is beneficial and causes no harm.
- Being honest about what Health Promotion is, and what it can and cannot achieve.
- Seeking the best available information and evidence needed to implement effective policies and programmes that influence health.
- Collaboration and partnership as the basis for Health Promotion action.
- The empowerment of individuals and groups to build autonomy and self-respect as the basis for Health Promotion action.
- Sustainable development and sustainable Health Promotion action.
- Being accountable for the quality of one's own practice and taking responsibility for maintaining and improving knowledge and skills.

Source: IUHPE Health Promotion Accreditation System. Retrieved from www.iuhpe.org/index.php/en/the-accreditation-system

There are also a variety of ethical frameworks that have been advanced in recent years to inform health promotion, including the Nuffield Council on Bioethics (2007) "intervention ladder" (see box 20.4) that seeks to determine whether a health policy is acceptable by determining whether or not the policy is "proportionate." For example, this approach offers opportunities to ask, Will the benefits of the measure be enough to justify the interference in people's lives and the financial cost? And how likely is it that the measure will achieve its aim? The "intervention ladder" suggests that the higher up the ladder, the more intrusive an intervention, which therefore requires stronger justification. Importantly, the Nuffield Council also argues that "doing nothing" is also a choice and has critical ethical implications and, as such, both action and inaction require justification.

Box 20.4: Nuffield Council on Bioethics "Intervention Ladder"

Nuffield Bioethics Intervention Ladder argues that intervention options can be thought of as a "ladder" of choices, with each step up taking away individual freedom and therefore requiring increasing justification. The ladder of policy actions is as follows:

- Eliminate choice
- Restrict choice
- Guide choice through disincentives
- Guide choice through incentives
- Guide choice through changing the default policy
- Enable choice
- Provide information
- Do nothing or simply monitor the situation

Source: Nuffield Council on Bioethics. (2007). *Public health: Ethical issues.* London: Nuffield Council on Bioethics. Retrieved from nuffieldbioethics.org/wp-content/uploads/2014/07/Public-health-ethical-issues.pdf

CONCLUSION

The field of health promotion is compelled to minimize social inequities in health through the application of an interdisciplinary set of skills that includes both normative deliberation and applied decision-making. In doing so, there are opportunities to make progress in the field by engaging in ongoing philosophical reflection of many of the issues raised in this chapter, as well as other issues that will undoubtedly arise as the field continues to advance (e.g., as new technologies and evidence emerge). It may be, after all, a very difficult task to "do the right thing" without engaging in careful and transparent approaches to the ethical interrogation of the various issues that arise in the practice of health promotion.

CRITICAL THINKING QUESTIONS

1. Drawing on the discussions presented in this chapter (as well as using other resources if needed), develop your argument either "for" or "against" a proposed health promotion intervention in your area of expertise or interest. Be sure to indicate how you arrived at your moral conclusion. Consider the following in your discussion: What ethical theories and/or health promotion principles are you drawing on? How are you considering the interests of individuals among those of the broader population?

    As you answer these questions, consider/identify what additional evidence might be missing and that you might want or need to have in order to make a more informed decision. Describe how you would acquire that evidence, and how you would assess the extent to which the evidence you are using is "value-laden."

2. What do you feel should be the limit of paternalistic policies that limit free choice within the practice of health promotion?

3. Is it ethical to design health promotion policy that accepts health inequity is unjust and the result of "upstream" factors (e.g., socio-economic deprivation), while continuing to intervene on "downstream" risk factors (e.g., smoking, drinking, exercise)? Describe how you came to your decision. For example, how do the values that inform health promotion align or clash with the mainstream political discourses of society? How can potential tensions in this area best be reconciled?

RESOURCES

Further Reading

Canadian Institutes of Health Research—Institute of Population and Public Health. (2012). *Population and public health ethics: Cases from research, policy and practice.* Toronto: University of Toronto Joint Centre for Bioethics. www.jcb.utoronto.ca/publications/documents/Population-and-Public-Health-Ethics-Casebook-ENGLISH.pdf

This book provides in-depth cases of different ethical dilemmas that are often faced by those practising health promotion in Canada. This is a good source for advancing one's normative reasoning and applied skills regarding issues that are relevant in health promotion ethics.

Relevant Websites

Globethics.net
www.globethics.net

Globethics.net is a network of those interested in the application of ethics, including the application of issues that are relevant in health promotion. Globethics.net provides resources on ethics, including a global digital ethics library.

National Collaborating Centre for Determinants of Health
www.nccdh.ca/

The NCCDH's mission is to provide tools and methods to promote and improve the use of scientific research and other knowledge, with a particular emphasis on acting on the social determinants of health and advancing health equity through practice and policy.

Nuffield Council on Bioethics, "Public Health: Ethical Issues"
nuffieldbioethics.org/project/public-health/

This report considers issues that are relevant to health promotion, including what various sectors (e.g., government) should do to enable people to lead a healthy life. Specifically, it draws on several case studies to illustrate the various ethical issues that can arise, including infectious diseases, obesity, alcohol, and smoking.

NOTE

1. *Lifestyle drift* refers to the tendency for health promotion interventions to intervene on "downstream" determinants of health (e.g., "risk" behaviour), rather than the "upstream" factors and life conditions in which health behaviour occurs (e.g., social determinants of health).

REFERENCES

Bayer, R., & Fairchild, A. L. (2004). The genesis of public health ethics. *Bioethics, 18*(6), 473–492.

Bayer, R., & Moreno, J. D. (1986). Health promotion: Ethical and social dilemmas of government policy. *Health Affairs, 5*(2), 72–85.

Baylis, F., Kenny, N. P., & Sherwin, S. (2008). A relational account of public health ethics. *Public Health Ethics, 1*(3), 196–209.

Beauchamp, T. L., & Childress, J. F. (2008). *Principles of biomedical ethics*. New York: Oxford University Press.

Benach, J., Malmusi, D., Yasui, Y., & Martinez, J. M. (2013). A new typology of policies to tackle health inequalities and scenarios of impact based on Rose's population approach. *Journal of Epidemiology & Community Health, 67*(3), 286–291.

Brassolotto, J., Raphael, D., & Baldeo, N. (2014). Epistemological barriers to addressing the social determinants of health among public health professionals in Ontario, Canada: A qualitative inquiry. *Critical Public Health, 24*(3), 321–336.

Bull, T., Riggs, E., & Nchogu, S. N. (2012). Does health promotion need a code of ethics? Results from an IUHPE mixed method survey. *Global health promotion, 19*(3), 8–20.

Canadian Institutes of Health Research. (2012). *Population Health Ethics*. Retrieved from www.cihr-irsc.gc.ca/e/41867.html

Carter, S. M., Cribb, A., & Allegrante, J. P. (2012). How to think about health promotion ethics. *Public Health Reviews, 34*(1), 1–24.

Dawson, A. (2010). The future of bioethics: Three dogmas and a cup of hemlock. *Bioethics, 24*(5), 218–225.

Doxiadis, S., & Blaney, R. (Eds.). (1987). *Ethical dilemmas in health promotion*. Chichester: John Wiley & Sons Ltd.

Frohlich, K. L., & Potvin, L. (2008). Transcending the known in public health practice: The inequality paradox: The population approach and vulnerable populations. *American Journal of Public Health, 98*(2), 216–221.

Goldberg, D. S. (2009). In support of a broad model of public health: Disparities, social epidemiology and public health causation. *Public Health Ethics, 2*(1), 70–83.

Government of Canada. (2014). *Tri-Council Policy Statement 2: Ethical conduct for research involving humans.* Retrieved from www.pre.ethics.gc.ca/eng/policy-politique/initiatives/tcps2-eptc2/Default/

Knight, R. (2016). Empirical population and public health ethics: A review and critical analysis to advance robust empirical-normative inquiry. *Health, 20*(3), 274–290.

Lorenc, T., Petticrew, M., Welch, V., & Tugwell, P. (2012). What types of interventions generate inequalities? Evidence from systematic reviews. *Journal of Epidemiology & Community Health, 67*(2), 190–193.

Mill, J. S. (1859). *On liberty* (2nd ed.). London: J. W. Parker.

Nuffield Council on Bioethics. (2007). *Public health: Ethical issues.* London: Author. Retrieved from nuffieldbioethics.org/wp-content/uploads/2014/07/Public-health-ethical-issues.pdf

Nussbaum, M. (2011). *Creating capabilities: The human development approach.* Boston: Harvard University Press.

Nys, T. R. V. (2008). Paternalism in public health care. *Public Health Ethics, 1*(1), 64–72.

O'Neill, O. (2011). *Broadening bioethics: Clinical ethics, public health and global health.* Presented at Nuffield Council's Annual Lecture at the Royal Society of Arts.

Powers, M., & Faden, R. (2006). *Social justice: The moral foundations of public health and health policy.* Oxford: Oxford University Press.

Sen, A. (1989). Development as capability expansion. *Journal of Development Planning, 19*, 41–58.

CHAPTER 21

Participatory Practice and Health Promotion in Canada

Jane Springett and Jeff Masuda

LEARNING OBJECTIVES

1. Understand the underpinnings of participatory practice in health promotion in the context of contemporary Canada
2. Apply a practical rubric for engaging in participatory practice

> *To be denied the capacity for potentially successful participation is to be denied one's humanity.*
> —Doyal & Gough, 1991, p. 184

INTRODUCTION

Participation is a fundamental principle that goes to the core of the democratic and social justice ethos of health promotion. Promoting individual and collective participation is a key practice competency that requires a careful and critical analysis of its techniques and contexts. There are as many approaches to participation as there are potential health benefits; from physical activity promotion programs that improve mental and physical health to global social movements in health that advocate for more social justice policies. But there are also risks to participatory approaches—from accusations of tokenism, to placing undue and unnecessary burdens on the lives of people who may already face disproportionate health inequities. In the wake of the *Ottawa Charter*'s call for action, the effective conduct of participatory health promotion has been a major research priority in Canada (Green et al., 1995) and beyond (Minkler, 2000). This chapter explores the basic tenets of participatory health promotion, demonstrating how, through the daily practice of authentic participation, we can encourage social changes that will create and support health and health equity. In the first section we discuss how encouraging authentic participation is a product both about how we think and how we act. In the second section we outline a rubric that distills key elements of effective participatory practice. In the final section we present three real-world examples of participatory practice in a Canadian context.

THINKING AND ACTING PARTICIPATIVELY

Participation is not just a process; it is a mindset, a philosophy of being and acting in the world ecologically, organically, and holistically, and in health promotion, with the ultimate aim of improving the conditions for optimal health and social justice. Following (although not always recognizing) Indigenous ways of knowing, participation in health promotion encourages a way of seeing health and wellbeing not as a matter of causes and effects but rather as an inherently relational and cyclical process of questioning answers rather than answering questions (Brown, McPherson, Peterson, Newman, & Cranmer, 2012; Castleden, Garvin, & Nation, 2009; Ledwith & Springett, 2010). For example, while most know that daily exercise reduces their chance of developing chronic diseases, taking a participatory approach in health promotion may provide an avenue to go beyond simply implementing physical activity programs, but also includes examining and addressing how our society has become so accepting of sedentary forms of work, transportation, and life-style habits. When we encourage people to think in this way, they begin to recognize that we are all a part of an interconnected world of people, ideas, and things that are in constant flux and that influence our daily lives. To promote health participatively is to engage in a process of continual learning where, when, and how to intervene justly and effectively within the changing world around us. Furthermore, with this orientation, we soon realize that we are constantly in need of mutual support and the collective wisdom of others in and beyond our own communities who share our struggles (although often in more challenging circumstances than us) as well as our aspirations for a good life.

Unfortunately, many approaches to participatory practice in health promotion have adopted a utilitarian ethic that sees participation largely in functional or hierarchical terms in the contexts where health activities take place. The focus is often on ways of establishing lay actors as targets of health promotion intervention and working to initiate and organize participation to achieve predetermined health or lifestyle outcomes (Marent, Forster, & Nowak, 2012) against which success can be readily measured. Even so-called participatory evaluation, which has long been advocated in health promotion (Springett, 2001), adopts what Cousins and Whitmore (1998) call a *practical* rather than a *transformational* approach; evaluators and project staff make the decisions, and the targeted community simply responds to externally imposed encouragements and incentives (Nitsch et al., 2013).

More effective and transformative health promotion approaches have tried to move the field beyond this programmatic focus, starting instead where people are, rather than where we want them to be. In many ways, the onus to participate begins with the health promoter: listening to stories, entering into respectful dialogue, and engaging in critical reflection together. A more participatory practice encourages a cyclical process of reflection and action that is designed to uncover and address the conditions that undermine health and perpetuate health inequities. Rather than focus narrowly on individual behaviours such as smoking, healthy eating, or physical activity, the reflection/action cycle begins with an aspiration for a flourishing life connected to the rhythms and tempos of the world, and on the social action needed to change social, economic, and political conditions that prevent a flourishing life. This approach has been referred to as a salutogenic model of health, a practice that enables people to become more whole (Lindström & Eriksson, 2006).

Being participative is thus inherently political rather than procedural; collective health is undermined by environmental and social injustices that exist everywhere in the world and requires addressing unequal power relations within particular contexts, whether at the local or global level, or anywhere in between. Participatory health promotion puts relational power at the centre of the work for social change, valuing trust, reciprocity, diversity, mutual respect, dignity, and equality, as well as focusing on the processes of co-learning and consciousness-raising to shift power relations. In many cases, participatory health promotion begins with taking a supportive, subordinate role within existing processes that have been generated from within communities already mobilizing for change. In other cases, a health promoter may draw from their own institutional power and/or resources to create a new space for communities that are otherwise immobilized due to socio-economic distress or political oppression to come together, to co-learn, and to act collectively according to their own terms. In both cases, participatory practice focuses on goals of collective education through the deepening of knowledge about the underlying social, political, or economic circumstances that have undermined the community.

While there is always a concern with power and democracy and their interactions, the craft of participation is to set the stage for encounters and not to explain things as *we* see them, or direct outcomes that *we* desire. Rather, we are impelled to work alongside and at the behest of the community, who are the experts and change agents of their own lives. Following Blencow, Brigstocke, and Noorani (2015), our role is to move away from the arts of inclusion (which can be seen as coercive and hierarchical) to the arts of making new collective egalitarian and emancipatory spaces in which we can inquire together into the issues that affect everyday lives and explore ways in which we can combat existing alienation and co-create alternative shared worlds.

A RUBRIC FOR PARTICIPATORY PRACTICE IN HEALTH PROMOTION AND EVALUATION

In this section, we translate the principles reviewed above into specific tools for social change that lie in a rubric of three interlinked participatory practices that interweave in any context of health promotion. This rubric involves (1) listening to stories, (2) engaging in respectful dialogue, and (3) engaging in critical reflexivity (Ledwith & Springett, 2010). By orienting our health promotion efforts around these practices, we may start to make sense of how to go about creating the spaces for change that are central to social transformation (Cornwall, 2008).

The first elements of the rubric are the *stories* that capture life experiences. People are storytellers by nature; stories capture our experiences and express our feeling, intellectual, physical, and spiritual selves. As Bolton describes, "narratives express the values of the narrator; they also develop and create values in the telling" (2014, p. 104). Through the active encouragement to tell their story, people start to understand their world and their place in it. Through a story we can discover new ways of knowing, exposing the assumptions, contradictions, and paradoxes of everyday life. By listening to each other's stories, we start a process of collective story-making as we recognize the similarities and differences in our experiences (Labonté, 2011). Story fuses reason and emotion and touches people in a holistic way and facilitates connections between the storytellers' pasts and imagined futures (Treleavan, 2001). Such stories can be told in conventional ways or through more creative means such as art, music, drama, and dance. Whatever the medium, telling stories and listening to them respectfully creates spaces for mutual exchange of wisdom and the process of connection to a world created in common and the route to a community's process of self-inquiry and self-knowledge.

While story marks the beginning of the transformative process towards new stories, the second element of *dialogue* encapsulates the heart of participatory practice. Participation in health promotion inherently involves a dialogical relationship between the practitioner and the community within which they work. This dialogical relationship also extends into the wider world, including both human and non-human influences. The participatory practitioner creates what Kemmis (2006) calls communicative spaces, playing the mediating midwife of true dialogue and deliberation. Shotter and Katz (1999) have demonstrated how authentic dialogue creates a sense of moving forward as people co-create meanings in their lives through which they can transcend their differences and relate to one another in mutual, reciprocal, and trusting ways. Creating the conditions of dialogue means also paying attention to ways in which existing agendas and social conditions have contributed to current challenges. Conflict often occurs as most transformative processes have a stage in which confusion sets in and health promoters facilitating participation just need to hold the space as new meanings and pragmatic solutions emerge. For Freire, such a process cannot exist "in the absence of a profound love for the world and for people" (1973, p. 70).

Through dialogue we achieve the third element of transformation, a *critical reflection* that permits us to collectively question taken-for-granted assumptions that emerge in the process of dialogue based on story. Reflection is a cornerstone of adult learning (Kolb, 2014). For people to change their "meaning schemes" (specific attitudes, beliefs, and emotional reactions) they need to engage in an ongoing process of critical questioning, not just as an intellectual exercise but as a whole feeling, intuitive, and creative person so that these meaning schemes become embodied. Through critical questioning we might start to see how meta-narratives built upon myths have marginalized certain groups and manipulated public consciousness. Senge, Scharmer, Jaworski, and Flowers

(2005) argue that such reflection needs to involve what they call "presencing," a process whereby participants develop the capacity to let go and let come. Transformation comes from digging below the surface, questioning assumptions about the world and one's place within it. Critical reflection involves reflection back and forth between whole and part, subject and object, process and product to reveal contradictions and new constructive thinking and action to address them (McLaren, 2003). This means focusing not just on the individual or local action but linking it to wider issues in society. It is a collective process of social learning and true empowerment (for additional advice regarding "reflective" practice, see chapter 17).

In summary, these elements of transformative participatory practice—story, dialogue, and reflection—link people together within a community to connect across their differences, which in turn raises the possibility of forging new connections that extend well beyond the community. To think and act participatively is ultimately a socio-ecological endeavour, a means to *becoming whole*. Thus, initial dialogue focusing on the action that needs to happen to address immediate and pressing issues faced by the community is inevitably linked by a myriad of connective pathways to a larger vision for social justice, sustainability, and collective health and wellbeing. It is this recognition that inspires projects to reach beyond the boundaries of community (however defined), to see that everything about community life is part of an interconnected whole system of life on earth. The resulting practical projects that are developed in community are inevitably diverse, but always identified in dialogue with people as relevant to their needs. In a given community, strategies may range from anti-poverty initiatives such as economic community development corporations, to housing projects, such as increasing insulation or damp reduction, to identity politics, such as women's projects, anti-racist projects, and youth projects, to safety, health literacy, and many more. Through a commitment to participatory practice, single-issue mobilization can become interlinked through cycles that give more and more people voice and the confidence to "speak to power" to address common conditions that undermine them. What we are conditioned to think of as separate issues and actions come to be seen as interdependent and interconnected, encouraging further rounds of collective thinking and action. The collective dimension builds steadily outwards, from issue to project, from project to alliances/networks, gathering momentum towards a movement for change. Participatory strategies that help to support this level of organizing may include community-wide democratic bodies, such as forums, as well as efforts beyond the community, including regional and national campaigns, networks, and other connections.

THE CHALLENGES FOR PARTICIPATORY PRACTICE

Of course, there are a number of serious challenges to participatory practice in health promotion. These stem, to a great extent, from an ideology of neo-liberalism that has infused health promotion practices as well as societies more broadly, a process that began as early as the late 1970s but really took hold in the field after the 1980s. Neo-liberalism, in a nutshell, is a political doctrine, economic formulation, and cultural representation that gives primacy to the individual (rather than the collective) as the archetype upon which society is built. Neo-liberalism emphasizes the competitive spirit of the individual as the driving force of social change, abetted by a politics of small government that relinquishes social wellbeing to the free market (i.e., "non-intrusive") economics.

Since at least the 1990s, health promotion practitioners have found themselves effectively working in a "non-participatory world." In fact, the past 25 years has seen much of health promotion falling victim to, rather than challenging, neo-liberal orthodoxy (Ayo, 2012). For instance, the emphasis on competition that is a core feature of neo-liberalism has resulted in the closing down of spaces for reflection by creating a culture of doing and of focusing on short-term outcomes. This creates the conundrum we often face in health promotion where calls for participatory engagement are made to satisfy instrumental aims of consultation and funding criteria meant to secure the legitimacy of pre-established institutional agendas. However, engagement does not just happen because we ask for it. Relationships take time: to build trust, establish dialogue, align purposes, and establish roles that honour the value and constraints of all participating actors, especially those under precarious financial circumstances, political oppression, or social marginalization. Similarly, just as one person's ability to participate is constrained in specific ways, so too are the degrees of openness to different forms of engagement from sector to sector and jurisdiction to jurisdiction. Particularly in historically closed, elite-dominated policy spaces, like health care, such new engagements run in tandem beneath a deeper network of powerful actors and interests. Engaging under-resourced and undercompensated groups in health promotion activities within such spaces often instead leads to the reconstitution of "structural lacks" as "individual/community problems" (Ledwith, 2015). The burden of the "will to improve" (Li, 2007) is felt only by those targeted by health promotion programs, rather than on those doing the targeting.

Participation within a neo-liberal framework is very much an anathema to the ethos described earlier in this chapter—the coming together of communities to effect transformative collective change. Rather, neo-liberal notions of participation tend to define people as consumers and to encourage them as atomized individuals to liberate themselves from government-imposed constraints, encouraging them to compete (and win) in a world, to maximize their own economic position and individual health, and most importantly, to uphold the stratified social status quo by quelling dissent, resistance, and alternative ways of knowing. As one British prime minister and admirer of neo-liberal architect Friedrich Hayek once famously declared, "there is no such thing as society. There are individual men and women, and there are families. And no government can do anything except through people, and people must look to themselves first" (Thatcher, 1987). In fact, it has been argued that the past three decades has been a long and sordid history in which the profession of health promotion itself has fallen victim to this neo-liberal agenda (Ayo, 2012), due to the insistence of at least some of its proponents (i.e., those who abide by the *Ottawa Charter*) that there very much *is* such a thing as society, that social justice *is* a matter of life and death (Commission on Social Determinants of Health, 2008), and that collective (not individual) action *is* the only way that we can begin the process of addressing the so many complex problems that confront us in the world today, in order to build a more just world.

HOW CAN WE IMPLEMENT PARTICIPATORY HEALTH PROMOTION IN A CANADIAN CONTEXT? THREE EXAMPLES

Canadian health promotion practice has long been characterized as a field that has struggled to advance progressive, participatory approaches at the community level within a broader context of conservative, lifestyle-based governmental health agendas (Legowski & McKay, 2000). But within, and despite, this conservative arena are many participatory health promotion champions whose combined work has had a considerable impact within communities and on major health inequities that have only grown with rising levels of inequality and ecological disruption brought about by our increasingly neo-liberal society. However, much of this work does not find its way into academic papers (Harris, Croot, Thompson, & Springett, 2015). Rather, activity occurs under the radar and often outside the formal health care sector (which unfortunately much of health promotion is embedded within). In this section, we share three examples of participatory practice that we have encountered in our roles as academic contributors and observers that serve to provide a brief illustration of how it is possible to advance participation in a counter–neo-liberal way. The first case demonstrates the importance of the relational and connection in participatory practice, the second, the inherent nature of emergence in constructing solutions with communities to local issues, and the final case the importance of transformation for connecting to the wider whole.

Case #1: The Multicultural Health Brokers Cooperative

The Multicultural Health Brokers Cooperative is a unique workers' cooperative in Edmonton established by a group of health promoters to address health and social issues experienced by immigrant and refugee families. It is also unique in its longevity and the central role that participatory practice plays in how it undertakes its work and its unerring focus on the relational as a key to change. Through a variety of participatory processes, it has been able to engage immigrants/refugees in making their struggles and aspirations visible for the purpose of community actions and social change.

The Multicultural Health Brokers Cooperative's roots began in 1991 with an Edmonton Board of Health three-year project to identify which populations were not being well served by the health system, conducted by a radical team working in the Health Promotion Division. The scan found how isolated immigrant women felt and revealed how services were perceived and experienced. As a result, 12 women, who were nominated as natural leaders and community mobilizers by their communities, were trained in prenatal care. The training was based on a mutual learning framework, where both teachers and students learned from each other. The training gave the women credibility, and the women also formed strong friendships.

The curriculum's focus was to teach the women how to be childbirth educators, so they could deliver prenatal classes in their own languages. But soon it became clear that because mothers were being discharged early from hospitals, there was a need to also incorporate post-natal care. The Brokers also realized that it wasn't just about health education—to be truly holistic, they had to look at the whole family and focus on community development and building mutual support groups so families could be connected to help each other. Over the years, this role has expanded to serve the youth and senior communities as well. The Brokers formed a cooperative in 1998, seeing this governance structure as most consistent with their participatory, flexible, non-hierarchical approach. The core values of mutual care, self-help, self-responsibility, democracy, equality, equity, and solidarity drive the way their work is done. These are reflected in the warm and friendly ambience of their base in an old school in Edmonton's McCauley area.

There are now more than 75 brokers who are the eyes, ears, and witnesses of what is happening in the system for families new to Canada. Many started as volunteers in their communities and were identified as natural leaders, moving on to a paid capacity within the Cooperative. They represent 25 different cultural and linguistic communities in Edmonton, and at the time of writing, serve more than 2,000 families. They use participatory practices sensitive to diverse cultures to close the gap between systems and families, and build capacity by teaching cultural competency for those who work in the mainstream system. For example, in 2003 they helped to enable an experiment in participatory policy-making, bringing the government and agencies together with the local multi-cultural community (Multicultural Health Brokers Cooperative, 2004). Story, dialogue, and critical reflexivity drive their daily practice, starting where people are at and ensuring dignity and respect in understanding cultural differences and similarities, believing that immigrants have unique resources of value to Canada as a whole but experience barriers to making a difference (Ortiz, 2011; Torres, Spitzer, Labonté, Amaratunga, & Andrew, 2013).

One issue for the brokers is that marginalized populations suffer from lack of political power on the one hand and invisibility on the other, so their stories are not heard—creating a lack of understanding between the different cultural groups and the general population. The cooperative uses the five levels of empowerment (Labonté, 1993) in its work with creating relationships and connection at the core. In the first level of empowerment, co-op members interview families to develop a holistic understanding of what's in the way of achieving their visions for the future. They take family members to service providers who can help them overcome the barriers they face, and provide tools that empower them to achieve their goals. In this work, they strive to develop an equitable relationship between each family and service provider. At the second and third levels of empowerment, the co-op members engage in community organizing. On one level, they create spaces for people facing similar challenges to come together for mutual support and collective learning and, at a broader level, they work to build awareness and mobilization around common issues affecting their community. The final two areas of empowerment involve advocacy for systemic change. At the fourth level, the co-op creates a network of service providers that cooperate and coordinate efforts to provide the holistic support that newcomer families need. Finally, the last level of empowerment involves advocating for a greater voice with the organizations providing services. "The singular mission as a workers' co-op is to build relationships that remove the 'us versus them' mentality between communities and service providers. And, so, almost every single initiative that we have is either partnering with a public institution or a government entity, or bringing diverse partners together to illustrate the power of the collective, and the need to work together" (Chiu, Ortiz, & Wolfe, 2009). Working as they do at the interface between institutions and community and in a funding system of short-term "projectism," their longevity bears witness to the effectiveness of the shared vision and participatory practices of the culture brokers.

Case Study #2: From Aging to Saging: Intergenerational Community Connections in Alberta

This case has many of the contextual elements identified by Kar, Lundstrom, and Adkins (1997) that support participation: a political environment characterized by democracy and decentralization; support of a local leadership for changing their institutions, by relearning and realizing the capability of "lay" people and the richness of local resources; and the facilitation capacity for community-based planning and management, with sufficient participatory practitioners to undertake this work. Such contextual elements provide a supportive environment for participatory practice in Edmonton where there has been a coming together across many communities to address poverty, the product of a changing consciousness that has been gradually taking place over many years. The Multicultural Health Brokers Cooperative referred to above has, along with others, contributed to that change, resulting in the development of an Anti-Poverty Strategy, approved by the city council in December 2015. The strategy development process actively involved the Indigenous community, giving them a central role, but also sought to engage those in poverty, young and old. "There is a word in Cree, kîyânaw, which means 'for all of us.' By firmly believing that we are all in this together, our capacity to build relationships of trust with one another will form the foundation of community cohesion" (Edmonton EndPoverty, 2016, p. 26). The implementation plan has a wheel-like participatory governance structure of five community tables and adopts a stewardship approach. As a community resident at an Aboriginal workshop said, "The wheel represents balance and is not meant to be static—it is always moving. We are all part of the wheel, the more we learn about it the more we become selfless" (Edmonton EndPoverty, 2016).

   This second example from Edmonton is one of a number of initiatives within the city that are taking a new approach to old problems through facilitated citizen action and a focus on relationships and process. It addresses a central determinant of health, social connection, the key to living a healthy life in the later years as well as playing a crucial role in promoting and maintaining health throughout the life-course. It began in a very different place from where it ended but has had a transformative effect within the originating community and beyond. It demonstrates how, starting with any tangible project, people will begin to connect and move things forward in an unexpected but appropriate way.

The seeds for change started in a neighbourhood where a group of local parents wanted to experiment in creating local naturescapes adjacent to the local elementary school. The co-creation of a public space for people to come together gradually drew people in as, over time, the building of the space created an opportunity for people to contribute and also connect. Not only were local schoolchildren involved but also men from the local seniors' centre. The latter initially helped to build a bird house and then a bench. The bench then encouraged seniors to sit in the newly created space, which in turn encouraged further connections. Participation was facilitated using the principles outlined above, story, dialogue, and reflection.

Over time, people self-organized to connect with local agencies and successfully obtain small community grants. However, the idea of intergenerational connecting, of involving seniors in the local school and community, did not remain in that community. It was carried across to another more socially challenging community in another part of Edmonton where not only were there many seniors, but also—due to the influx of refugees and an urban Indigenous population—many families living in poverty. In this community, seniors were invited to share their ideas about how they might support children living in poverty. As they explored their gifts and resources in dialogical circles, they overcame their initial concern that they had nothing to offer and decided they wanted to get involved with local schools. In discussions with a local school principal they explored together what the school needed and what they felt they could offer in terms of knowledge and experience to help children living in poverty. In this school, over 25 percent of children were Indigenous, many others from refugee families suffering trauma, with parents experiencing mental health issues and addictions. The initial solution was an open house half-day, to which seniors came to teach skills such as knitting and indoor gardening on a one-to-one basis. As they taught the skill, they also provided emotional support for the children. Over time, a number of other activities were developed by the seniors, including the revamping of the school library as well as building a community garden as a public space in which to connect. The impact spiralled beyond the immediate school, as seniors gained confidence and moved beyond the school to connect to local agencies. Such efforts ranged from exploring housing needs to finding space for seniors to engage in local "jam" sessions.

The role of the health promotion practitioner in this example was to create the dialogical space and enable the process through connecting people to local resources. The ongoing process surfaced hidden resources, ways of knowing, deep caring, and a sense of belonging, all of which are essential to collective health and wellbeing (Mears & Sabo, 2015). The role of seniors in the community was transformed through a sharing of knowledge that started a process of social change that will help local families, but also the seniors themselves. At the time of writing, the same participatory processes to engage local seniors at the neighbourhood level are being taken to new neighbourhoods.

Case #3: The Canadian Partnership for Children's Health and Environment: Embracing Equity-Focused Health Promotion to Address Unhealthy Housing for Tenants on Low Income in Ontario

The story of the Canadian Partnership for Children's Health and Environment provides a useful illustration of a health promotion organization that has taken on the challenge of becoming transformative in its efforts to promote healthy environments for all children in Canada. Launched in 2001, CPCHE is an Ontario-based partnership of several local to national organizations that came together out of shared concern about the harmful effects of toxic chemicals and pollution on the developing fetus and child. CPCHE partners and affiliates include organizations working in public health, medicine, environmental protection, law, disability advocacy, and child care.

Much of the early work of CPCHE followed a health education model, translating toxicological and epidemiological research on environmental exposures into readily understandable and actionable messages for parents to understand in order to protect children from exposure to household toxicants (e.g., BPA) and contaminants (e.g., heavy metals). This translational work focused on generating resources for service providers who routinely interact with families (e.g., public health nurses, child care professionals) to include children's environmental health protection in routine practice. For example, the partnership developed its evidence-based "Top Five Tips" on how to create healthy home environments for kids, including a brochure, plain-language tip cards, and a video intended for use in prenatal classes and other educational programming for expectant and new parents (CPCHE, 2011).

In addition to its work translating scientific evidence about toxins into usable health education messages for service providers and parents, CPCHE has also established a track record of national leadership in influencing federal policy on regulation of chemicals, consumer products, and environmental protection. This policy advocacy has been motivated by the belief that the fulsome protection of child health can only be realized through precautionary policies that don't allow known and suspected toxicants into the market and consumer products in the first place.

While CPCHE's efforts in health education and policy advocacy have been well received by both policy and practice communities, recent efforts by the partnership have focused on prioritizing health inequities related to children's environmental health. Health inequities fall along two lines: first, the recognition that health education may be less effective among families in socio-economically precarious situations. The ability to make consumer choices around safe food and household products often relies upon financial resources that are too costly or requires the ability to purchase products that are not readily accessible in lower-income neighbourhoods. Second, policy development and decisions have often been made on the basis of "population based" arguments, thus neglecting the many structural inequities associated with the non-random distribution of risks in housing quality, air quality, and other environmental conditions.

To address these gaps, several CPCHE partners joined a participatory equity-focused capacity-building program in 2012, which began the process of engendering a more participatory stance within CPCHE's overall orientation to their practice. From this experience, which involved leaders from educational, research, and community sectors from across the country, CPCHE members began to acknowledge that much of their work seemed to have been done without the presence—or voices—of those whom they were working to support. A desire to align CPCHE's priorities with the community meant that more of their work needed to be done alongside these individuals rather than just for them.

The next few years were a transformative experience for CPCHE, as the partnership took steps, often beyond its comfort zone, to establish a new mode of operation that would see an emphasis on listening to first-hand experiences of poverty, unhealthy housing, food insecurity, and environmental exposures. New projects began to be formulated that would place families experiencing environmental health inequities centrally within processes of inquiry and grassroots knowledge translation, seeing them as "experts" capable of helping CPCHE partners to see the social injustices within the policy environment that lay at the root of exposure inequities.

These early explorations culminated in 2014 in a decisive shift in the orientation of the organization to focus on addressing the gaps in support for tenants living in substandard housing conditions. This culminated in the emergence of Rentsafe, providing an opportunity to work participatively, not on "fixing" housing problems (especially by making people more aware of the problems they already know about) but on fixing a housing system that has often failed communities—fragmentation, assumptions, and lack of recognition and reconciliation.

While still adhering to a partner formula, through Rentsafe, CPCHE has actively sought to connect, through new partnerships, to the concerns and expertise within the community. Community food centres, progressive public health practitioners, and Indigenous friendship centres took centre stage within CPCHE's work early on, and importantly these partners included, and were often constituted by, people acting in leadership roles for their communities.

The ongoing partnership development and advocacy tied to the Rentsafe project has led CPCHE to invest in relationship-building across sectors, to integrate the practical wisdom within communities into their overall strategic planning and policy advocacy efforts, and most importantly to take a more critical and reflexive stance in their practice, opting for developing processes in which professional actors within and beyond the CPCHE partnership begin to see the main interventions in addressing health equities as change occurring within themselves and their institutions, rather than the "objects" of their concern.

This new configuration has helped to foster new kinds of stories within and about CPCHE and its priorities, often uncovered through facilitated conversations among people living in low-income housing conveying very diverse lived experiences of service gaps within policy roundtables. By investing in the creation of safe and inclusive spaces, these stories have generated a more critical and reflexive dialogue among intersectoral actors; often these dialogues occur outside of the "epistemologically secure" spaces of academia and professional practice and into the more "uncomfortable" spaces of politically persecuted and socially marginalized communities.

Ultimately, this re-orientation of CPCHE has led the partnership to readily embrace the challenge of taking on the "wicked problems" that lay at the root of children's environmental health and to begin the process of personal and organizational transformation that will inform its future work. For CPCHE partners, this has led to a sense of becoming whole, of seeing CPCHE as a support system for critical thinking and action that is a fundamentally different state of affairs than the prevailing service provision and poverty amelioration practices that still dominate the environmental health promotion field. In the context of housing, CPCHE, with the voices of community leaders at the forefront, sees the right to a healthy home as fundamental—and recognizes that its role is in the alleviation of social injustice as an essential pathway for improved practice, with an end result being more equitable relationships among landlords, government officials, tenants, and service providers.

CONCLUSION

The continuation of neo-liberal, patriarchal, and colonial regimes in Canada and around the world poses a huge challenge for participatory health promotion practice. The majority of current institutional arrangements and funding systems focus on projects and products that aim for clear and instrumental outcomes rather than changed processes and relationships. The orientation of health and social systems remains focused on parts rather than wholes, on mitigating specific diseases rather than promoting socio-ecological wellbeing. Moreover, engagement of the marginalized will mean encountering conflicting viewpoints and hidden political agendas with strong resistance to changing the status quo. This is not unsurprising, for as Bourdieu has argued, everyday practice is purpose-built to maintain the unequal structure of society. For Bourdieu, social relations are "battles" in which, while the underprivileged may be working to develop their resources, the privileged are working as hard to maintain their advantage (Stephens, 2010).

Certainly, there is a need to develop the capacity of health promotion organizations to work in more participatory ways. There are increasing signs that this is happening in different places, mostly outside of the health care sector. This is not necessarily a problem, but an opportunity for health promotion. For too long, health promotion has been subordinated to a biomedical paradigm of health that has dominated medicine, allied health care, and population and public health—a paradigm that has been sustained, in part, by its facile alignments with neo-liberalism. But where health promotion has felt squeezed in its efforts to co-exist within these sectors, it has also thrived in other places, including social sciences and interdisciplinary health departments at universities, and in non-profit organizations pursuing positive community change and social justice.

The rubric for a participatory practice process suggested here is not just for others, it is one in which we as practitioners must be a part. For all of us involved, personal conscious-ness leads to transformative autonomy and in turn leads to collective autonomy that is a precursor to transformative collective action (Doyal & Gough, 1991). It is a process that is, of course, not without its risks. Speaking truth to power or unwelcome truths requires some "ducking and diving" and "flying below the radar" (Mayo, 2009; Griffiths, 2003). Risk-taking, however, is part of growth. As someone (unattributed) once said, "if you do what you have always done you get what you have always got." We can change the story of health promotion by changing ourselves.

CRITICAL THINKING QUESTIONS

1. What impact would thinking and acting participatively have on the types of health promotion programs that currently operate in public health units in Canada?
2. In what ways do participatory practices align, or not, with Indigenous perspectives and priorities related to health and social justice?
3. How has neo-liberalism influenced your own perspective on what constitutes the relational and collective and their value in creating health?
4. In thinking about a situation, project, or program in your own professional or stu-dent life, how would a more participatory stance have influenced your objectives, approach, and outcomes?

RESOURCES

Further Readings

Baldwin, C., & Linnea, A. (2010). *The circle way: A leader in every chair*. San Francisco: Berrit-Koehler.
This is an introduction to one of the most ancient of social practices, the circle, based on the authors' experiences of implementing this practice in organizations and communities. Through illustrative stories the authors provide detailed instructions for starting conversations that matter and using story, dialogue, and deep reflection to generate innovative social change.

Green, L. W., George, M. A., Daniel, M., Frankish, C. J., Herbert, C. J., Bowie, W. R., & O'Neill, M. (1995). *Study of participatory research in health promotion: Review and rec-ommendations for the development of participatory research in health promotion in Canada*. Vancouver: Institute of Health Promotion Research, University of British Columbia and the B. C. Consortium for Health Promotion Research, Royal Society of Canada.

This landmark report, published at the pinnacle of health promotion's influence and institutional status in the wake of the *Ottawa Charter*, sets out principles and guidelines for effective participatory practice in health promotion research. It was meant to inform funders and applicants alike of acceptable and non-acceptable forms of participatory research.

Ledwith, M., & Springett, J. (2010). *Participatory practice. Community-based action for transformative change.* Bristol: The Policy Press.
This book on community development expands on some of the ideas presented in this chapter. It explores story, dialogue, and critical reflection in greater detail. There are also two chapters on a participatory worldview and participatory practice in a non-participatory world that use examples from the field of health.

Relevant Websites

Art of Hosting
www.artofhosting.org/
    This international website supports the participatory practice outlined in this chapter and provides the training and skill development required to fully engage in the practice, alongside a wealth of resources including books and papers.

Community Tool Box
www.ctb.ku.edu
    The Community Tool Box is supported by the Work Group for Community Health and Development at the University of Kansas. It is a free online resource that contains more than 7,000 pages of practical information for promoting community health and development, and is a global resource for both professionals and grassroots groups engaged in the work of community health and development.

National Coalition for Dialogue and Deliberation
ncdd.org
    The National Coalition for Dialogue and Deliberation is an excellent resource centre of participatory practice. Although based in the US its materials are of value in a Canadian context.

Participatory Analysis Tool
www.powercube.net
    A key element in understanding action for change is through a participatory analysis of power within a particular situation. This tool, developed by John Gaventa, who has worked extensively in the area of development, provides a useful starting point for deliberation.

Participatory Research at McGill

www.pram.mcgill.ca

Participatory Research at McGill (PRAM) is a centre dedicated to promoting participatory research and community engagement in health care. It follows the Royal Society of Canada's approach to participatory action research (PAR) and provides a space for the dissemination of PAR-related policies, guidelines, and practices in the Canadian context.

Tamarack

www.tamarackcommunity.ca/

Tamarack remains the go-to place for everything on working with communities. Values and principles underpin its ways of working and it has a wealth of resources and tools as well as books and articles.

World Café

www.theworldcafe.com

This website introduces one of the most common tools used to encourage dialogue by facilitating open and intimate discussion, and then linking ideas within a larger group to access the collective wisdom and knowledge.

REFERENCES

Ayo, N. (2012). Understanding health promotion in a neoliberal climate and the making of health conscious citizens. *Critical Public Health, 22*(1), 99–105.

Blencowe, C., Brigstocke, J., & Noorani, T. (2015). Theorizing participatory practice and alienation in health research: A materialist approach. *Social Theory and Health, 13*, 397–417.

Bolton, G. (2014). *Reflective practice: Writing and professional development* (4th ed.). London: Sage.

Brown, H. J., McPherson, G., Peterson, R., Newman, V., & Cranmer, B. (2012). Our land, our language: Connecting dispossession and health equity in an indigenous context. *Canadian Journal of Nursing Research, 44*(2), 44–63.

Canadian Partnership for Children's Health and Environment (CPCHE). (2011). *Creating healthy environments for kids.* Retrieved from www.healthyenvironmentforkids.ca/resources/creating-healthy-environments-kids

Castleden, H., Garvin, T., & Nation, H. A. A. F. (2009). "Hishuk Tsawak" (everything is one/connected): A Huu-ay-aht worldview for seeing forestry in British Columbia, Canada. *Society and Natural Resources, 22*(9), 789–804.

Chiu, Y., Ortiz, L., & Wolfe, R. (2009). Beyond settlement: Strengthening immigrant families, communities and Canadian society through cultural brokering. *Our Diverse Cities.* Edmonton: Metropolis.

Commission on Social Determinants of Health (CSDH). (2008). *Closing the gap in a generation: Health equity through action on the social determinants of Health.* Geneva: World Health Organization.

Cornwall, A. (2008). Unpacking "participation": Models, meanings and practices. *Community Development Journal, 43*(3), 269–283.

Cousins, J. B., & Whitmore, E. (1998). Framing participatory evaluation. *New Directions for Evaluation, 1998*(80), 5–23.

Doyal, L., & Gough, I. (1991). *A theory of human need.* Basingstoke: Palgrave Macmillan.

Edmonton EndPoverty. (2015). *EndPoverty strategy.* Edmonton: Edmonton City Council.

Edmonton EndPoverty. (2016). *EndPoverty implementation strategy.* Edmonton: Edmonton City Council.

Freire, P. (1973). *Education for critical consciousness (Vol. 1).* London: Bloomsbury Publishing.

Green, L. W., George, M. A., Daniel, M., Frankish, C. J., Herbert, C. J., Bowie, W. R., & O'Neill, M. (1995). *Study of participatory research in health promotion: Review and recommendations for the development of participatory research in health promotion in Canada.* Vancouver: Institute of Health Promotion Research, University of British Columbia and the B. C. Consortium for Health Promotion Research, Royal Society of Canada.

Griffiths, M. (2003). *Action for social justice in education: Fairly different.* Milton Keynes: Open University Press.

Harris, J., Croot, L., Thompson, J., & Springett, J. (2015). How stakeholder participation can contribute to systematic reviews of complex interventions. *Journal of Epidemiology and Community Health, 70,* 207–214.

Kar, K., Lundstrom, T., & Adkins, J. (1997). *Who will influence the institutionalisation of participation and on whose terms? Recent experiences in institutionlaising participatory approaches to development from Lindi and Mtwara Regions, Rural Integrated Programme Support Tanzania.* Brighton: Institute for Development Studies, University of Sussex.

Kemmis, S. (2006). Participatory action research and the public sphere. *Educational Action Research, 14*(4), 459–476.

Kolb, D. A. (2014). *Experiential learning: Experience as the source of learning and development* (2nd ed.). Upper Saddle River: FT Press.

Labonté, R. (1993). *Health promotion and empowerment: Practice frameworks Promotion Series #3.* Toronto: Centre for Health Promotion, University of Toronto and ParticipACTION.

Labonté, R. (2011). Reflections on stories and a story/dialogue method in health research. *International Journal of Social Research Methodology, 14*(2), 153–163.

Ledwith, M. (2015). *Community development in action: Putting Freire into practice.* Bristol: Policy Press.

Ledwith, M., & Springett, J. (2010). *Participatory practice. Community based action for transformative change.* Bristol: Policy Press.

Legowski, B., & McKay, L. (2000). *Health beyond health care: Twenty-five years of federal health policy development.* Ottawa: Canadian Policy Research Networks.

Li, T. M. (2007). *The will to improve: Governmentality, development, and the practice of politics.* Durham: Duke University Press.

Lindström, B., & Eriksson, M. (2006). Contextualizing salutogenesis and Antonovsky in public health development. *Health Promotion International, 21*(3), 238–244.

Marent, B., Forster, R., & Nowak, P. (2012). Theorizing participation in health promotion: A literature review. *Social Theory & Health, 10*(2), 188–207.

Mayo, P. (2009) Flying below the radar: Critical approaches to adult education. In M. W. Apple, W. Au, & L. Gandin, *The Routledge international handbook of critical education* (pp. 268–280). London: Routledge.

McLaren, P. (2003). Critical pedagogy: A look at the major concepts. In A. Darder, M. Baltodano, & R. D. Torres (Eds.), *The critical pedagogy reader* (pp. 69–96). Hove: Psychology Press.

Mears, S., & Sabo, S. (2015). *From age-ing to sage-ing report June 2015*. Edmonton: Seniors Association of Greater Edmonton (SAGE).

Minkler, M. (2000). Using participatory action research to build healthy communities. *Public Health Reports, 115*, 191–197.

Multicultural Health Brokers Cooperative. (2004). *All together now: A multicultural coalition for equity in health and well-being: Final report*. Edmonton: Author.

Nitsch, M., Waldherr, K., Denk, E., Griebler, U., Marent, B., & Forster, R. (2013). Participation by different stakeholders in participatory evaluation of health promotion: A literature review. *Evaluation and program planning, 40*, 42–54.

Ortiz, L. (2011). Advocacy and social support: The Multicultural Health Brokers Co-op's journey towards equity of access to health. In D. L. Spitzer, *Engendering migrant health: Canadian perspectives* (pp. 169–192). Toronto: University of Toronto Press.

Senge, P. M., Scharmer, C. O., Jaworski, J., & Flowers, B. S. (2005). *Presence: An exploration of profound change in people, organizations, and society*. London: Nicholas Brealey Publishing.

Shotter, J., & Katz, A. (1999). Living moments in dialogical exchanges. *Human Systems, 9*, 81–93.

Springett, J. (2001). Appropriate approaches to the evaluation of health promotion. *Critical Public Health, 11*(2), 139–151.

Stephens, C. (2010). Privilege and status in an unequal society: Shifting the focus of health promotion research to include the maintenance of advantage. *Journal of Health Psychology, 15*(7), 993–1000.

Thatcher, M. (1987). Transcript from interview with Douglas Keay for *Woman's Own*. Retrieved from www.margaretthatcher.org/document/106689

Treleavan, L. (2001). The turn to action and the linguistic turn: Towards an integrated methodology. In P. Reason & H. Bradbury (Eds.), *Handbook of action research: Participative inquiry and practice*. London: Sage.

Torres, S., Spitzer, D. L., Labonté, R., Amaratunga, C., & Andrew, C. (2013). Community health workers in Canada: Innovative approaches to health promotion outreach and community development among immigrant and refugee populations. *The Journal of Ambulatory Care Management, 36*(4), 305–318.

CHAPTER 22

Population Health Promotion in the Anthropocene

Trevor Hancock

LEARNING OBJECTIVES

1. Understand what the Anthropocene is and why it is a threat to population health
2. Understand the forces that are driving global ecological change
3. Understand the societal and community-level changes that we need to create to ensure a sustainable, just, and healthy future for all
4. Understand the role that public health and health promotion workers and organizations need to play in bringing about these changes

INTRODUCTION

We live at the dawn of a new, human-made geological epoch—the Anthropocene. So large is our impact on the planet that Earth scientists suggest our presence will show up in the geologic record far into the future. The global ecological changes we are creating include not only climate change, but ocean acidification, pollution and ecotoxicity, resource depletion, and the loss of biodiversity that threatens a sixth "Great Extinction." These changes pose a significant—indeed profound—threat to the health of current and future generations, and in some parts of the world, to their very existence.

But while the Anthropocene is at one level simply a geological marker of the changes we are creating in global ecosystems, it should also be viewed as an indicator of the scale of human activity that is causing those changes, a warning of the present and future impacts of these changes on human and other life forms, and a sign that we have to change our values and our way of life.

The Anthropocene is not simply an ecological phenomenon, but at the same time a sociological phenomenon, and thus is best understood and addressed as an eco-social system. It is our present way of life that has caused the changes we call the Anthropocene, and thus it is only through changing our present way of life—our values, our economy, our communities, and our societies—that we can hope to change the present ecologically unsustainable course we are on.

The importance of the Anthropocene for the health of the population is simple, but profound. The ultimate determinants of our health are not in fact the social determinants of health, but the ecological determinants that underlie them and that underpin our society, our economy, our way of life, and indeed our very survival. The air we breathe, the water we drink, and the food we eat all come from nature, as do the materials with which we build our infrastructure and products, and the fuels with which we power them. Natural processes remove and detoxify many of our wastes, shield us from harmful UV radiation, and have given us a fairly stable and warm climate for the past 11,000 years, during which time agriculture was developed and cities emerged, creating the basis for our entire modern civilization.

What the Anthropocene shows us is that we have become a force of nature in our own right, and that we are disrupting and damaging these and other "ecosystem goods and services" that are the ecological determinants of not only our health (Millennium Ecosystem Assessment, 2005a) but the health of many other species with whom we share the planet. Indeed, we are creating a sixth "Great Extinction," and since we are part of the great web of life, when we undermine that web of life, we undermine ourselves (to paraphrase the mid-nineteenth-century Duwamish Chief Seattle[1]).

We Have Been Ecologically Blind

One would think that these threats to health would prompt the health promotion professions and public health organizations to pay serious attention to this issue, but sadly that has largely not been the case. While certain pioneers such as the late Tony McMichael (author, among many other things, of the landmark 1993 book *Planetary Overload*) and our own John Last (author of the 1987 book *Public Health and Human Ecology*) have pointed out the challenges we face and proposed solutions, and while the Canadian Public Health Association's Task Force on the Implications for Human Health of Global Ecological Change reported on this issue in 1992 (CPHA, 1992), the topic has received little serious attention until very recently.

This is strange—and frustrating—since the *Ottawa Charter for Health Promotion* (WHO, 1986) included within the list of prerequisites for health "stable ecosystems and sustainable resources," called for a socio-ecological approach to health, and included a pledge to "address the overall ecological issue of our ways of living." But in the early 1990s, the progressive, action-oriented, socio-ecological, and socio-political movement that is health promotion was supplanted by a new concept—population health (see chapter 1); in fact, from 1993 to 2003, "health promotion went largely unnoticed. It was not positioned as a serious strategy within the health system" (Jackson & Riley, 2007).

While population health was criticized for many things (Labonté, 1997) it is relevant to note that "Population health arguments are largely silent on ecological issues" (Labonté, 1995). A search through the index of the foundational text for population health (Evans,

Barer, & Marmor, 1994) reveals no mention of ecology or ecosystem. It is, when you stop and think about it, an astonishing omission; how can one possibly write about "the determinants of the health of populations"—the subtitle of their book—without recognizing that air, water, and food—the most fundamental determinants of our health—along with materials, fuels, and many other essentials, come from nature?

Instead, the discourse on the determinants of health quickly became a discourse on the social and economic determinants of health, culminating of course in the work and the report of the WHO Commission on Social Determinants of Health (2008). Without diminishing in any way the importance of the work of the Commission, nor the importance of the social determinants of health, we need to recognize that in our focus on the social and economic determinants, mainstream population and public health—including health promotion—has become largely ecologically blind.

This cannot and must not continue, for if it does, we will have failed in our mission of protecting and improving the health of the population. Nor is it simply a matter of rejecting the social and economic determinants of health in favour of the ecological determinants, because the detrimental ecological changes we are witnessing are driven by socio-economic change. Instead, we need to go back to what the *Ottawa Charter* said and adopt a socio-ecological approach to health, or what is now more often called an eco-social approach.

Dropping the Blinkers

Fortunately, and perhaps due to the increasing severity and immediacy of the global ecological crises we face, that understanding is slowly (re)emerging. The Canadian Public Health Association established a Task Force on Global Change and Public Health in 2012, which I led, and after three years of intensive work our "brief" report and a CPHA Discussion Document were released in May 2015 (Hancock, Spady, & Soskolne, 2015; CPHA, 2015). We identified natural systems as the source of what we called "the ecological determinants of health," called for an integration of the social and ecological determinants in an eco-social framework, and explored the implications for public health, ending with a comprehensive set of recommendations.

Our report was shortly followed by the report of the Rockefeller Foundation–Lancet Commission on Planetary Health (Whitmee et al., 2015), and there is an emerging literature now on the health implications of the Anthropocene and the public health response that is required (McMichael, 2014; Hancock, 2015a; Butler, 2016). Indeed, the University of Sydney in Australia recently established the world's first Chair in Planetary Health, *The Lancet* launched a new journal, *Lancet Planetary Health*, in April 2017, and a new Planetary Health Alliance (planetaryhealthalliance.org) has been established, further indication that these issues are going mainstream.

In the rest of this chapter, I will very briefly describe the Anthropocene and its health implications, and discuss the role that health promotion, and public health more generally, must play. In doing so, I will draw heavily on the work of the CPHA Task Force, whose members (listed in the report) I gratefully acknowledge for their significant contributions to my thinking and our work.

Information specific to Canada is provided, where appropriate, but it is important to recognize that the issue of ecological change and its health impacts is a global one, not simply a Canadian issue, and needs to be addressed in those terms. We cannot only—or even primarily—think about the health implications for Canada, for two reasons:

- First, as a large, resource-rich, and wealthy country, we are better able than most to protect ourselves from the worst, at least in the early and middle stages of many of these changes.
- Second, as a large, resource-rich, and wealthy country, we contribute disproportionately to these global ecological changes, so we bear an added burden of responsibility for those elsewhere in the world who are affected by our actions here in Canada.

Finally, it is important to understand that this is not all about doom and gloom, crisis and disaster. Yes, there are challenges, some of them massive challenges, but an essential characteristic of health promotion is that it is positive and hopeful; it holds out the promise of a better, healthier way of life, with healthier people living in healthier communities in a healthy world. So while there is much that is troubling in what follows, it is worth noting that the CPHA Task Force report includes chapters on finding hope and imagining and creating an alternative, better future; there is no more important task facing health promotion today than to help create a more just, sustainable, and healthy future for all (CPHA, 2015; Hancock, Spady, & Soskolne, 2015).

WELCOME TO THE ANTHROPOCENE

What follows is only a high-level overview of this very large and complex issue. For more detailed information see Hancock, Spady, and Soskolne (2015).

The concept of the Anthropocene was proposed only recently by Crutzen and Stoermer (2000), who noted that "mankind [sic] will remain a major geological force for many millennia, maybe millions of years, to come." As with volcanoes, earthquakes, or meteor strikes, evidence of human impacts will be present in the geological record for all time.[2]

Waters et al. (2016) identify a range of geologic changes that "render the Anthropocene stratigraphically distinct from the Holocene and earlier epochs," and suggest that a starting time for this new epoch is the mid-twentieth century. This coincides with what Steffen, Broadgate, Deutsch, Gaffney, and Ludwig (2015) call "The Great Acceleration"; beginning around 1950 there was a dramatic surge across a wide array of social and economic system indicators, and a concomitant decline across a range of Earth system indicators.

One way to understand the scale of human demand on the planet is the ecological footprint (EF). First developed by Bill Rees and Mathis Wackernagel at UBC in

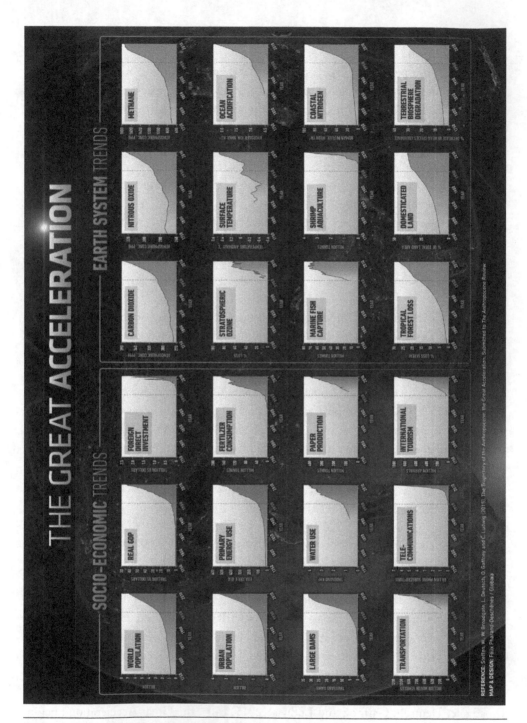

Figure 22.1: The Great Acceleration

Source: Steffen, W., Broadgate, W., Deutsch, L., Gaffney, O., & Ludwig, C. (2015). The trajectory of the Anthropocene: The great acceleration. Submitted to *The Anthropocene Review*. Map and design by: Félix Pharand-Deschênes / Globaïa. Used by permission.

the 1990s, it "represents the productive area required to provide the renewable resources humanity is using and to absorb its waste" (Global Footprint Network, n.d.). Globally we used about 1.6 planets' worth of bio-productive capacity in 2012, which is clearly unsustainable (WWF, 2016). Wealthier countries and wealthier populations have larger footprints than poorer ones; if the entire world lived at the same level of demand as does the US or Denmark, our global footprint would be the equivalent of almost four planets.

The Canadian EF is large, consistent with its status as a high-income country. But there are marked differences in EF within Canada, based on income, with the EF of the richest 10 percent of the population being nearly 2.5 times larger than that of the poorest 10 percent (Mackenzie, Messinger, & Smith, 2008). In fact, the footprint of the richest 10 percent of Canadians in 2002 was 25 percent greater than that of the country with the largest footprint in 2009.

Earth System Changes

While there is an understandable tendency to focus on the increasingly evident indications of climate change we see all around us, it is important to understand that the Anthropocene is much more than simply climate change. One key approach refers to

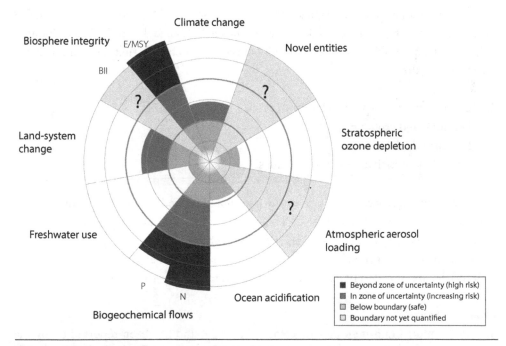

Figure 22.2: Safe Operating Boundaries

Source: Steffen, W., Richardson, K., Rockström, J., Cornell, S. E., Fetzer, I., Bennett, E. M., ... Sörlin, S. (2015). Planetary boundaries: Guiding human development on a changing planet. *Science, 347*(6223), 1259855. doi: 10.1126/science.1259855. Used by permission.

changes in nine key Earth systems (a couple of which are subdivided), only one of which is climate change; the other eight are biodiversity loss (a couple of which are subdivided), biogeochemical flows (both the nitrogen and phosphorus cycles), land system change, freshwater use, atmospheric aerosol loading, novel entities,[3] stratospheric ozone depletion, and ocean acidification (Steffen, Richardson, et al., 2015).

The authors also propose boundaries for change that should not be exceeded if we are to remain within what they call a "safe operating space" for humanity (see figure 22.2). Of these nine they find

- We have passed the boundaries for five: rate of biodiversity loss (extinctions per million species-years, E/MSY) and disruption of the nitrogen and phosphorus biogeochemical flows (for both we are in a high-risk zone), and land system change and climate change (for both we are in a zone of increasing risk).
- For three of the key Earth system processes (loss of functional biodiversity, atmospheric aerosol loading, and novel entities), we lack sufficient knowledge or data to even determine the boundaries.
- In only three areas—stratospheric ozone depletion, ocean acidification, and freshwater use—do they find we are operating within safe boundaries.

Based on a paper Kate Davies and I prepared for the Royal Society of Canada's Global Change Program some 20 years ago (Davies & Hancock, 1997), I have found it helpful to think of four broad areas of global ecological change that have implications for human health:

1. Climate and atmospheric change
2. Pollution and ecotoxicity
3. Resource depletion
4. Loss of biodiversity, species extinctions

Those four, plus ocean acidification, an issue not identified back then but now also underway, were used in our report for CPHA on the health implications of global ecological change (Hancock, Spady, & Soskolne, 2015). Some brief highlights from that report that illustrate the extent of the changes underway in these key global systems, updated where appropriate, are provided here. For a more detailed review, see the report itself.

Climate Change

This is the most prominent global ecological change, and has been reported on by the Intergovernmental Panel on Climate Change (IPCC) since 1988. Their reports have become increasingly specific and pointed as the evidence becomes ever more clear. In 2014, the IPCC reported that "human influence on the climate system is clear, and recent anthropogenic emissions of greenhouse gases are the highest in history" (IPCC, 2014).

The US National Oceanic and Atmospheric Administration reported in August 2016 that "the January–July 2016 global land and ocean temperature was the warmest such period on record at 1.03°C (1.85°F) above the 20th century average, besting the previous record set in 2015 by 0.19°C (0.34°F)" (NOAA, 2016). In Canada, "the national average temperature for the winter of 2015/2016 (December 2015, January 2016, and February 2016) was 4.0°C above the baseline average (defined as the mean over the 1961–1990 reference period)" (Environment and Climate Change Canada, 2016).

The main impacts of global warming include warming oceans, melting of glaciers and polar icecaps, rising sea levels, more frequent and severe extreme weather events, droughts, flooding, wildfires, changes to food agro-ecosystems, and changes in the distribution of many plants and animals. The main health impacts of climate change (discussed later) arise from these environmental changes (IPCC, 2014).

Pollution and Ecotoxicity

We massively pollute the air, water, soil, and food chains, harming ourselves and other species we depend upon or value. Such pollution is for the most part site-specific or regional in nature. On the whole, high-income countries have largely controlled many of these forms of pollution, although pollution remains a concern in many places, but the situation is in general much worse in middle- and low-income countries.

One of the most insidious and least understood forms of pollution is ecotoxicity (Hall & Chant, 1979). We have created many novel and toxic persistent organic pollutants (POPs) in the past century, for which there are no natural detoxifying mechanisms.[4] These pollutants spread widely in the environment, before becoming bio-concentrated up the food chain, reaching levels in top predators (including humans) millions of times higher than in the source water (Gilbertson, 1998). As a result, almost every person born or living since World War II—and many other life forms on Earth—carry a lifelong body burden of multiple POPs, the lifetime health consequences of which are unknown. In one troubling Canadian example, Inuit women, who live thousands of miles away from heavy industrial plants, have among the highest levels of PCBs and other POPs in their breast milk (Dewailly, 2006).

Resource Depletion

We use natural resources to meet our basic needs. Some resources, such as water, forests, soil, and fish, are renewable as long as their exploitation does not exceed the rate of renewal and as long as the necessary ecosystem services can enable that renewal.

Other resources, particularly metals and fossil fuels, are non-renewable on any scale relevant to humans; there is a finite supply of retrievable/extractable resources. We may be reaching limits in the global production of some of these non-renewable resources (Heinberg, 2007; Seppelt, Manceur, Liu, Fenichel, & Klotz, 2014).

Among the major concerns are the depletion of water, soil, foodlands, and fisheries, since they provide the most basic requirements for life and health.

- *Fresh water supply* is threatened by a combination of climate change and the drawing down of aquifers in many parts of the world.
- *Agriculture*: World food production will need to double within the next 50 years, yet it is threatened not only by inadequate water supply but by soil degradation and loss (Myers & Patz, 2009). One-quarter of agricultural land is highly degraded (FAO, 2011) and soil has been called a threatened natural resource (International Soil Research Information Centre, n.d.).
- *Marine and freshwater ecosystems* are under threat, leading to the collapse of some fisheries (McCauley et al., 2015). Acidification of the oceans could have significant consequences in altering species composition, disrupting marine food webs and ecosystems, thus affecting marine-based diets of people worldwide (UNEP, 2010).

Species Extinction

The Living Planet Index (LPI) assesses the trend in population abundance for 14,152 populations of 3,706 vertebrate species (mammals, birds, reptiles, amphibians, and fish) monitored across the globe between 1970 and 2012. The LPI has declined 58 percent since 1970, with the freshwater ecozone LPI declining a frightening 81 percent (WWF, 2016). The rapid loss of species we are experiencing is between 1,000 and 10,000 times higher than the natural extinction rate (WWF, n.d.). The combination of all the human-driven ecological changes outlined above, as well as human intrusion and destruction of habitats, is creating the sixth mass extinction of species—but the first to be induced by humans (WWF, n.d.).

Socio-Economic Aspects of the Anthropocene

The scale of human impact on the planet has grown rapidly over the past 50 years, and even more so since about 1950. It can best be understood, in a famous equation put forward by Ehrlich and Holdren (1972), as a function of population growth, affluence, and technology: $I = P \times A \times T$; the interaction of these three elements can have a powerful impact.

For example, a child born in Canada today, with a life expectancy of about 80 years, would see an increase in impact during their lifetime of more than 23 times the starting point, if current population and economic growth conditions prevail (Hancock, Spady, & Soskolne, 2015). This is clearly unsustainable, given that we are already exceeding the Earth's carrying capacity, as noted earlier.

Some point to technology as a way out of this problem, although our technology has generally tended to have the opposite effect. But even if our technology could deliver a fivefold increase in efficiency, as some have suggested (von Weizsäcker, Hargroves, Smith, Desha, & Stasinopoulos, 2009), this would still be an increase of more than four times our current impact for that infant over their lifetime, which remains both unsustainable and unachievable.

Clearly a key factor is economic growth, which is generally linked to material consumption and the ecological footprint. But this points to a wider and deeper issue: our way of life, our values, and our belief in the importance of rising levels of wealth and material goods. It is the underlying values of our modern Western industrialized society, and the economic system based on those values, that lies at the heart of the Anthropocene, and to which I turn next.

Values and the Economy

First, it is important to recognize that the economy is a social construct. We created it, we imbued it with the values that drive it, and we can change those values and we can change the economic system—indeed, we must. The biggest challenge is the very idea of growth, which is equated with progress and development; "economic growth as the central defining feature of an industrial … economy" (Kumar, n.d.).

This is not to say that economic development is a bad thing; indeed it—not health care—has largely been the source of the high level of health we enjoy in high-income countries. However, Wilkinson and Pickett (2010) have shown convincingly that in high-income countries it is the degree of social equity, not the level of GDP, that best correlates with a wide range of health and social outcomes.

In fact, data from 2012 show that above $30,000 USD GDP per capita "the relationship between income and life expectancy becomes non-significant. For countries where income exceeds US$40,000, the relationship becomes inverse" (Biciunaite, 2014).

So the clear implication is that we do not need a high GDP to have a high life expectancy at birth—countries such as Anguilla (81.2 years), Greece (81.01), Malta (80.67), and Costa Rica (79.59) do almost as well as Canada (82.14) and better than the US, at 79.16 years, with a much lower GDP per capita, ranging from $12,200 to $29,200 USD PPP compared to $43,100 in Canada and $52,800 in the US (Index Mundi, n.d. a & b). What higher-income countries are purchasing is more consumption, more "stuff," but to very little actual benefit, and at considerable expense to the environment.

As Gandhi said, "Earth provides enough to satisfy every man's need, but not every man's greed." That will need to become part of the health promotion credo in the twenty-first century, if we are all to live safely and equitably on this one small blue planet that we call home.

HEALTH IN THE ANTHROPOCENE[5]

As noted earlier, we depend upon natural systems for the very stuff of life—air, water, food, materials, and fuels, for example. These natural ecosystem goods and services, which also include a stable climate, protection from UV radiation, and the nitrogen and phosphorus cycles that underpin plant growth, are the most fundamental determinants of health; in our CPHA report we described them as the ecological determinants of health.

So at its most fundamental level, changes to natural systems on the scale described above will alter the conditions under which modern humans and their civilizations have emerged. One of the characteristics of natural systems when they are perturbed is that they may settle down in an alternate stable state (such as an ice age, or a hothouse planet). However, the alternate state cannot necessarily be predicted, and the transition can be rapid, as natural systems are capable of rapid non-linear change, or state-shift (Barnosky et al., 2012). Those changes may not be compatible with the continued existence of many of our societies and communities—and that, clearly, will have massive health implications.

The report from the UN's Millennium Ecosystem Assessment (2005a) found that "approximately 60% (15 out of 24) of the ecosystem services examined during the Millennium Ecosystem Assessment are being degraded or used unsustainably." In summation, the Board of the Millennium Ecosystem Assessment wrote, "At the heart of this assessment is a stark warning. Human activity is putting such strain on the natural functions of Earth that the ability of the planet's ecosystems to sustain future generations can no longer be taken for granted" (Millennium Ecosystem Assessment, 2005b).

The more recent report of the Rockefeller-Lancet Commission on Planetary Health (Whitmee et al., 2015) is equally blunt:

> Far-reaching changes to the structure and function of the Earth's natural systems represent a growing threat to human health. And yet, global health has mainly improved as these changes have gathered pace. What is the explanation? As a Commission, we are deeply concerned that the explanation is straightforward and sobering: we have been mortgaging the health of future generations to realise economic and development gains in the present. By unsustainably exploiting nature's resources, human civilisation has flourished but now risks substantial health effects from the degradation of nature's life support systems in the future.

Yet it is hard to be precise in estimating the potential future health impacts, in part because there has been insufficient attention paid to this issue until very recently. For example, the Rockefeller-Lancet report (Whitmee et al., 2015) notes that a 2006 WHO report on the burden of disease from environmental factors "did not include the effects of global environmental change," while a 2007 report from the Earth System Science Partnership noted that "to date there has been little formal description and study of the relationships between global environmental changes and human health" (Confalonieri & McMichael, 2007, p. 1).

Ten years later, this is still largely the case. The most recent WHO report on the environmental burden of disease attributable to environmental risks comments, "It should be noted that many of the potential health implications of climate change, acting through food supply and migration, could unfortunately not be accounted for by the methods used in the report" (Prüss-Ustün, Wolf, Corvalán, Bos, & Neira, 2016).

However, both the CPHA report (Hancock, Spady, & Soskolne, 2015) and the report of the Planetary Health Commission (Whitmee et al., 2015) provide recent up-to-date overviews of the health impacts of global ecological change, and readers should look to them for details. Moreover, Whitmee et al. (2015) note that "Although better evidence is needed to underpin appropriate policies than is available at present, this should not be used as an excuse for inaction. Substantial potential exists to link action to reduce environmental damage with improved health outcomes for nations at all levels of economic development."

Some key points for the main health impacts of the main forms of global ecological change are presented below.

Health Impacts of Climate Change

Climate change has been called "the biggest global health threat of the 21st century" by the first Lancet Commission on Health and Climate Change (Costello et al., 2009), while the second Lancet Commission stated, "The effects of climate change are being felt today, and future projections represent an unacceptably high and potentially catastrophic risk to human health" (Watts et al., 2015).

The most recent report on health impacts by the Intergovernmental Panel on Climate Change (IPCC, 2014) assesses the probability of major increases in ill-health by mid-twenty-first century due to climate change as follows:

- Very high confidence
  - Greater risk of injury, disease, and death due to more intense heat waves and fires
  - Increased risks of food- and water-borne diseases

- High confidence
  - Increased risk of under-nutrition resulting from diminished food production in poor regions
  - Consequences for health of lost work capacity and reduced labour productivity in vulnerable populations

- Medium confidence
  - Increased risks of vector-borne diseases

One estimate is that climate change already directly causes 400,000 deaths annually, while another 4.5 million deaths annually are linked to air pollution, hazardous occupations, and cancer associated with the carbon-intensive energy system that is the main driver of climate change; this could rise to 700,000 and 6 million annual deaths respectively by 2030 (DARA and the Climate Vulnerable Forum, 2012).

Health Impacts of Pollution and Fossil-Fuel–Based Energy Systems

According to an assessment published by WHO (Prüss-Ustün & Corvalán, 2006) the most important health effects at a global level that arise from pollution are diarrhoeal disease (94 percent of which is due to unsafe drinking water and poor sanitation) and indoor and outdoor air pollution; an estimated 42 percent of lower respiratory tract infections (LRTIs) in developing (sic) countries, and up to 20 percent of LRTIs in developed countries are due to indoor air pollution (largely from burning biomass indoors for cooking and heating) and to a lesser extent outdoor air pollution.

Smith et al. (2013) report that energy use accounts for roughly 80 percent of particulate matter (PM) air pollution worldwide, and that in 2010 PM pollution resulted in 3.1 million premature deaths. Overall, it is estimated that energy systems directly cause "perhaps as many as five million premature deaths annually and more than 5% of all ill health (measured as lost healthy life years)" (Smith et al., 2012), meaning that "the direct effects of energy systems alone exceed the global health impact of most other risk factors except malnutrition, rivalling the global impacts of tobacco, alcohol, and high blood pressure" (Smith et al., 2013).

Health Impacts of Resource Depletion

The main concern here focuses on the depletion of water and both land- and water-based food resources; the over-use by humans will be compounded in many cases by climate change. The health effects could be catastrophic, at least locally, and potentially more widely. As with other global changes, the health impacts of resource scarcity will be felt most in low-income countries and among low-income and disadvantaged populations around the world.

The unavailability of an adequate supply of clean, safe water is a major concern. The WHO (2016) reports that "over 1 billion people lack access to safe water supplies" and that "water-associated infectious diseases claim up to 3.2 million lives each year, approximately 6% of all deaths globally."

Water is also important for food production, but the International Food Policy Research Institute (n.d.) reports that

> In 2010, 36 percent of the global population, 39 percent of the world's grain production and 22 percent of global GDP were at risk due to water stress. Under business-as-usual, 52 percent of the global population, 49 percent of global grain production, and 45 percent of total GDP will be at risk due to water stress by 2050.

In addition to water scarcity, we also face the challenges of land degradation and over-fishing already noted. The combination of all these effects on global food supply and thus on health is very troubling. Myers and Patz (2009) note that "at least one-third of the burden of disease in poor countries is due to malnutrition and roughly 16% of the global burden of disease is attributable to childhood malnutrition," and that world food production will need to double within the next 50 years, in part because of a growing shift to a high-meat diet.

Yet an animal-based diet is a more ecologically harmful way of providing food than a plant-based diet, requiring more inputs in terms of energy, water, and other resources and a less efficient conversion of plant calories to calories consumed by humans than direct consumption of the plants (Foley, 2014). Moreover, a high-meat diet is a less healthy diet. In a recent review, a low-meat or vegetarian diet was found to be associated with reduced risk of coronary heart disease, type 2 diabetes, and cancer (McEvoy, Temple, & Woodside, 2012).

While we face the challenge of dramatically increasing global food supply, a switch to a low-meat diet will make agriculture more environmentally sustainable and our diet more healthy.

Health Impacts of Species Extinction

Biodiversity contributes to important ecological determinants of health, including water and air quality, food security, microbial diversity in the human microbiome, infectious disease control, pharmaceuticals and traditional medicines, and mental, physical, and cultural wellbeing (Secretariat of the Convention on Biological Diversity and WHO, 2015). Species extinction represents perhaps the most profound and yet the least understood threat to human health.

IMPLICATIONS FOR HEALTH PROMOTION

What would it mean for health promotion—and public health more generally—if we took seriously the advent of the Anthropocene and an understanding of the ecological determinants of health, and adopted an eco-social approach that integrated the ecological and social determinants of health?

The CPHA report (Hancock, Spady, & Soskolne, 2015) identifies a set of specific challenges we need to address, which include the following:

- Integrate the ecological and social determinants of health in our thought and work, recognizing that each shapes both the other and the health of the population.
- Change population and public health curricula to incorporate this approach.
- Undertake research on the health implications of global and local ecological change.
- At a societal and policy level, challenge the prevailing economic model that creates unsustainable and unjust development—and help create the new healthy, just, and sustainable economic model we need.
- Include measures of ecosystem health and ecologically sensitive health indicators in population and community health reports.
- Undertake integrated impact assessments that include ecological and human health impacts.

- Protect people and communities from harm.
- Use the powers of public health to oppose developments that harm ecosystems and human health.
- Work with partners at the local level to create healthy, sustainable, and just communities.

These will be briefly reviewed here, but for a fuller discussion, see the report.

A Shift in Our Thinking and Our Values

As a profession that prides itself on being holistic in its thinking, we need to stop the artificial separation of the ecological and the social in our minds and in our work. In our report, we proposed a simple conceptual framework (figure 22.3) that illustrates that the ecological and social/economic determinants interact with each other: Social and economic factors drive ecological change, but ecological changes will impact adversely on social and economic development, and both sets of changes will impact the health of the population. Moreover, failing population health will further adversely affect social and economic development.

Underlying this shift in viewpoint, and the resultant shift in the focus of our work, lies a necessary shift in our ethical frameworks and thinking. The CPHA report specifically refers to a number of ethical precepts that should guide our work in the future: Two of the key ones are to take into account the wellbeing of non-human species with whom we share this planet, and also the wellbeing of future generations, to whom we also have an obligation.

> Considering justice for both future generations and non-human life necessitates a new ethical perspective in public health, which recently has been very clear in the area of social determinants of health, but now needs to consider equally the ecological determinants of health. (Hancock, Spady, & Soskolne, 2015, p. 80)

The report has a number of other ethically based suggestions for policy and practice.

Change Population and Public Health Curricula to Incorporate an Eco-social Approach

We need to update Canada's set of Core Competencies for Public Health to give greater prominence to the ecological determinants of health, ensuring that public health practitioners have the ability to address the determinants of health using an eco-social approach.

This will also require a restructuring of the population and public health curriculum to frame it around an eco-social approach to health, guided by the ethical principles noted above. In addition, considerable effort will need to be put into continuing professional development (CPD) to upgrade the knowledge and skills of existing public health staff.

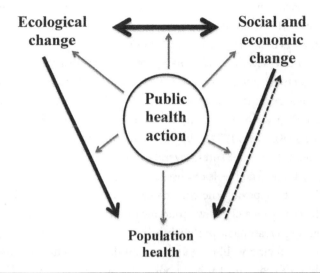

Figure 22.3: An Eco-social Framework for Public Health Action

An important part of both formal education and ongoing CPD will be to learn with and from other disciplines, including ecologists, urban planners and other design professionals, energy and transportation planners, food system workers, social entrepreneurs who are building the new economy, and many others.

Undertake Research on the Health Implications of Global and Local Ecological Change

The Canadian government, either through the CIHR (which, scandalously, lacks an Institute for Environmental Health) or some other mechanism, needs to establish a program of research into the health implications of global ecological change. This needs to occur at all levels from the local to the global, and should include research on changing ecological and health conditions in Canada and globally, so that we can monitor change and—hopefully—progress.

Challenge the Prevailing Economic Model—and Help Create the New Healthy, Just, and Sustainable Economic Model

As already noted, the current economic model of endless growth, consumption, and pollution has created the Anthropocene. We need an alternate approach if we are to successfully transition to the future we need to secure. In our report, we include an extensive discussion of the challenges of the existing economic system and an exploration of alternatives.

It makes no sense to make economic growth and development the central pillar of public policy. The focus must be on ensuring human and social development in a manner that is compatible with sustaining in perpetuity the natural systems that are the fundamental underpinnings of human wellbeing. Or as the 1992 CPHA report put it, "Human development and the achievement of human potential require a form of economic activity that is socially and environmentally sustainable in this and future generations" (p. 3).

Central to the argument for a new economics is the need to find better measures of progress than GDP; it was never intended as a measure of social welfare, according to one of its architects (Kuznets, 1934), although only too often that is what it has become. There are a number of better measures, several of which are discussed in the report; one of them—the Happy Planet Index—is discussed in chapter 12.

But in addition to opposing the current harmful economic model, we also need to be supporting the emergence of a new economic model, one rooted in sustainable human development, making a reasonable profit while improving the environment, strengthening community, and enhancing wellbeing and human development. One useful concept is that of the steady state economy. In their book about such an economy, *Enough is Enough*, Dietz and O'Neill (2012) "explore specific strategies to conserve natural resources, stabilize population, reduce inequality, fix the financial system, create jobs, and more—all with the aim of maximizing long-term well-being instead of short-term profits."

Include Measures of Ecosystem Health and Ecologically Sensitive Health Indicators in Population and Community Health Reports

It has become commonplace to include social and economic conditions as health determinants in population health reports. Now we need to go further: Public health reports at all levels should include indicators of ecological determinants of health in their routine reports, and should report specifically on the ecological determinants of health on a regular basis, reflecting local, regional, provincial, national, Indigenous, and global contexts.

To do this, we need to revise and update the core set of indicators of health used in Canada in line with the socio-ecological model of health, by including indicators of the state of key ecological determinants of health, the socio-ecological system, and sentinel health conditions associated with ecological change.

Undertake Integrated Impact Assessments that Include Ecological and Human Health Impacts

These indicators can be used to monitor and report on these issues across all four orders of government (i.e., federal, provincial, municipal, and First Nations) and can also be used to guide more comprehensive impact assessments of the ecological, social, health, and economic impacts of major public policies and private sector developments, as discussed below.

A good place to begin is energy policy. There has never been a full health impact assessment of Canada's energy systems, or the alternative energy policy options open to us; it is time there was, especially given the significant health impacts of energy systems described earlier.

Protect People and Communities from Harm

The best strategy for protecting people is primordial prevention—preventing the ecological changes that may harm human wellbeing. But realistically, ecological damage has already been sustained, and we cannot avoid further ecological changes that will harm our health. Given the momentum in our socio-economic systems, the decline in the functioning of key ecosystem components and the availability of key resources will continue.

This means we will need to be prepared for disasters, and ecological decline or even collapse, by developing resilient physical and social infrastructure able to cope with changing and potentially unstable environmental conditions. Part of this infrastucture is the health care system, which needs to be prepared to handle failure in other components of infrastructure (e.g., electical or water supply, telecommunications) in disasters, while managing casualties effectively.

We also need flexible, adaptable, and resilient people and communities able to manage the necessary societal changes and "bounce forward" to a better future. It will be particularly important to identify vulnerable populations, reduce their vulnerability, and protect them from harm.

Use the Powers of Public Health to Oppose Developments that Harm Ecosystem and Human Health

Historically, public health has been granted and has used extraordinary powers to protect the health of the public, and many of these powers remain in public health legislation to this day. Now we need to use this legislation to address issues where harmful impacts on natural systems are occurring that might harm human health. Where appropriate, we should request the Minister, Provincial Health Officer, or other appropriate public health officials to initiate an inquiry or investigation using the powers under the Public Health Act; for example, we should seek a comprehensive study into the health impacts of fossil-fuelled energy systems.

Public health also has a duty to advocate (Hancock, 2015b) and act in the public interest, challenging corporate and government power, where that power is harmful to ecosystems, societies, communities, and the health of the population. To do so we should ally ourselves with others, especially environmental groups, that are also acting in the public interest.

Naming and shaming, ethical purchasing and investments, boycotts, legal challenges, divestment, and civil disobedience in the form of demonstrations and blockades are some of the legitimate tools and strategies to which those who seek to protect the health of the public and the Earth's natural systems have had to resort in the past, and will have to resort in the future.

Work with Partners at the Local Level to Create Healthy, Sustainable, and Just Communities

"Think globally, act locally" was a rallying cry for environmental activists in the 1970s, and it remains excellent advice today. But we also need to think positively: Indeed, in our report we have two entire chapters on finding hope and imagining and creating a more positive future.

Health promotion is or should be hopeful, focused on a positive and future-oriented approach that recognizes the importance of the environmental, social, economic, cultural, and political determinants of health and that builds on existing capacity, assets, and strengths to improve the health of the entire population, while at the same time placing special emphasis on reducing inequalities in health.

Since the basis of much public health and health promotion work is local, the experience gained over the past few decades in asset-based community development and the creation of healthier and more sustainable communities, in Canada and around the world, is one of the most important building blocks we have.

In virtually every policy area one can think of, from the municipal to the national level, improved health and ecological sustainability can work hand in hand. At the government level, this calls for a "whole-of-government" approach at all levels in which various departments collaborate within a guiding framework of a commitment to a more just, sustainable, and healthy society (see chapter 18 for further discussion on whole-of-government approaches).

But beyond government, the process of governance requires that all sectors of society also collaborate and contribute what they can to this task, which thus becomes a "whole-of-society," or "whole-of-community" approach. There are many social movements—locally, nationally, and internationally—that are working to achieve the same objectives as are we. These movements are our natural allies, especially as their work is often rooted in place—in local communities and local action (see chapter 12 for a more extensive discussion of these issues).

An emerging approach to this is the concept of a "One Planet" community or region (Hancock, Capon, Dooris, & Patrick, 2017), which brings together the concepts of both healthy and sustainable communities. The challenge that health promoters and others must address is how we are to live a life in good health and of high quality, in a socially just way, while reducing our ecological footprint from the three- to five-planet ecological footprint of today to one planet.

CONCLUSION: HEALTH PROMOTION HAS AN OBLIGATION TO RESPOND TO THE ANTHROPOCENE

I am convinced that the global ecological changes discussed here represent the greatest threat to population health in the twenty-first century. While Canada is a wealthy country and may be able to stave off or ameliorate some of these impacts, we nonetheless have an ethical duty to the rest of humanity, to future generations, and to the myriad other species with whom we share the planet to dramatically reduce our contribution to these ecological changes. As ethical professionals imbued with a sense of social justice and a concern for health and wellbeing, health promotion and public health professionals need to be committed to playing their part in the transformative changes we need.

In writing about the report of the Second Lancet Commission on Climate Change, Dr. Margaret Chan, Director-General of the World Health Organization, wrote, "the health community has a vital part to play in accelerating progress to tackle climate change … I endorse the call for the health community to support the growing movement for a cleaner, more sustainable, and healthier future" (Chan, 2015). But she was only talking about one aspect of the Anthropocene—climate change; as I have shown here, global ecological change is a much larger phenomenon. Addressing the health implications of the Anthropocene is the greatest challenge facing health promotion and public health workers today.

We alone cannot create the massive cultural, social, and economic changes that are needed. Just as was the case in the nineteenth century, when public health faced the appalling conditions of the industrial slums in Europe and North America, we need to find and engage with partners across society, and we need to mobilize communities and society as a whole to address this issue. Together with those partners, we must work to create the more sustainable, just, and healthy future we need for all the people of the Earth.

CRITICAL THINKING QUESTIONS

1. Is it possible to live within the constraints of the Earth's resources and ecosystems within our current economic system? If not, what needs to change and how can we help create the necessary changes?

2. How will we ensure that people living in low-income countries get their fair share of the Earth's resources, and thus a fair opportunity to live long, healthy lives?

3. How can health promotion and public health workers and organizations prepare for and support adaptation to the social, environmental, and health implications of global and regional/local ecological change?

4. What are the local examples of social/green/sustainable entrepreneurship in your community, and how can health promotion and public health workers and organizations encourage and support these entrepreneurs?

RESOURCES

Further Readings

Hancock T., Spady, D. W., & Soskolne, C. L. (Eds.). (2015). *Global change and public health: Addressing the ecological determinants of health: The report in brief.*
www.cpha.ca/uploads/policy/edh-brief.pdf
This 100-page report was prepared by a CPHA Working Group between 2012 and 2015. It is a comprehensive overview of the Anthropocene, its socio-economic drivers, and its population health implications. It also includes a chapter on finding hope, a chapter on imagining a better future, and an action agenda for public health professionals and organizations. A shorter version, a 30-page CPHA Discussion Paper, is also available at www. cpha.ca/uploads/policy/edh-discussion_e.pdf.

McMichael, A. (1993). *Planetary overload.* Cambridge: Cambridge University Press.
A now-classic early examination of the health implications of what we now call the Anthropocene.

Whitmee, S., Haines, A., Beyrer, C., Boltz, F., Capon, A. G., Ferreira de Souza Dias, B., ... Yach, D. (2015). Safeguarding human health in the Anthropocene epoch: Report of The Rockefeller Foundation–Lancet Commission on Planetary Health. *The Lancet, 386*(1007), 1973–2028.
dx.doi.org/10.1016/S0140-6736(15)60901-1
Dr. Richard Horton, the editor of *The Lancet*, coined the term *planetary health* in a presentation in Beijing on the challenges facing the Rockefeller Foundation as it enters its second century. This high-level Commission was established by *The Lancet*, funded by the Rockefeller Foundation, and reported in summer 2015, covering much of the same ground as the CPHA's Workgroup.

Relevant Websites

UNEP Environmental Data Explorer
geodata.grid.unep.ch/
The Environmental Data Explorer is the authoritative source for data sets used by UNEP and its partners in the Global Environment Outlook (GEO) report and other integrated environment assessments. Its online database holds more than 500 different variables, as national, subregional, regional, and global statistics or as geospatial data sets (maps), covering themes like freshwater, population, forests, emissions, climate, disasters, health, and GDP. Display them on-the-fly as maps, graphs, and data tables or download the data in different formats.

Welcome to the Anthropocene

www.youtube.com/watch?v=-cJYXlfjADE

This is a three-and-a-half-minute video made for a 2012 conference on Planet Under Pressure organized by a number of the world's leading international scientific bodies concerned with Earth science and related issues. It is a powerful introduction to the topic that makes a great starting point for discussion.

WWF Living Planet Report

wwf.panda.org/about_our_earth/all_publications/lpr_2016/

Global biodiversity is declining at an alarming rate, putting the survival of other species and our own future at risk. The latest edition of WWF's Living Planet Report brings home the enormity of the situation—and how we can start to put it right.

NOTES

1.   Chief Seattle was a Duwamish Chief in the Pacific Northwest. The text of his speech, some time around 1854, was written down much later, and after several translations, so his precise words are not certain.

2.   For a succinct but powerful introduction, see the three-and-a-half-minute video produced for the Planet Under Pressure conference in London in 2012. Available at www.youtube.com/watch?v=-cJYXlfjADE

3.   Includes "new forms of existing substances and modified life-forms that have the potential for unwanted geophysical and/or biological effects," e.g., persistent organic pollutants, POPs, heavy metals, nano-particles, and genetically engineered organisms.

4.   In addition, we have created nano-particles and genetically modified organisms, collectively described as "novel entities," which are also widespread in the global environment (Steffen, Richardson, et al., 2015).

5.   The issue of health care in the Anthropocene is discussed in Hancock (2016) and Hancock, Capon, Dietrich, and Patrick (2016), and will not be further discussed here.

REFERENCES

Barnosky, A. D., Hadly, E. A., Bascompte, J., Berlow, E. L., Brown, J. H., Fortelius, M., ... Smith, A. B. (2012). Approaching a state shift in Earth's biosphere. *Nature, 486*, 52–58.

Biciunaite, A. (2014). Economic growth and life expectancy—Do wealthier countries live longer? *Euromonitor International*. Retrieved from blog.euromonitor.com/2014/03/economic-growth-and-life-expectancy-do-wealthier-countries-live-longer.html

Butler, C. (2016). Sounding the alarm: Health in the Anthropocene. *International Journal of Environmental Research and Public Health, 13*(7), 665. doi:10.3390/ijerph13070665

Canadian Public Health Association (CPHA). (1992). *Human & ecosystem health: Canadian perspectives, Canadian action*. Ottawa: Author. Retrieved from www.cpha.ca/uploads/policy/human-ecosystem_health_e.pdf

Canadian Public Health Association (CPHA). (2015). *Global change and public health: Addressing the ecological determinants of health.* Ottawa: Author. Retrieved from www.cpha.ca/uploads/policy/edh-discussion_e.pdf

Chan, M. (2015). Achieving a cleaner, more sustainable, and healthier future. *The Lancet.* Retrieved from dx.doi.org/10.1016/S0140-6736(15)61080-7

Confalonieri, U., & McMichael, A. (Eds.). (2007). *Global environmental change and human health: Science plan and implementation strategy.* Earth System Science Partnership (DIVERSITAS, IGBP, IHDP, and WCRP) Report No. 4.

Costello, A., Abbas, M., Allen, A. Ball, S., Bell, S., Bellamy, R., ... Patterson, C. (2009). Managing the health effects of climate change. *Lancet, 373,* 1693–1733.

Crutzen, P. J., & Stoermer, E. F. (2000). The "Anthropocene." *International Geosphere-Biosphere Program Newsletter, 41,* 17–18.

DARA and the Climate Vulnerable Forum. (2012). *Climate vulnerability monitor* (2nd ed.). *A guide to the cold calculus of a hot planet.* Madrid: DARA.

Davies, K., & Hancock, T. (1997). *The health implications of global change: A Canadian perspective.* Paper for the "Rio + 5" Forum prepared for Environment Canada. Ottawa: The Royal Society of Canada, Canadian Global Change Program.

Dewailly, É. (2006). Canadian Inuit and the Arctic Dilemma. *Oceanography, 19*(2), 88–89.

Dietz, R., & O'Neill, D. (2012). *Enough is enough: Building a sustainable economy in a world of finite resources.* San Francisco: Berrett-Koehler Publishers.

Ehrlich, P., & Holdren, J. (1972). Impact of population growth. In R. G. Riker (Ed.), *Population, resources, and the environment* (pp. 365–377). Washington, DC: U.S. Government Printing Office.

Environment and Climate Change Canada. (2016). *Climate trends and variations bulletin—winter 2015–2016.* Retrieved from www.ec.gc.ca/sc-cs/default.asp?lang=En&n=55965A8C-1

Evans, R., Barer, M., & Marmor, T. (Eds.). (1994). *Why are some people healthy and others not? The determinants of the health of populations.* New York: Adeline de Gruyter.

FAO. (2011). *The state of the world's land and water resources for food and agriculture (SOLAW): Managing systems at risk.* Rome: Food and Agriculture Organization of the United Nations and London: Earthscan.

Foley, J. (2014). A five-step plan to feed the world. *National Geographic, 225*(5), 27–47.

Gilbertson, M. (1998). Linking water quality to wildlife and human health. *Focus, 23*(3), 18–19.

Global Footprint Network. (n.d.). *Footprint basics.* Retrieved from www.footprintnetwork.org/en/index.php/GFN/page/footprint_basics_overview/

Hall, R., & Chant, D. (1979). *Ecotoxity: Responsibilities and opportunities.* Ottawa: Canadian Environmental Advisory Council.

Hancock, T. (2015a). Population health promotion 2.0: An eco-social approach to public health in the Anthropocene. *Canadian Journal of Public Health, 106*(4), e252–e255. doi: 10.17269/CJPH.106.5161

Hancock, T. (2015b). Advocacy: It's not a dirty word, it's a duty. *Canadian Journal of Public Health, 106*(3), e86–e88.

Hancock, T. (2016). Healthcare in the Anthropocene: Challenges and opportunities. *Health Care Quarterly, 19*(3), 17–22. doi:10.12927/hcq.2016.24870

Hancock, T., Capon, A., Dietrich, U., & Patrick, R. (2016). Governance for health in the Anthropocene. *International Journal of Health Governance, 21*(4), 1–20. Retrieved from www.emeraldinsight.com/doi/pdfplus/10.1108/IJHG-08-2016-0041

Hancock, T., Capon, A., Dooris, M., & Patrick, R. (2017). One planet regions: Planetary health at the local level. *Lancet Planetary Health, 1*, e92–e93. Retrieved from www.thelancet.com/pdfs/journals/lanplh/PIIS2542-5196(17)30044-X.pdf

Hancock T., Spady, D. W., & Soskolne, C. L. (Eds.). (2015). *Global change and public health: Addressing the ecological determinants of health: The report in brief.* Retrieved from www.cpha.ca/uploads/policy/edh-brief.pdf

Heinberg, R. (2007). *Peak everything: Waking up to the century of declines.* Gabriola, BC: New Society Publishers.

Index Mundi. (n.d. a). *GDP per capita, as of 1 January 2014.* Retrieved from www.indexmundi.com/g/r.aspx?v=67

Index Mundi. (n.d. b). *Life expectancy at birth in 2015.* Retrieved from www.indexmundi.com/facts/indicators/SP.DYN.LE00.IN/rankings

Intergovernmental Panel on Climate Change (IPCC). (2014). Summary for policymakers. In C. B. Field, V. R. Barros, D. J. Dokken, K. J. Mach, M. D. Mastrandrea, T. E. Bilir, … L. L. White (Eds.), *Climate change 2014: Impacts, adaptation, and vulnerability. Part A: Global and sectoral aspects. Contribution of Working Group II to the Fifth Assessment Report of the Intergovernmental Panel on Climate Change.* Cambridge.

International Food Policy Research Institute. (n.d.). *Water futures.* Retrieved from www.ifpri.org/project/water-futures

International Soil Research Information Centre. (n.d.). *Soil threats.* Retrieved from www.isric.org

Jackson, S., & Riley, B. (2007). Health promotion in Canada: 1986 to 2006. *Promotion Education, 14*, 214–218. doi:10.1177/10253823070140040601

Kumar, K. (n.d.). Modernization. *Encyclopedia Britannica.* Retrieved from www.britannica.com/EBchecked/topic/387301/modernization

Kuznets, S. (1934). *National income, 1929–1932.* 73rd US Congress, 2nd session, Senate document no. 124, p. 7.

Labonté, R. (1995). Population health and health promotion: What do they have to say to each other? *Canadian Journal of Public Health, 86*(3), 165–168.

Labonté, R. (1997). The population health/health promotion debate in Canada: The politics of explanation, economics and action. *Critical Public Health, 7*(1–2), 7–27. doi:10.1080/09581599708409075

Last, J. (1987). *Public health and human ecology.* East Norwalk: Appleton & Lange.

Mackenzie, H., Messinger, H., & Smith, R. (2008). *Size matters: Canada's ecological footprint, by income.* Ottawa: Canadian Centre for Policy Alternatives.

McCauley, D. J., Pinsky, M. L., Palumbi, S. R., Estes, J. H., Joyce, F. H., & Warner, R. R. (2015). Marine defaunation: Animal loss in the global ocean. *Science, 347*(6219). DOI: 10.1126/science.1255641

McEvoy, C. T., Temple, N., & Woodside, J. V. (2012). Vegetarian diets, low-meat diets and health: A review. *Public Health Nutrition, 15*(12), 2287–2294.

McMichael, A. (1993). *Planetary overload.* Cambridge: Cambridge University Press.

McMichael, A. (2014). Population health in the Anthropocene: Gains, losses and emerging trends. *The Anthropocene Review, 1*(1), 44–56.

Millennium Ecosystem Assessment. (2005a). *Ecosystems and human well-being: Synthesis.* Washington, DC: Island Press. Retrieved from www.millenniumassessment.org/documents/document.356.aspx.pdf

Millennium Ecosystem Assessment. (2005b). *Living beyond our means: Natural assets and human well-being.* Washington, DC: Island Press. Retrieved from www.millenniumassessment.org/documents/document.429.aspx.pdf

Myers, S. S., & Patz, J. A. (2009). Emerging threats to human health from global environmental change. *Annual Review Environmental Resour*ces, *34*(1), 223–252.

New Economics Foundation. (2016). *The Happy Planet Index 2016.* London: Author. Retrieved from happyplanetindex.org

NOAA National Centers for Environmental Information. (2016). *State of the climate: Global analysis for July 2016.* Retrieved from www.ncdc.noaa.gov/sotc/global/201607

Prüss-Ustün, A., & Corvalán, C. (2006). *Preventing disease through healthy environments: Towards an estimate of the environmental burden of disease (Executive summary).* Geneva: WHO.

Prüss-Ustün, A., Wolf, J., Corvalán, C., Bos, R., & Neira, M. (2016). *Preventing disease through healthy environments: A global assessment of the burden of disease from environmental risks.* Geneva: WHO.

Secretariat of the Convention on Biological Diversity and WHO. (2015). *Connecting global priorities: Biodiversity and human health, summary of the state of knowledge review.* Montréal: Author.

Seppelt, R., Manceur, A. M., Liu, J., Fenichel, E. P., & Klotz, S. (2014). Synchronized peak-rate years of global resources use. *Ecology and Society, 19*(4), 50.

Smith, K., Frumkin, H., Balakrishnan, K., Butler, C., Chafe, Z., Fairlie, I., … Schneider, M. (2013). Energy and human health. *Annual Review of Public Heath, 34,* 159–188.

Smith, K. R., Balakrishnan, K., Butler, C., Chafe, Z., Fairlie, I., Kinney, P., … Schneider, M. (2012). Chapter 4: Energy and health. In *Global energy assessment—Toward a sustainable future* (pp. 255–324). Cambridge and New York: Cambridge University Press; and Laxenburg, Austria: International Institute for Applied Systems Analysis.

Statistics Canada. (2013). *Canada's total population estimates, 2013.* Retrieved from www.statcan.gc.ca/daily-quotidien/130926/dq130926a-eng.htm?HPA

Steffen, W., Broadgate, W., Deutsch, L., Gaffney, O., & Ludwig, C. (2015). The trajectory of the Anthropocene: The great acceleration. *The Anthropocene Review, 2*(1), 81–98.

Steffen, W., Richardson, K., Rockström, J., Cornell, S. E., Fetzer, I., Bennett, E. M., … Sörlin, S. (2015). Planetary boundaries: Guiding human development on a changing planet. *Science, 347*(6223), 1259855. DOI: 10.1126/science.1259855

UNEP. (2010). *Environmental consequences of ocean acidification: A threat to food security.* Retrieved from www.fao.org/fileadmin/user_upload/fsn/docs/HLPE/Environmental_Consequences_ of_Ocean_Acidification.pdf

UNEP. (2012). *Keeping track of our changing environment: From Rio to Rio+20 (1992–2012).* Retrieved from ourworld.unu.edu/en/the-environment-in-numbers-1992-2012/

Von Weizsäcker, E., Hargroves, C., Smith, M., Desha, C., & Stasinopoulos, P. (2009). *Factor 5: Transforming the global economy through an 80% increase in resource productivity.* London: Earthscan.

Waters, C., Zalasiewicz, J., Summerhayes, C., Barnosky, A. D., Poirier, C., Gałuszka, A., ... Wolfe, A. P. (2016). The Anthropocene is functionally and stratigraphically distinct from the Holocene. *Science, 351*(6269). DOI: 10.1126/science.aad2622

Watts, N., Adger, N., Agnolucci, P., Blackstock, J., Byass, P., Cai, W., ... Costello, A. (2015). Health and climate change: Policy responses to protect public health. *Lancet.* Retrieved from dx.doi.org/10.1016/S0140-6736(15)60854-6

Whitmee, S., Haines, A., Beyrer, C., Boltz, F., Capon, A. G., Ferreira de Souza Dias, B., ... Yach, D. (2015). Safeguarding human health in the Anthropocene epoch: Report of The Rockefeller Foundation–Lancet Commission on Planetary Health. *The Lancet, 386*(1007), 1973–2028. Retrieved from dx.doi.org/10.1016/S0140-6736(15)60901-1

World Health Organization (WHO). (1986). *Ottawa Charter for Health Promotion.* Copenhagen: WHO/Europe.

World Health Organization (WHO). (2016). *Water services for health.* Retrieved from www.who. int/globalchange/ecosystems/water/en/

WHO Commission on Social Determinants of Health. (2008). *Closing the gap in a generation: Health equity through action on the social determinants of health. Final Report of the Commission on Social Determinants of Health.* Geneva: WHO.

Wilkinson, R., & Pickett, K. (2010). *The spirit level: Why equality is better for everyone.* London: Penguin.

WWF. (2016). *Living Planet Report 2016: Risk and resilience in a new era.* Gland, Switzerland: WWF International.

WWF. (n.d.). *Biodiversity.* Retrieved from wwf.panda.org/about_our_earth/biodiversity/ biodiversity/

CHAPTER 23

Globalization: The Perils and Possibilities for an Equitable Health Promotion

Ronald Labonté

LEARNING OBJECTIVES

1. Understand the meaning and drivers of contemporary globalization, and how global-ization affects health
2. Examine income, wealth, and health inequality trends globally, and in Canada
3. Explore the two main ways in which capitalist countries can reduce inequalities
4. Understand the economic meaning of neo-liberalism, and how its three phases since the 1980s have affected health and health equity
5. Examine the available policy options at national and global scales that can reduce wealth and health inequalities, and the role of the new Sustainable Development Goals in advancing action on these policy choices

INTRODUCTION

When the first edition of this book appeared in 1994 most of us writing about health pro-motion were concerned with several persisting tensions in practice: unhealthy lifestyles/living conditions; top-down/bottom-up programming; individual change/collective mo-bilization; and professional knowledge/community wisdom. Our locus for grappling with these tensions was the community, and our major challenge was scaling up to those policy reaches that condition and constrain health opportunities. The limited geography of our terrain was not parochial. It was merely a product of its time. These health promotion tensions and challenges still define the territory for most practitioners—the important "ordinary" of our work that needs to be celebrated, extended, and sustained into the future. But, although necessary, health promotion's empowering localism—even its nationalism—is no longer sufficient. As the 2005 *Bangkok Charter for Health Promotion* stated more than a decade ago, "Health promotion must become an integral part of domestic and foreign policy and international relations" (WHO, 2005). What changed?

THE GLOBALIZATION OF HEALTH AND DISEASE

The most obvious intrusion into national health complacency has been the continuing wave of infectious outbreaks, some new or newly global in reach: from SARS to Ebola to chikungunya to Zika, with pandemic influenza an almost regular health security alert. The awareness that previously local outbreaks can be a short air flight to almost anywhere with pandemic impact has created a new "global health security" discourse, in which unchecked or poorly controlled disease outbreaks in distant lands are seen as inherently global health risks. With climate change expanding the geography of such pathogens, and with the rise of anti-microbial resistance in those infections with which most of the world is already familiar (from E. coli to golden staph to tuberculosis), the local has become unavoidably global.

The global, of course, also instantiates itself in the local, with few better examples than the corporate diffusion of unhealthy Western commodities across developing countries (from tobacco, to sugar-sweetened beverages, to obesogenic foods), aided and abetted by an increasing array of "free" trade and investment treaties. The high-income epidemics of non-communicable diseases (NCDs) have become global pandemics, outpacing even infectious disease risks in all corners of the world except sub-Saharan Africa. Our health promotion terrain is no longer just the local community, but a global village of communities, and our healthy public policies are no longer confined to "making healthy choices the easier choices," but must encompass the new international rules that govern who wins and who loses (and whose choices are healthier and whose are not) in an increasingly globalized world.

Let's first consider the term *globalization*. Kelley Lee, one of the early thinkers on the globalization/health linkage, considers it broadly as a function of technology, culture, and economics leading to a compression of time (everything is faster), space (geographic boundaries begin to blur), and cognition (awareness of the world as a whole) (Lee, 2003). This is undoubtedly true, although these have been societal qualities for as long as there have been written records of societies, just as diseases have a long history of following trade routes and population movements. The qualitative shift we experience today lies in the intensity of these changes. Others have argued (convincingly) that "economic globalization has been the driving force behind the overall process of globalization" (Woodward, Drager, Beaglehole, & Lipson, 2001, p. 876), and when the term *globalization* began its popular ascendency in the early 1980s it was used first to describe the international integration of economic markets. Changes in our global economy, particularly since the 1980s, have been the source of contemporary globalization's intensification, bringing with it new challenges to health and its promotion.

Globalization's Positive Health Claims

When the Globalization Knowledge Network that I chaired for the World Health Organization's Commission on Social Determinants of Health (2005–2008) completed its tasks, our final report included a brief synopsis of some of the positive health gains over the recent decades of rapid and intensified globalization (Labonté et al., 2008). Prime amongst these was coined the "child health revolution": the global diffusion of low-cost health technologies promoted by UNICEF (and others) under the moniker of GOBI-FFF (Growth monitoring, Oral rehydration, Breastfeeding promotion, Immunization, Female education, Family spacing, and Food supplementation). Together with the spread of anti-malarial bed nets, these interventions are credited with saving some 90 million children's lives since 1990 (UNICEF, 2013). There have been modest declines in maternal mortality in many low-income countries, attributed in part to expanded health extension programs and community health workers in rural areas. The net impact of these improvements has been an increase in global life expectancy, which had fallen rapidly in the 1990s due, in part, to HIV/AIDS and the negative economic and social impacts in Eastern Europe that followed the collapse of the Soviet Union. These losses reversed between 2000 and 2015, with global life expectancy rising by five years, and by over nine years in the African region, attributed to the child health revolution and improved access to anti-retrovirals for HIV (WHO, 2016). Although these gains are impressive, and in the case of access to ARVs in Africa only arose when civil society opposition forced down the costs of patented drugs, they remain highly skewed, with inequalities in health and health care access worsening within many countries (global or national averages tell us little about how equitably such health benefits are shared). As one example: the maternal mortality risk is 1 in 3,300 in high-income countries, but jumps to 1 in 41 in low-income countries, with even greater risks in under-resourced rural areas (UNICEF, 2016).

Moreover, two critical questions remain:

- How sustainable are our recent health gains?
- What role did globalization (via its economic market integration and global economic growth) play in them?

In the first instance, considerable credit for recent health improvements has gone to increased donor funding for the eight Millennium Development Goals (MDGs), a consolidation of development commitments made in the 1990s and announced in 2000 with the promise that the poorest in the world should not lack for resources to attain these goals by 2015. Although substantial new funds for many of the MDGs did flow as a result, especially for the three so-called health goals (MDGs 4, 5, and 6, on reducing child mortality, improving maternal health, and reducing HIV, malaria, and other diseases, respectively), the rhetoric was not matched by the generosity required, and most of the goals fell far short of their 2015 targets. Official development assistance (ODA or simply "aid") remains the principal form of public wealth transfers from rich to poor countries. For more than 30 years, most of the world's wealthier donor nations have pledged to contribute at least 0.7 percent of their gross national income (GNI) to ODA. As of 2014, only five have: Luxembourg, Denmark, Sweden, Norway, and the UK. Global ODA is stuck at just 0.29 percent, lower than it has been in past years (Development Initiatives, 2014). The European Union countries had pledged to reach the 0.7 percent target by 2015; they managed to reach 0.42 (Organisation for Economic Co-operation and Development [OECD], 2015). Canada does remarkably poorly, with our ODA declining to only 0.24 percent in 2014 (OECD, 2015)—a dismal 16th place among the top donor countries. Development assistance, although still important and especially for the world's poorest countries, is a weak and arbitrary means for the global resource redistributions needed to create and sustain equitable global health (more on other options later in this chapter).

One of the key health arguments defending the past 40 years of globalization has had little to do with ODA, and focuses instead on the "trickle down" health benefits associated with global economic growth. Its proponents hold that liberalization (the removal of border barriers on the flow of goods, services, and capital) increases trade, which perforce increases growth that in turn decreases poverty; and any decline in poverty is good for people's health (Dollar, 2001). Economic growth also provides revenue for investments in health care, education, women's empowerment programs, and so on. Improved health increases economic growth (WHO Commission on Macroeconomics and Health, 2001) and the circle closes virtuously upon itself. Although a compelling narrative, the evidence behind it is weak to non-existent. As one example: A study undertaken for the Globalization Knowledge Network examined trends in life expectancy at birth (LEB), contrasting a continuation of trends from 1960 to 1980 (the pre-contemporary liberalization-globalization era) through to 2005 with actual LEB outcomes from 1980 to 2005. Compared to this counterfactual trend line, there has actually been a slowdown in health gains, equal to a loss in potential global LEB of 1.23 years with much greater losses in potential gains in the former Soviet Union and sub-Saharan Africa. These losses are attributed to liberalization-globalization policies (the independent variables in the regression equations) associated with the post-1980s period, with the authors concluding that the "negative association found between [these] policies, poor economic performance and unsatisfactory health trends [are] quite robust" (Cornia, Rosignoli, & Tiberti, 2008).

Poverty Reduction: Globalization's Great Deceit?

Although the evidence so far gives us pause to query the extent of globalization's health benefits, the greatest indictment against it lies in the global chorus applauding the accomplishment of MDG 1's extreme poverty target, poverty being the single greatest risk condition for poor health. According to the World Bank and its $1.25/day extreme poverty measure (since adjusted to $1.90/day), we have done very well since the 1980s, with more than a 50 percent drop in extreme poverty between 1990 and 2015 (World Bank, 2016). But progress has been very uneven, with China accounting for most of this decline and with the numbers in sub-Saharan Africa as high now as they were in the 1980s (Hickel, 2016). This poverty decline also occurred during a period when global economic product (one measure of global wealth) increased by more than 400 percent. More importantly, poverty at the not so extremely poor level has exploded, with relative poverty (~$2.90/day global average) increasing rapidly (Ravaillion, 2012), characterized by informal, low-pay, no-benefit, insecure, and precarious employment—conditions that describe most of the new jobs created since the mid-1990s (International Labour Organization [ILO], 2015).

We now have a more ambitious poverty goal with the post-2015 Sustainable Development Goals (SDGs): eliminate extreme poverty ($1.90/day) by 2030. There is already concern that, given current rates of poverty reduction, we will not make this new goal. Even if we did, most analysts now agree that it is a singularly *unambitious* poverty goal. Studies that estimate the level of daily consumption required for people to live, on average, to around 70 years (which is still more than a decade less than wealthier folks can expect to live) put it at $5/day (Hickel, 2016; Edward, 2006). The United Nations Conference on Trade and Development (UNCTAD) suggests that the $5/day level should be accepted as a minimum acceptable poverty line, and estimates that at this level, 90 percent of South Asia and sub-Saharan Africa would still be poor in 2030. A more recent re-evaluation of this $5/day level places it at $7.40/day (Hickel, 2016). Based on historic growth rates under the prevailing business-as-usual global economic model, eliminating poverty

- At $1.90/day would take 100 years
- At $5.00/day would take 200 years
- At $7.40/day would take more than 300 years (Woodward, 2015)

Stated simply: the growth model of poverty reduction (and better health) is not working; rather, as UNCTAD concluded, reducing inequalities matters. Reducing income/wealth inequalities is increasingly accepted by governments, multilateral agencies, and think tanks around the world as one of the world's most important imperatives, if not for the sake of health equity, then as essential to reducing the threat of social conflict and the pace of refugee movements regrettably fomenting a xenophobic backlash rather than a cosmopolitan embrace. It is also underscored by the sheer extent of global wealth inequalities that have grown to such an extent that a mere 62 people now own as much wealth as the rest of the world combined (OXFAM, 2016), with their wealth (and the political power and influence it brings) rising by 44 percent since just 2010, while the bottom 3.5 billion of our planetary neighbours saw theirs drop by 41 percent (OXFAM, 2016).

REDUCING WEALTH INEQUALITIES TO IMPROVE HEALTH EQUITY

Most of the world is still under the thrall of capitalism; and in our 300-year experience with this highly resilient political economic model only two means of reducing the inequalities it invariably generates have so far been found:

1. Reduce market income inequalities through more equitable distribution between capital and labour.
2. Reduce post-market income inequalities through taxes, income transfers, universally

accessible public services (e.g., education and health care), and/or subsidized essential goods and services (e.g., food and housing).

The first requires regulating markets for a fairer allocation of benefits between those who work and those who invest; while the second captures the post-market adjustments that have become the hallmarks of the so-called welfare (well/fair) state. Both means are needed and are interrelated. They are also both best captured in the aphorisms of two Americans (apologies: two white, middle-aged males) of a few generations back: Henry Ford's comment that "I have to pay my workers enough to buy the cars they make for me" (US Senate, 2005), and the statement by the American jurist Oliver Wendell Holmes engraved in granite over the entrance to the US Internal Revenue Service, "Taxes are the price we pay for a civilized world" (Internal Revenue Service, 2016). Our modern era of neo-liberal globalization has failed resoundingly in both.

Box 23.1: The Three Phases of Disequalizing Neo-liberalism

Neo-liberalism was first propounded in the 1940s by the economist Friedrich von Hayek. Concerned with the rise of communism in the immediate post-war era, Hayek argued that the economy is too complex for governments to manage, and that it was best to let markets regulate themselves through free trade, strong property rights, and minimal government interference, governed by the "rational" choice of a world of sovereign individual producers and consumers (Hayek, 1945). The competing model at the time, Keynesianism, prevailed in high-income countries for the next "thirty golden years" of economic growth (Hall, 1989), including progressive taxation, new social protection programs, strong labour rights and unionization rates, and sharp declines in income inequalities (Atkinson & Leigh, 2010). By the 1970s high inflation rates and low economic growth created a political space for neo-liberal economics to enter. It became more firmly entrenched with the election in the 1980s of conservative governments in the US, the UK, and Germany, then the three most powerful economies in the world.

Neo-liberalism began globalizing in the 1980s when the developing world debt crisis (the result of reckless bank lending and oil price shocks) threatened to collapse the nascent global banking industry. To prevent this, the International Monetary Fund (IMF) and World Bank began making emergency loans and grants to heavily indebted developing countries to ensure they could continue meeting their obligations to international creditors, but with conditionalities attached.

These conditionalities marked the beginning of neo-liberalism 1.0: structural adjustment programs, which required countries to privatize state assets, deregulate markets, lower taxes, charge user fees for public services, and engage in rapid trade and financial liberalization (Labonté, Schrecker, Sanders, & Meeus, 2004). According to neo-liberal economic theory, these measures would return countries to healthy economic growth. But they did not; although

continued

they did succeed in increasing income inequalities and slowing or reversing previous health gains (Structural Adjustment Participatory Review International Network, 2004; Breman & Shelton, 2001; United Nations [UN], 2006; Cornia, Jolly, & Stewart, 1987).

Even as neo-liberalism 1.0 was "rolling back" the state (reducing government spending in health and social protection programs), neo-liberalism 2.0 was "rolling it out" in the form of liberalized financial markets. Aided by deregulated banking rules, new digital technologies, and the removal of capital controls restricting the flow of money in and out of countries, investors (often banks themselves) found that it was easier and faster to make huge sums of money from money, rather than lending to the "real economy" of production and consumption that actually employs people. The scale of this leveraged, speculative investing is unprecedented in human history. In 1980 the value of all financial assets was roughly equal to the world's Gross Economic Product (the planet's entire "real economy"). By 2012 the value of outstanding derivatives alone (investment contracts in which value is "derived" from underlying financial assets) exceeded $710 trillion, or almost ten times the total value of the world's Gross Economic Product (figure 23.1). This unregulated "shadow banking" system was one of the key drivers behind the global financial crisis in 2008.[1] The 2008 near-global collapse put a temporary brake on such speculation, but within a few years this "casino capitalism," as the international political economist Susan Strange (1997) presciently named it several years ago, continues apace.

The 2008 global financial crisis led to a global recession (from which the world has yet to fully recover), with predictable negative health impacts associated with increased unemployment and "relative poverty." In an effort to stave off global financial collapse, the world's richest nations organized unprecedented public bailouts of failing banks, estimated as high as $15 trillion (Haldane, 2010; Ortiz & Cummins, 2012), in the hopes that banks would lend this to producers and consumers so the traditional economic growth game could re-ignite. Many governments also engaged in counter-cyclical public spending in a brief moment of neo-Keynesianism, hoping to stimulate their domestic economies through public spending on employment-generating infrastructure projects. But this moment of government re-engagement with economic stimulus lasted barely two years before neo-liberalism 3.0 (austerity) entered stage right. Once again promoted as a way for indebted governments to pay international creditors and to re-start their economies, austerity measures are almost identical to the discredited structural adjustment programs of the 1980s. But unlike earlier structural adjustment, these measures have gone global, affecting most of the world's countries and 90 percent of the human population (Ortiz & Cummins, 2013).

WHAT TO DO: HEALTHY PUBLIC POLICY FOR GLOBAL HEALTH EQUITY AND A LIVEABLE ENVIRONMENT

There are policy options that can reverse our present neo-liberal downward spiral, which returns us to the aphoristic wisdom of Henry Ford and Oliver Wendell Holmes: strengthening labour markets, and increasing national and global progressive taxation.

Strengthening Labour Power

One of the striking features of our post-1980s neo-liberal globalization has been the decline in the share of economic product going to labour, with a concomitant surge in share being captured by capital (in classical Marxist terms, those who own the means of production, and in our post-industrial economy, those who control global finance). There was a drop of almost 11 percent in labour's income share of global output between 1980 and 2010 (United Nations Conference on Trade and Development [UNCTAD], 2013), one of the reasons for the startling rise of the "1 percent." This decline in labour income was associated with steep declines in union membership (Labonté & Stuckler, 2016) and parallel increases in low-paying, hazardous, and insecure informal employment in developing countries, and (generally health-damaging) precarious employment in high-income countries (Standing, 2011; Helmore, 2013; Connolly & Osborne, 2013; Caldbick, Labonté, Mohindra, & Ruckert, 2014; Jaumotte & Buitron, 2015). As unionization rates fall, income inequality rises and with it the negative health and social externalities, argued, somewhat contentiously, the 2010 book *The Spirit Level* (Wilkinson & Pickett, 2010). In Canada, between 1980 and 2010 the Gini index of income inequality rose from 0.34 to almost 0.40 (the higher the number the greater the inequality), with studies finding that anything above 0.3 is associated with an almost 10 percent increase in preventable premature mortality (Kondo et al., 2009). When aggregate labour income shrinks, especially when it also grows more unequal between a small cadre of "knowledge" or "hi-tech" workers and the rest, consumption spending by the majority becomes increasingly debt-financed, often by borrowing against rising real estate prices—the "tipping point" that sparked the 2008 global financial crisis.

These findings tell us that stronger organized labour is a prerequisite to greater income equality and the positive health externalities that would create, as well as likely creating greater financial market stability. Even central banks in high-income countries are now arguing for centralized collective bargaining to raise wages, albeit less from a concern for fairness than as a means to spark some inflation and consumer demand to get the sclerotic economy growing again. Rather than the precarious "labour market flexibilization" countries have pursued over the past several decades in the name of global competition, we need stronger labour organizations with the power to negotiate a fairer share of economic output (Reich, 2015). But even as we might support such an effort, we also face a global structural problem: We now live in a world of too many workers chasing too few jobs and producing too many goods for too few consumers (to say nothing of technology replacing human labour, and productivity creating more value from less work). Thus, the US government in 2016 is lobbying China to reduce its "excess capacity" (making too much stuff more cheaply than what the US can manufacture, thanks to outsourcing by American companies that began in 1990s), while China needs to continue to create more employment for its billion-plus citizens to avoid their own disenfranchisement and discontent. This global labour conundrum underscores the importance of the second, redistributive means:

Reducing post-market income inequalities through taxes, transfers, universally accessible public services (e.g., education and health care), and/or subsidized essential goods and services (e.g., food and housing).

Increasing Taxation

Post-market redistribution relies upon the willingness and ability of governments to appropriate through taxation some of the wealth generated by markets for investment in national and global public goods, including those goods that are essential to health. Unfortunately, we are failing badly here as well. Our current austerity era simply reflects and deepens a longer-term trend in tax competition and reforms in Anglo-American and some Eurozone countries associated with neo-liberal economic policies: a shift from corporate to individual taxation, and from taxation of high income earners to median, low-income earners. Across the OECD, the average top income tax rate fell from 66 percent in 1981, the dawn of neo-liberalism, to a low of 41 percent in 2008 (OECD, 2008). Just since 2005, there's been a steep drop globally in taxes as a percentage of corporate profit, from around 55 percent to just 40 percent (World Bank, 2016), although a more nuanced study by a major corporate accounting firm found the average tax actually paid was closer to 23 percent (PWC, 2012). A study in the US, where the official corporate tax rate sits at around 35 percent (and is the subject of continual complaint from the business sector as being too high), found that the use of that country's colander of tax "loopholes" meant that the effective rate paid in 2008 was only 12.6 percent (Johnston, 2012), rising slightly to a paltry 13 percent in 2012 (Orszag, 2013).

Canada has stumbled down the same path, with declines in our top income and corporate tax rates since the 1990s, and especially at the federal level. We have seen our combined federal and provincial government spending (only some of which is for health and social protection programs) fall from 50 percent of GDP in 1991 to 42 percent in 2011 (OECD, 2015; Canadian Centre for Policy Alternatives, 2014). Federal tax cuts since 2006 under the Conservative government led to a loss of $220 billion in foregone revenue. Once commending ourselves for being the Scandinavia of the Americas, Canada now ranks near the bottom of the OECD pack in our tax/GDP ratio (24th of 34 countries)—with consequent cutbacks across many of our health-promoting social programs, perhaps one reason why we've seen no change at all in the mortality gap between top and bottom income quintiles over the past 15 years (Tjepkema, Wilkins, & Long, 2013).

To put this abandonment of progressive taxation into global context: using monetized (constant dollars) value of the Global Economic Product and the amount captured by the effective global tax rate, the amount of private capital falling outside the bounds of taxation jumped from USD 28 trillion in 2004 to USD 58 trillion in 2012, more than doubling in just eight years. This is not to suggest that all wealth should be taxed, but the sheer scale of what has slipped through public hands into the private stashes of the uber-rich is stunning—and avoidable.

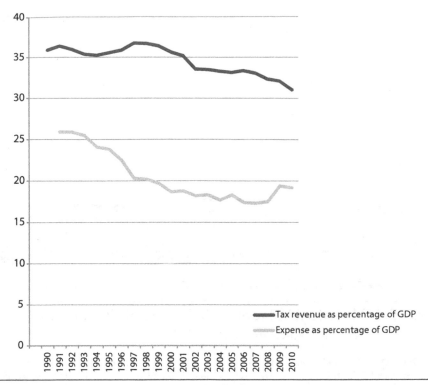

Figure 23.1: Canada's Declining Tax Revenues and Social Spending, 1991–2009

Sources: Data from (1) Organisation for Economic Co-operation and Development. (2014). *Revenue Statistics.* Retrieved from www.oecd.org/ctp/tax-policy/table2totaltaxrevenueasofgdp1965-2012en.htm; (2) The World Bank. (n.d.). *Expense (% of GDP).* Retrieved from http://data.worldbank.org/indicator/GC.XPN.TOTL.GD.ZS (expenses include social protection spending).

What does this free-fall in taxation mean for health? Oxfam crunched the numbers for low-income countries, finding that a tax of just 1.5 percent on billionaires could save 23 million lives (OXFAM, 2014). While it is simplistic to directly equate an increase in tax revenue with funding for health services that save lives, it is even more naïve to assume that health-promoting public policies that create supportive environments can arise out of the blue without an increase in public resources to finance them. And there is enormous health and economic benefit in public spending, through a little-known measure called the "fiscal multiplier," which applies to all countries regardless of their per capita income or development level. The fiscal multiplier is a measure of how government spending affects economic growth through its impact on employment, provision of public programs, and the purchase of goods and services. For every new dollar in government spending, the economy would grow by, on average, $1.60 (Labonté & Stuckler, 2016). Not all forms of government spending are so economically generous. Defence spending robs the economy, while spending in health, education, infrastructure, and environmental protection all contribute substantially to economic growth (Labonté & Stuckler, 2016).

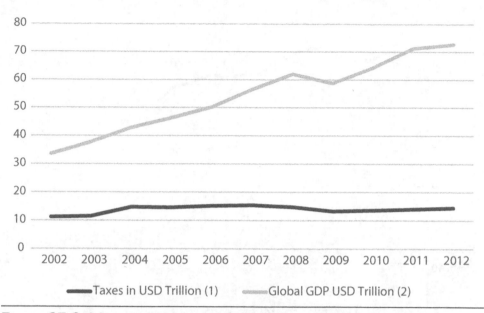

Figure 23.2: Monetized Value of Global Economic Product and Taxation Revenue, 2002–2012

Sources: Data from (1) The World Bank. (n.d.). *Tax revenue (% of GDP).* Retrieved from http://data.worldbank.org/indicator/GC.TAX.TOTL.GD.ZS/countries/1W?display=graph; (2) The World Bank. (n.d.). *GDP (current US$).* Retrieved from data.worldbank.org/indicator/NY.GDP.MKTP.CD/countries/1W?display=graph.

When Canada's federal government argued the economic wisdom of its deep austerity cuts in 2010, its own finance department forecast that every new dollar in public spending for infrastructure, housing, or measures for low-income households and the unemployed would boost the economy by between $1.30 and $1.50. Individual and corporate tax cuts, the option the Conservatives took, would actually shrink the economy, with business tax cuts the worst of all, shrinking the economy by up to 90 cents for every dollar of tax cut (Labonté & Stuckler, 2016).

Despite the (usually conservative) rhetoric that increased taxation will harm the economy, a US study found that raising the top income tax rate from its present level of 35 percent to 68 percent (where it once was before neo-liberalism took sway) would have no impact on factors driving economic growth, but would reduce poverty and inequality, and stimulate growth through public spending (the fiscal multiplier) (Fieldhouse, 2013). The IMF, a little more cautiously, suggested a top rate of 60 percent as posing no economic harm. Yet another study suggested that a 90 percent tax rate on incomes above $300,000 might lead to some small loss in GDP growth, but would also lead to greater overall well-being and happiness (Kindermann & Krueger, 2014).

Increasing taxation and its progressivity will not be easy given the hypermobility of capital, unless a number of countries reach an agreement to do so in tandem. It will also require real, and not merely token, efforts to close down offshore financial centres, better known as "tax havens." Estimates of the amount of tax revenue lost each year (through "legal" avoidance or illegal evasion) range between USD 200 billion for developing countries, and USD 300 billion for governments worldwide (Crivelli, De Mooij, & Keen, 2015). So far, efforts to close such havens have been ineffectual, although investigative journalists and leaks are beginning to shed more light on the rich and famous who make use of them. The OECD and the G20 (group of 20 richest countries) have committed to develop a single identity tax system to ensure taxes are paid where economic activity takes place, but as of 2017 without any real action. Since most of the tax haven countries are in the G20 or OECD groups of nations (or are under their protectorate), this raises the rhetorical question, Why haven't they done so already?

There is an equally urgent need for better and more accountable tax authorities in many low- and middle-income countries, and to increase taxes on the forms of capital that are less mobile (such as natural resources) and inequitably owned. Capital flight and tax evasion hurt all countries, but are particularly devastating on the fiscal revenues of poorer nations. Developing countries lose $2.40 for every $1 they gain in aid, remittances, and investment, inadvertently contributing to the growth of the global 1 percent (Ooms, Stuckler, Basu, & McKee, 2010).

Efforts to improve the domestic self-financing of development goals are important for low-income countries, to avoid the trap of "aid dependency" and, more importantly, to allow for greater citizen engagement in setting their own health and social development priorities. But even as some low-income country governments are attempting to increase their domestic revenue generation, tax holidays to attract foreign investment, illicit capital flight, high unemployment rates, and low GDP means that many countries will be unable to self-finance sufficient health and social protection measures, and certainly not achievement of the new Sustainable Development Goals (SDGs). The lowest estimate of the amount of new development financing needed to reach these goals is over $3 trillion annually, which governments (high- or low-income) still under the yoke of austerity are reluctant to finance. Yet a simple mechanism does exist: financial transaction taxes (FTT).

The 2008 financial crisis re-invigorated interest in FTTs, once known as Tobin taxes, after the economist who first proposed them. Originally intended to act as a damper on the form of speculative investing that eventually led to the 2008 crisis, FTTs are now more widely seen as a fair and reasonable way to finance international development and global public goods (such as climate change mitigation). More than 60 countries have signalled in recent years their support for such a tax; nine countries of the EU have agreed to enact a FTT by the end of 2017. The potential revenue of such a tax, if applied globally and on all currency exchanges (including the "shadow banking" world of derivatives), and at the paltry rate of 0.05 percent (5 cents on every 100 dollars), could raise over $8.6 trillion annually (McCulloch & Pacillo, 2011)—more than enough to fund all 17 SDGs with considerable change left over. There are even internationally agreed mechanisms to aid in a progressive redistribution of such revenues, such as the global health funds (or the proposed and less disease-specific Global Fund for Health), the Green Climate Fund, and a proposed Global Social Protection Fund.

There is no lack of fiscal resources to make the world fairer and healthier; simply an absence of political decisions to begin tackling the wealth and power of a small global elite, whose individual and corporate practices are putting all of us in peril. Harnessing this potential is all the more critical since we cannot continue endlessly growing the "real economy" of production and consumption (Sustainable Development Commission [SDC], 2009), at least not without destroying the environmental basis of life (see chapter 22 in this book).

FROM MDGS TO SUSTAINABLE DEVELOPMENT GOALS—THE LOCAL IS THE GLOBAL, AND VICE VERSA

In 2015, 193 of the world's countries agreed to a sweeping set of new global development goals, the Sustainable Development Goals (SDGs) mentioned earlier in this chapter. The SDGs have been criticized as too ambitious (the 17 goals have 169 targets); and they have many flaws, most notably in their paltry poverty reduction goal and their blithe acceptance of the unsustainable and dis-equalizing business-as-usual global growth machine as the means to solve the very inequalities and environmental degradations the growth machine has generated over the past 40 years (and which the SDGs are supposed to correct). Notwithstanding these flaws, which can and should be critiqued and challenged, the SDGs nonetheless represent one of the most comprehensive visions of the kind of world we could live in, a vision to which hundreds of thousands of people contributed through a very open and public process of consultations.

Unlike the MDGs, the SDGs apply to all countries (including Canada) and are nominally indivisible, meaning that countries cannot cherry-pick their favourite goal to the exclusion of the others. Although some in the global public health community were upset that "health" (by name) is now only one of 17 goals, from a determinants of health vantage almost all of the SDGs can be considered health goals. Considered as a set, the SDGs afford the strongest case yet for a "health in all policies" approach (see chapter 18 in this book), one in which health promoters may be uniquely placed to contribute, given their post–*Ottawa Charter* efforts to strengthen intersectoral efforts around the social determinants of health.

Box 23.2: SDGs and Health: The Short List

Goal 1: End poverty in all its forms: Its importance to UN member states is signalled by its position as the first goal, and poverty is certainly the greatest single "risk condition" for poor health. But the goal requires a meaningful metric and not the World Bank's "extreme" measure.

Goal 2: End hunger, achieve food security and improved nutrition, and promote sustainable agriculture: Undernourished people cannot be healthy or economically and politically well-functioning citizens. Apart from malnutrition targets, the goal calls for "sustainable food production systems ... that increase productivity and production [and] that help maintain ecosystems," emphasizing assistance for small-scale producers.

Goal 3: Ensure healthy lives and promote wellbeing for all at all ages: "Achiev[ing] universal health coverage," including "affordable essential medicines and vaccines for all," is important, if weakened by disagreements over how it can be financed (public or private or both?). "Universal access to sexual and reproductive health-care services" is equally important for its positive health impacts on women's and children's health, and its ability to keep population growth within ecological limits. But most of the targets concern reductions in mortality and morbidity rates, with little discussion of how this might be achieved.

Goal 4: Ensure inclusive and equitable quality education and promote lifelong learning opportunities for all: The link between education and good health is well-established, particularly for women and girls in low- and middle-income countries (LMICs) (Population Reference Bureau, 2011). An important related target emphasizes development of knowledge and skills related to "sustainable lifestyles, human rights, gender equity ... and global citizenship," which could help to build a stronger activist base essential to moving governments forward on the SDGs.

Goal 6: Ensure availability and sustainable management of water and sanitation for all: No water, no health; poor sanitation, much disease. This goal is the mainstay of historic public health, but its prioritization needs to be tempered with some critique. The first target references "affordable drinking water," code for engaging private markets in water supply or user fees for public provision. Recent history in both approaches has not been sanguine for equitable access (Kishimoto, Lobina, & Petitjean, 2015). With diminishing supply and increasing population (and agricultural/industrial) demand, water access is becoming a source of conflict and a driver of refugee populations.

Goal 10: Reduce inequality within and among countries: Given the impossibility of meaningful poverty reduction through economic growth alone, the reducing inequality goal assumes paramount importance. It targets sustained income growth for the bottom 40 percent at a rate greater than the national average, but says nothing about the distortion of accumulating wealth at the top, without which inequalities could continue to rise. A disappointment was removal of a proposed global financial transaction tax, long opposed by the US, the UK, and other countries with vested interests in footloose global capital (Labonté, Baum, & Sanders, 2015).

Goal 12: Ensure sustainable consumption and production patterns: The implication of this goal is more profound than its targets, which recycle most of the tropes of "sustainable development" that first made the global rounds with the 1987 publication of the Bruntland Report, *Our Common Future* (World Commission on Environment and Development, 1987), adding ecology to the 1986 *Ottawa Charter*'s sociology (Labonté, 1991). Weak on reducing fossil-fuel subsidies (another sovereign escape clause, "in accordance with national circumstances"), the goal itself needs a syntax inversion: not "sustainable consumption" (in which *sustainable* is a second-place adjective to the primary nouns of *consumption* and *production*), but "consume sustainably" (which can only be achieved by reducing current global levels of our material gorging). This recasting of the goal implies a reduction in demand, especially in HICs, at a time when conventional economics is calling for an increase in demand to get the growth economy back on track, underpinning again the foundational importance of an appropriately calibrated inequality goal.

CONCLUSION: TOWARDS AN OPTIMISM OF THE WILL

The Italian Marxist Antonio Gramsci is credited with the phrase "pessimist of the intellect, optimist of the will." The actual quotation is worded slightly differently, but the intent is the same. Our evidence and our knowledge of our present state almost demand an analytical pessimism; yet we are challenged to remain almost hopelessly optimistic. I have believed for many years that optimism isn't simply a personality characteristic; following from Gramsci's insight, I consider it to be a studied act of political resistance. I also believe that most, if not all, people working in public health and health promotion are as hopelessly optimistic as I am; it is an essential prerequisite to the work that we do.

On a somewhat optimistic note, then, neo-liberalism, the economic model that has predominated and characterized the past 40 years of globalization, may be on the way out, with voices from within its former bastions of promulgation (such as the IMF) now explicitly critiquing its excesses and failures (Ostry, Loungani, & Furceri, 2016). But neo-liberalism is simply the latest iteration of our 300-plus-year-old (and wholly globalized) capitalist economic system. And so we are left with an older political dilemma, drawn more sharply since the 2008 financial crisis but deepening with each passing year: How can we tame capitalism and its predatory market logic to support human equity and (now) a liveable planet? Or, if it cannot be tamed (its resilience—and this is a good instance in which to invoke that term—is remarkable), how might capitalism be transformed into something better fit for human social and ecological survival into a twenty-second century?

As I concluded in an article marking the *Ottawa Charter*'s 25th anniversary, and which remains pertinent today,

> The deeply structural forms of health-promoting change we so urgently need are only likely to arise in the wake of even more profound crises. Our task, as we continue our quotidian and localized best health promoting efforts, all the time supporting those attempting to leverage change at national and global levels, is to nurture the blueprint for what a social order could look like, if human, animal and ecological health formed its core rather than being relegated to its periphery. (Labonté, 2011)

This task is now slightly easier, with the SDGs providing such a blueprint upon which we can—and must—build.

CRITICAL THINKING QUESTIONS

1. What are some of the ways in which contemporary globalization might affect your own health?
2. Is a return to nationalism (a retreat from globalization) something that will be healthier for people? Why or why not?
3. Should we develop global rules for multi-national enterprises—and the smaller companies from which they source their materials—to ensure healthier and fairer

working conditions? Or are voluntary codes enough? If we had global rules instead, what should they be?

4. Can the new Sustainable Development Goals help us to promote the idea of global health equity? Why or why not?

5. What steps could Canadian health promoters take to reduce global inequalities in health and its political and economic determinants?

RESOURCES

Further Readings

Labonté, R. (2016). Health promotion in an age of normative equity and rampant inequality. *International Journal of Health Policy and Management, 5*(12), 675–682. www.ijhpm.com/article_3243_9cfe55f382f6c9876bd955b41b2c9007.pdf
This open access article reviews the challenge of global health inequalities, and describes in more detail the Sustainable Development Goals, and the priority goals that should be the focus of health promotion advocacy at national and global scales.

Labonté, R., & Laverack, G. (2008). *Health promotion in action: From local to global empowerment.* London: Palgrave Macmillan.
This short book attempts to move from the local terrain of health promotion work to the global scales of necessary engagement. It is a useful text for health promoters engaging in "acting and thinking (both) locally and globally" for the first time.

Labonté, R., Schram, A., & Ruckert, A. (2016). The Trans-Pacific Partnership: Is it everything we feared for health? *International Journal of Health Policy and Management, 5*(8), 487–496.
www.ijhpm.com/article_3186_0.html
Using the recent (and as of 2016 still to be ratified) Trans-Pacific Partnership agreement as the example, this article provides a health impact assessment of new regional trade and investment agreements, outlining the risks they pose for public health.

Labonté, R., Schrecker, T., Packer, C., & Runnels, V. (Eds.). (2009). *Globalization and health: Pathways, evidence, and policy.* London: Routledge.
This book is a consolidation of 12 extensive background papers and a final report on various aspects of globalization as a health determinant, prepared by the Globalization Knowledge Network of the World Health Organization's Commission on Social Determinants of Health. The book's chapters are now free online at www.globalhealthequity.ca, where a link also takes one to all of the background research papers. The site also has links to numerous other articles and reports on global health.

Labonté, R., & Stuckler, D. (2016). The rise of neoliberalism: How bad economics imperils health and what to do about it. *Journal of Epidemiology and Community Health*, *70*(3), 312–318.

jech.bmj.com/content/70/3/312.full

This article describes in greater detail the evolution of neo-liberalism's three phases, and the policy options that could confront its ongoing political dominance.

Lee, K. (2003). *Globalization and health: An introduction*. London: Palgrave Macmillan.

As the title suggests, this short text provides an introductory overview of globalization and health. It is particularly useful for its focus on global health policy.

People's Health Movement, Medact, Global Equity Gauge Alliance, UNISA Press, & Zed Books. (2014). *Global Health Watch 4: An alternative world health report*. London: Zed Books. Also available: *Global Health Watch 3* (2012), *Global Health Watch 2* (2008), and *Global Health Watch 1* (2005–2006).

The product of hundreds of health activists and organizations around the world, these four volumes examine health in a globalizing world, with foci on health systems and vulnerable populations, development assistance and migration, and global health governance. An entire multi-chapter section is devoted to holding countries and multi-national institutions accountable for improving global health. Available free online at www.ghwatch.org.

Schrecker, T., & Bambra, C. (2015). *How politics makes us sick: Neoliberal epidemic*. London: Palgrave MacMillan.

This book argues that the obesity, insecurity, austerity, and inequality that result from neo-liberal (or "market fundamentalist") policies are hazardous to our health, asserting that these neo-liberal epidemics require a political cure.

Relevant Websites

Canadian Coalition for Global Health Research

www.ccghr.ca

Research is only one of many pathways to improving global health, but it is an important one. The Canadian Coalition was formed on the fateful day of 9/11 (quite by chance) and is committed to harnessing global health research evidence to policy action.

Canadian Society for International Health

www.csih.org

The CSIH is a non-governmental organization that undertakes international health promotion activities and other health development projects around the world. It also hosts an annual international health conference in the fall, one of the best ways for health promoters interested in global health to learn and network.

Global Health Watch

www.ghwatch.org

This site provides up-to-date information on global health campaigns, solicits inputs for future Global Health Watches, and offers useful advice and materials for global health promoting campaigners.

Globalization and Health

www.globalizationandhealth.com

This open access journal publishes important peer-reviewed research and commentary.

People's Health Movement

www.phmovement.org

The PHM is an activist group dedicated to the cause of "health for all" through a combination of national actions and international mobilizations. Its *People's Charter for Health* is the most widely publicized, translated, and endorsed statement on international health since the *Alma-Ata Declaration on Primary Health Care*.

NOTE

1. The immediate cause of the 2008 global financial crisis was the collapse of real estate bubbles, primarily in the US and southern Europe. As low- and middle-income families in both regions saw their incomes erode as manufacturing jobs were outsourced to lower-wage countries, banks increasingly pushed home ownership as a means of obtaining cash through low-interest mortgage loans. Such loans helped to spark a real estate bubble, prompting banks to promote ever more risky loans. To protect themselves against defaults, the banks bundled these high-risk loans into so-called residential mortgage–backed securities, which were then sold to individuals, pension funds, and other banks worldwide as safe and secure investments—even though the banks knew full well that they were not. When the real estate bubble burst, trillions in financial assets were wiped out, many smaller banks started to fail, and individual savings disappeared. Most of the banks involved in this scandal have been fined billions of dollars for their collusion, although none of the individuals responsible has faced criminal charges or jail, and these penalties have had little impact on the persisting "bonus culture" of extremely high pay to investment bankers and asset fund managers (Marriage & Mooney, 2016).

REFERENCES

Atkinson, A. B., & Leigh, A. (2010). *The distribution of top incomes in five Anglo-Saxon countries over the twentieth century* (Discussion paper DP No 4937). Bonn: Institute for the Study of Labor. Retrieved from ftp.iza.org/dp4937.pdf

Breman, A., & Shelton, C. (2001). *Structural adjustment and health: A literature review of the debate, its role-players and presented empirical evidence* (Working paper No WG6:6). Geneva:

Commission on Macroeconomics and Health, WHO. Retrieved from library.cphs.chula.ac.th/Ebooks/HealthCareFinancing/WorkingPaper_WG6/WG6_6.pdf

Caldbick, S., Labonté, R., Mohindra, K. S., & Ruckert, A. (2014). Globalization and the rise of precarious employment: The new frontier for workplace health promotion. *Global Health Promotion, 21*(2), 23–31. doi: 10.1177/1757975913514781

Canadian Centre for Policy Alternatives. (2014, February 5). *Alternative federal budget 2014: Striking a better balance.* Retrieved from www.policyalternatives.ca/sites/default/files/uploads/publications/National%20Office/2014/02/AFB2014_MainDocument.pdf

Connolly, K., & Osborne, L. (2013, August 30). Low-paid Germans mind rich-poor gap as elections approach. *The Guardian.* Retrieved from www.theguardian.com/world/2013/aug/30/low-paid-germans-mini-jobs

Cornia, G. A., Jolly, R., & Stewart, F. (1987). *Adjustment with a human face.* London: Clarendon Press.

Cornia, G. A., Rosignoli, S., & Tiberti, L. (2008). *Globalization and health: Pathways of transmission and evidence of its impact* (Report). Globalization Knowledge Network, World Health Organization Commission on Social Determinants of Health. Retrieved from www.who.int/social_determinants/resources/gkn_cornia_al.pdf

Crivelli, E., De Mooij, R., & Keen, M. (2015, May). *Base erosion, profit sharing and developing countries* (Working paper). International Monetary Fund (IMF). Retrieved from www.imf.org/external/pubs/ft/wp/2015/wp15118.pdf

Development Initiatives. (2014, March 25). *Global aid trends–ODA: What you need to know.* Retrieved from devinit.org/#!/post/global-aid-trends-need-know

Dollar, D. (2001). *Globalization, inequality, and poverty since 1980.* Washington, DC: World Bank.

Edward, P. (2006). The ethical poverty line: A moral quantification of absolute poverty. *Third World Quarterly, 27*(2), 377–393. doi: 10.1080/01436590500432739

Fieldhouse, A. (2013, April 2). A review of the economic research on the effects of raising ordinary income tax rates. *Economic Policy Institute.* Retrieved from www.epi.org/publication/raising-income-taxes/

Haldane, A. (2010, March 30). *Bank of England: The $100 billion question* (Proceedings). Hong Kong: Institute of Regulation and Risk North Asia (IRRNA). Retrieved from www.bis.org/review/r100406d.pdf

Hall, P. A. (1989). *The political power of economic ideas: Keynesianism across nations.* Princeton, NJ: Princeton University Press.

Hayek, F. A. (1945). *The road to serfdom.* London: George Routledge & Sons.

Helmore, E. (2013, August 10). US fast-food workers in vanguard of growing protests at "starvation" wages. *The Guardian.* Retrieved from www.theguardian.com/world/2013/aug/10/us-fast-food-protests-wages

Hickel, J. (2016). The true extent of global poverty and hunger: Questioning the good news narrative of the Millennium Development Goals. *Third World Quarterly, 37*(5), 749–767. doi: 10.1080/01436597.2015.1109439

Internal Revenue Service. (2016, September 23). *Tax quotes.* Retrieved from www.irs.gov/uac/tax-quotes

International Labour Organization. (2015). *World employment social outlook.* Geneva: Author. Retrieved from www.ilo.org/wcmsp5/groups/public/@dgreports/@dcomm/@publ/documents/publication/wcms_337069.pdf

Jaumotte, F., & Buitron, C. O. (2015, March). Power from the people. *Finance & Development, IMF, 52*(1). Retrieved from www.imf.org/external/pubs/ft/fandd/2015/03/jaumotte.htm

Johnston, D. C. (2012). Nine things the rich don't want you to know about taxes. In D. Starkman, M. M. Hamilton, & R. Chittum (Eds.), *The best business writing 2012* (pp. 190–207). New York: Columbia University Press.

Kindermann, F., & Krueger, D. (2014, November 15). High marginal tax rates on the top 1%. *VOX CEPR's Policy Portal.* Retrieved from voxeu.org/article/high-marginal-tax-rates-top-1

Kishimoto, S., Lobina, E., & Petitjean, O. (Eds.). (2015). *Our public water future: The global experience with remunicipalisation.* Amsterdam, London, Paris, Cape Town, Brussels: Transnational Institute (TNI), Public Services International Research Unit (PSIRU), Multinationals Observatory, Municipal Services Project (MSP), European Federation of Public Service Unions (EPSU). Retrieved from www.municipalservicesproject.org/sites/municipalservicesproject.org/files/publications/Kishimoto-Lobina-Petitjean_Our-Public-Water-Future-Global-Experience-Remunicipalisation_April2015_FINAL.pdf

Kondo, N., Sembajwe, G., Kawachi, I., van Dam, R. M., Subramanian, S. V., & Yamagata, Z. (2009). Income inequality, mortality, and self-rated health: Meta-analysis of multilevel studies. *British Medical Journal, 339.* doi: dx.doi.org/10.1136/bmj.b4471

Labonté, R. (1991). Econology: Integrating health and environment. *Health Promotion International, 6*(1), 49–65.

Labonté, R. (2011). Toward a post-*Charter* health promotion. *Health Promotion International, 26*(S2), ii183–ii186. doi: 10.1093/heapro/dar062

Labonté, R., Baum, F., & Sanders, D. (2015). Poverty, justice and health. In R. Detels, C. C. Tan, Q. A. Karim, & M. Guilliford (Eds.), *Oxford textbook of public health.* Oxford: Oxford University Press.

Labonté, R., Blouin, C., Chopra, M., Lee, K., Packer, C., Rowson, M., … Woodward, D. (2008). *Towards health-equitable globalisation: Rights, regulation and redistribution.* Ottawa: Globalization Knowledge Network, University of Ottawa. Retrieved from www.who.int/social_determinants/resources/gkn_report_06_2007.pdf

Labonté, R., Schrecker, T., Sanders, D., & Meeus, W. (2004) *Fatal indifference: The G8, Africa and global health.* Cape Town: University of Cape Town Press.

Labonté, R., & Stuckler, D. (2016). The rise of neoliberalism: How bad economics imperils health and what to do about it. *Journal of Epidemiology and Community Health, 70*(3), 312–318. doi: 10.1136/jech-2015-206295

Lee, K. (2003). *Globalization and health: An introduction.* London: Palgrave Macmillan.

Marriage, M., & Mooney, A. (2016, September 4). Bonus culture in asset management "out of control." *Financial Times.* Retrieved from www.ft.com/content/72a733a2-7111-11e6-a0c9-1365ce54b926?mhq5j=e3

McCulloch, N., & Pacillo, G. (2011, May). The Tobin tax: A review of the evidence. *Institute of Development Studies, 68,* 1–77. doi: 10.1111/j.2040-0217.2011.00068_2.x

Ooms, G., Stuckler, D., Basu, S., & McKee, M. (2010). Financing the Millennium Development Goals and beyond: Sustaining the "Big Push." *Globalization and Health, 6*(17). doi: 10.1186/1744-8603-6-17

Organisation for Economic Co-operation and Development (OECD). (2008). *Growing unequal? Income distribution and poverty in OECD countries.* Retrieved from darp.lse.ac.uk/resources/books/GrowingUnequal_OECD.pdf

Organisation for Economic Co-operation and Development (OECD). (2015). *Official development assistance 2015.* Retrieved from www.oecd.org/dac/financing-sustainable-development/development-finance-data/

Orszag, P. (2013, January 22). As foreign profits rise, corporate tax rates fall. *Bloomberg View.* Retrieved from www.bloomberg.com/view/articles/2013-01-22/as-foreign-profits-rise-corporate-tax-rates-fall

Ortiz, I., & Cummins, M. (Eds.). (2012). *A recovery for all? Rethinking socio-economic policies for children and poor households.* New York: UNICEF.

Ortiz I., & Cummins, M. (2013, March). *The age of austerity: A review of public expenditures and adjustment measures in 181 countries* (Working paper). New York & Geneva: IPD and South Centre. Retrieved from policydialogue.org/files/publications/Age_of_Austerity_Ortiz_and_Cummins.pdf

Ostry, J. D., Loungani, P., & Furceri, D. (2016). Neoliberalism: Oversold? *IMF Finance & Development, 53*(1), 38–41. Retrieved from www.imf.org/external/pubs/ft/fandd/2016/06/pdf/ostry.pdf

OXFAM. (2014, October). *Even it up: Time to end extreme inequality* (Report). Retrieved from www.oxfam.org/sites/www.oxfam.org/files/file_attachments/cr-even-it-up-extreme-inequality-291014-en.pdf

OXFAM. (2016, January 18). *An economy for the 1%: How privilege and power in the economy drive extreme inequality and how this can be stopped* (Briefing paper). Retrieved from www.oxfam.org/sites/www.oxfam.org/files/file_attachments/bp210-economy-one-percent-tax-havens-180116-en_0.pdf

Population Reference Bureau. (2011, August). *The effect of girls' education on health outcomes* (Fact sheet). Retrieved from www.prb.org/Publications/Media-Guides/2011/girls-education-fact-sheet.aspx

PWC. (2012). *Corporate income tax: A global analysis* (Report). Retrieved from www.pwc.com/gx/en/paying-taxes/pdf/pwc-corporate-income-tax-report.pdf

Ravaillion, M. (2012, July). *More relatively: Poor people in a less absolutely-poor world* (Public Lecture). UTS, Sydney: Development Economics, World Bank. Retrieved from siteresources.worldbank.org/DEC/Resources/GlobalPovertyUpdate-MartinR-SydneyLecture-July2012.pdf

Reich, R. (2015, September 28). Why we must end upward pre-distribution to the rich. *Common Dreams.* Retrieved from www.commondreams.org/views/2015/09/28/why-we-must-end-upward-pre-distribution-rich

Standing, G. (2011). *The precariat: The new dangerous class.* London: Bloomsbury.

Strange, S. (1997). *Casino capitalism.* Manchester: Manchester University Press.

Structural Adjustment Participatory Review International Network. (2004). *Structural adjustment: The SAPRI report: The policy roots of economic crisis, poverty, and inequality.* London: Zed Books.

Sustainable Development Commission. (2009). *Prosperity without growth? The transition to a sustainable economy* (Report). Retrieved from www.sd-commission.org.uk/data/files/publications/prosperity_without_growth_report.pdf

Tjepkema, M., Wilkins, R., & Long, A. (2013). Cause-specific mortality by income adequacy in Canada: A 16-year follow-up study. *Health Reports, 24*(7), 14–22. Retrieved from www.statcan.gc.ca/pub/82-003-x/2013007/article/11852-eng.pdf

UNICEF. (2013, September 12). *Ninety million children's lives saved since 1990, says UNICEF* (Press release). Retrieved from www.unicefusa.org/press/releases/ninety-million-childrens-lives-saved-1990-says-unicef/8285

UNICEF. (2016, April). *Maternal mortality fell by almost half between 1990 and 2015* (Press release). Retrieved from data.unicef.org/topic/maternal-health/maternal-mortality/

United Nations. (2006). *World economic and social survey: Diverging growth and development* (Report). New York: United Nations Department of Economic and Social Affairs, Development Policy and Analysis Division. Retrieved from www.un.org/en/development/desa/policy/wess/wess_archive/2006wess.pdf

United Nations Conference on Trade and Development (UNCTAD). (2013, November). *Growth and poverty eradication: Why addressing inequality matters* (Policy Brief Series, No. 2). Retrieved from unctad.org/en/PublicationsLibrary/presspb2013d4_en.pdf

US Senate. (2005, November 1). *Congressional Record, 109th Congress, 1st session, 151*(142), 24375.

Wilkinson, R., & Pickett, K. (2010). *The spirit level: Why more equal societies almost always do better.* London: Penguin Books.

Woodward, D. (2015). *Incrementum ad absurdum*: Global growth, inequality and poverty education in a carbon-constrained world. *World Economic View, 4*, 43–62. Retrieved from wer.worldeconomicsassociation.org/files/WEA-WER-4-Woodward.pdf

Woodward, D., Drager, N., Beaglehole, R., & Lipson, D. (2001). Globalization and health: A framework for analysis and action. *Bulletin of the WHO, 79*, 875–881.

World Bank. (2016). *Total tax rate (% of commercial profits)* (Data file). Retrieved from data.worldbank.org/indicator/IC.TAX.TOTL.CP.ZS

World Commission on Environment and Development (WCED). (1987). *Our common future.* Oxford: Oxford University Press.

World Health Organization (WHO). (2005). Commitments to health for all. In *The Bangkok Charter for Health Promotion in a Globalized World*. Retrieved from www.who.int/healthpromotion/conferences/6gchp/bangkok_charter/en/index.html

World Health Organization (WHO). (2016). Life expectancy. In *Global Health Observatory (GHO) Data*. Retrieved from www.who.int/gho/mortality_burden_disease/life_tables/situation_trends_text/en/

World Health Organization Commission on Macroeconomics and Health. (2001). *Macroeconomics and health: Investing in health for economic development* (Report). Geneva: World Health Organization. Retrieved from apps.who.int/iris/bitstream/10665/42435/1/924154550X.pdf

CHAPTER 24

Reflections on the Future of Health Promotion in Canada

Ann Pederson, Irving Rootman, Katherine L. Frohlich, and Sophie Dupéré

LEARNING OBJECTIVES

1. Understand the connections between health promotion in Canada and globally
2. Describe the evolution of the contents of *Health Promotion in Canada*
3. Identify potential directions for the future of health promotion in Canada

We can only see a short distance ahead, but we can see plenty there that needs to be done.

—Alan Turing[1]

This quotation captures the challenge we face as editors and health promotion advocates: to summarize what this book is about and to use those ideas to offer some thoughts on a possible future for the field. But it is much easier to shine the light on the path we have already taken than it is to illuminate the way ahead. The first task may take fortitude and self-awareness, but the second demands farsightedness. As noted in chapter 1, the field of health promotion has continued to evolve with successive government policies and directions, technological change, and evidence on effective interventions. The contents of this book reflect many of the most recent changes and developments, but because the chapters are written from the perspective of particular contributors and we are constrained by space limits, this is necessarily a selective collection of ideas about what we believe are important features of the current health promotion landscape. We also try in this final chapter to reflect the totality of the book and to offer our thoughts on what the future of health promotion may look like. In keeping with Turing, we can only see part of the path ahead for health promotion in Canada but we are convinced that there are significant problems in need of attention, both here and globally, and that health promotion could have an important role to play in addressing them.

HEALTH CONCERNS IN CANADA WITHIN THE GLOBAL CONTEXT

Looking back over the contributions in this and earlier editions, we can see that the field of health promotion continues to develop intellectually and practically in Canada. Today, there are nearly 40 master's programs available alone that offer some sort of introduction to the field—a vast difference from 30 years ago when there were only two schools of public health in the entire country.[2] These programs offer the opportunity to develop a relatively large new generation of public health researchers, policy makers, and practitioners to tackle the complex health and social challenges we face in Canada and abroad. These challenges include the continuing fallout of the global financial crisis of 2008, for example, which led to un- and underemployment, mental illness, and social disruption; climate change and its transformation of the planet; our colonial history and its contemporary manifestations; continuing struggles for human rights and social equality; and the turbulence of armed conflict, civil wars, and displacement. More and better-trained health promoters will help in dealing with these growing disruptions to population health, as well as the trials yet to come.

An important current example is the migrant crisis of northern Africa, the Middle East, and Europe that has reached Canada. Over the past year, the federal government and private sponsors have brought to this country some 38,000 Syrian and numerous other refugees from the war-ravaged Middle East and elsewhere. While there was tremendous excitement among some as these newcomers arrived, we know that their paths to settlement vary and that they face countless challenges as they seek a home, a community, employment, and safety. As individuals and families come to the one-year point in their migration journey, many face new challenges such as managing on diminished financial resources as their support shifts from federal to provincial support. Some are struggling to find adequate, appropriate employment given credentialing, language difficulties, and a less-than-vibrant economy in many regions. And some will struggle to adjust to living in this vast country, with its linguistic variations, history of colonialism and racism, and various political divides. While it is likely that most of these individuals will find their way through this maze into a new and hopefully full and peaceful life, there will be some who find it alienating and frightening and who will require more support than is currently on offer to them, particularly in terms of support for healing from trauma, the atrocities of war, and displacement. These developments imply, among other things, that health promoters in Canada will need to face the critical issue of reconciliation with the country's colonial and racist past (and present), develop and promulgate skills in working across diversity without "othering," and form new partnerships (such as with the settlement sector) in recognition that health affects settlement (e.g., the healthy immigrant effect), but settlement also affects health (e.g., the nutritional and mental health of immigrants often deteriorates over time spent in Canada). (For more discussion of these issues, see chapter 11.)

A second example concerns the effects of climate change on population health. The Paris Agreement on climate change, adopted in December 2015, came into force on November 4, 2016, mere days before the United States federal election.[3] As of mid-January 2016, 125 out of the 197 Parties to the Convention, including Canada, China, and the United States, had ratified the agreement. However, the withdrawal from the treaty by the United States in May 2017 may severely undermine its effectiveness.[4] As Trevor Hancock reminds us in chapter 22, the threats of climate change to human health—indeed human existence—demand that health promoters engage with climate scientists, activists, and communities to uphold the obligations set out in Paris.

But climate change and the environment are complex health and socio-economic problems, with some solutions creating potential new problems. For instance, in a recent issue of the Canadian Communicable Disease Report (October 2016)[5] efforts to "green" and "blue" Canadian cities and the promotion of healthy transport and active living were described as potentially having the unintended effect of increasing exposure to vector-borne diseases, notably Lyme (tick-borne) and West Nile (mosquito-borne). Thus, though it is commonplace to speak of countries such as Canada as having undergone the epidemiological transition from communicable to chronic diseases as the major causes of mortality, new diseases can and will emerge. This will happen in part as a consequence of climate change, globalization and its economic impacts, deforestation, and changes in the water level, but also from genetics—all of these influenced by changes in social structures, fractures, and politics.

This was the case, for example, with the sudden and unexpected emergence of the Zika virus, which threatened the cancellation of the 2016 Summer Olympic Games in Rio de Janeiro. The identification of the Zika virus as the culprit behind a sudden rash of infants born with microcephaly in Brazil reminds us that any organism can mutate from benign to lethal under the right conditions and that the threats to health known today are not necessarily the threats of tomorrow. While much attention has been directed towards understanding the specific mosquito that has been spreading the infection, and the mechanisms through which infection with the virus leads to brain malformations, this epidemic has also raised questions about the other usual suspects in public health: poverty, powerlessness, and gender, to name a few. This is, in part, a poverty issue as the mosquitoes involved breed in stagnant water and are therefore more often found in environments lacking plumbing and sanitation, hallmarks of poverty. It is a gender issue because in many Latin American countries, access to abortion is limited or non-existent, leading health officials to advise women to not become pregnant. In a thought-provoking commentary, Alicia Ely Yamin, policy director of the Harvard FXB Center, wrote, "The speed with which the Zika virus appears to be spreading is only surpassed by the speed at which structural political failures in Latin America have been transformed into apparent personal deficiencies."[6] The health promotion advice to avoid pregnancy assumes that women and girls have control over their sexual relations and/or access to secure, effective contraception or abortion—when this is most certainly not the case for millions of women at risk. Instead of focusing only on vector control, Yamin calls on public health leaders to work on the social conditions that put poor and marginalized women at risk, including discrimination and women's lack of rights.

Canada is also not able to escape the threats to health and wellbeing that arise from climate change, vectors, gender-based inequities, and civil war, even when the actual events occur far from our shores. In the globalized world we live in today, such problems are our problems as well—or may become so with time. While a particular organism may not yet threaten our health, we have witnessed the devastation caused by an infectious illness with the SARS crisis, and vectors continue to move across the North American continent with each passing year. Further, every day there are people in Canada who suffer because of lack of sanitation and limits to their human rights. Indeed, the United Nations Human Rights Committee has called out Canada for failing to address violence against women and girls; the gender wage gap; the disproportionate experiences of violence, homicide, and disappearance among Indigenous women and girls; and the use of force by law enforcement officers during mass arrests, such as student protests and Indigenous land claim protests.[7] Health promoters cannot avoid these fundamental issues of social justice, environmental safety, and inequity but must, instead, participate in partnerships to address them and seek ways to minimize the likelihood that programs and policies will sustain or exacerbate them.

Health promotion *in* Canada cannot be understood by looking only at the infrastructures of government and universities, at budgets for public health and acute care, or the number of individuals with formal health promotion credentials. These are but indicators of the potential resources available to address the problems of this country. What they do not tell us is how well we are doing at improving the conditions for health for those living in Canada or how health-promoting activities here compare with those in other countries. While we have not included an international comparative chapter in this edition, the chapters by Labonté, Hancock, and McCall and Laitsch each challenge us to engage at multiple political, geographic, and institutional levels to effect needed change.

TWENTY-FIVE YEARS OF *HEALTH PROMOTION IN CANADA*

The first edition of this book was published in 1994, just short of a decade after the *Ottawa Charter* was released and 20 years after the publication of the Lalonde Report, both landmark events in the evolution of health promotion in Canada. The Lalonde Report signalled that the federal government understood that what influences health includes environmental conditions and daily health practices, in addition to biology and the organization of health care. The *Ottawa Charter* established a global dialogue on the actions required to enable people to increase control over and improve their health. Both documents served as key reference points in the first edition, a socio-historical assessment and reflection of the state of health promotion in Canada. That book identified a mix of conditions—fiscal, political, epidemiological, and social—that accounted for the emergence and form of health promotion research, policy, and practice across the country. These conditions included an increase in the rates of chronic diseases, rising expenditures on health services, continued support for the welfare state, and the emergence of various social movements (feminist, gay rights, environmental, and/or civil rights). Though the conditions were the same across the country, we observed differences in the concrete manifestations of health promotion with respect to policy, education/training, and research/implementation, depending upon the particular politics and histories of jurisdictions.

This new edition retains the same concerns as the first, namely to assess the state of the field in Canada. The jurisdictional emphasis on federal, provincial, and territorial government institutionalization of health promotion, however, has been replaced by a focus on how the field has evolved with respect to theory, research, and practice, independent of place. Indeed, "place" has been an aspect of health promotion theorizing, as would be expected of research and practice that recognizes the importance of context in the identification of health problems and their possible solutions. An ecological approach to understanding health and health problems leads to highly contextualized, multi-factorial interventions informed by an understanding of the deeply social nature of health. Such an understanding does not apply only to the health of Canadians. Accordingly, the critical reflections in this book, while telling about the state of the art and science of health promotion in this country, could be of service to anyone concerned with improving health on this planet. Indeed, we see greater emphasis than ever on the link between health promotion *in* Canada with health promotion *beyond* Canada—a question we have pursued through all editions of the book. Perhaps it is time to move past the phrase coined in the 1950s and embraced by environmentalists worldwide—"think globally, act locally"—to "think globally *and* locally, act globally *and* locally"?

Canada and Canadians continue to influence the field of health promotion at an international level. Researchers, practitioners, and politicians participated, for example, in major recent global events, including the 9th Global Conference on Health Promotion in Shanghai in November 2016. Canadians were the second-largest group of participants at the International Union of Health Promotion and Education (IUHPE) conference in Curitiba, Brazil, in May of that same year (Brazil had the largest number of delegates) and we hosted the Global Forum on Health Promotion in Charlottetown, PEI, in October 2016. These events—all of which engaged wide audiences and long-time and emerging leaders in the field—demonstrate the continuing role that health promoters in Canada play on the global stage. Indeed, the IUHPE Board is considering moving the head office from Paris to Montréal, a significant move for an organization that is more than 65 years old. Such a move could offer many opportunities for Canada and Canadians to influence the practical, educational, and policy agenda of this leading health promotion NGO.

This book is also an example of critical reflexivity, a practice advocated among leading theorists and practitioners for decades (see chapter 17). Developing the book meant adopting a self-critical stance regarding the nature of the field and its intended and unintended effects. Reflecting on the final contents of the book, we would argue that they demonstrate continued concern with social justice and health inequities, both within Canada and more broadly, as well as their determinants and the actions that might reduce them. This suggests that this aspect of the health promotion agenda is as important as ever.

Box 24.1: Reflections on the 9th Global Conference on Health Promotion in Shanghai, China—November 2016

Suzanne Jackson, PhD

Every global conference in the *Ottawa Charter* series has engaged the participants in debate and discussion towards writing a declaration or statement. The five strategies for health promotion that were identified in the *Ottawa Charter* have stood the test of time and after 30 years, still serve as a guide for health promotion practice around the world. The Shanghai conference also produced a declaration, but through comments online before the conference itself. This is symbolic of the direction of health promotion in China, where there is attention to health in all policies and health education but lesser attention to community and civil society participatory processes. That was a disappointing aspect of the conference. However, Dr. Margaret Chan, Director-General of the WHO, and Ilona Kickbusch stated that we are at a political watershed where politicians have to take courage to affect commercial interests (e.g., tobacco, sugar, soda industries) at a global level. The significance of the 9GCHP in Shanghai was to raise the profile of health promotion as a cornerstone for achieving the Sustainable Development Goals, the major determinants of health with support by UN member states. Communities have to be involved and heard and the health promotion field is in the best position to support politicians to link citizens at the local level to organizations working at the level of civil society to policies at all governance levels. Health promoters know how to work across sectors, engage everyone in planning and decision-making using participatory processes, recognize the different contexts in which people live, and connect multiple strategies at multiple levels in complex environments.

Within Canada we continue to witness changes in the organizational and operational dimensions of health promotion within government, the academy, and public health practice. What has remained constant, however, are the core principles that animate health promotion in Canada. The *Ottawa Charter* continues to be a touchstone in the field, encouraging strengthening community action, building healthy public policy, creating supportive environments, developing personal skills, and re-orienting health services. In the academy, however, we are witnessing a debate among universities about whether there should be programs and degrees in health promotion (indicative of the field as a discipline) or just courses in health promotion (suggesting it is a more generalist area of knowledge or that it can be learned in piecemeal fashion). Though not a new debate, the decision to take one path or the other will, as it has for the past three decades, continue to have implications for employment, further education, and organizational sustainability as individuals and funders grapple with issues of identity, credentialing, and legitimacy. Always the poor cousin of public health—itself the poor cousin of medicine—health promotion practitioners, in particular, continue to be challenged to demonstrate their value within the health system. Perhaps this explains why so many of health promotion's leaders have found their way into the academy, as it remains a setting that offers, to some degree, the opportunity for engagement in advocacy and service as legitimate alternatives to research and teaching.

These patterns are consistent with comments by several contributors regarding the constraints that health promotion practitioners face with respect to autonomy, flexibility, resources, and support for engaging in innovative practices. It speaks also to the limitations on advocacy activities that challenge organizations to speak truth to power regarding injustice and the questioning of policy priorities. The entrenchment of neo-liberalism means, more than ever, that individuals need local, provincial, and national organizations like the Canadian Public Health Association to raise issues of concern, offer spirited public health feedback, and maintain pressure on government and public health leadership to take principled, evidence-informed actions.[8] Critical health promotion researchers and surveillance experts have continued to develop theories, models, and methods for understanding the significance of income as a determinant of health and how much more meaningful it is at explaining health inequities than health behaviour. Explaining the persistence of the social gradient in health and championing the social determinants of health must be priorities for health promoters. And we must continue to study and seek to understand the impact on health of other aspects of social location that shape everyday life, including gender inequalities, racialization, and poverty.

On the positive side, there are a number of developments that give one hope for the future of health promotion in Canada. One is the emergence of energetic younger leaders who have a strong commitment to, and knowledge of, health promotion and are willing to step into leadership roles. An example is Rebecca Fortin, a graduate of the health promotion program at the University of Toronto, who has led the development of a new Pan-Canadian organization called Health Promotion Canada.[9] So far, under her leadership, several provincial chapters or provincial communities of practice have been formed or are in the process of forming. This organization has the potential to provide badly needed leadership for the field from the non-governmental sector.[10] As made evident in chapter 14, new leadership has also stepped forward from the university sector, which has contributed to the success of "Healthy University" initiatives and their spread across the country using university-based resources. As noted in chapter 14, an unintended outcome of the healthy university initiatives may be that universities as institutions become important "change agents" for the promotion of health with reach across various disciplines outside of health. As noted in chapter 15, on clinical care, students in clinical programs are also being exposed to knowledge about the social determinants of health and their relevance for the practice of clinicians in clinical settings and the community—a change from earlier models of health professional education.

Another example of involving younger leaders in health promotion is an initiative developed by Bridge for Health, a newly established Canadian health promotion cooperative, and the Public Health Association of British Columbia under the leadership of Paola

Ardiles. Called "Youth Leadership in Health Promotion Global Policy," the initiative involved preparing and submitting a briefing report on participation of youth to the Scientific Committee for the 2016 WHO Global Conference on Health Promotion. The report was based on two participatory activities with Canadian youth: a 90-minute discussion with a diverse group of 11 student leaders about why it is important for youth voices to be heard in conferences such as the one on health promotion, and a social media campaign (using the hashtag #EngagewithWHO) with the aim of giving youth a platform to share their opinions regarding health promotion issues. The campaign reached 6601 individuals and/or organizations (in Canada and other countries). The methods were co-designed, facilitated, and analyzed by young-adult Bridge for Health network members. For example, the youth leaders chose the four questions posed on the social media site, and also supported the analysis of results and the discussion and recommendations.[11]

The briefing report was taken up by the conference steering committee and led to the creation of a youth symposium at the WHO conference in Shanghai in November 2016. In addition, a video entitled "Engaging the Leaders of Tomorrow"[12] that specifically linked health promotion and youth leadership to the UN Sustainability Goals was developed and launched at the 22nd IUHPE World Conference on Health Promotion in Brazil. In October 2016, the youth engagement lead at Bridge for Health had the opportunity to co-host a public leadership pre-conference event and present the video at the 6th Global Health Promotion Forum held in Charlottetown, PEI, in October 2016. These examples suggest that the health promotion torch is being passed on and received by a younger generation.

Another encouraging sign is a merging of health promotion with "population health." This is not only signified by the use of the term *population health promotion* by people who were, and still are, identified with "health promotion" (see chapters 19 and 22) but by people in health promotion supporting population health initiatives (see chapters 8 and 23) and people identified with population heath adopting ideas from health promotion. An example of the latter is the prominent use of wording from the *Ottawa Charter* in the report of the WHO Commission on *Social* Determinants of Health (Kickbusch, 2012, emphasis added). Hopefully, Hancock's chapter in this book will persuade our colleagues in population health to include elements of the physical environment as determinants of the health of populations (see chapter 22). Beyond toxicology, or other areas of public health that traditionally focus on the physical environment, recognizing that climate change is a result of human activity makes action through policy possible. Economic and social policies need to take health into account—which has been the long-standing rationale for healthy public policy and health in all policy.

A third important area in which we see valuable progress being made involves work with other sectors. For example, over the past few years the Public Health Association of British Columbia has held annual conferences in partnership with other sectors including the private, education, and recreation sectors. These conferences have produced ongoing relationships with members of these sectors—though perhaps not yet to the extent we had hoped. On the other hand, it is encouraging that other provinces are organizing continuing education opportunities related to health promotion that include other sectors, such as the Atlantic Summer Institute on Healthy and Safe Communities (see box 24.2). As a national level example, there has been a remarkable, greater-than-35-year continuing relationship between the public health and literacy sectors. More recently, there have been several encouraging developments in work on health literacy, including the establishment of several health literacy networks in BC along with an intersectoral steering committee that meets monthly. Also, the Ministry of Health and Long-Term Care in Ontario recently established a working group on health literacy that bridges several sectors including health

Box 24.2: Atlantic Summer Institute on Healthy and Safe Communities

The Atlantic Summer Institute on Healthy and Safe Communities (ASI) is a bilingual not-for-profit organization established in 2003, responding to the need for a health promotion summer institute in Atlantic Canada. The mission of ASI to increase capacity to take action on determinants of health and to serve as a catalyst for social change, ultimately leading to the creation of healthier, safer, more inclusive, and sustainable communities in Atlantic Canada. ASI organizes learning institutes, symposia, and workshops focused on health promotion, intersectoral collaboration, and leadership.

ASI programs strengthen collaboration between community groups, educators, health practitioners and researchers, government representatives, parents/caregivers, and youth, and reflect the diverse perspectives of communities and individuals who have a stake in health promotion. The curricula are guided by the belief that policy and programs benefit from three sources of evidence: research, best practice, and lived experience.

ASI programs are organized around themes connected to regional issues in health promotion, including inclusion; literacy; gender and community leadership; democracy and social justice; and child and youth mental health. The Circle of Health—a collaborative teaching tool that includes the *Ottawa Charter*, the determinants of health, and the Aboriginal Medicine Wheel—serves as the curriculum and planning framework.

ASI was incorporated in Prince Edward Island in 2008, and is managed by a Board of Directors with representatives from all four Atlantic Provinces. ASI is committed to mentoring leadership in the next generation and offers a youth leadership and children's program each summer. Since 2004 its programs have reached more than 1,000 registrants from health, education, and justice sectors, as well as community and multi-cultural groups. The annual summer programs have served as an incubator of innovative curricula that are evaluated, further refined, and disseminated regionally.

Contact: Malcolm Shookner, ASI President: mshookner@eastlink.ca or Patsy Beattie-Huggan, Coordinator: patsy@thequaich.pe.ca.

promotion and health care. And in Québec, since the 2002 adoption of the Québec Public Health Act's section 54, Québec government bodies proposing laws or regulations must first go through a health impact assessment (HIA) process—a strong demonstration of intersectoral action.

Another example that is taking health promotion values, principles, and strategies to work collaboratively with the business sector to advance social innovation and sustainability is Bridge for Health, mentioned above. The Bridge for Health model uses design thinking and systems approaches to address the root causes of illness in the workplace. The co-op model itself is designed to encourage engagement, interdisciplinary approaches, as well as shared power and ownership. Based on this example, the creator of Bridge for Health has suggested that health promotion in Canada needs to evolve outside of "health-care" by promoting (1) new models that support increased public participation and interdisciplinary collaboration; (2) new partners across sectors in order to join collective societal efforts that are calling for a more just, safe, and sustainable planet; and (3) new organizational structures that support innovative funding mechanisms (Ardiles, 2017).

Finally, we believe that this book in itself is an encouraging sign for the future of health promotion in Canada. Many new and younger scholars have contributed excellent new chapters to this edition, based on innovative developments in health promotion in Canada over the past five years, and have provided us with many suggestions regarding how the field could move forward, as does a selection of key suggestions from each of the preceding chapters noted below.

1.   There are new opportunities for health promotion to collaborate with other sectors such as engineering, environmental science, education, economics, political science, and social welfare to address the social, political, and economic barriers to health and health equity in Canada and elsewhere (see chapter 1).

2.   Key concepts in health promotion (e.g., empowerment, health literacy, and quality of life) have provided, and can continue to provide, bridges to other fields (see chapter 2).

3.   The use of social theory in health promotion can substantially enhance its intellectual resources for engaging in broader societal debates beyond the narrow health sector (see chapter 3).

4.   In using behavioural change theories and models, practitioners and researchers should consider applying those that, in addition to addressing individual behaviour, include intrapersonal and environmental/social factors such as the Behaviour Change Wheel (see chapter 4).

5.   Health promotion practitioners and researchers need to continue efforts to undertake comprehensive evaluations of ecological programs and knowledge transfer and exchange activities. Research on the identification of factors associated with greater levels of integration of the ecological approach in real-world programming is also a promising avenue for future efforts (see chapter 5).

6. Health promotion practitioners and researchers need to address social context as a potential of intervention using the collective lifestyles framework, as well as issues relating to power and reflexivity (see chapter 6).

7. Health promotion must recognize gender-based violence as a health issue and work to prevent violence in the first place; improve the health sector's awareness of this issue; and help the sector respond to violence in effective ways (see chapter 7).

8. The best means of reducing health inequities involve health promoters and their agencies and organizations informing citizens about the political and economic forces that shape the health of a society (see chapter 8).

9. Health promotion practitioners and researchers in partnership with communities need to lobby for dedicated resources and infrastructure for mental health promotion at all levels (see chapter 9).

10. Non-Indigenous health promotion professionals should only undertake work with Indigenous communities if they have an understanding and appreciation of Indigenous history, concepts, contexts, and processes. Additionally, it is important that clear consent be established at the front-end from community members, that the possibility to guide the process be offered to community members, and that trust is continually sought out and co-constructed (see chapter 10).

11. Policy makers at multiple levels need to develop health promotion strategies targeted and tailored to meet the unique needs of an increasingly diverse immigrant/refugee population and make suggestions for specific interventions (see chapter 11).

12. In partnership with municipalities, health promoters must create a vision of a more just, sustainable, and healthy future in order to co-create cities, towns, and villages compatible with that vision (see chapter 12).

13. Leaders in school health and health promotion need to shift to systems-based approaches and implement and maintain that shift in policy and practice (see chapter 13).

14. Health promotion practitioners and researchers need to work with universities and colleges to build the evidence base for "healthy university" initiatives and the capacities of students, faculty, and administration to act as health promotion change agents for the community at large (see chapter 14).

15. Health care professionals need to become more engaged in the health and wellbeing of the populations and communities they serve. More work can be done to educate students from various health care fields to transition their knowledge of health promotion into clinical practice in both acute and community care settings, and to strengthen their understanding of the social and ecological determinants of health (see chapter 15).

16. Health promotion practitioners need to seriously consider the evidence on the strengths and limitations of using "digital health promotion" (see chapter 16).

17. Although collaborative reflection is part of the health promotion reflective process, each individual health promotion initiative will be unique according to the diversity of individual interests, organizations, values, personalities, and goals involved (see chapter 17).

18. Health promotion practitioners and researchers need to work together to encourage and undertake research in the relative effectiveness of *health in all policies* and encourage managers and politicians to consider trying and evaluating this approach (see chapter 18).
19. Health promotion researchers and practitioners need to continue to work with colleagues committed to population health intervention research (see chapter 19).
20. Health promotion practitioners need to engage in careful and transparent approaches to the ethical interrogation of the various issues that arise in the practice of health promotion (see chapter 20).
21. There is a need to develop the capacity of health promotion organizations to work in more participatory ways (see chapter 21).
22. Health promotion needs to engage with issues confronting the planet's environment based on the notion of Anthropocene. This will require shifting thinking in health promotion, bringing an end to the separation of the ecological from the social, and encouraging more interdisciplinary work with areas such as ecology and urban planning (see chapter 22).
23. Health promotion should lead the way in being reflexive about how the political economy affects the health of our population (including the widening of inequities) and work towards a more equitable and salubrious society (see chapter 23).

Based on these developments, it would be fair to say that the field of health promotion has been strengthened to some degree over the past five years. On the other hand, it is important that we recognize some of the forces that will likely impede future development in the field in Canada.

One of these is the downgrading of two more of the university-based centres for health promotion. The Atlantic Centre for Health Promotion has been absorbed into a new Institute and the University of Alberta's Centre for Health Promotion Research has been incorporated into the School of Public Health. These changes mean that there are no longer *any* freestanding centres for health promotion research in Canada. While the incorporation of health promotion into entities with broader mandates may facilitate research within other areas of study, the elimination or downgrading of such centres reduces the strength and autonomy of research in health promotion in Canada as well as capacity-building in the field.

Another key factor that may constrain the development of health promotion in Canada is the continuing priority given to "health *care*" services by policy makers and the public. This focus may continue to limit the resources available for health promotion unless there is a significant recognition that health promotion can help reduce health care costs. Sadly, there are not many champions for this point of view, nor is there enough strong evidence to make the case. Perhaps "population health intervention research," discussed in chapter 19, will ultimately generate the required evidence?

Finally, given these and other implications mentioned in this book, it does appear as if there is indeed "plenty there that needs to be done." The question that remains is, do practitioners, researchers, policy makers, and others that resonate with the values, objectives, and strategies of health promotion have the energy, resolve, and resources to get it done? We hope that this book will make a contribution to enabling them to do so.

CRITICAL THINKING QUESTIONS

1. What can health promoters in Canada learn from health promotion issues and approaches in health promotion in other countries and globally?
2. What do you think is the most important lesson about health promotion that you have learned from this book? Why do you think this is most important?
3. Which chapter in the book do you like most? Why?
4. What do you think is the future of health promotion in Canada?

RESOURCES

Further Readings

PEI Health Promotion Declaration. (2016).
    globalforumpei-forummondialipe.com/en2016/pei-declaration/
This declaration was produced at the 6th Global Forum on Health Promotion held in Charlottetown in October 2016. It was submitted for consideration at the 9th Global Conference on Health Promotion and is currently being used as a tool for programming and advocacy by the Global Alliance for Health Promotion.

Shanghai Declaration on Promoting Health in the 2030 Agenda for Sustainable Development.
    www.who.int/healthpromotion/conferences/9gchp/shanghai-declaration.pdf?ua=1
This declaration was developed and released at the 9th Global Conference on Health Promotion in Shanghai, China, in November 2016.

Relevant Websites

Affiliation of Multicultural Societies and Service Agencies of BC (AMSSA)
www.amssa.org/resources/videos/e-symposia/collaborative-approaches-to-promoting-newcomer-health/
    A series of videos are available from an e-symposium on Collaborative Approaches to Promoting Newcomer Health that took place in Vancouver in the winter of 2016. These materials offer some ideas about the links between settlement and health discussed in this chapter.

Health Promotion Canada
www.healthpromotioncanada.ca

Established in 2017, Health Promotion Canada is a national association to enhance the capacity of Canadian health promoters to promote health and health equity among communities, empowering people to achieve their full life potential. Through the website you will be able to access resources to enhance your capacity to understand and engage in health promotion.

International Union for Health Promotion and Education (IUHPE)
www.iuhpe.org/index.php/en/

The IUHPE's mission is to promote global health and wellbeing and to contribute to the achievement of equity in health between and within countries of the world. The IUHPE fulfills its mission by building and operating an independent, global, professional network of people and institutions to encourage the free exchange of ideas, knowledge, know-how, and experiences, and the development of relevant collaborative projects, both at global and regional levels. Learn more about the IUHPE and the opportunities it provides for networking, collaboration, and global action at this website.

NOTES

1.   Alan Turing, English mathematician, logician, cryptanalyst, and computer scientist. Retrieved from www.goodreads.com/author/quotes/87041.Alan_Turing

2.   Based on the list of Educational Programs in Public Health maintained by the Public Health Agency of Canada. Retrieved from www.phac-aspc.gc.ca/php-psp/master_of_php-eng.php

3.   See Framework Convention on Climate Change at unfccc.int/paris_agreement/items/9485.php

4.   See: www.nationalobserver.com/2016/10/05/news/canada-officially-ratifies-historic-paris-climate-agreement

5.   Public Health Agency of Canada. (2016). *Canada communicable disease report. Emerging challenges of vector-borne disease and cities. Volume 42-10*. Retrieved from www.phac-aspc.gc.ca/publicat/ccdr-rmtc/16vol42/dr-rm42-10/assets/pdf/16vol42_10-eng.pdf

6.   Alicia Ely Yamin on Health, Human Rights and the Zika Virus. Retrieved from fxb.harvard.edu/4941-2/

7.   See the United Nations Human Rights Office of the High Commissioner, International Covenant on Civil and Political Rights, 13 August 2015. Retrieved from tbinternet.ohchr.org/_layouts/treatybodyexternal/Download.aspx?symbolno=CCPR%2fC%2fCAN%2fCO%2f6&Lang=en

8.   Disclaimer: Ann Pederson is currently a member of the Board of Directors of the Canadian Public Health Association.

9.   See www.healthpromotioncanada.ca

10. One issue that may affect the ability of Health Promotion Canada to offer leadership is the question of the professionalization of health promotion that was recently raised in a letter to the

editor of *Health Promotion and Chronic Disease Prevention in Canada* (Graham, 2017). According to the author "the more HP is professionalized, the less it will be integrated across all areas of public health practice" (Graham, 2017), although two editorials challenging to this view were published in subsequent issues (Gagné, Lapalme, & Leroux, 2017; Machado, 2017).

11.   The results from these two activities are captured in Bridge for Health's *Engaging the Leaders of Tomorrow*: a briefing report on youth engagement for the 9th Global Conference on Health Promotion. Retrieved from www.bridgeforhealth.org/www/bridge/youth-engagement-report/

12.   Video retrieved from www.youtube.com/watch?v=Ux0-L_uspqc

REFERENCES

Ardiles, P. (2017). *Bridge for Health Co-operative case study.* Bridge for Health, Vancouver. Retrieved from www.bridgeforhealth.org.

Gagné, T., Lapalme, J., & Leroux, J. (2017). Letter to the editor: The implications of the professionalization of health promotion in Canada: A response to JR Graham's letter to the editor. *Health Promotion and Chronic Disease Prevention in Canada: Research, Policy and Practice*, 37(5), 172–173. doi:10.24095/hpcdp.37.5.05

Graham, J. R. (2017). Letter to the editor: Who benefits from the professionalization of health promotion? *Health Promotion and Chronic Disease Prevention in Canada: Research, Policy and Practice*, 37(1), 32. www.phac-aspc.gc.ca/publicat/hpcdp-pspmc/37-1/index-eng.php.

Kickbusch, I. (2012). Understanding the rhizome effect: Health promotion in the twenty-first century. In I. Rootman, S. Dupéré, A. Pederson, & M. O'Neill (Eds.), *Health promotion in Canada: Critical perspectives on practice* (3rd ed.) (pp. 308–313). Toronto: Canadian Scholars' Press.

Machado, S. (2017). Letter to the editor: The professionalization of health promotion in Canada: A student perspective. *Health Promotion and Chronic Disease Prevention in Canada: Research, Policy and Practice*, 37(6), 201–202. doi:10.24095/hpcdp.37.6.04

AFTERWORD

To Go Much More Boldly Where We Have Gone Before

Ronald Labonté

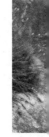

I have spent over 40 years working under the umbrella of "health promotion"—a term I have never liked much, but a practice nonetheless imbued with the core values of social justice and ecological sustainability that are the necessary foundations for anyone who finds themselves working in the broader playing field we call "public health." Being sufficiently long-toothed, I plead forgiveness for some historical nostalgia in this Afterword.

In this book's first edition, I mused that the health promotion envisioned by the *Ottawa Charter* was, at least in part, a response to progressive social movements arising in high-income countries in the 1970s and 1980s: the New Left, feminist, environmental, labour, anti-racist, and pro-gay (today's pro-LGBTQ2) movements, to name a few. The socially critical ideals of these movements challenged the individualist, health behaviourist models that still persist in much of our practice, with "lifestyle drift" becoming once again a lament in many parts of the global health promotion community. In this book's second edition I launched my first salvo at the global/globalization dimensions of health, as my past work in localized health empowerment projects confronted the disequalizing practices of a neo-liberal economic orthodoxy that could undo years of progressive small-scale health promotion progress with the brush of a finance minister's pen or the conclusion of a secretly negotiated trade and investment treaty. The third edition updated this analysis; and in this newest fourth edition I have crafted a wholly new analysis of the global health landscape and its contemporary meaning for health promoters worldwide.

For health promotion quickly became a global phenomenon, attracting practitioners from most of the world's countries for the salience of its values and the centrality of good health and wellbeing in most people's life priorities. As recently as the 9th Global Conference on Health Promotion, convened in Shanghai in November 2016, Ilona Kickbusch (one of health promotion's godmothers) argued that promoting health has become the centre of a global agenda, with a clear recognition that this is a *political* agenda, and not simply an exercise in improving our practice's technical skills. The final *Shanghai Declaration* is perhaps the most politically explicit in health promotion's 30 years of international rhetoric. As my own contribution to this present volume posits, the new Sustainable Development Goals (however flawed in some respects) offer health promotion the strongest invitation yet to the *Charter*'s call for advocacy on "healthy public policy" (today's "health in all policies"). It is there for us to seize.

I admire Ilona's Shanghai optimism as I, too, am afflicted with the same pathological hopefulness, a personality trait that I have long regarded as a prerequisite to anyone working in public health for the simple reason that without such a disposition we would be immobilized by the weight of the challenges we confront, and the more so today than just 30 years ago.

Climate change. Rampant economic inequality. The greatest movement of refugees and environmental or economic migrants the world has experienced. A retreat from liberal democracy, the rise of "strongman" or "strong woman" politics (not restricted to the surprise election of Donald Trump to the US presidency), and an "alt-right" return to a misogynist and racist xenophobia not seen since the "dirty 30s" decade that was prelude to World War II. It is hard to square the politics of increased surveillance and repression in many parts of the world with the circle of "bold political choices for health" to which the *Shanghai Declaration* commits our leaders.[1]

We are left, then, with the appropriately clichéd Chinese word for crisis: danger and opportunity. The dangers are obvious, the opportunities perhaps less so. To elaborate on just four:

First, we must avoid concluding that the increasing global rejection of a politics of elitism means the abandonment of the values of fairness, conviviality, and healthful living that have long guided our own work (which remains captured in many of the chapters in this volume), and that are regularly reiterated in opinion polls, research findings, and international meetings. There is both space and an urgent need for a progressive and inclusive political populism, based on the ideals inherent in the Sustainable Development Goals. This is a task to which the quotidian and locally empowering practices of health promotion can make a valued contribution.

Second, as we continue whatever (non-victim-blaming) form our health promotion work takes, we need to ensure it is undertaken in a way that challenges the many discriminatory "ism's" that our right-wing political populism is feeding. I recall years ago working in the City of Toronto Public Health Department, where complaints about racism in the city were rising. I was not surprised that racism existed, but that it was less than what might have been, given Toronto's long-standing recognition as the most ethnically diverse city on the planet[2]—an imperfect accomplishment I attributed then, and attribute now, to the efforts of federal and local governments, local community workers, and local health promoters to explicitly advance and support an inclusive politics of tolerance and respect in every program, policy, or public engagement they undertook. Let us re-embrace that recent, emancipatory history and the political collaboration with progressive civil society movements it demands.

Third, as Trevor Hancock (this volume) reminds us, we now reside in an Anthropocene era, where our planetary ecosystems are governed (unhealthily) by our human activities. Climate change, resource depletion, and toxic pollution are leading us headlong into a probable mass extinction, one that includes human life. Amongst the imperatives this creates for health promotion are a concerted campaign to reduce our own "hyper consumption," an end to fossil fuel subsidies and new infrastructure (balancing sustainability with economic growth is no longer an option), a rejection of the population Ponzi scheme in which we are told that we need to keep growing the base of the working-age population to support long-toothed elders such as Trevor and me, blind to what happens when the enlarged bottom half of the demographic pyramid reaches its own retirement age, and, as my own contribution to this volume argues, a vigorous defence of commercial and labour market regulation and national systems of redistribution (there is more than enough wealth to go around to shift to a green, de-growth economy).

Fourth, our corporate and elite opponents (local, national, and global) will not change their unhealthy wealth accumulation or commodity production and marketing behaviours without strong and committed vigilance and push-back on our parts. Our health promotion successes in tobacco control should embolden us to advance a similar approach to regulation in other domains of health-harmful practices and commodities. Food labelling and content requirements for processed foods and beverages are just one of the many new health promotion frontiers, with the international food oligopolies not keen to see the profits of their obesogenic practices diminish. One of health promotion's greatest (albeit still frequently counter-challenged) accomplishments since the first edition of this book was published has been its shift in focus from individuals to settings and, more recently with the imprimatur of the WHO Commission on Social Determinants of Health, to "a toxic combination of the poor social policies and programmes, unfair economic arrangements and bad politics" that "are killing people on a grand scale" (CSDH, 2008, pp. 4, 26).

I am writing this Afterword as 2016 enters its twilight. It has been a perilous and disrupting year, with little clear idea of what 2017 will bring given the unpredictability of those who are now leading the world's most powerful countries, whether they be in China, India, Russia, the US, or any of a score of other nations. What we can proclaim is that the values that have long informed health promotion as a practice, dating at least as far back as those that underpinned the social medicine movement of the mid-nineteenth century in Europe, are as vital today as they have ever been. It is those values that will both gird us for the challenges ahead and guide us in the policy, programmatic, and political choices we make, not only as health promoters but as citizens with responsibilities to each other and to generations to come.

As we exercise these value-based (and, yes, evidence-informed) choices, we bring an awareness that what we have learned from our recent health promotion past demands a much bolder future. Our efforts, and our voices, must be stronger now than they have ever been, and should be expressed with hope and without fear. As Naomi Klein wrote earlier this year (2016) about climate change, but which applies to all of the health-challenging depredations in our socio-ecological global commons, "There are no non-radical options left before us."[3]

December 15, 2016

NOTES

1.   Go to www.who.int/healthpromotion/conferences/9gchp/shanghai-declaration/en/
2.   Go to www.metronews.ca/news/toronto/2016/05/16/toronto-the-diverse.html
3.   Go to www.salon.com/2016/02/04/naomi_klein_there_are_no_non_radical_options_left_before_us_partner/

REFERENCE

Commission on Social Determinants of Health (CSDH). (2008). *Closing the gap in a genera-tion: Health equity through action on the social determinants of health*. Geneva: World Health Organization.

ABOUT THE CONTRIBUTORS

Paola Ardiles is a Lecturer in Health Sciences at Simon Fraser University, Founder of Bridge for Health co-op, and past President of the Public Health Association of BC. Paola received the 2012 Dr. Nancy Hall Public Policy Leadership Award of Distinction in recognition of her innovative, collaborative, and upstream approaches in mental health promotion.

Michelle Aslan has a strong passion for teaching, knowledge translation, and the communication of ideas. She has a Master's in Education and Curriculum Planning from Simon Fraser University (SFU), and a PIDP (Provincial Instructor Diploma). Currently she is the Director of Education and Training for HM|HC Student Network, which is part of the Provincial Leadership Council.

Ariane Bélanger-Gravel is an Assistant Professor at the Department of Information and Communication at Université Laval and a research associate at the Centre de recherche de l'Institut universitaire de cardiologie et de pneumologie de Québec. Her main interests reside in the understanding of theoretical processes underlying behaviour change, with particular reference to physical activity and in the examination of the effects of individually based interventions on health-related behaviour change. She completed a CIHR-funded post-doctoral fellowship at the School of Public Health of the Université de Montréal and the Centre de recherche du Centre Hospitalier de l'Université de Montréal to study the impact of population-based interventions aimed at promoting physical activity. She is also interested in reducing social inequalities in health.

Katherine Bertoni is an Assistant Teaching Professor in the Faculty of Human and Social Development at the University of Victoria and a family nurse practitioner at the Jack Petersen Health Clinic, with expertise in diabetes education. She has published in the areas of maternal-child nursing care in Canada, and better access to health care through system navigation. Her contribution to research and teaching includes diabetes education, best practice guidelines for diabetes triage, and medication reconciliation.

Tara Black is the Associate Director, Health Promotion at Simon Fraser University. She has a Master of Science in Health Promotion and specializes in socio-ecological action for building healthy higher-education settings. She co-chaired the development of the *Okanagan Charter* and is chairing the Canadian Health Promoting Universities Network.

Joan L. Bottorff is a Professor in the School of Nursing, Faculty of Health and Social Development and the Director of the Institute for Healthy Living and Chronic Disease

Prevention at the University of British Columbia's Okanagan campus. She is a Fellow of the Canadian Academy of Health Sciences and a Fellow of the American Academy of Nursing. Her research program focuses on the influence of gender-related factors on health behaviour, and using technologies to design and evaluate gender-sensitive health promotion approaches.

Marie Boutilier conducts research in health policy, organizations, professionals, and the communities they serve. She has used participatory and qualitative research strategies in local communities, health services, professional organizations, and different levels of government, both in Canada and internationally.

Simon Carroll is an Assistant Teaching Professor in the Department of Sociology at the University of Victoria. A sociologist by training, he has had a long interest in the health promotion research field, completing his doctoral work on alternative approaches to assessing the effectiveness of complex health interventions. He is currently developing a variety of social theory approaches to assessing the effectiveness of complex public health interventions.

Rosie Dhaliwal has practised in Health Promotion at Simon Fraser University since 2007. She brings together her diverse experiences as a clinician and educator to create a healthy campus community. Her passion for teaching and learning drove her to pursue her Master of Education degree in Curriculum and Instruction at SFU. This is an asset in co-leading the Well-being in Learning Environments Project.

Geneviève Dubé has a Master's in Nursing from the University of Victoria and currently works as a family nurse practitioner in British Columbia. Her clinical focus is in the provision of primary care to marginalized populations in urban areas. Geneviève has experience in remote nursing with Aboriginal populations and she led program development and implementation in Québec remote First Nations. Her contribution to teaching includes preceptorship and work as an instructor for the University of British Columbia (Okanagan).

Sophie Dupéré has been an Associate Professor in the Faculty of Nursing at Université Laval since 2011. She has been involved in community health/health promotion in Canada and internationally for the last 20 years, working as a nurse, consultant, researcher, and activist. She is the co-editor of five books, two of which were the second and third editions of *Health Promotion in Canada*. Her research interests include poverty, social inequities, participatory approaches, equity in health care, and innovative professional practices.

Katherine L. Frohlich is an Associate Professor in the Département de médicine sociale et préventive at the Université de Montréal and a Research Associate at the Université de Montréal Public Health Research Institute (IRSPUM). She also holds a Canadian

Institutes of Health Research (CIHR) New Investigator Award. She has published widely in the areas of health promotion, social theory in public health, social inequities in health, as well as in the sociology of smoking.

Lise Gauvin is a Full Professor in the School of Public Health at the Université de Montréal and a Researcher and Associate Scientific Director for Population Health Research at the Centre de recherche du Centre Hospitalier de l'Université de Montréal (CRCHUM). In addition to her current academic position, she has held positions at Queen's University in Kingston, Ontario, and Concordia University in Montréal, Québec. In September 2015, she was named a Fellow of the Canadian Academy of Health Sciences. Her research focuses on socio-environmental and individual determinants of involvement in physical activity and the reach, acceptability, and impact of interventions to promote physical activity and prevent eating disorders. In addition to publishing her work in the peer-reviewed scientific literature, she is actively engaged in knowledge transfer and exchange activities developed in partnership with researchers, policy makers, and practitioners.

Lorraine Greaves is Senior Investigator at the Centre of Excellence for Women's Health. She is a medical sociologist, writer, and speaker with a focus on integrating sex, gender, and equity into health research, programs, and policies. She has worked in leadership positions across Canada in government, hospital, education, and research sectors.

Rebecca J. Haines-Saah is an Assistant Professor in the Department of Community Health Sciences, Cumming School of Medicine, University of Calgary. Trained as a Health Sociologist, her research focuses on adolescent mental health and substance use through the lens of a critical public health approach that prioritizes harm reduction, social justice, and the lived experiences of persons that use drugs and/or live with mental illness. She is especially interested in using qualitative, arts-based, and participatory methods as research tools for ensuring the meaningful involvement and inclusion of participants in the context of policy forums.

Trevor Hancock is a public health physician and Professor and Senior Scholar at the School of Public Health and Social Policy at the University of Victoria. He is one of the founders of the now-global Healthy Cities movement, co-authoring the original background paper for WHO/Europe in 1986, and has a strong interest in healthy urban governance. He also has a long-standing interest in the links between human and ecosystem health and the health impacts of our current unsustainable system of economic activity. He was a founder of the Green Party of Canada (and was its first leader), the Canadian Association of Physicians for the Environment, and the Canadian Coalition for Green Health Care. He more recently led a CPHA workgroup that produced a major report on the ecological determinants of health in 2015. He was awarded Honorary Fellowship in the UK's Faculty of Public Health in 2015 for his contributions to public health and the R. D. Defries Award (the highest award of the Canadian Public Health Association) in 2017 for his significant influence on public health and health promotion in Canada and globally.

Natalie Hemsing is a Research Associate at the Centre of Excellence for Women's Health. She specializes in research on addictions, tobacco use, and health promotion among girls and women, and has extensive experience in conducting knowledge syntheses and systematic reviews.

Crystal Hutchinson is a Health Promotion Specialist at Simon Fraser University. She has worked in the field of Health Promotion since 2013. Within her current role at SFU, Crystal draws on her professional and academic background in Education, where she specialized in Indigenous perspectives, health education, and contemplative pedagogy.

Mushira Mohsin Khan is a PhD candidate in the Department of Sociology and a Student Affiliate with the Institute on Aging and Lifelong Health at the University of Victoria. Her research primarily focuses on transnational ties and intergenerational relationships within mid- to later-life diasporic South Asian families, ethnicity and immigration, aging, and health and social care. She is particularly interested in exploring the complex dynamics and everyday negotiations around care and kin-work within Canada's immigrant families. Her work has been published in an edited volume on health care equity for ethnic minority older adults (SFU, 2015); the *Population Change and Lifecourse Strategic Knowledge Cluster Discussion Paper Series* (2015), and peer-reviewed journals including *Current Sociology* (2016) and the *International Journal of Migration, Health, and Social Care* (2017; 2015). She is also the recipient of the Social Sciences and Humanities Research Canada (SSHRC) Joseph-Armand Bombadier Canadian Doctoral Scholarship (2015–2018).

Rodney Knight is a Post-Doctoral Fellow at the British Columbia Centre for Excellence in HIV/AIDS where he is housed in Simon Fraser University's Faculty of Health Sciences. Rod is a recognized expert in the social determinants of young people's sexual health as well as a scholar in the realm of population and public health ethics. Rod is supported by a Post-Doctoral Fellowship from the Canadian Institutes of Health Research (CIHR) and the Michael Smith Foundation for Health Research.

Karen Kobayashi is an Associate Professor in the Department of Sociology and a Research Affiliate at the Institute on Aging and Lifelong Health at the University of Victoria. She is a social gerontologist who has published widely in the areas of family and intergenerational relationships, ethnicity and immigration, dementia and person-hood, and health and social care. The majority of her research has been developed and carried out collaboratively in interdisciplinary and intersectoral teams with colleagues at the University of Toronto, McMaster, McGill, the University of British Columbia, and

Simon Fraser University, the BC Ministry of Health, and multiple health authorities. She has been nominated to and held positions in the Canadian Sociological Association, the Canadian Association on Gerontology, and with two large NCE networks focused on aging and health, the National Initiative for the Care of the Elderly (NICE) and Aging Gracefully Across Environments Using Technology to Support Wellness, Engagement, and Long Life (AGE-WELL).

Ronald Labonté is Canada Research Chair in globalization and health equity at the Institute of Population Health; Professor in the Faculty of Medicine, University of Ottawa; and Adjunct Professor in the Department of Community Health and Epidemiology, University of Saskatchewan. He worked in public health and health promotion for over 25 years with municipal and provincial governments and internationally before becoming a full-time, university-based researcher in 1999. Recent co-edited or co-authored books include *Globalization and Health: Pathways, Evidence, and Policy* (2009), *Health Promotion in Action: From Local to Global Empowerment* (2008), and *Critical Perspectives in Public Health* (2007). Many of his writings are available on his website: www.globalhealthequity. ca/content/ronald-labonte

Daniel Laitsch is an associate professor with the Faculty of Education at Simon Fraser University. He is a researcher with the SFU Centre for the Study of Educational Leadership and Policy and his primary teaching area is in Educational Leadership. Dr. Laitsch's research interests include the use and misuse of research in teaching, policy-making, and issue advocacy; the impact of high-stakes accountability and assessment programs on educational systems; and school health–related approaches to systemic education reform.

Charlotte Loppie is a Professor in the School of Public Health and Social Policy, Faculty of Human and Social Development, and Director of the Centre for Indigenous Research and Community-Led Engagement, University of Victoria. Dr. Loppie teaches and conducts research on issues related to Indigenous peoples' health, health promotion, and health inequities, as well as the social determinants of health and HIV/AIDS among Indigenous people.

Robin Mason is a Research Scientist at Women's College Research Institute and the Scientific Lead of Women's Xchange, a women's health research knowledge and exchange centre at Women's College Hospital. She is also an Assistant Professor at the Dalla Lana School of Public Health, and the Department of Psychiatry, at the University of Toronto. She works in health education and research, with a focus on issues of violence, abuse, and trauma.

Jeff Masuda is Canada Research Chair in Environmental Health Equity and Associate Professor in the School of Kinesiology and Health Studies at Queen's University where he teaches health promotion at undergraduate and graduate levels. Jeff blends his training as a social geographer and interdisciplinary health promotion scholar within participatory researcher partnerships that aim to understand and contest health inequities associated with capitalist and colonialist urbanization. Since obtaining his MSc in Health Promotion in 2001 and PhD in Geography 2005, Jeff has worked across the country, following his own career path in Hamilton, Toronto, Vancouver, Winnipeg, and Kingston. He has published on themes of critical health promotion, environmental justice, the right to the city, participatory research, knowledge translation, and health equity. He is a senior editor of the *Canadian Journal of Public Health* and an editor of *Global Health Promotion*.

Douglas McCall is a scholar affiliated with the Centre for the Study of Educational Leadership and Policy at Simon Fraser University. He has worked in school health promotion since 1985, serving as Executive Director of the Canadian Association for School Health and, more recently, as the Executive Director for the International School Health Network. He has written numerous manuals, manuscripts, and peer-reviewed journal articles, as well as pioneered work in Web-based knowledge exchange.

Michel O'Neill retired in 2011 as Professor in community health and health promotion in the Faculty of Nursing of Université Laval and is currently Professor Emeritus of the same university. Michel received his PhD in sociology from Boston University, and has been involved in health promotion at the local, national, and international levels since 1974 as a community health worker, professor, researcher, consultant, and activist. His long-standing teaching and research interests relate to the history as well as to the political and policy dimensions of health promotion, with a special interest in the Healthy Cities movement in Québec, Canada, and internationally. He is author or co-editor of numerous books, including the first three editions of *Health Promotion in Canada*, has published extensively in the scientific and professional literature, and has presented numerous papers in various scientific and professional meetings in Québec, Canada, and all over the world.

Ann Pederson is currently the Director of Population Health Promotion at BC Women's Hospital & Health Centre in Vancouver, BC. She studied health promotion at the University of Toronto, earning a Master's of Science in Community Health, and at UBC, where she completed doctoral studies on sex, gender, and health promotion. She has participated in all four editions of *Health Promotion in Canada* to date, as an editor and contributor, and has contributed to numerous other books, most recently *Women's Health: Intersections of Policy, Research, and Practice* (Women's Press) and *Making it Better: Gender-transformative Health Promotion* (CSPI). Ann is active in the Canadian Public Health Association and International Union of Health Promotion and Education and serves as a preceptor and mentor to students in the public health and health promotion programs at several universities.

Blake Poland is a professor in the Dalla Lana School of Public Health at the University of Toronto, Director of the Collaborative Graduate Program in Community Development, Co-lead of the Healthier Cities and Communities hub, Director of the PhD program in Social and Behavioural Health Sciences at DLSPH, Co-director of the WHO Collaborating Centre in Health Promotion, and former Interim Director of the Transformative Learning Centre at OISE. From 1999 to 2007 Blake was the Director of the MPH program in Health Promotion at U of T. His areas of specialization include community resilience, social change, qualitative and dialogical methods, the settings approach in health promotion, ecological determinants of health, social movements, community development as an arena of practice for health and social care professionals, and the relationship between inner and outer change. His current research includes the emergence of the Transition movement in Canada, and the role of civil society in healthy public policy-making (and implementation) on active transportation. Blake currently teaches courses in generative dialogue, community development in health, and building community resilience.

Louise Potvin holds the Canada Research Chair in Community Approaches and Health Inequalities at the School of Public Health, Université de Montréal. Her main research interest concerns the development, implementation, impact, sustainability, and scaling up of health promotion programs and interventions that address social health inequalities. She is a member of the Canadian Academy of Health Sciences and the Vice-President for Scientific Affairs of the International Union for Health Promotion and Education (IUHPE). She is the Editor-in-Chief of the *Canadian Journal of Public Health*.

Dennis Raphael is a professor at the School of Health Policy and Management at York University. The most recent of his over 150 scientific publications have focused on the health effects of income inequality and poverty, the quality of life of communities and individuals, and the impact of government decisions on Canadians' health and wellbeing. Dr. Raphael is editor of *Social Determinants of Health: Canadian Perspectives* and *Health Promotion and Quality of Life in Canada: Essential Readings*; co-editor of *Staying Alive: Critical Perspectives on Health, Illness, and Health Care*; and author of *Poverty in Canada: Implications for Health and Quality of Life* and *About Canada: Health and Illness*.

Lucie Richard is a Professor in the Faculty of Nursing at the Université de Montréal. A FRSQ national scholar, she is currently affiliated with the Institut de recherché en santé publique de l'Université de Montréal (IRSPUM) and the Centre de recherche de l'Institut universitaire de gériatrie de Montréal. Over the last ten years, she has conducted many projects pertaining to disease prevention and health promotion. She is currently Deputy Director of the IRSPUM.

Irving Rootman is an Adjunct Professor in the Faculty of Human and Social Development at the University of Victoria and a Visiting Professor at Simon Fraser University. He has worked as a researcher, research manager, program manager, and educator in the field of health promotion for more than 30 years in the federal government, the World Health Organization, the University of Toronto, and the University of Victoria. He has published widely in health promotion, including as an author of several chapters and as an editor of the first three editions of *Health Promotion in Canada*. He is a Fellow of the Canadian Academy of Health Sciences. He recently joined the Executive Committee of Health Promotion Canada.

Ketan Shankardass is an Associate Professor in the Department of Health Sciences at Wilfrid Laurier University and an Associate Scientist at the Centre for Urban Health Solutions (St. Michael's Hospital). He is social epidemiologist and educator with an interest in health-promoting equity interventions. He is an active member of Health Promotion Ontario.

Martine Shareck is a CIHR-funded Post-Doctoral Research Fellow at the London School of Hygiene and Tropical Medicine, UK. Martine holds a PhD in Public Health (specializing in health promotion) from the Université de Montréal and has multi-disciplinary training, with an undergraduate degree in Environmental Sciences from McGill University and a Master's in Community Health (specializing in epidemiology) from the Université de Montréal. Her broad research interest is in the socio-spatial determinants of health and health equity. Her current research is focused on under-standing how the places where people live, work, and play (i.e., their activity space) influence their health behaviours. She is currently involved in a study of social inequal-ities in eating behaviours in adolescents in London, UK, and in smoking among young adults in Montréal, Canada. More details on Martine's past and current research can be found at www.martineshareck.weebly.com.

Jean Shoveller is a Professor at UBC's School of Population and Public Health and Program Director, Epidemiology and Population Health & Drug Treatment Program, British Columbia Centre for Excellence in HIV/AIDS. She is widely recognized for her contributions to the social determinants of young people's sexual health inequities. In 2015, Professor Shoveller was inducted into the Canadian Academy of Health Sciences.

Jane Springett is a Professor in the School of Public Health at the University of Alberta. She is a former Director of the Centre for Health Promotion Studies at the University of Alberta and teaches graduate students taking health promotion programs at that univer-sity. With a PhD in Geography from the University of Leeds, UK, she came to health promotion through involvement in the WHO Healthy Cities Project in Liverpool 30 years ago. She has a long-standing interest and experience in participatory research and evaluation and is currently a member of the International Collaboration on Participatory Health Research. She has extensive international experience, has published widely in the field of health promotion, and is a founding member of Health Promotion Canada, a pan-Canadian association supporting health promotion practitioners.

Alisa Stanton has a Master's of Public Health from Simon Fraser University, and is currently working on a PhD that combines studies in Education and Health. Alisa has worked as a Health Promotion Specialist at SFU since 2011, where she co-leads the Well-being in Learning Environments project.

Laura L. Struik recently received a PhD in Interdisciplinary Graduate Studies from the University of British Columbia. She has expertise in the areas of population health and chronic disease prevention, with a particular focus on eHealth initiatives. Her innovative doctoral research was funded by highly competitive awards including two CIHR-funded training fellowships: the Population Intervention for Chronic Disease Prevention (PICDP) fellowship and the Psychosocial Oncology Research Training (PORT) fellowship. She has published her research in several peer-reviewed journals and presented at various national and international conferences.

COPYRIGHT ACKNOWLEDGEMENTS

BOXES

TABLES

FIGURES

PHOTOGRAPHS

INDEX